Regulation of
Matrix Accumulation

Biology of Extracellular Matrix:
A Series

Editor

ROBERT P. MECHAM

A list of books in this series is available from the publisher on request.

REGULATION OF MATRIX ACCUMULATION

Edited by **ROBERT P. MECHAM**

Pulmonary Disease and Critical Care Division

Department of Cell Biology and Physiology

Washington University School of Medicine

Jewish Hospital

St. Louis, Missouri

1986

ACADEMIC PRESS, INC.

Harcourt Brace Jovanovich, Publishers

Orlando   San Diego   New York   Austin
London   Montreal   Sydney   Tokyo   Toronto

ACADEMIC PRESS, INC.
Orlando, Florida 32887

United Kingdom Edition published by
ACADEMIC PRESS INC. (LONDON) LTD.
24–28 Oval Road, London NW1 7DX

Library of Congress Cataloging in Publication Data

Regulation of matrix accumulation.

(Biology of extracellular matrix)
Bibliography: p.
Includes index.
1. Ground substance (Anatomy)   2. Cellular control
mechanisms.   3. Collagen—Metabolism.   4. Connective
tissues.   I. Mecham, Robert P.   II. Series.
QP88.23.R44   1986   611'.0182   86-3418
ISBN 0–12–487425–8 (alk. paper)

PRINTED IN THE UNITED STATES OF AMERICA

86 87 88 89   9 8 7 6 5 4 3 2 1

Contents

REFLECTIONS ON A CAREER IN CONNECTIVE TISSUE RESEARCH

S. M. PARTRIDGE

INTRACELLULAR TURNOVER OF COLLAGEN

RICHARD A. BERG

THE BIOLOGICAL REGULATION OF COLLAGENASE ACTIVITY

JOHN J. JEFFREY

FEEDBACK REGULATION OF COLLAGEN SYNTHESIS

PETER K. MÜLLER, ANDREAS G. NERLICH,
JOACHIM BÖHM, LUU PHAN-THAN, and
THOMAS KRIEG

STEROID HORMONE REGULATION OF EXTRACELLULAR MATRIX PROTEINS

KENNETH R. CUTRONEO, KENNETH M. STERLING,
JR., and SUSAN SHULL

CONTROL OF ELASTIN SYNTHESIS: MOLECULAR AND CELLULAR ASPECTS

JEFFREY M. DAVIDSON and M. GABRIELLA GIRO

ELASTASES: CATALYTIC AND BIOLOGICAL PROPERTIES

JOSEPH G. BIETH

CHARACTERIZATION AND REGULATION OF LYSYL OXIDASE

HERBERT M. KAGAN

MATRIX ACCUMULATION AND THE DEVELOPMENT OF FORM: PROTEOGLYCANS AND BRANCHING MORPHOGENESIS

BRIAN S. SPOONER and HOLLY A. THOMPSON-PLETSCHER

Contributors

Numbers in parentheses indicate the pages on which the authors' contributions begin.

RICHARD A. BERG, *Department of Biochemistry, University of Medicine and Dentistry, Rutgers Medical School, Piscataway, New Jersey 08854* (29)

JOSEPH G. BIETH, *INSERM Unité 237, Faculté de Pharmacie, Université Louis Pasteur, 67048 Strasbourg Cedex, France* (217)

JOACHIM BÖHM, *Max-Planck-Institut für Biochemie, 8033 Martinsried, Federal Republic of Germany* (99)

KENNETH R. CUTRONEO, *Department of Biochemistry, College of Medicine, University of Vermont, Burlington, Vermont 05405* (119)

JEFFREY M. DAVIDSON,[1] *Department of Pathology, University of Utah School of Medicine, and Research Service, Veterans Administration Medical Center, Salt Lake City, Utah 84148* (177)

M. GABRIELLA GIRO,[2] *Department of Pathology, University of Utah School of Medicine, and Research Service, Veterans Administration Medical Center, Salt Lake City, Utah 84148* (177)

[1] Present address: Department of Pathology, Vanderbilt University School of Medicine, and Research Service, Veterans Administration Medical Center, Nashville, Tennessee 37203.

[2] Permanent address: Istituto di Istologia–Embriologia, Università di Padova, 35100 Padova, Italy.

JOHN J. JEFFREY, *Division of Dermatology, Departments of Medicine and Biological Chemistry, Washington University School of Medicine, St. Louis, Missouri 63110* (53)

HERBERT M. KAGAN, *Department of Biochemistry, Boston University School of Medicine, Boston, Massachusetts 02118* (321)

THOMAS KRIEG, *Dermatologische Klinik, Ludwig-Maximilians-Universität, 8000 München, Federal Republic of Germany* (99)

PETER K. MÜLLER, *Max-Planck-Institut für Biochemie, 8033 Martinsried, Federal Republic of Germany* (99)

ANDREAS G. NERLICH, *Max-Planck-Institut für Biochemie, 8033 Martinsried, Federal Republic of Germany* (99)

S. M. PARTRIDGE, *Millstream House, Cheddar, Somerset BS27 3N6, England* (1)

LUU PHAN-THAN, *Max-Planck-Institut für Biochemie, 8033 Martinsried, Federal Republic of Germany* (99)

SUSAN SHULL, *Department of Biochemistry, College of Medicine, University of Vermont, Burlington, Vermont 05405* (119)

BRIAN S. SPOONER, *Division of Biology, Kansas State University, Manhattan, Kansas 66506* (399)

KENNETH M. STERLING, JR.,[3] *Department of Biochemistry, College of Medicine, University of Vermont, Burlington, Vermont 05405* (119)

HOLLY A. THOMPSON-PLETSCHER, *Department of Chemistry, University of Montana, Missoula, Montana 59812* (399)

[3] Present address: Division of Pediatric Gastroenterology, Mount Sinai School of Medicine, New York, New York 10029.

Preface

More than two decades have passed since the first publication of the *International Review of Connective Tissue Research*. Under the editorship of Dr. David Hall, later joined by Dr. David Jackson, the series has published timely reviews which highlight the tremendous developments in connective tissue research. Moreover, the *International Review* has helped to encourage interactions between diverse disciplines, a goal stated by Dr. Hall in the first preface.

With this volume, the *International Review of Connective Tissue Research* undergoes a change of editorship and, with this, major changes in format. The most obvious format change is a new title: *Biology of Extracellular Matrix*. The title was selected to emphasize the new breadth of connective tissue studies; once limited principally to the biochemical characterization of individual connective tissue components, the field has grown to include, indeed ordain, research on the interactions between cells and extracellular macromolecules.

A second, more substantial change in format is that most volumes in the series will be devoted to a particular theme, rather than covering diverse, unrelated subjects. To ensure that the volumes have cohesion and appropriate editorial review, editors and co-editors will be selected who are leaders in the various areas of study reviewed. For example, Dr. Thomas Wight will be co-editor of the second volume of this series, devoted to the biology of proteoglycans. Drs. Richard Mayne and Robert Burgeson will edit the third volume, which will address the genetic diversity of collagen, emphasizing the "new" collagen types IV–X.

Another feature of the new series will be autobiographical reminiscences from investigators who have greatly influenced our progress in understanding extracellular matrix biology. This first volume of *Biology of Extracellular Matrix* opens with a personal retrospective by Miles Partridge. Those who read the article surely will acquire a keener appreciation for the creative insights that people like Dr. Partridge brought to the field.

While most volumes of this series will explore specific subjects, we expect to publish occasional collections that are not unified by a single theme, believing that this practice will encourage new lines of research and new perspectives on basic knowledge not always conducive to discussion in a rigidly topical survey. In some ways this first volume might be viewed as such a collection. Although each review is appropriate for the topic "Regulation of Matrix Accumulation," each also draws attention to the possibilities of the subject when looked at in new ways.

The article by Jeffrey presents an analysis of collagenolytic degradation of extracellular collagen, but its larger purpose is to raise a more fundamental question about the relationship between collagenolytic proenzymes and enzyme–inhibitor complexes and the role of this relationship in the regulation of collagen turnover. Similarly, Berg proposes that degradation of newly synthesized intracellular collagen provides a tightly controlled mechanism for cells either to sort or to modulate the amount of collagen which is available for extracellular transport. Müller *et al.* hypothesize that degradation fragments of collagen have biological activity; specifically, that fragments of collagen molecules liberated during extracellular processing of procollagen feed back to the cell to alter specifically the collagen synthetic rate. This feedback system may be an exquisite example of reciprocal interaction between a cell and the macromolecules that it secretes to form a structurally intact matrix.

To view regulation of matrix accumulation by cells in isolation is almost certainly to see the process too narrowly. Cutroneo *et al.* point to the role of humoral factors as potent regulators. The broad dimensions of the subject are suggested by considering the varied responses of the cell to multiple signals in the extracellular environment. The inhibitory or stimulatory effects of steroid hormones on the synthesis of matrix macromolecules may lead to altered composition or architecture of the extracellular matrix or result in abnormal biochemical functions of cells.

The use of modern experimental techniques to answer difficult biological questions is illustrated in the review of elastin by Davidson and Giro. Elastin has been a difficult protein to study because of its unusual biochemical and physical properties. Yet recent advances in molecular and cellular biology and the application of useful model systems have contributed greatly to understanding the synthesis, deposition, and turnover of this unique protein. Equally detailed and impressive information on elastin degradation is presented by Bieth. Looking closely at the proteases that degrade elastin, Bieth seeks to define the circumstances under which a proteolytic enzyme can be properly called an elastase. This analysis leads also to questions regarding the relationships between elastase and proteolytic inhibitors in serum and disease.

Accumulation of functional collagen or elastin in the extracellular space necessitates an enzymatically catalyzed joining of individual molecules to form a highly cross-linked polymer. Kagan addresses the problem of forming an insoluble matrix from soluble macromolecules in an analysis of the complex enzyme system that catalyzes cross-link formation. Spooner and Thompson-Pletscher, in the final article in this volume, summarize the important interrelationship between matrix accumulation and the development of form. Spooner and Thompson-Pletscher discuss how a wide variety of matrix components act as morphogenetic substrates and as cues for cellular differentiation in branching morphogenesis. As embryonic cells organize to form tissues and organs, it is clear that matrix accumulation—which includes remodeling as well as synthesis—is subject to direct regulation by the reacting cells.

It is hoped that the *Biology of Extracellular Matrix* will serve to focus current and future research in the biochemistry and cell biology of extracellular matrix. This series cannot thrive without a large measure of enthusiasm and active participation from contributors and readers. Comments including suggestions of topics will be gratefully received. Indeed, nothing could be more useful in this endeavor than to know from those who are interested how they would have us proceed.

ROBERT P. MECHAM

Reflections on a Career in Connective Tissue Research

S. M. Partridge

Somerset, England

I was born in Whangarei, New Zealand, on August 2nd, 1913. My father emigrated from Warwickshire, England, in 1912 and, among rumours of the coming war joined the New Zealand army as a Sergeant Instructor. My mother was born in Kent and joined him for marriage in New Zealand soon after her nineteenth birthday. She had very happy recollections of New Zealand, but unfortunately their time together was short: my father was killed in action with the ANZAC expeditionary force soon after the fateful landing at Gallipoli in April, 1915. Having little to keep her in New Zealand, my mother returned with me to her parents' home in Dover.

My early schooling was supported by and conducted under the supervision of the New Zealand High Commissioner's Office in London, but at the end of the war this arrangement changed because my mother married again. My stepfather was Lt. Charles McCarthy R.N.V.R., a "Wireless Officer" posted with the mine-sweeping trawlers of the Dover Patrol. As soon as the war was over and he was demobilized, my stepfather joined with two ex-naval colleagues to establish a business in London. This was still in existence when he died in 1952 but underwent all sorts of varying fortunes in the meantime. As it was, my mother was needed to help establish the new business, and at the age of seven I went to live with my grandmother who had retired to live near her family in a country cottage in the village of Heckington in Lincolnshire.

I lived in the village until the age of twelve, and still have happy memories of what seems like an almost idyllic experience, moving freely around the various farms occupied by my grandmother's family, and witnessing the interesting operations of the wheelwright, the

1

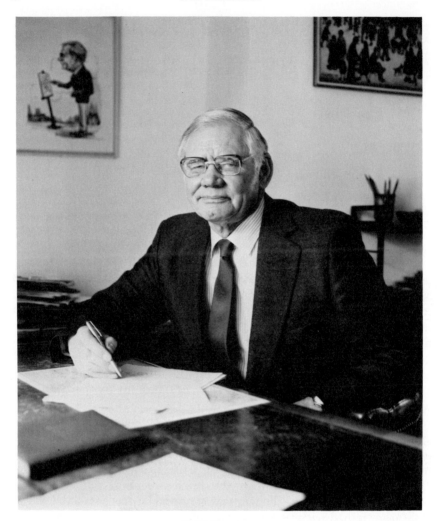

S. M. Partridge

blacksmith, the saddler and half-a-dozen other tradesmen, some prac-
tising trades that are no longer pursued. My formal education, however, was very attenuated: I attended the two-roomed village school,
where the pace was necessarily set by the slowest learners.

Inevitably this had to come to an end and I rejoined my parents in a
London suburb, this decision being taken mainly, I believe, because of
the necessity of finding a good school. This proved successful, and with
a good recommendation from my village school master I was accepted
by a school of "grammar school" standing in West London. However, I

stayed at this school only 3 years, and, as the family home moved to Yorkshire, I completed my secondary education at Roundhay School, Leeds. Both these schools had very able and dedicated science masters, and during this period I made up my mind to become a chemist.

However, as it happened, by another quirk of chance, my stepfather's business again called him to London, so we returned and this time set up in a very comfortable house in Surrey.

BRIEF EXPERIENCE AS A SCIENTIFIC APPRENTICE

I still had a strong urge to be a chemist, but neither I nor my stepfather knew if this was really a good idea, or how to go about it. However, I noticed an advertisement by the drug house May & Baker for a "scientific apprentice" and resolved to try my luck. The post was for work in a very antiquated and run-down factory in Wandsworth, soon to be closed. I decided that here was the way to find out about chemistry and applied for the post. This really turned out to be rather exciting since most of the reactions seemed to be carried out in the open air in the yard; in the 4 months I stayed at Wandsworth I witnessed one or two spectacular chemical events such as a 500-liter-scale bromination getting way out of control and a fire caused by digitalis leaves soon after extraction with benzene. This seemed to me to be a heroic sort of chemistry, but I was tired after my days work in the laboratory, and I realised that it was scarcely possible to make any headway working all day, travelling long distances and studying at nights.

The senior chemical staff did not take much interest in a "lab boy", but for a week or two I worked for Dr. A. J. Ewins (later FRS) who was to become famous for his part in the development of drugs of the sulphanilamide series and the discovery of sulphapyridine (M & B 693). During this short period I formed a great respect for Dr. Ewins and asked if he would talk to my stepfather on the subject of my career, as neither of us had much idea of how I should become a chemist. This meeting took place, and Dr. Ewins was quite firm that I should apply for a free place in Battersea College of Technology and work for a degree full time.

This was decided on, but I soon met a snag: a visit to Battersea disclosed that my entry qualifications for the Northern Universities would not be accepted as Matriculation for London University. This seemed a considerable set-back; however, I found a correspondence course for London Matriculation, and in the 4 months remaining before University entry that year I managed to prepare for the London Matriculation examination and was successful.

FIRST DEGREE AT BATTERSEA

There followed a normal and fairly uneventful full-time honours degree course with organic chemistry as the major subject and physical chemistry the subsidiary. Here I met my future wife, but both of us knew that marriage was unlikely to be conveniently possible before the age of 25 or 26 so we were prepared to wait without exchanging any reckless promises. In due course I passed the degree examination with upper second class honours, and so became qualified to register for a Ph.D. degree in organic chemistry.

During the 3-year first degree course the head of the chemistry department, Dr. Joseph Kenyon (afterwards FRS), gave the main lecture on organic chemistry every Monday afternoon. These lectures were a model of simplicity and precision. They were designed simply to teach and certainly not to display Dr. Kenyon's own erudition. The Monday afternoon lectures finally confirmed my own love for the simplicity and elegance of organic chemistry, although it had to be admitted that teaching by other lecturers on specific groups of compounds was probably more useful for covering the syllabus and revising for examinations.

C. W. Davies (afterwards Professor in the University of Wales) gave the lectures in physical chemistry, and here again his interpretation of the subject was clear and intellectually satisfying. Thanks to his good teaching, I was much more interested in physical chemistry at the end of the course than I believed I would be at the beginning.

The prospect of 3 or 4 more years as a student without any source of income apart from that provided by my parents was rather daunting, however, and it became imperative to find an activity that would give some financial independence. As it happened I was able to rent about a half-acre of land from a near neighbour and during the summer set to work to build chicken houses for about 120 head of poultry, according to the latest designs from various library books. I purchased day-old chicks of the best laying strain available and in due course had a thriving concern selling eggs in returnable dozen boxes to the neighbours. This enterprise was apparently timely and produced an income which allowed me to run a motor bicycle for the daily journeys to Battersea.

The next step, inevitably, was to join Joseph Kenyon's research laboratory as a Ph.D. student. The subject of most of the work under Dr. Kenyon's direction was to study prototropic and anionotropic reactions by resolving the less-stable reactant into its optical enantiomers and, by measuring the rate of change in optical activity, to follow the course of the tautomeric reaction under various physical conditions.

SYNTHETIC ORGANIC CHEMISTRY WITH DR. J. KENYON

The problem given to me was to study the tautomeric pair: phenylvinylcarbinol (1), the unstable isomer, and methylstyrylcarbinol (2), the product of the anionotropic reaction

$$(-)\text{-Ph}\cdot\overset{*}{C}\text{H(OH)CH}{=}\text{CH}\cdot\text{Me} \rightleftharpoons \text{Ph}\cdot\text{CH}{=}\text{CH}\cdot\overset{*}{C}\text{H(OH)Me}$$
$$(1) \qquad\qquad (2)$$

This was done by Grignard synthesis of both carbinols, purification and crystallization, followed by preparation of the hydrogen phthalic ester and salt formation with various alkaloids. The resolution was carried out by counter-current crystallization of the alkaloid salts and yielded both enantiomers of both isomers. The course of the tautomeric change was then studied under various solvent conditions and temperatures and with various carbinol esters, in each case by following the change in optical rotation using a jacketed polarimeter tube. Since some of the compounds were new (i.e., not in Beilstein), each compound was carefully purified, several crystalline derivatives prepared and three or four physical parameters recorded for each (1,2).

The type of work exemplified organic chemistry as it then was, and demonstrated the very high degree of certainty that could be attained simply by applying the rules as they were known in laboratories of the time, such as those of Kenyon, R. Robinson and C. K. Ingold—and many others since Perkin. It is interesting that in the laboratory at the same time the prototropic system

$$\begin{array}{ccc} \text{Me} & & \text{Ph} \\ \diagdown & & \diagup \\ & \text{C(H)}\cdot\text{N:C} & \\ \diagup & & \diagdown \\ \text{Ph} & & \text{C}_6\text{H}_4\text{Cl-}p \end{array} \rightleftharpoons \begin{array}{ccc} \text{Me} & & \text{Ph} \\ \diagdown & & \diagup \\ & \text{C:N}\cdot\text{C(H)} & \\ \diagup & & \diagdown \\ \text{Ph} & & \text{C}_6\text{H}_4\text{Cl-}p \end{array}$$

was under investigation (3). This was to prove the source of an important idea in later work on elastin cross-links.

The work on the retention of asymmetry during aniotropic change led to a further development in which $(+)$-γ-phenyl-α-methylallyl alcohol (3) was dibrominated to give a mixture of two methyl-α,β-dibromo-β-phenyl ethyl carbinols (4) which by fractional crystallization could be separated into a $(+)$ and a $(-)$ isomer: mp 112–113 and 87–88°C, respectively. Oxidation of the alcohol of higher melting point yielded a (+) ketone, and that of lower melting point a (−) ketone, both of mp 127°C. Since the rotatory powers of the two ketones, although of opposite sign, were of equal magnitude, it is very probable that they were optically pure substances. The explanation given for this type of asym-

$$Me\cdot\overset{*}{C}H(OH)\cdot CH:CH\cdot Ph \rightarrow Me\cdot\overset{*}{C}H(OH)\cdot\overset{*}{C}HBr\cdot\overset{*}{C}HBr\cdot Ph \rightarrow Me\cdot CO\cdot\overset{*}{C}HBr\cdot\overset{*}{C}HBr\cdot Ph$$
$$\text{(3)} \qquad\qquad\qquad\qquad \text{(4)} \qquad\qquad\qquad\qquad \text{(5)}$$

metric synthesis was that the two dibromo alcohols were different compounds (with different melting points) and were therefore associated with a different energy of activation at the same temperature (2). As was expected, variation of the temperature of the bromination reaction resulted in wide variation in rotatory powers of the ketones obtained by oxidation of the mixtures of dibromo alcohols.

At this time heavy water (D_2O) became available commercially, and in collaboration with J. M. B. Coppock I made an attempt to reduce (−)-phenylvinylcarbinol with deuterium in order to try to resolve phenyl-α,β-dideuteroethyl ketone by asymmetric synthesis. However, any optical activity resulting was too small to be measured by us (4,5).

Joseph Kenyon had a particular delight in careful recrystallization of these low-melting unstable aliphatic compounds. He would spend the afternoon carefully drying solutions in low boiling solvents such as methylene chloride and adding dry petrol ether of what he thought was the most promising boiling grade. He would finally filter the solution into a conical flask with a suitable sized neck and deposit it in his favourite position on the polished teak bench top with a circle of filter paper arranged symmetrically underneath. His students could be sure that by next morning the flask would contain a heavy crop of large highly refractive rhombs or glistening needles!

The aesthetic satisfaction of organic chemistry, both in practice and theory, had the same appeal for me; after spending 4 years in Kenyon's laboratory, however, I began to realize that this type of synthetic organic chemistry, even though exemplifying a working theory, could not offer a life's work for students of my generation. So much of the results of our labours did no more than fill the pages of Beilstein (already too large) and add meat to the bones of theories already in existence. For this reason, half-way through my research studies I asked Dr. Kenyon's permission to attend a London University course of lectures in biochemistry, given at the nearby Chelsea College of Technology.

He seemed rather shocked at this idea and earnestly persuaded me to finish off the job I was doing, saying there would be time enough to study biochemistry when I had secured my doctorate. This was undoubtedly good practical advice, but I have always been a little sorry I followed it. I certainly felt that the most rewarding outlet would lie in biochemistry, as a new subject for making worthwhile discoveries and because of its obviously important role in supporting medical science. As it turned out this was my last chance to acquire a systematic background to physiological chemistry as it existed at the time, and for many years in my later career I fell into at least temporary pitfalls, and made mistakes, because of the lack of some piece of information that was everyday knowledge to those who had a thorough grounding in biochemistry and physiology.

A TEMPORARY POST IN MANUFACTURING INDUSTRY, 1937–1939

In due course, having completed most of the work towards my thesis, it became necessary to think seriously about finding the right sort of employment, preferably to lead to a permanent career. However, the employment situation was in every way as difficult in the late 1930s as it is in the 1980s. Further, no young man seeking a professional career would consider accepting the "dole" even for a brief period.

After having looked at various rather unlikely prospects I decided to accept, as a temporary measure, a post of "chemist" to a newly incorporated company who had become the owners of a German patent for the manufacture of glass-beaded screens for the cinemas which were then proliferating at a high rate and converting to "talking pictures". The proposition was to manufacture a white "leather cloth" in 4-ft wide rolls to coat this material with fine glass beads and then to perforate it with a pattern of 1-mm diameter holes to allow the sound to pass through from loud-speakers behind the screen. The screen was then fabricated by sewing these 4-ft panels together. These screens, when well made, behaved very well in the long, narrow halls which were then popular as cinemas—but there were many technical problems, and the company was experiencing great difficulty in producing a product to a satisfactory standard. The demand, however was very brisk and the prospect looked encouraging.

The only technical man in the company was the works manager, who claimed experience in wallpaper manufacturing and who had set up the production line using largely wallpaper technique and machinery. Unfortunately, after 6 months, this man engaged in a furious quarrel with the directors over financial matters and resigned on the spot. I was left to bring my new formulation into production, with no more help than that of the foreman and the senior men.

Fortunately the new product turned out quite well and I was almost tempted to make this kind of work my career; however, after nearly 2 years with the screen company a post became available which really did correspond with my long-standing desires and ambitions. I was asked to call on Dr. W. T. J. Morgan (later FRS) at the Lister Institute to discuss the possibility of my filling a studentship offered by the Grocers' Livery Company to sponsor some aspect of medical research. This was offered at a substantial reduction in salary, but it was exactly the kind of work for which I had always hoped, and I accepted it gratefully without any hesitation at all.

THE LISTER INSTITUTE 1939–1942

Morgan had already discovered that the somatic antigen of *Bacteroides dysenterae* (Shiga) could be separated into three discrete parts by heating in a water bath for 1 h in 1% acetic acid. The parts were a polysaccharide which carried the immunospecificity, a protein which was necessary for active antigenicity in animals, and a lipid material which seemed to be concerned with the formation of micelles in watery suspensions. This seemed to show a clear promise for a research effort designed to elucidate the chemical structure of the antigen. The situation in a biochemical laboratory such as Morgan's, studying the structure of proteins, polysaccharides and lipids and the large macromolecules they can form when they interact, was totally different from a synthetic organic chemistry laboratory. In Kenyon's laboratory there were well-tried methods for performing almost any task and even well-trodden paths for elucidating chemical mechanisms. The reverse was the case in the study of biochemical macromolecules: but there seemed to be more valid reasons for making the effort. To study the antigens of "Shiga dysentery" we felt we needed to know the amino acid composition of the protein part and the sugar composition and structure of the polysaccharide. However, at that time one might hope to secure a partial amino acid analysis after 2 years' work and the expenditure of several hundred grams of "pure" antigen. Similarly, structural studies on polysaccharides required equally large quantities of material and a similar time scale. This problem was very well understood by Morgan, who indoctrinated me with the belief that it was worthwhile to spend years, if necessary, to refine a useful analytical method. A case in point was the "Elson and Morgan" specific colorimetric method for hexosamine. This was used and quoted by innumerable authors and was a corner stone in the study of glycosaminoglycans.

Lacking methods for a more penetrating approach to structure it seemed that the most that could be done in a few years was to elucidate the gross structures of the macromolecular complexes forming the biologically active antigens of the *Bact. dysenteriae* organisms and to try to define the role played by the various constituents. We were fortunate in having the collaboration of Dr. David Henderson (afterwards Director of the Microbiological Research Establishment at Porton) who prepared for us enormous (100 g) batches of dry, acetone-killed "Shiga" or "Typhosum" organisms, sometimes at the rate of about one batch per week.

The work on the somatic antigens of *Bact. dysenteriae* (Shiga) and *Bact. typhosum* was published in four papers (6–9) which we regarded as a preliminary skirmish into the structural matters we wanted to know about. However, a promising line emerged when we found that we could recombine the protein part of the antigen with foreign polysaccharides to make good precipitating antigens with agar, gum acacia or cherry gum specificity (10).

I worked as the "Grocers' Scholar" for 2 years and was then offered a Beit Memorial Research Fellowship in October, 1940. This latter was at a good salary, and I was able to marry Ruth Dowling and set up house in a pleasant apartment on Harrow Hill, overlooking the school playing fields.

The work at the Lister Institute, however, was not to last long. The cold war became a very hot war, and the Lister Institute was bombed, probably by accident, by a single plane in day time. The work on the dysentery antigens was designed to support vaccine manufacture under war conditions, but the "TAB" vaccination was brought to a high pitch of efficiency by the Elstree Laboratories of the Lister Institute and elsewhere, and was offering no practical problems. The Institute at Chelsea was obliged to destroy all its experimental animals, and most of the staff left for other laboratories. For my own part, I was sent to the Elstree Laboratories for a few months, but when the Institute was approached by Dr. E. C. Bate-Smith for my services in a more urgent war-time investigation, there could be no objection.

The Low Temperature Research Station, Cambridge, Northern Ireland and India

The work at the Low Temperature Station was applied war-time research, undertaken at high speed, with little chance to investigate interesting phenomena not considered to be in the main stream. The part I was asked to play was to design a process for the dehydration of lean meat. It was supposed that this would be useful for shipping meat into the United Kingdom from Argentina, Canada, Australia and New Zealand where the great reduction in weight and bulk would be a valuable feature in view of the very heavy losses of ships by enemy action. Dehydrated foods compressed into cans would also provide a concentrated form of ration for the feeding of troops in far-distant fields of battle.

At first some very sophistocated ideas (for the time) were investigated, including freeze drying, which was a very new technique. However, in the end, oven drying of partly cooked mince meat was adopted as the only thing that could be done in time. With my collaborators A. J. Ede (a physicist), R. G. Westall and W. E. Lear the essential experimental work for designing the process was carried out, using laboratory-scale recirculating ovens in which airspeed, temperature and relative humidity could be controlled. As a pilot-scale drying oven, the "Torry Kiln", originally designed by J. K. Hardy for the controlled smoking of herring, was adapted to take 1-ton loads of mince meat. The pilot-scale work was done at Torry Research Institute at Aberdeen, and the first fully organized pilot-scale production plant was set up at the premises of New Forge Ltd. in Belfast. This was run for 4 months in the winter of 1943, and almost immediately R. G. Westall and I were asked to join the Food Department, Government of India, at New Delhi in order to advise on the installation of five similar plants at various centres of goat and sheep production in India. These plants were only just being brought into commission when the war in South-East Asia ended.

In spite of the considerable pressure of work, I found much to interest me as a scientific adviser in India. The civil departments of the Government of India were at the time about half Indian and half British, so far as staff was concerned, and the whole operation was characterized by courtesy and helpfulness but perhaps not much sense of urgency. My immediate superior was Dr. B. C. Guha, a kindly academic who had worked extensively in both England and the United States. The department had dehydration plants operating or being built in Peshawar, Amritsar, Delhi, Madras, Poona and many other places in India, so that I travelled the subcontinent extensively.

I found Indian small business men always courteous and surprisingly easy to get along with; it was even taken in good part when I had to explain that the Food Department was no longer interested in buying meat that had been sliced by hand and dried in the sun on the roofs of the workers' houses! I also had one or two rather unpleasant and difficult jobs to do: I had to close down a land disposal site for animal wastes because it was in the jungle near a village where bubonic plague was reported. I also inspected and closed down one of our new dehydration factories because of an outbreak of anthrax. I was never certain if there was actually anthrax in the factory, but the department allowed it to be reopened after about 2 months to allow every inch of the walls and floors to be sterilized with blow-torches!

On the whole I enjoyed the experience of India in spite of the fact that I had to work very hard to keep in touch with what was going on over so large an area. I spent two hot seasons in the plains with only 10 days holiday in the hills the whole time. Quite suddenly the work came to an end with the unexpected end of the war in the East, and my contract was terminated on the day appointed for the withdrawal of British forces.

It was probably a mistake to stay so long, but I felt I wanted to leave a clear desk. During the last few months I had been surprised and shocked to find that my Muslim assistants were convinced that civil war would break out as soon as the British left India. I did not take this too seriously as there was no sign of any concentrations of Muslims in the Delhi area. However, when I finally left Delhi on the last train before transfer of power the war-like preparations of the Sikhs around the railway station at Amritsar made it perfectly obvious what was to come. There was a hushed air of gloom throughout the rest of the journey, and my fellow ex-Indian civil servants had nothing to say and did not want to speak. The following morning I set sail from Bombay on a troop ship to England. During the train journey my metal trunks had been off-loaded and I thought they were lost; however, 3 months later they turned up at my house in Cambridge, unharmed and unopened!

CAMBRIDGE, 1945–1967

On returning to England I was disappointed that the unexpired part of my Beit Memorial Fellowship was no longer available to me. The Lister Institute had already restaffed with some able young chemists and biochemists, who had been able to continue with fundamental investigations during the war. However, I got in touch again with Dr. C. S. Hanes, FRS who was now Director of Food Investigation and Dr. E. C. Bate-Smith at the Low Temperature Station, Cambridge, and was offered the post of head of a new section to study animal connective tissues. This position pleased me as it implied continuing study of physiologically important polysaccharides and proteins. However, I made it quite clear that I did not see any future in such studies until new techniques became available for amino acid and sugar analysis, preferably at the microanalytical scale. I had become impressed with the chromatographic methods studied systematically by A. Tiselius (11) and S. Claesson (12) in Sweden and expressed my wish to spend part of my time, for some years if necessary, in trying to develop various systems of chromatography. This was received well, particularly by Bate-Smith: indeed I am very much indebted to him for his constant support and encouragement during a time when there could be little to guarantee a successful outcome.

With the collaboration of J. Bendall and R. G. Westall the first experiments on displacement chromatography of water-soluble bases and amino acids got under way and gave encouraging results that were later published (14). However, by this time, I had become interested in the paper chromatographic method for amino acids developed by Consden, Gordon and Martin (13) and visited them in Leeds in order to discuss the possibility of applying similar methods to sugars. They said they had tried it, but there was little possibility of success, since the sugars were far too soluble in water and had very little solvent solubility.

Returning in the train, however, I remembered some experiments I had done previously on the solubility of oligosaccharides in 90% phenol and became convinced that sugars would migrate in a phenol–water system. I became very excited about this and could scarcely wait until I had collected enough gear to run a chromatogram with spots of various reducing sugars in a phenol–water system. The only way I could think of to visualize the spots was to spray the paper with ammoniacal silver nitrate. Needless to say, this produced a very black chromatogram, but some difference in migration was immediately obvious.

In later developments of the method, ammoniacal silver nitrate was replaced by a butanolic solution of aniline hydrogen phthalate, and the ammoniacal phenol solvent largely replaced by butanol–acetic acid–water. This greatly improved the cleanliness of the chromatograms and the ease of operation (15–18).

The two paper methods were very valuable for qualitative and semiquantitative investigations of the sugar and amino acid compositions of polysaccharides and proteins and also of extracts of various kinds, but I felt that they should be backed up by a method for large-scale isolation so as to permit the determination of physical constants, elementary analysis etc. In taking this sort of view it should be explained that I believed that there should be many more amino acids in the world besides the 20 or so commonly found in proteins. At that time molecular genetics was unknown and there seemed to be no reason to think that the missing members of homologous series of α-amino acids should not turn up as a result of closer investigation, even if at a lower concentration. This was a mistaken idea, but it led us to devise a systematic ion-exchange displacement procedure which could be used to enrich any of the known amino acids with respect to the others in the mixture. Naturally, the same procedure would show up any new α-amino acid that happened to be present.

This work on displacement chromatography was published as a series of eight papers (19–27). My co-authors in these investigations were R. G. Westall, R. C. Brimley and K. W. Pepper. The scale of the methods could quite easily be increased to 200–300 g of amino acids and organic bases using only laboratory apparatus, and quite a number of extracts and waste liquids arising from the food industry were fractionated in this way. However, no hitherto unknown amino acids were discovered in the course of this survey, and despite various attempts in small pilot-scale work, new viable processes did not immediately arise.

One point is of interest: in this kind of work we had great difficulty in evaporating frothy solutions, and our method was to sit on the bench near a water pump and pull off the vapour from a flask by rotating it between thumb and finger in a hot water bath. About this time I conceived the idea of an apparatus in which the flask was driven by a motor and the vapour pulled off through a hollow trunion. We used this for several years and then published it in the *Journal of Scientific Instruments* (1951) under the title "Rotary film evaporator for laboratory use" (32). Soon afterwards Dr. L. C. Craig wrote to me with details of a piece of apparatus that looked very like mine. Almost the same thing had happened to him and his publication was submitted at almost the same time. Of course these rotary evaporators are in common use nowadays.

This kind of work was pursued partly in collaboration with the National Research Development Corporation because it was believed to offer prospects for advances in the food industry. A number of patents were granted, and the work was extended to the use of ion-exchange membrane cells on a pilot scale. These processes became competitive with traditional procedures, and some of them have since been incorporated piecemeal into commercial practice. Ion-exchange membrane cells have still a long way to go, particularly in the chemical design of membranes with specific properties. Perhaps considerable further advances will yet be made in this technology.

STUDY OF THE PROTEOGLYCANS

While the applied work in the field of ion-exchange separations was going on a certain amount of progress was also being made in the study of connective tissues. A start was made with cartilage, perhaps because it had features in common with the bacterial antigens with which I had been involved at the Lister Institute. Bovine nasal septum cartilage was the tissue of choice because it was easy to acquire in large quantities and was reasonably homogeneous. After some preliminary exploration designed to assess the possibility of separating the mucopolysaccharide part of the cartilage from collagen without degrading either too seriously, it was decided to make a start with the method of Einbinder and Schubert which consisted in the use of a 30% aqueous solution of potassium chloride containing 1% of potassium carbonate. This mildly alkaline reagent was effective in separating the bulk of the polysaccharide-containing material from the residual collagenous structures without causing observable degradation. The residual soluble collagen in the extract was removed by treatment with an ion-exchange resin and checked by hydroxyproline determination. It was found that the remaining clear solution contained, in addition to glycosaminoglycan, a non-collagenous protein which could not be separated from the polysaccharide part by a variety of fractionation techniques. However the new protein could be recovered after mild acid or alkaline hydrolysis.

It should at this point be mentioned that while we were working on ion-exchange displacement chromatography as a large-scale preparative method for amino acids, Stanford Moore and William Stein were developing elution chromatography on ion-exchange resins as a very accurate micromethod for amino acid analysis (28). Stanford Moore visited Cambridge for a year in 1951, and since he was without assistance my colleague D. F. Elsdon volunteered to assist him in setting up the first amino acid analytical columns to be constructed in England. Needless to say it was very valuable to us to be in possession of this instrument at such an early date. One of its first uses was to analyse the noncollagenous protein prepared from cartilage extracts by dilute acid or alkaline hydrolysis of the complex with undegraded chondroitin sulphate.

In order to get some idea of the gross structure of the protein–chondroitin sulphate complex it was necessary first to estimate the molecular weight of the whole complex and then the molecular weight of the protein and polysaccharide fractions prepared under the mildest conditions of degradation possible. Osmometry was the only method of molecular weight determination available at the time, and this offered a difficult problem, first because of the very large size of the complex and thus the very small osmotic pressure to be measured, and second because at low salt concentrations the potassium salt of chondroitin sulphate had a false high osmotic pressure due to the K^+ counter-ions. In pure water the molecular weight measured was 520! Dr. Gilbert Adair, FRS (who died in 1979) had a laboratory in the Low Temperature Research Station and came to our rescue with his usual kindness and concern. He commenced by making a whole series of osmotic pressure determinations simply in order to estimate the characteristics of the membrane required.

His habit was to make the membranes by hand by pouring solutions of cellulose nitrate in a mixture of a poor solvent and a good solvent over a rotating glass boiling tube fixed on the shaft of a gear box coupled with an electric motor. The experimental equipment had to be set up at a fixed distance from an open window and an open door in order to control the air-speed, and the membrane casting was performed at a set time of the day in order to control the temperature. Nevertheless, he consistently made thin membranes with the required porosity! The results of the osmotic pressure experiments led to the description of the chondroitin sulphate–protein of beef nasal septum cartilage as a brush-like structure of molecular weight $1–5 \times 10^6$ containing 20–100 chondroitin sulphate chains linked together by protein (29, 31). It was first thought that the chondroitin sulphate chains were connected to the protein core by a linkage which did not involve the terminal reducing residue; this was because approximately 60% of a single reducing residue in each chain was detected by the Somogyi–Nelson copper-reduction method when applied to the protein–polysaccharide from fresh cartilage. It later became clear that this fraction of a reducing residue was liberated by the reagent during the course of copper reduction.

During the early 1950s a number of very able biochemists were attracted to work in my laboratory by the chromatographic opportunities. Among these were A. Gottschalk of the Walter and Eliza Hall Institute of Medical Research, Melbourne. Dr. Gottschalk wanted to extend his study of the interaction of reducing sugars with bases and amino acids; the so-called "Browning Reaction". The first product of the reaction of glucose with lysine gave a good spot on paper chromatograms and proved to be an N-glycoside: dilute acids then catalysed isomerization to a ketone derivative (Amadori rearrangement) (30). The study of these reactions was again of great help later in understanding the cross-linking reactions of elastin.

Another visitor from Australia was N. K. Boardman (now FRS) who came to qualify for a Cambridge Ph.D. He chose to study the separation of neutral proteins on ion-exchange resins and made use of the commercial availability of a monofunctional carboxylic acid cation exchanger "Amberlite IRC 50". He proved to be successful in separating several interesting proteins (33, 34) and developed a useful theoretical background for the behaviour of polyions on cation exchange resins (35). Here again the experience of Gilbert Adair was very valuable in suggesting strategies for separations in the hemoglobin series. With help from Gilbert Adair, Boardman was able to affect a good separation of sheep fetal CO-hemoglobin from bovine CO-hemoglobin. Boardman's examiner for the Cambridge Ph.D. was A. J. P. Martin (afterwards Nobel Laureate) who in my opinion was the genius of chromatography. During the examination a fierce argument developed between Boardman and Martin over the mass-action characteristics of the reaction of soluble polycations with insoluble polyanions. I do not think that either convinced the other, but Boardman got his Ph.D.!

WORK ON THE STRUCTURE OF ELASTIN

About 1950 H. F. Davis and I made the chance discovery that many proteins, when heated at 100°C with acetic or oxalic acid, preferentially released a single amino acid, aspartic acid. This appeared as a single spot on paper chromatograms after precipitation of the remaining protein and large peptides with 75% ethanol (36). We were very interested in this because we thought the reaction might have some useful degree of peptide-bond specificity, and we were then looking for some way in which large proteins could be degraded specifically into polypeptides small enough to allow sequencing by the dinitrophenyl (DNP) end-group method of Sanger (37). We knew that elastin had a very low content of the dicarboxylic amino acids and thought that it might well be degraded into some large peptides which could be isolated by one of the methods we had available at the time.

When we treated purified elastin fibres with 0.25 N oxalic acid for successive periods of 1 hr at 100°C, we were delighted to find that the whole protein went smoothly into solution (38). It was noted that the soluble protein, after dialysis to remove oxalic acid and small peptides, formed a liquid precipitate or "coacervate" on raising the temperature a few degrees, and this passed back into clear solution on cooling under the water tap. Osmotic pressure experiments showed that the initial solutions, after dialysis in cellophane, gave molecular weights of 60,000–65,000. However, when the initial solution was dialysed against buffer using a highly permeable collodion membrane, the non-diffusible fraction (which represented 60% of the whole) gave a mean molecular weight of 84,000. This was disappointing as it indicated a rather considerable degree of inhomogeneity. Nevertheless, the approach did seem promising, and thereafter we turned our attention increasingly to the study of elastin.

There had been work done on elastin previously by many authors, but as usual this had been hampered by the lack of technique, particularly amino acid analysis (for review up to 1962, see ref. 39). One of the early difficulties met with was that elastins from the same species but from different tissues, on purification by the same procedures, gave widely different compositions.

The word "elastin" (as distinct from elastic tissue) was defined as the insoluble protein that remained after removal of all the other proteins and polysaccharides of elastic tissue by treatment with reagents such as hot alkali. What was obviously required was to isolate the elastins from tissues such as *ligamentum nuchae,* aorta, skin and elastic cartilage under fairly mild conditions, and then to continue with purification procedures of increasing severity until all the samples reached constant composition, as determined by Moore and Stein amino acid analysis. If the samples reached not only constant composition but also the *same composition* we would know that all the elastin fibres in all the tissues of the same animal contained the same unique protein, which could be justly named "elastin". This offered the prospect of a considerable effort for a small team, but we were fortunate at that time to have a prolonged visit from Dr. (now Professor) Lorenzo Gotte from Padua University, Italy. He took charge of the investigation and in fact was able to isolate elastins of almost identical composition from bovine *ligamentum nuchae,* aorta and ear cartilage (40). There was some hydrolytic damage during the purification of the most resistant elastic tissues, and this was investigated by isolating and estimating the newly formed N-terminal residues by the FDNB technique of Sanger (37).

For the main line of the constitutional studies, we chose the elastin derived from bovine *ligamentum nuchae,* as this could be obtained in plentiful amounts and could be purified with minimum damage. It was already known that in solvents such as 30:70 ethylene glycol:water elastic fibres behaved as almost perfect elastomers of the classical type, the stress–strain behaviour and the elastic recoil being attributable to entropic changes only (41).

This structure of a classical elastomer implies long flexible peptide chains with very little mutual interaction, but stabilized at intervals by covalent cross-bonding to form polymeric gels with units large enough to be insoluble. We already knew that partial hydrolysis of purified elastin fibres gave rise to a soluble protein which we called α-elastin. This protein had the characteristic property of forming a gel-like coacervate on raising the temperature in dilute salt solutions, and had a mean molecular weight in the region of 60,000–84,000, in different preparations. However, further fractionation and investigations with the ultracentrifuge suggested that α-elastin was itself polydisperse.

In spite of this inhomogeneity it still seemed possible to determine the mean molecular weight of a sample osmometrically and then to determine the average chain length by end-group assay using the quantitative FDNB technique of Sanger. This was done (42, 43) and led to the description of α-elastin as being composed of 17 peptide chains containing (as an average value) 35 amino acid residues each. These results, together with the physical properties of α-elastin, clearly implied that the 17 or so peptide chains were linked together by some kind of chemical cross-link (43). The only type of cross-link that had so far been proved to exist in proteins was the —S—S— bridge in cystine residues. In elastin, however, cystine represented no more than 0.4% of the protein dry weight, and this content would not provide sufficient cross-links to account for the stability of the structure. Further, elastin powder, treated with performic acid did not go into solution. However, it was observed that only approximately 95% of the protein dry weight could be accounted for by amino acid analysis and it was believed that an unidentified substance was involved in cross-bond formation. During this investigation advantage was taken of the opportunity of having elastin in clear water solution, to determine the ultraviolet adsorption spectrum. The spectrum showed the expected presence of tyrosine, but there was another peak present (not due to tryptophane, which is absent in elastin) due to some other, probably aromatic, substance. The thought occurred that this may be an indication of the nature of the cross-link.

This looked very exciting, but a long search to find the cross-link was envisaged and clearly our small team needed reinforcement. Dr. J. Thomas from the University College of South Wales, who was already in the department, offered to join us, and accordingly we agreed to tackle it together with Don Elsden in general charge of the amino acid analysis and chromatography.

Although we had noticed one or two unidentified slow-moving spots on paper chromatograms from hydrolysates of various elastin fractions we did not think it enough merely to isolate new amino acids from elastin: we wanted to identify the structures concerned with the cross-bridging points in the most unambiguous way possible. We set out with the idea that if elastin were broken down to the smallest possible peptides by the successive action of a variety of enzymes, then the peptides bearing the cross-links should on the whole be larger than the straight-chain peptides. In fact we were delighted when we found that a fraction of the peptides bearing most of the ultraviolet absorption could be sifted out by using short columns of sulphonated polystyrene resins with decreasing divinylbenzene content and thus increasing pore size. These resins we made under the tutorledge of our old colleague Dr. K. W. Pepper at the Chemical Research Laboratory, Teddington. This crude peptide fraction was estimated to have a minimum molecular weight of about 1,000 and showed the presence of at least two α-carboxy groups and two α-amino groups which in the protein could be engaged with two independent peptide chains. Further chemical work on this peptide material showed it to be a mixture of a number of closely related multichain peptides containing mainly glycine, alanine and proline. Unfortunately we could not isolate homogeneous compounds from this mixture. However, we found that the peptide mixture gave on acid hydrolysis and further purification two hitherto unknown amino acids in very high yield.

These new amino acids were at first designated A and M and were provisionally assigned the empirical formulae $C_{26}H_{45}N_5O_8$ and $C_{26}H_{41}N_5O_8$ respectively. It was deduced from the titration curves that both compounds contained four charged α-amino and four charged α-carboxy groups and a very strongly basic group, probably quarternary ammonium, which titrates above pH 11.5 (44).

The two compounds were then isolated on a larger scale directly from the acid hydrolysis products of 1,000 g of purified elastin from bovine *ligamentum nuchae*. In the process of purification most of the acidic and neutral amino acids were removed from the mixture by use of our existing semitechnical-scale ion-exchange displacement columns, and the final purification was by the same procedure as before.

With the larger quantity of purified A and M available (nearly 1 g of each) we were able to secure better titration curves and elementary compositions (45). The best fitting empirical formula for both compounds (as chlorides) was $C_{24}H_{40}N_5O_8Cl$. From this and the titration results it was concluded that A and M were isomers. Good ultraviolet absorption spectra were also obtained. It was here that some previous experience of J. Thomas became invaluable. He obtained from a friend, Mr. H. G. Willcock of Midland Tar Distillers, Ltd., authentic specimens of the three possible trimethylpyridines. From these he made the *N*-methyl quarternary derivatives and compared them with A and M. The ultraviolet spectrum of compound A matched 1,3,4,5-tetramethylpyridinium and compound M matched 1,2,3,5-tetramethylpyridinium, thus establishing the steric relationship of the isomers. We proposed the name "desmosine" for compound A and "iso-desmosine" for compound M. Desmosine denotes some sort of link or rivet in the armour of an ancient Greek soldier.

At this point I should digress a little to explain something about Cambridge biochemistry that may not have been apparent to short-term visitors. This was the existence in Downing Street of a rather broken-down lease-expired pub with the unlikely name of "The Bun Shop". This edifice has long since been pulled down, but in its time it had a particular and benign influence on the members of the laboratories roundabout. Many formed the habit of calling in on the way home (usually by bicycle) at about 6 pm and spending half an hour or more with a glass of beer. The point is that, apart from winding down after the day's work, one could always be sure of finding somebody in a receptive mood for idle scientific chat.

I do not know what codes we use to store thoughts and memories in our brains or what causes ideas to congeal and erupt in English, but I do know it is a potent process that happens only when there is not much else going on, and it is stimulated all the more when two people engage in general part scientific and part nonscientific chat together. I noticed this particularly when J. Thomas, Don Elsden and I were engaged with the work on elastin cross-links. This work took quite a time—about a year—because we all three had other duties, but we kept in touch mainly in the evenings in The Bun Shop. Mainly because of this we were able to share the intellectual satisfaction of the research as well as the hard work. Perhaps this is what the ancient Greeks meant by their word "symposium".

I feel that this kind of arrangement has a genuine value in scientific research. Too often young researchers are given a defined project, probably supported by a specific grant, and they thereupon find themselves in an isolated world of their own: isolated from chat or the random exchange of ideas. When the laboratory left Cambridge for a fine new building on the outskirts of Bristol there were all the facilities we needed—but J. Thomas went off to fill a senior teaching post in Cardiff, and for some reason we were never able to establish another long-running symposium. Most scientists now have working wives, and too many young men feel they have to rush off home at 5:30.

The empirical formulae of the desmosines made it immediately prob-able that they arise from four molecules of lysine (47). This could cause no surprise to anybody because so many of the plant alkaloids arise from similar lysine condensations. It was obviously necessary to seek formal proof of this origin by isotopic labelling. However, we had no skill at these techniques and no apparatus for counting. Accordingly, I took advantage of a visit to Chicago to put the matter before Albert Dorfman. He immediately took the point and we arranged to feed young rats with [U-^{14}C]lysine in Chicago and to isolate the aortic elas-tin and fractionate the hydrolysate in Cambridge. The labelled sam-ples were then counted in Chicago. The results showed that at least two molecules of lysine (and possibly four) are incorporated during the synthesis of both desmosine isomers (48).

About the same time Miller, Martin, and Piez showed clearly that the elastin from the aortae of 12-day-old chick embryos contained much more lysine and less desmosine than elastin from full-grown birds. Over the age range investigated the sum of lysine and quarter-desmo-sine remained constant, and there was a smooth transition of the ly-sine/quarter-desmosine ratio with increase in age. The same authors reported that, in tissue culture experiments with chick embryo aorta, the amount of lysine incorporated into desmosine and isodesmosine increased steadily for some days after the culture had been allowed to take up a quantity of radioactive lysine from the medium.

In a further collaboration with Albert Dorfman's team, young rats were killed 0.5, 5 and 17 days after an injection of [U-^{14}C]lysine. The elastin was isolated from the aortae and counted as before. After allow-ance for growth during the course of the experiment the results sug-gested the incorporation of four molecules of lysine into both desmo-sine and isodesmosine and also that the cyclization process is a slow one, occupying up to 17 days after the uptake of the lysine (49).

The same year Dr. Boyd O'Dell spent a sabbatical leave with us from the University of Missouri and set up a study of the effects of copper deficiency and lathyrism induced by BAPN feeding on the composition of purified chick aorta elastin. In the case of copper deficient elastin, the lysine content was nearly five times that of the controls, while the desmosines averaged only 60% of the control values (50). The result of the lathyritic diet was not quite so marked. The BAPN-fed elastin showed no change in desmosine and had only twice the normal lysine content. However, the failure to observe more significant differences in the desmosine content was doubtless due to the mild nature of the lathyrism induced. Aortae from young ducklings, 1–7 days old, were grown in organ culture and the effect of BAPN on the incorporation of lysine into desmosine examined. It was found that the specific activities of desmosine and isodesmosine were depressed to about one-tenth or less of the value found for the controls (51).

ATTEMPTS TO STUDY THE PHYSICAL PROPERTIES OF ELASTIN AND ELASTIC TISSUE

From about 1965 onwards I was beginning to feel that quite a useful amount of knowledge had been collected about the chemistry and biosynthesis of elastin by teams around the world, but that its physical properties had been neglected: of course it is the changes in the physical properties of elastic fibres that are directly responsible for the failures of elastic tissue that give rise to disease. I began to take every opportunity to talk to physicists and to try to persuade them to use any available modern methods in the study of elastin and the changes brought about in elastin fibres by disease.

On our own account we were much interested in the state of water in purified elastin and the size and distribution of the water-filled pores in it. Having spent a great part of my working life with chromatographic methods it was natural that I should look to the behaviour of columns packed with water-swollen elastin fibres as a way of studying the pore-size and absorptive behaviour of purified elastins from various sources.

Obviously we made a start with the very pure and very regular elastin fibres that can be made from *ligamentum nuchae* of cattle. We packed a large column of this material and then carefully demineralized it by allowing 1% acetic acid to percolate through for about 2 months during a vacation. The final ash content was so low that no increase of weight could be measured in 1 g of dry elastin fibres after ashing in a large platinum crucible.

These very regular fibres proved to be an almost perfect column packing for "molecular exclusion chromatography". In order to determine the "effective radius" of the pore systems in water-swollen elastin fibres a number of solutes of known Stokes radius were chromatographed to find the respective values of the elution volume (V_e) for each solute, and from these values of the distribution coefficients (K_D) were calculated. This allowed the pore size in elastin to be calculated from the data for each solute.

The values of the effective pore diameter calculated for sugars and glycols ranging in molecular weight from 60 to 1,000 were almost constant, at 30–33 Å. I took the precaution of sending the draft paper to Prof. T. C. Laurent in Uppsala before publication and almost immediately received a reply that he had plotted the chromatographic data according to the equation of Siegel and Monty (52) and that the points fell on a rather good straight line, indicating that the data were also valid for a gel consisting of a system of parallel hydrated molecular rods of 8 Å radius (46). We were rather disappointed that no clear discrimination between the two models was possible with the data available—however, the probability is that under the experimental conditions (high water activity) the structure of elastin contains elements of both models.

We and various colleagues have made a number of other attempts to show structure in elastin at the molecular level, and to us it seems clear that such ordered structure is a reality provided the swollen gel has unrestricted access to water. If access is restricted either by blotting off the experimental fibre or by doing the experiments under conditions of low water activity (i.e., in 20% ethylene glycol), the evidence of structure at the molecular level disappears and elastin fibres behave as though composed of a truly random network. At a much lower water content (around 30% of water) the structure changes again and the fibres become rigid and glass-like.

I believe these points are important if only because of the perverse behaviour of elastin fibres in atherosclerotic tissue. In order to try to throw more light on the subject I talked to Professor Weis-Fogh (unfortunately now deceased) who, when he took up his appointment at Cambridge University, found himself in possession of a very sensitive (and very large) calorimeter, made by a predecessor. Torkel Weis-Fogh decided to use the calorimeter to measure heat exchanges during stretching and relaxation of elastin fibres in contact with water or various aqueous solutions. The expectation, with a random polymer, was to find that the heat exchange would be very small and equivalent to the potential energy stored in the stretched fibre. It was found, however, that, in water and dilute buffers at room temperature, the heat produced and absorbed when the fibre is extended or relaxed was very considerable (53). When the water was partly replaced by solvents that reduced the water activity (ethylene glycol, formamide, ethanol) the heat produced and absorbed was much reduced. Indeed, in pure formamide the heat exchange was reduced to the value expected for a wholly entropic system.

It has been pointed out that the heat exchange observed can be regarded as arising from the bulk transfer of water to and from the fibre as it is stretched or relaxed. This implies that the water content of the fibre changes during stretching under conditions of free water access. Attempts have been made to measure the water content of fibres,

but they are all rather crude. The usual procedure at present is to blot
the fibres quickly and then weigh them. An alternative procedure is to
centrifuge a fibre preparation in a tube fitted with a scintered glass
plate and a rubber or plastic closure, but this is subject to error because
the centrifugal pressure forces water from the cross-linked gel. The
matter is obviously one of importance and would be worth studying by
making duplicate runs at different values of G and extrapolating to
zero G.

To avoid getting into difficulties due to changes in water of swelling
it has become customary to carry out measurements of stress–strain
relations, heat-exchanges, and the molecular weight of chain between
the cross-links in solvents such as 20:80 ethylene glycol:water in
which water activity is low and migration of swelling water is at a
minimum. This, however, also avoids the whole problem of hydrophobic bonding: the structures at the molecular level that are seen to occur
in the presence of free water. These structures have been reported by
very many workers using different experimental techniques and are
apparent under a wide variety of experimental circumstances when
access to water is unlimited.

MEASUREMENT OF THE MOLECULAR WEIGHT BETWEEN
CROSS-LINKS (M_c)

Rigorous work on this subject has been described by D. P. Mukherjee
in his Doctoral Thesis, 'The Viscoelastic Properties of Elastin' at the
Massachusetts Institute of Technology (1969). Specimens of purified
elastin were swollen in different aqueous and nonaqueous solutions,
and the elastic creep behaviour was studied in the swelling solutions in
order to obtain the molecular weight between cross-links (M_c) by the
application of the theory of rubber elasticity. The solvent systems were
chosen as suitable to study the role of hydrogen bonding, hydrophobic
interactions and ionic interactions in the stability of possible secondary structure in elastin.

Formamide–water systems at higher concentrations of formamide
are good swelling agents for elastin, giving swollen volumes up to
three times that for water. The M_c value increases with addition of
formamide to water, reaching a maximum around the concentration of
44% v/v (M_c 7900 compared to 3400 in deionised water). On the other
hand, alcohols (methanol, ethanol and butanol) are poor swelling
agents for elastin; however, the M_c value increases with the addition of
alcohols to water, reaching a maximum (M_c 6000) at around 10% v/v
methanol in water. These two solvent systems have very different

swelling properties, but both reduce the water activity of the system, both reduce hydrophobic bonding and both almost double the kinetically free chain between the cross-links.

Electron Microscopy. Of all the strategems devised for studying protein structure in the presence of free water, negative-staining for electron microscopy is perhaps the most elegant. The sample, suspended in water, is blotted with filter paper and the liquid phase replaced with the suspension of electron-opaque particles. Thus, in skilful hands, the negative image is produced without disturbing the state of swelling. Very thin sections of water swollen elastin can be good specimens to display this kind of technique, and several groups of workers, particularly Professor L. Gotte and his colleagues (cf. Ref. 54), have advanced the study over many years. Their work shows that, in aqueous suspensions of elastin fragments, a system of oriented beaded filaments of 3.5–4.0 nm diameter is very prominent. The periodicity along the axis of the fibres is also about 3.5–4.0 nm. The spaces occupied by the negative stain form parallel arrays of very considerable length and appear to be about 2.5–3.5 nm thick. I am of the opinion that these structures are only to be seen at high values of water activity and that they arise mainly in response to the formation of regions of hydrophobic interaction: that is to say, hydrophobic regions are squeezed out from the water continuum. From a different viewpoint, the primary driving force for the hydrophobic interactions can be regarded as the exclusion of water from the interacting hydrophobic surfaces, estimated at 10 kJ nm^{-2} (55).

The structures formed by hydrophobic bonding at high water activity arise equally when soluble degradation products of elastin, such as α-elastin or κ-elastin, are allowed to coacervate by raising the temperature a few degrees. Indeed, as early as 1966 Professor L. Robert and his colleagues pointed out the critical role of hydrophobic forces in the structure of elastin and its soluble derivative prepared by partial alkaline hydrolysis, κ-elastin (56).

It is pleasant to be able to record here the many visits my wife and myself have paid to and received with Leslie Robert and his family during the past 20 years. Our talks together have done much to clarify my own thinking on many questions of elastin structure, some of which are still not yet fully resolved.

The work of Gotte and others has left us with subfilaments about 1.5 nm in diameter as the smallest unit of structure in water-swollen elastin, and two or three of these units may be linked together to give what appears to be beaded filaments about 4.0 nm in diameter. This kind of structure forms flakes and has shear planes. Passing down-

wards through the hierarchy, the preferred secondary structure of the
1.5-nm subfilaments at the molecular level has been discussed by Urry
and his collaborators (57). Elastin contains repetitions of runs of identical or similar sequences containing predominantly glycine, proline
and valine (58). Typical repeat peptides are Val_1-Pro_2-Gly_3-Gly_4, Val_1-
Pro_2-Gly_3-Val_4-Gly_5 and Ala_1-Pro_2-Gly_3-Val_4-Gly_5-Val_6, all of which
contain Pro in the second position and Gly in the third position. Proton
and carbon-13 magnetic resonance spectra of synthetic polymers containing these peptide sequences have been studied in a variety of solvents, and extensive conformational energy calculations have been
made. All of the peptides were found to contain a predominating conformational feature called the β-turn which used prolyl and glycyl
residues to produce almost right-angle bends in the peptide chain. At
elevated temperature (above 50°C) in water, the dominant structure is
of the cross-β type. This increase in intramolecular order with increase
in temperature in water is a temperature transition typical of elastin
peptides generally.

The dimensions of the α-spiral conformations of the polypentapep-
tide and the polyhexapeptide are such that association in pairs or
threefold units could readily provide the "beaded" 4.0 nm filaments
observed in electron micrographs of coacervates of α-elastin, soluble
elastin precursors or native elastin. The repetitive pattern formed by
such a combination of subfilaments during the coacervation of tropoelastin could well account for an organized distribution of cross-
linking points formed as a result of the apposition of lysine residues
(47).

From my viewpoint it seems that a large part of the biophysical
effort that has been expended on elastin over the past 10 years has
really sprung up under the stimulus of the letter to *Nature* from Weis-
Fogh and Anderson in 1970 (53). In the light of hindsight I think these
authors were rather imprudent to describe the elasticity of elastin as
"of a new type" because of course the accepted theory of rubber-like
elasticity is based on fundamental considerations only and assumes
nothing except the gas laws. Nevertheless, having discussed this with
Torkel Weis-Fogh many times before he died, I can fully understand
what he meant, and wish only that he were with us again to defend his
model. Before he became interested in elastin he spent many years
studying "resilin", a structural rubber-like protein found only in ar-
thropods. Particularly favourable samples of resilin can be prepared
from the elastic tendon of dragonflies, but during the course of his
studies he encountered very thin structures indeed, such as me-
chanoreceptors which had very stable elastic properties (i.e., did not

creep or flow) and which seemed to have dimensions too small to be regarded as comprised of a three-dimensional random net.

Of course Weis-Fogh's structure for elastin, consisting of hydrophobic globules connected by short peptide chains and cross-links, could form very thin structures without sacrificing stability, and indeed could consist of single chains of "hydrophobic globules" of molecular size. Such very thin rubber-like threads are making their appearance in other tissues, and it would be interesting to know how "titin", a new major constituent of mammalian muscle (59), compares with resilin and elastin.

Finally, perhaps I should say that on re-reading this manuscript I realize that I have not written of my wife and family since I mentioned our marriage in 1940. This is because since then we have been almost uniformly happy, thanks to my wife, and I have received all the help and encouragement I could have hoped for. We have four healthy and pretty daughters and, to date, three granddaughters and two grandsons, equally a source of pleasure and satisfaction to their grandparents.

REFERENCES

1. Kenyon, J., Partridge, S. M., and Phillips, H. (1936). *J. Chem. Soc.* 85.
2. Kenyon, J., and Partridge, S. M. (1936). *J. Chem. Soc.* 1069.
3. Kenyon, J., Partridge, S. M., and Phillips, H. (1937). *J. Chem. Soc.* 207.
4. Coppock, J. B. M., and Partridge, S. M. (1936). *Nature (London)* 1313.
5. Coppock, J. B. M., and Partridge, S. M. (1938). *J. Chem. Soc.* 1069.
6. Morgan, W. T. J., and Partridge, S. M. (1940). *Biochem. J.* **34**, 169.
7. Morgan, W. T. J., and Partridge, S. M. (1941). *Biochem. J.* **35**, 1140.
8. Partridge, S. M., and Morgan, W. T. J. (1940). *Br. J. Exp. Pathol.* **21**, 180.
9. Partridge, S. M., and Morgan, W. T. J. (1942). *Br. J. Exp. Pathol.* **23**, 84.
10. Morgan, W. T. J., and Partridge, S. M. (1842). *Br. J. Exp. Pathol.* **23**, 151.
11. Tiselius, A. (1943). *Ark. Kem. Min. Geol.* **16A** (18).
12. Claesson, S. (1946). *Ark. Kem. Min. Geol.* **23A** (1).
13. Consden, R., Gordon, A. H., and Martin, A. J. P. (1944). *Biochem. J.* **38**, 224.
14. Bendall, J. R., Partridge, S. M., and Westall, R. G. (1947). *Nature (London)* **160**, 374.
15. Partridge, S. M. (1948). *Biochem. J.* **42**, 238.
16. Partridge, S. M. (1948). *Biochem. J.* **42**, 251.
17. Partridge, S. M. (1949). *Biochem. Soc. Symp.* **3**, 52.
18. Partridge, S. M. (1949). *Nature (London)* **164**, 443.
19. Partridge, S. M., and Westall, R. G. (1949). *Biochem. J.* **44**, 418.
20. Partridge, S. M., and Brimley, R. C. (1949). *Biochem. J.* **44**, 513.
21. Partridge, S. M. (1949). *Biochem. J.* **44**, 521.
22. Partridge, S. M. (1949). *Biochem. J.* **45**, 459.
23. Partridge, S. M., Brimley, R. C., and Pepper, K. W. (1950). *Biochem. J.* **46**, 334.
24. Partridge, S. M., and Brimley, R. C. (1951). *Biochem. J.* **48**, 313.
25. Partridge, S. M., and Brimley, R. C. (1951). *Biochem. J.* **49**, 153.
26. Partridge, S. M., and Brinley, R. C. (1952). *Biochem. J.* **51**, 628.

27. Partridge, S. M. (1949). *Discuss. Faraday Soc.* (7), 296.
28. Moore, S., and Stein, W. H. (1951). *J. Biol. Chem.* **192,** 663.
29. Partridge, S. M., Davis, H. F., and Adair, G. S. (1961). *Biochem. J.* **15,** 79.
30. Gottschalk, A., and Partridge, S. M. (1950). *Nature (London)* **165,** 684.
31. Partridge, S. M., and Elsden, D. F. (1961). *Biochem. J.* **79,** 26.
32. Partridge, S. M. (1951). *J. Sci. Instrum.* **28,** 28.
33. Boardman, N. K., and Partridge, S. M. (1953). *Nature (London)* **171,** 208.
34. Boardman, N. K., and Partridge, S. M. (1954). *J. Poly. Sci.* **12,** 281.
35. Boardman, N. K., and Partridge, S. M. (1955). *Biochem. J.* **59,** 543.
36. Partridge, S. M., and Davis, H. F. (1950). *Nature (London)* **165,** 62.
37. Sanger, F. (1945). *Biochem. J.* **39,** 567.
38. Adair, G. S., Davis, H. F., and Partridge, S. M. (1951). *Nature (London)* **167,** 605.
39. Partridge, S. M. (1962). *Adv. Protein Chem.* **17** (Review).
40. Gotte, L., Stern, P. L., Elsden, D. F., and Partridge, S. M. (1963). *Biochem. J.* **87,** 344.
41. Hoeve, S. A. J., and Flory, P. J. (1958). *J. Am. Chem. Soc.* **80,** 6523.
42. Partridge, S. M., Davis, H. F., and Adair, G. S. (1955). *Biochem. J.* **61,** 11.
43. Partridge, S. M., and Davis, H. F. (1955). *Biochem. J.* **61,** 21.
44. Partridge, S. M., Elsden, D. F., and Thomas, J. (1963). *Nature (London)* **197,** 1297.
45. Thomas, J., Elsden, D. F., and Partridge, S. M. (1963). *Nature* **200,** 651.
46. Partridge, S. M. (1963). *Biochim. Biophys. Acta* **140,** 132.
47. Partridge, S. M., Elsden, D. F., and Thomas, J. (1966). *Proc. NATO Advanced Study Inst.* pp. 88–92.
48. Partridge, S. M., Elsden, D. F., Thomas, J., Dorfman, A., Telser, A., and Ho, Pei-Lee (1964). *Biochem. J.* **93,** 30c–33c.
49. Partridge, S. M., Elsden, D. F., Thomas, J., Dorfman, A., Telser, A., and Ho, Pei-Lee (1966). *Nature (London)* **209,** 399–400.
50. O'Dell, B. L., Elsden, D. F., Thomas, J., and Partridge, S. M. (1965). *Biochem. J.* **96,** 35P.
51. O'Dell, B. L., Elsden, D. F., Thomas, J., and Partridge, S. M. (1966). *Nature (London)* **209,** 401.
52. Siegel, L. M., and Monty, K. J. (1966). *Biochim. Biophys. Acta* **112,** 346.
53. Weis-Fogh, T., and Anderson, S. O. (1970). *Nature (London)* **227,** 718.
54. Gotte, L., Volpin, D., Horne, R. W., and Mammi, M. (1976). *Micron (London)* **7,** 95.
55. Clothia, C. (1974). *Nature (London)* **248,** 338.
56. Robert, L., and Poullain, N. (1966). *Arch. Mal. Coeur* **59** (Suppl. 3), 121–127.
57. Urry, D. W., and Long, M. N. (1976). *C.R.C. Crit. Rev. Biochem.* **4,** 1.
58. Sandberg, L. B., Weissman, N., and Gray, W. R. (1971). *Biochemistry* **52.**
59. Trinick, J. A., Knight, P. J., and Whiting, A. H. (1984). *J. Mol. Biol.* **180,** 331.

Intracellular Turnover of Collagen

Richard A. Berg

Department of Biochemistry, University of Medicine and Dentistry Rutgers Medical School, Piscataway, New Jersey

I. Introduction

Collagen is the major protein of vertebrate organisms and is the structural protein which is vital to the maintenance of the extracellular matrix. It contributes tensile strength to tissues such as bone or tendon which bear weight or transmit forces. Collagen is responsible for the structural integrity and compartmentation of all major organ systems (Bornstein and Traub, 1979) and may play a critical role in the control of cellular differentiation and embryogenesis (Hay, 1981). Although collagen performs a structural role it is continuously turned over in the extracellular matrix of all organ systems including soft

REGULATION OF MATRIX ACCUMULATION

organs such as the lung and kidney and hard organs such as tendon and bone.

II. BIOSYNTHESIS

Collagen biosynthesis is a complex process consisting of several specific intracellular steps. Since collagen is composed of a unique repeating sequence and contains the posttranslationally derived imino acid hydroxyproline, many of the steps in collagen biosynthesis have been identified (Davidson and Berg, 1981). Collagen is subject to several posttranslational modification reactions including both synthetic and proteolytic steps, so there are numerous potential sites for regulating the amount of final product that eventually becomes incorporated into the extracellular matrix (Fig. 1).

A. Gene Selection

There are at least 10 types of collagen, comprised of at least 17 polypeptide chains which have been identified in a variety of connective tissues (Bornstein and Traub, 1979; Bornstein and Sage, 1980; Burgeson, 1982; Bentz *et al.*, 1983; Sage *et al.*, 1983; Crawford *et al.*, 1985; van der Rest *et al.*, 1985; Schmid and Linsenmayer, 1985). The collagens differ from one another in the primary sequence of their constituent polypeptides, in the extent of posttranslational modifications, and in their tissue distribution. In mature collagen molecules, three α chains are associated into triple helical trimers having distinct properties and tissue distributions (Bornstein and Traub, 1979). For types I, II, and III collagens the collagenous polypeptides are synthesized as high molecular weight precursors known as procollagen proα chains (Prockop *et al.*, 1976; Fessler and Fessler, 1978). These precursor forms are characterized by the presence of additional polypeptide extensions located at the amino and carboxy termini of the collagen α chains that increase the molecular weight of the α chains by as much as 50%. The remaining types of collagen differ from the first three types. These contain either shorter or interrupted helical segments or longer helical segments than the more common types of collagens (Schuppan *et al.*, 1980; Gibson *et al.*, 1983; Bentz *et al.*, 1983). Types I, II, and III collagens readily polymerize to form fibrils and fibers and serve primarily in organs requiring transmission of forces, mechanical support, and stress control. Type IV collagen forms a network structure in basement membranes which separate cell types having distinct functions in every organ system (Timpl *et al.*, 1981; Yurchenco and

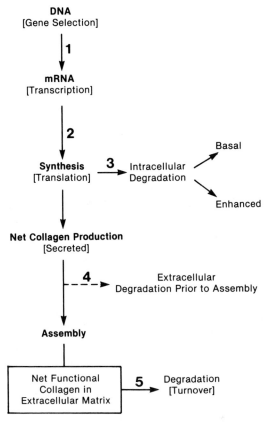

FIG. 1. Collagen biosynthesis: biosynthetic steps at which collagen production may be regulated. The level of collagen production may be controlled by the transcription of MRNA (1), posttranscriptional processing of mRNA (2) and adjustment of translation rates (2). In addition, it has been shown that the rapid intracellular degradation of newly synthesized collagen is an important posttranslational control mechanism (3). After secretion collagen may be degraded prior to assembly into functional collagen fibrils since defective collagen is not completely degraded prior to secretion (4). Collagen in the extracellular matrix is degraded by a family of extracellular collagenases that are responsible for collagen turnover in both tissue homeostasis and remodeling (5). Dotted line indicates unproven event.

Furthmayr, 1984). A structural role for the other collagens is less well established than for types I, II, III, and IV although from their distribution in extracellular and pericellular matrices they must have specific structural functions.

The triple helical conformation of collagen is unique to collagen and is due to the presence of a unique primary sequence, in which the repeating tripeptide Gly-X-Y comprises the triple helical portion of the collagen molecule (Prockop *et al.*, 1976). Approximately 15–30% of the X and Y positions are occupied by proline and the posttranslationally derived imino acid hydroxyproline, with proline often in the X position and hydroxyproline in the Y position (Bornstein and Traub, 1979). The triple helical conformation confers on the collagen molecules the ability to assemble into supramolecular structures and be resistant to most proteinases.

B.   Translation

Collagen synthesis and secretion follow a well-characterized sequence of events (Prockop *et al.*, 1976) similar to that summarized for other secretory proteins (Palade, 1975; Walter *et al.*, 1984). Like most other secretory proteins, collagen is synthesized on membrane-bound polysomes and contains a signal sequence at the amino terminus of the growing polypeptide. This preprocollagen form has been demonstrated in cell-free translations of collagen proα(I) message (Palmiter *et al.*, 1979; Graves *et al.*, 1979). The signal sequence has been shown to be removed proteolytically coincident with transport into the rough endoplasmic reticulum (RER) (Palmiter *et al.*, 1979) and is unique for α_1 (I), α_2 (I), and α_1 (III) chains (Liau *et al.*, 1985). Cleavage of this signal sequence from procollagen is similar for most known secretory proteins (Blobel and Dobberstein, 1975) which have been shown to require the participation of a signal recognition particle (for review, see Walter *et al.*, 1984).

C.   Modifications

In the lumen of the RER, newly synthesized procollagen undergoes hydroxylation of specific proline and lysine residues by the actions of prolyl-4-hydroxylase, prolyl-3-hydroxylase, and lysyl hydroxylase (Kivirikko and Myllyla, 1981). Although three separate enzymes mediate these activities, all three share the requirement for the presence of molecular oxygen, Fe^{2+}, ascorbate, and α-ketoglutarate as cofactors (Kivirikko and Myllyla, 1981). The hydroxylation of specific residues is sequence specific (Bornstein and Traub, 1979).

Underhydroxylation of prolyl residues can be accomplished by incubating fibroblasts in the presence of the iron chelator α,α'-dipyridyl, and early results suggested the accumulation of underhydroxylated procollagen in the cells (Jimenez *et al.*, 1973). In contrast to fully hydroxylated collagen, underhydroxylated collagen is nonhelical at 37°C (Berg and Prockop, 1973); as a consequence such collagen does not polymerize into fibrils. It is not secreted from cells at the same rate as helical collagen and is susceptible to a wide variety of proteinases. The incorporation of proline analogs such as cis-4-hydroxyproline which sterically interferes with collagen triple helix formation (Inouye et al., 1976) also causes both lack of triple helicity, slower secretion from the cells (Kao et al., 1979), and collagen that is susceptible to proteinases.

The glycosylation of specific hydroxylysine residues is begun in the RER through the activities of hydroxylysylgalactosyltransferase and galactosylhydroxylysylglucosyltransferase (Prockop et al., 1976; Kivirikko and Myllyla, 1981). These enzymes share with prolyl hydroxylase and lysyl hydroxylase the requirement that the procollagen substrate be nonhelical to be recognized and modified. Therefore, these modifications must occur before procollagen undergoes triple helical formation. Since there is evidence that carbohydrate transfer may continue as the substrate travels from the RER into the Golgi apparatus (Harwood et al., 1975; Kivirikko and Myllyla, 1979; Oohira et al., 1979), the location of triple helical folding of collagen is not known with certainty. Additionally, it has been shown that an N-acetylglucosamine and mannose-containing asparagine-linked oligosaccharide are present on the carboxy terminal propeptide of the proα1 and proα2 chains of type I procollagen (Murphy et al., 1975; Olsen et al., 1977; Clark, 1979). The function of these high mannose oligosaccharides on procollagen is currently unclear as their absence has been shown to either decrease the secretion from cells (Housley et al., 1980) or have no effect on secretion (Duksin and Bornstein, 1977). The absence of the high mannose oligosaccharide on the COOH propeptide has no effect on the conversion of procollagen to collagen (Duskin et al., 1978).

The three proα chains in type I procollagen are disulfide bonded through cystinyl residues present in the carboxy extension propeptides. The relationship between the formation of disulfide linkages and chain association is still uncertain, but it has been suggested that disulfide bond formation may serve to facilitate the triple helix formation of the three proα chains (Fessler and Fessler, 1978; Prockop et al., 1976; Bornstein and Traub, 1979; Bachinger et al., 1980). It has been shown that the prevention of triple helix formation does not inhibit the formation of disulfide linkages in types I or II procollagens (Prockop et al., 1976) or type III procollagen (Fessler et al., 1981), implying that disulfide bond formation occurs after association of the three carboxy terminal propeptides and may further stabilize that trimeric structure.

The carboxy extension peptide region of the procollagen molecule has been shown to be the site of interchain registration necessary for the triple helical folding to begin (Rosenbloom *et al.*, 1976).

D.   *Translocation and Secretion*

During transfer from the lumen of the RER to the extracellular space the procollagen molecule passes through the Golgi apparatus (Prockop *et al.*, 1976; Grant and Jackson, 1976; Fessler and Fessler, 1978; Bornstein and Traub, 1979) and into condensing granules and secretory vesicles en route to exocytosis (Weinstock and Leblond, 1974; Karim *et al.*, 1979). It has been shown that the secretion of procollagen requires cellular energy in the form of ATP (Kruse and Bornstein, 1975) and is dependent upon the formation of the triple helical conformation (Blank and Peterkofsky, 1975; Prockop *et al.*, 1976; Grant and Jackson, 1976; Fessler and Fessler, 1978; Kao *et al.*, 1977, 1979; Bornstein and Traub, 1979). The secretion of procollagen has been shown to require functional microtubules and microfilaments as it is inhibited by colchicine and vinblastine (Ehrlich *et al.*, 1974; Ehrlich and Bornstein, 1972). It can also be blocked at the level of the Golgi apparatus by the Na^+ ionophore monensin (Uchida *et al.*, 1980).

The collagen biosynthetic and secretory pathways are similar to those of other secretory proteins (Farquhar and Palade, 1981). However, collagen secretion differs from some secretory proteins in that collagen is secreted continuously by the cell, in a fashion similar to the secretion of immunoglobulins (Tartakoff and Vassalli, 1977; Palade, 1975) and albumin (Peters *et al.*, 1971). In contrast, hormones and some other secretory proteins are synthesized and stored in secretion granules which are released by the cell only upon the recognition of an appropriate signal. Examples of these proteins are parathyroid hormone (Morrissey and Cohn, 1979), insulin (Sando *et al.*, 1972), and prolactin (Farquhar *et al.*, 1978).

III.   PROTEOLYTIC PROCESSING OF SECRETORY PROTEINS

Proteolytic processing of secretory proteins may be divided into two classes: limited proteolytic processing and degradation. The first proteolytic event for secretory proteins is the removal of the signal peptide (Blobel and Dobberstein, 1975). This is followed by various degrees of proteolytic processing both prior to and coincident with secretion. Procollagen is proteolytically converted to collagen just at the moment of exocytosis or shortly thereafter by the actions of separate N- and C-propeptidases (Duskin *et al.*, 1978; Tuderman *et al.*, 1978; Leung *et al.*, 1979; Davidson *et al.*, 1979; Njieha *et al.*, 1982; Berger *et al.*, 1985; Tanzawa *et al.*, 1985; Hojima *et al.*, 1985) in cleavages which occur as separate events. Since each procollagen molecule is a trimer, the cleavages are characterized by the presence of intermediate forms (Davidson *et al.*, 1979; Morris *et al.*, 1979; Berger *et al.*, 1985). The enzymes responsible for this processing are believed to be calcium-activated metalloproteinases (Duskin *et al.*, 1978; Tuderman *et al.*, 1978; Leung *et al.*, 1979). It has been shown that similar activities may be attributed to intracellular acid proteinases (Davidson *et al.*, 1979; Helseth and Veis, 1983), but this may be coincidental as acid proteinases are capable of cleaving collagen in the telopeptide region at residues that are several residues removed from those residues acted on by N- and C-propeptidases (Burleigh, 1977).

Partial proteolysis has been shown to occur during the maturation of a number of secretory proteins (see Bienkowski, 1983, and Berg *et al.*, 1986, for reviews). Larger molecular weight precursors of insulin, lactin, parathyroid hormone, and albumin have been demonstrated. Although several possibilities exist (Dannies, 1982), it appears that the Golgi apparatus may be the site of partial proteolytic processing of some of these prohormones during subcellular transit. The processing of proinsulin to insulin has been shown to occur in Golgi fractions (Steiner *et al.*, 1970; Tager *et al.*, 1981; Orci *et al.*, 1984), as has the conversion of proparathyroid hormone to parathyroid hormone (Habener *et al.*, 1981). The conversion of proalbumin to albumin has been reported to occur in Golgi fractions as mediated by a cathepsin B-like acid proteinase (Quinn and Judah, 1978), while another report indicated that this conversion occurred only in secretory vesicles containing albumin (Redman *et al.*, 1978). The Golgi has been shown to be a complex organelle composed of membrane stacks having unique functions. Recently it has been suggested as an intracellular site for the sorting of macromolecules including lysosomal proteinases and secretory proteins (Brown and Farquhar, 1984), and it has been reported to be a site for the degradation of secretory proteins under certain conditions (Glaumann *et al.*, 1982).

IV. ROLE OF INTRACELLULAR PROTEINASES IN MAINTAINING COLLAGEN SYNTHESIS

Although at least three separate proteinases including signal peptidase, N-terminal proteinase, and C-terminal proteinase have been identified as important for the processing of type I procollagen molecules after translation on membrane bound polysomes to the release of functional collagen in the extracellular matrix, several lines of evidence indicate that heretofore uncharacterized cellular proteinases may be important for maintaining collagen production in fibroblasts. When chick fibroblasts are grown in the presence of the proteinase inhibitors leupeptin and pepstatin, TLCK, or lysosomotropic weak bases such as NH_4Cl or chloroquine, the production of collagen by the cells was reduced by as much as 50% with no effect on overall protein synthesis or the rate of secretion of collagen from cells. These effects were first evident in freshly isolated chick tendon cells (Neblock and Berg, 1982, 1984a) but have also been shown in primary cultures of chick tendon cells (Neblock and Berg, 1984b). Although the evidence for the involvement of cellular proteinases is indirect because inhibitors of proteinases were used, the presence of intracellular proteinases required for continual production of collagen may not be too surprising as it is unclear what signals are used to sort macromolecules to be secreted from cells as opposed to molecules that are not secreted from cells but are present in the secretory pathway. Perhaps intracellular proteinases are required at one or more points in the secretory pathway to sort secretory proteins correctly. It has been suggested that fragments of procollagen are capable of inhibiting translation of collagen (for review see Bornstein et al., 1982).

V. Degradation of Secretory Proteins: Collagen

In addition to the limited proteolysis of proteins en route to secretion, it has been also demonstrated that several newly synthesized secretory proteins are subjected to degradation intracellularly before secretion from the cell (Fig. 1). The intracellular degradation is very extensive in the proteins which have been examined: approximately 15% of all newly synthesized collagen is degraded before secretion in human fetal lung fibroblasts (Bienkowski et al., 1978a,b; Berg et al., 1980; Bienkowski and Engels, 1981; Bienkowski, 1984a,b). The milk protein casein is degraded intracellularly at levels of at least 55% (Razooki-Hassen et al., 1982), and it was demonstrated that parathyroid hormone may be degraded at levels of up to 70% (Morrisey and Cohn, 1979).

The intracellular degradation of newly synthesized collagen, like the degradation of cytoplasmic proteins, has been classified by subdivision into two major modes. These have been designated basal and enhanced degradation (Bienkowski, 1983; Berg et al., 1980, 1985). These modes of degradation have defined characteristics which depend upon the conditions of culture employed and the levels of degradation determined (Hershko and Ciechanover, 1982).

The phenomenon of intracellular degradation of secretory proteins has been most thoroughly characterized in collagen producing systems. Intracellular degradation of newly synthesized collagen has now been demonstrated for type I collagen (Bienkowski *et al.*, 1978a,b), type II collagen (Duchene *et al.*, 1981), type III collagen, and type IV collagen (Palotie, 1983) (see Table I). The observation of this phenomenon for a variety of collagens provides support for the concept that the degradation is universal in collagen producing cells. Also in agreement with this concept is the observation that the intracellular degradation of newly synthesized collagen has been demonstrated in a variety of collagen producing cells and tissues (see Table I). These include cultured human fetal lung cells (Bienkowski *et al.*, 1978a; Berg *et al.*, 1980), embryonic chick tendon fibroblasts in monolayer cultures (Duchene *et al.*, 1981) and in suspension cultures (Neblock and Berg, 1982b), cultured human skin fibroblasts and muscle cells (Imberman *et al.*, 1982), and cultured chick chondrocytes (Duchene *et al.*, 1981). Recently intracellular degradation of collagen has been observed in hepatoma cells and hepatocytes (Bienkowski, 1984b). Intact tissues such as lung (Bienkowski *et al.*, 1978a), bone (Sakamoto *et al.*, 1979), skin (Schneir *et al.*, 1982), gingiva (Schneir *et al.*, 1984), and tendon (Neblock, 1984) have been shown to degrade collagen intracellularly. The intracellular degradation of newly synthesized collagen has been observed in fibroblasts from patients with osteogenesis imperfecta (Steinmann *et al.*, 1979; Bateman *et al.*, 1984), in human tumor cells (Palotie, 1983), and in skins of streptozotocin-induced diabetic rats (Schneir *et al.*, 1982).

A. *Basal Level Degradation Is Nonlysosomal*

The basal level of degradation in cells has been shown to be insensitive to the presence of serum or to differences in pH from 6.8 to 7.8 in cultured human lung fibroblasts (Bienkowski, 1984c). The basal level of degradation has been shown to vary, however, with the labeling time in the cells from 16% for an 8-hr labeling period to 23% for a 24-hr labeling period. Since adding collagen back to culture medium of cells indicated that it was not taken up by cells and degraded (Bienkowski *et al.*, 1978a; Berg *et al.*, 1980), the results with increased labeling time point to the possibility that long times may be required to saturate all intracellular compartments capable of degrading newly synthesized collagen. Of interest is the observation that at least two cellular com-

TABLE 1

INTRACELLULAR DEDGRADATION OF NEWLY SYNTHESIZED COLLAGEN

Culture system	Principal collagen type	Mode of degradation	Special conditions	Level of degradation (%)	Refs.[a]
Human fetal lung fibroblasts	I, III	Basal	—	15–20	1, 2
		Enhanced	−Ascorbate	50	3
		Enhanced	+Azetidine-2-carboxylic acid	30	1
		Enhanced	Log growth	30	2
		Enhanced	+cis-4-Hydroxy-proline	30	2
		cAMP enhanced	PGE$_1$, PGE$_2$ isoproterenol	50	4, 5
Rabbit lung slices	I, III	Basal	—	20–40	6
Chicken embryo fibroblasts	I	Basal	Suspension	10	7, 8
		Basal	Cultured	25	9
		Enhanced	+cis-4-hydroxy-proline	25–35	7
Embryonic chick tendon	I	Basal	Organ culture	10	10
		Enhanced	Organ culture	25–35	10
Chicken chondrocytes	II	Basal	—	15–20	9
Human skin fibroblasts	I, III	Enhanced	Elevated temperature	50	11
		Enhanced	Log growth	50	11
Muscle cells	I, III	Basal	—	10	12
Osteogenesis imperfecta skin fibroblasts	I, III	Basal	(?)Abnormal chains	30	13
		Enhanced	Abnormal chains	30	14
Human tumor cells	IV	Basal	—	40	15

[a] 1, Bienkowski et al. (1978a); 2, Berg et al. (1980); 3, Berg et al. (1983); 4, Baum et al. (1980); 5, Berg et al. (1981); 6, Bienkowski et al. (1978b); 7, Neblock and Berg (1982b); 8, Neblock and Berg (1985a); 9, Duchene et al. (1981); 10, Neblock (1984); 11, Steinmann et al. (1981); 12, Imberman et al. (1982); 13, Steinmann et al. (1979); 14, Bateman et al. (1984); 15, Palotie et al. (1983).

partments containing intact molecules of the collagen precursor procollagen can be distinguished kinetically and that one of those compartments requires considerable time to become saturated (Kao et al., 1977).

Lysosomal proteolysis does not appear to be directly required for basal intracellular degradation, since inhibitors of lysosomal proteolysis such as NH_4Cl, chloroquine, leupeptin, and pepstatin A had no effect on basal levels of degradation in several systems. This was in marked contrast to the ability of lysosomal inhibitors to suppress the enhanced levels of degradation shown to occur when the synthesis of conformationally defective collagen had been induced (Berg et al., 1980, 1986; Neblock, 1984).

In addition to its insensitivity to lysosomal inhibitors, the basal level intracellular degradation mechanism has been shown to be uninhibited by a variety of agents in pharmacological studies. In human fetal lung cells, basal intracellular degradation continued at control levels in the presence of the microfilament disruptor cytochalasin B, and the microtubule disrupting agent colchicine (Berg et al., 1980). The results have been interpreted to indicate the lack of microfilament or microtubule involvement in the basal degradation mechanism.

B. Kinetics of Basal Intracellular Degradation

The precise cellular location for the basal degradation mechanism remains to be demonstrated. Also, it has not yet been directly shown that proteinases actually mediate the basal level intracellular degradation of newly synthesized collagen. However, recent data have revealed important clues pertaining to these questions. The earliest identification of products from the intracellular degradation of newly synthesized collagen in fibroblasts occurs within 15 min after the addition of label (Bienkowski et al., 1978b; Curran et al., 1983). In contrast to the kinetics for the intracellular translocation and secretion of collagen, a pathway which saturates within 45 min in chick tendon fibroblasts (Kao et al., 1979; Curran et al., 1983), the saturation for the pathway of intracellular degradation of newly synthesized collagen requires in excess of 90 min to achieve steady state (Curran et al., 1983). On the basis of these data, the basal degradation pathway appears to require a longer filling time than the major route for secretion of collagen from the cells. Further support for this concept has been obtained from studies which showed that levels of degradation could be increased by changing the length of the labeling time in HFL-1 cells (Bienkowski, 1984c). The basal level of degradation was shown to increase from 16% in cells labeled for 8 hr to 23% for a 24-hr labeling period.

The coexistence of both secretion and degradation processes suggests that there is a branch point on the secretory pathway and that degradation occurs in a kinetically distinct compartment from the major route of translocation and secretion from cells (Fig. 2). The exact loca-

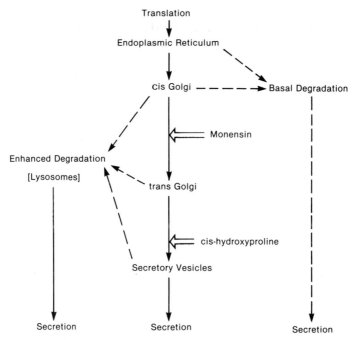

FIG. 2. Intracellular degradation of newly synthesized collagen: schematic representation of the proposed cellular mechanisms and location for the sorting of newly synthesized collagen into secretory and degradation pathways. It is postulated that a cellular mechanism exists which is responsible for the routing of newly synthesized collagen into the basal and lysosomal degradation mechanisms. Current evidence has suggested that the basal sorting mechanism may reside in the cis Golgi region of cells. It is unknown whether the routing of defective collagen to the lysosomes occurs in the Golgi apparatus or at other points in the secretory pathway. The products of intracellular degradation are known to accumulate in the extracellular space. Monensin and *cis*-hydroxyproline inhibit secretion where indicated. Dotted lines indicate unproven events.

tion of this point remains to be established, but, using the ionophore monensin, it has been suggested to occur between the endoplasmic reticulum and the Golgi apparatus (see below).

C. Role for the Golgi Apparatus in the Basal Degradation Mechanism

Pulse-chase analyses of basal intracellular degradation have also indicated that the collagen fated for degradation may be retained by cells for periods of time longer than required for secretion. After pulse labeling 1–2 rounds of procollagen synthesis in chick tendon fibroblasts for 15 min, 15–20% of the total amount of procollagen synthesized was degraded during the chase period (Curran *et al.*, 1983; Neblock and Berg, 1985b). The degradation was shown to continue for periods of 90–120 min, coincident with the saturation of the intracellular degradation pathway in continuous labeling studies (Curran *et al.*, 1983). Interrupting the secretion of newly synthesized collagen at the level of the Golgi apparatus using the ionophore monensin (Uchida *et al.*, 1980; Tartakoff, 1983; Ledger and Tanzer, 1984) caused the chick tendon cells to accumulate collagen with a concomitant increase in the amount of collagen degraded (Berg and Neblock, 1984; Neblock and Berg, 1985a,b). The increased degradation shown to occur in the monensin-treated cultures occurred over a longer period of time and did not vary with respect to the rate of degradation, suggesting that the secretory block increased the amount of substrate available for degradation (Fig. 2). Since the principal effect of low doses of monensin has been shown to be the inhibition of protein secretion at the level of cis Golgi cisternae (Tartakoff, 1983), the data point to the involvement of the Golgi apparatus as the site of the basal intracellular degradation mechanism or the site of the branch-point leading to it (Neblock and Berg, 1985b).

The Golgi apparatus has been predicted to be important for the sorting of secretory proteins and lysosomal enzymes. Brown and Farquhar (1984) have demonstrated that mannose-6-PO_4 receptors responsible for directing lysosomal proteins to the lysosomes are located in the cis region of the Golgi as well as coated vesicles which the authors interpret to be derived from the Golgi. They were not present in trans Golgi or GERL cisternae (Brown and Farquhar, 1984). Recently, Bienkowski (1984b) has put forth a model hypothesis that the entry of collagen into a basal degradation pathway is essentially a random selection of molecules that would normally be secreted. The hypothesis has merit in that it helps explain why basal degradation is ubiquitous in the collagen producing cells and tissues, but it is also possible that collagen chains are tagged in some way that is not yet understood. It has not been possible to isolate collagen destined for basal degradation to show that it is indistinguishable from completely normal collagen.

The Golgi apparatus has been implicated as the site for limited proteolysis of other secretory proteins (Bienkowski, 1983, 1984a). The processing of proinsulin to insulin has been shown to occur in Golgi fractions (Tager *et al.*, 1981), as has the conversion of proparathyroid hormone to parathyroid hormone (Habener *et al.*, 1981). The Golgi has been suggested as a site for the conversion of proinsulin to insulin using monensin (Orci *et al.*, 1984). In this case a clatherin-coated Golgi-derived compartment accumulated proinsulin which was not converted to insulin and was not transferred to secretory granules. The conversion of proalbumin to albumin has been reported to occur in Golgi fractions and may be mediated by a cathepsin B-like acid proteinase (Quinn and Judah, 1978). Another report suggested that this conversion occurred only in secretory vesicles (Redman *et al.,* 1978).

D. Enhanced Intracellular Protein Degradation

In contrast to basal degradation, enhanced proteolysis of cytoplasmic proteins was first recognized as the type of catabolism elicited by stress conditions, such as nutritional or hormonal deprivation (Warburton and Poole, 1977), the synthesis of conformationally defective proteins (Knowles and Ballard, 1976), and when secretion of certain proteins including collagen is inhibited (see Hershko and Ciechanover, 1982, and Bienkowski, 1983, 1984b, for reviews) (see Table I). Conformationally defective proteins produced by the incorporation of amino acid analogs or by the premature termination of puromycyl peptides or error-containing peptides which have arisen from specific mutations have also been shown to undergo enhanced intracellular degradation (see Goldberg and St. John, 1976, and Wilson and Hatfield, 1984, for reviews). The incorporation of canaverine and other amino acid analogs such as *p*-fluorophenylalanine has been shown to cause newly synthesized protein to be degraded much more rapidly than normal proteins in fibroblasts (Bradley *et al.,* 1976; Dean and Riley, 1978), L cells (Hendil, 1976), and reticulocytes (Etlinger and Goldberg, 1980). In several mutant lines of lymphocytes secreting IgM, increased degradation of chains occurred and was due to either changes in primary structure or glycosylation (Sidman *et al.,* 1981).

The enhanced level of intracellular degradation can be caused by several different and widely diverse phenomena. Enhanced intracellular degradation follows the incorporation of amino acid analogs into specific proteins, which may be either cellular or secretory proteins. Dean (1977) has observed that the increased catabolism of analog-containing proteins in murine macrophages was decreased by inhibitors specific for lysosomal proteinases.

Collagen containing amino acid analogs is known to be more susceptible to proteolysis than normal collagen (Uitto and Prockop 1975). The hypothesis that such abnormal collagen may be susceptible to intracellular degradation was tested in newly synthesized collagen made in the presence of the proline analog *cis*-4-hydroxyproline (Berg *et al.,* 1980, 1985; Neblock and Berg, 1982b). Incorporation of *cis*-4-hydroxyproline into newly synthesized collagen caused the level of degradation to increase from 10 to 30% of all newly synthesized collagens.

This hypothesis has also been supported by studies of intracellular degradation of collagen in cells incubated above the helix–coil transition temperature of collagen. Incubation of fibroblasts at 42–43°C caused the degradation of newly synthesized collagen to increase from 12 to 49% in human skin fibroblasts (Steinman *et al.*, 1981). Similar results have been demonstrated for type II collagen in chicken sternal chondrocytes and for type IV collagen in a human tumor cell line, HT-1080 (Palotie, 1983). The degradation of type IV collagen was increased from 38 to 62% when the incubation temperature was increased from 37 to 43°C (Palotie, 1983).

In addition to the enhanced intracellular degradation brought about by the incorporation of amino acid analogs and thermal denaturation, newly synthesized collagen also has been shown to undergo increased degradation when proline fails to be converted to hydroxyproline. This can be caused by incubating fibroblasts in the presence of the iron chelator α,α'-dipyridyl to inhibit prolyl hydroxylase (Prockop *et al.*, 1976; Kao *et al.*, 1979). Increased intracellular degradation of underhydroxylated collagen was also shown for fibroblasts grown in the absence of ascorbate (Berg *et al.*, 1983), a co-factor required by prolyl hydroxylase. Early log-phase fibroblasts contain reduced levels of prolyl hydroxylase (Berg *et al.*, 1976) and were shown to produce collagen which was underhydroxylated and subject to higher levels of degradation than that produced by confluent cells (Berg *et al.*, 1980; Tolstoshaev *et al.*, 1981).

These data emphasize the relationship between the stability of the collagen triple helix and the degree of intracellular degradation. In contrast to fully hydroxylated collagen, underhydroxylated collagen is nonhelical at 37°C, and thus may be considered to be defective (Berg and Prockop, 1973). It is secreted with a rate that is only one-tenth that shown for fully hydroxylated collagen (Kao *et al.*, 1979). The basal degradation level of approximately 10% has been shown to be increased to 40% or more by enhanced degradation under conditions which promote the synthesis of conformationally abnormal collagen.

E. Enhanced Intracellular Degradation of Collagen Occurs in Lysosomes

Aside from the involvement of the lysosomal system in the degradation of endocytosed particles and molecules (Dean and Barrett, 1976;

Livesey *et al.*, 1980), lysosomes also participate in the enhanced intracellular protein degradation seen in nutritional deprivation (Goldberg and St. John, 1976; Dean, 1978; Mortimore and Schworer, 1980; Hershko and Ciechanover, 1982; Ballard and Gunn, 1982). This phenomenon was first characterized by the extensive work of Mortimore and his co-workers (Mortimore, 1982). In experiments with perfused liver, it was shown that increased protein degradation in livers grown in unsupplemented medium (Mortimore and Mondon, 1970) was inhibited by physiological concentrations of amino acids and insulin (Woodside and Mortimore, 1972). This basic observation has been corroborated in a number of types of cultured cells (Hershko and Ciechanover, 1982) and has been correlated to lysosomal activity by demonstrating increased osmotic fragility of lysosomes isolated from the livers of starved animals (Neely *et al.*, 1974). Several lines of evidence indicate the presence of autophagic vacuoles in starved cells or livers perfused without amino acids (Mortimore and Schworer, 1977, reviewed by Mortimore and Pösö, 1984). Autophagic vacuoles are secondary lysosomes derived from the lysosomal engulfment of intracellular particles (Dean and Barrett, 1976) and have been correlated to enhanced protein breakdown (Mortimore *et al.*, 1973; Mortimore, 1982).

In both bacterial and eukaryotic systems, abnormal proteins arising from the incorporation of amino acid analogs from mutations or translational errors are much more susceptible to proteolysis than are normal proteins (Wilson and Hatfield, 1984). Several analog-containing proteins in mammalian systems have been shown to undergo rapid degradation. For example, incorporation of hydroxynorvaline for threonine in cathepsin D, a lysosomal protein, results in its increased degradation compared with controls in human fibroblasts (Hentze *et al.*, 1984). The authors indicated that the degradation was probably lysosomal as inhibitors of lysosomal proteinases inhibited the degradation.

The function of lysosomal proteinases has been shown to be required for the increased levels of degradation of conformationally defective collagen. The enhanced levels of degradation have been shown to be returned to basal or near-basal levels by the lysosomotropic amines chloroquine or NH_4Cl, and cathepsin-specific inhibitors such as leupeptin and pepstatin A in HFL-1 fibroblasts (Berg *et al.*, 1980; Bienkowski, 1984b) and chick tendon cells (Neblock, 1984).

This analysis was corroborated by the demonstration of the procollagen marker imino acid hydroxyproline in the lysosomes of fibroblasts whose function had been suppressed (Berg *et al.*, 1984). Thus, it may be asserted that enhanced degradation of analog-containing proteins is mediated at least in part by the lysosomal system.

Extracts of cultured human lung fibroblasts have been shown to possess proteolytic activity against purified ^{14}C-collagenous substrates. These activities were characterized by acidic pH optima, showed a 10-fold preference for denatured substrate, and were partially inhibited by leupeptin or pepstatin A individually (Berg et al., 1984). Leupeptin plus pepstatin A together inhibited proteolysis by more than 98% (Berg et al., 1984), indicating that cysteine and aspartic proteinases such as cathepsins B and D, respectively, can degrade nonhelical collagen in vitro. The effects of these agents on intracellular degradation in cultured cells indicate the probable involvement of these classes of proteinases in the enhanced degradation of newly synthesized collagen.

Together, these reports support a model in which the enhanced degradation of nonhelical collagen occurs in lysosomes. Whether lysosomal proteinases mediate the destruction totally, or in conjunction with another pathway (such as the basal degradation mechanism), is unknown. Similarly, it is unknown if the conformation of newly synthesized collagen is the sole recognition signal responsible for the routing of defective collagen to lysosomes. It is possible that an intracellular system similar to the phosphomannosyl receptor for lysosomal hydrolases (Sly and Fischer, 1982) may participate in the routing of newly synthesized collagen at some point in the secretory pathway. A summary of the known and unknown steps in the intracellular degradation of collagen is shown in Fig. 2.

It has been shown that not all types of enhanced degradation occur in the lysosomal system. Hershko and Ciechanover and others have demonstrated that existence of a proteolytic system present in the cytosol of reticulocytes which is dependent upon cellular energy in the form of ATP (Etlinger and Goldberg, 1977; Hershko et al., 1978) and is capable of degrading abnormal globin chains (see Hershko and Ciechanover, 1982, for review). The system may be necessary for the maturation of reticulocytes to erythrocytes (Muller et al., 1980) and has been shown to be active in reticulocyte lysates, as well as in intact cells (Etlinger and Goldberg, 1977). The lysate system has also been shown to require ATP and is inhibited by metal chelators, sulfhydryl blocking agents, and chloromethyl ketones (Etlinger and Goldberg, 1977). Neither of these ATP-dependent, nonlysosomal proteolytic mechanisms has been shown to be involved in the intracellular degradation of secretory proteins.

This is not an unexpected result since secretory proteins are confined to intracellular vesicles during their biosynthesis, transcellular movement, and secretion; they are not released at any point into the cytoplasm of cells. Proteins that are taken up by cells through endocytosis are transferred through vesicle systems to various organelles including receptosomes, Golgi, and lysosomes, and are not released into the cytoplasm. In support of the concept of two separate systems, one cytoplasmic and one lysosomal, for intracellular proteolytic degradation is the report that proteins, including secretory proteins such as bovine serum albumin, that are micoinjected into the cytoplasm of cells are degraded in the cytoplasm and not in lysosomes (Bigelow *et al.*, 1981).

VI.   REGULATION OF COLLAGEN PRODUCTION BY CHANGES IN INTRACELLULAR DEGRADATION

The intracellular degradation of newly synthesized collagen has been shown to be sensitive to various culture conditions and hormones and may be an important factor in the regulation of the net production of collagen by cells (Fig. 1). Basal degradation levels of 10% were shown to be increased to over 50% in cultured human lung fibroblasts treated with prostaglandins E_1 or E_2 or with the β-agonist isoproterenol (Baum *et al.*, 1980). In these studies, a corresponding increase in cAMP values was shown. Cyclic AMP and intracellular degradation were both reduced from the elevated levels caused by the presence of isoproterenol when the β-antagonist propanolol was also added (Berg *et al.*, 1981). Recently it has been shown that in mice administration of propranolol caused an increase of lung collagen as measured by hydroxproline content above that obtained when mice were treated with agents that increased lung collagen or caused lung fibrosis (Lindenschmidt and Witschi, 1985). Regulation of intracellular degradation by cAMP is not limited to collagen and indeed may be of major physiological significance in the regulation of protein degradation in the muscle (Goldberg *et al.*, 1984). It has been shown that prostaglandin E_2 stimulated proteolysis in isolated muscles (Rodemann and Goldberg, 1984).

In studies of streptozotocin-induced diabetes in rats, it was observed that collagen degradation was increased severalfold relative to that shown for control animals (Schneir *et al.*, 1982). It was not determined if the soluble hydroxyproline measured in these experiments resulted from the intracellular degradation of newly synthesized collagen or if it was derived from the turnover of recently deposited matrix collagen. However, the possibility that hormones which affect intermediary metabolism may influence intracellular degradation of newly synthesized collagen should receive further attention. Insulin and amino acids have been shown to cause a reduction in the enhanced proteolysis caused by nutritional deprivation or the presence of glucagon (Mortimore *et al.*, 1973; Mortimore and Mordon, 1970). Since elevated cAMP levels have been correlated to increased intracellular collagen degradation, it should be considered that hormonally altered intracellular degradation of newly synthesized collagen may contribute to the connective tissue complications associated with long-term diabetes (Foster, 1983).

Insulin deficiency has been shown to be accompanied by increased proteolysis of muscle tissue to provide amino acids for glyconeogenesis (Dice and Walker, 1980; Ballard and Gunn, 1982). Since collagen is also known to be degraded in insulin deficiency this may provide a clue to the trigger for proteolysis. A central question is whether intracellular degradation is due to increased cAMP mediated by glucagon or is caused by the insulin deficient state itself (Spencer *et al.*, 1978) as has been suggested by Schrier *et al.* (1982).

In additional studies with lung tissue it has been observed that bleomycin produces lung fibrosis in several species, including man (Snider *et al.*, 1978; Kelley *et al.*, 1980). It was observed that in normal rabbit lungs about 30% of all newly synthesized collagen was degraded shortly after synthesis. After treatment of the rabbits with bleomycin the level of intracellular degradation of newly synthesized collagen decreased by 30%, and collagen synthesis increased to account for a net increase in collagen production in this fibrotic condition (Laurent and McAnulty, 1983).

The extracellular matrix protein collagen performs functions which are necessary for the organization of differentiated cells into tissues and organs. Its presence is required to provide structural support and a selective barrier in tissue organization (Bornstein and Traub, 1979) as well as a probable signal for the differentiation and migration of cells during embryogenesis (Hay, 1981). Collagen production must be rigorously controlled to ensure the formation of functional extracellular matrix; many clinically important connective tissue disorders are characterized by the deposition of improper amounts of collagen, or collagen which is structurally abnormal (Prockop and Kivirikko, 1984; Ramirez *et al.*, 1985). In addition, the mechanism responsible for the control of this normally stable protein must be capable of adjusting to requirements for altered levels of synthesis and degradation, as in periods of rapid growth or during the tissue remodeling which follows injury. It is therefore of interest to understand the molecular mechanisms responsible for control of collagen production. In addition to the more well-characterized control mechanisms (Fig. 1), a rapid intracellular degradation of newly synthesized collagen may provide another important way that cells either sort or modulate the amount of collagen which is available for extracellular matrix formation.

ACKNOWLEDGMENTS

The authors gratefully acknowledge the assistance of Mrs. Moira Schneider and Ms. Pat Clark for their invaluable help in preparing this review. The original work from the author's laboratory was supported by NIH research Grants AM 31839, AM 16516, and by NIH Training Grant HL 07467.

REFERENCES

Bachinger, H. P., Bruckner, P., Timpl, R., Prockop, D. J., and Engel, J. (1980). *Eur. J. Biochem.* **106,** 619–632.

Ballard, F. J., and Gunn, J. M. (1982) *Nutr. Rev.* **40,** 33–42.

Bateman, J. F., Mascara, T., Chan, D., and Cole, W. G. (1984). *Biochem. J.* **215,** 103–115.

Baum, B. J., Moss, J., Breul, S. D., Berg, R. A., and Crystal, R. G. (1980). *J. Biol. Chem.* **255,** 2843–2847.

Bentz, H., Morris, N. P., Murray, L. W., Sakai, L. Y., Holister, D. W., and Burgeson, R. E. (1983). *Proc. Natl. Acad. Sci. U.S.A.* **80,** 3168–3172.

Berg, R. A., and Neblock, D. S. (1984). *Fed. Proc.* **43,** 1851.

Berg, R. A., and Prockop, D. J. (1973). *Biochem. Biophys. Res. Commun.* **52,** 115–120.

Berg, R. A., Kao. W. W.-Y., and Prockop, D. J. (1976). *Biochim. Biophys. Acta* **444,** 756–764.

Berg, R. A., Schwartz, M. L., and Crystal, R. G. (1980). *Proc. Natl. Acad. Sci. U.S.A.* **77,** 4746–4750.

Berg, R. A., Moss, J., Baum, B. J., and Crystal, R. G. (1981). *Clin. Invest.* **67,** 1457–1462.

Berg, R. A., Steinmann, B., Rennard, S. I., and Crystal, R. G. (1983). *Arch. Biochem. Biophys.* **226,** 681–686.

Berg, R. A., Schwartz, M. L., Rome, L., and Crystal, R. G. (1984). *Biochemistry* **23,** 2134–2138.

Berg, R. A., Neblock, D. S., and Curran, S. F. (1986). *Biomaterials,* in press.

Berger, J., Tanzawa, K., and Prockop, D. J. (1985). *Biochemistry.* **24,** 600–605.

Bienkowski, R. S. (1983). *Biochem. J.* **214,** 1–10.

Bienkowski, R. S. (1984a). *Arch. Biochem. Biophys.* **229,** 455–458.

Bienkowski, R. S. (1984b). *Coll. Related Res.* **4,** 399–412.

Bienkowski, R. S. (1984c). *J. Cell. Physiol.* **121,** 152–158.

Bienkowski, R. S., and Engels, C. (1981). *Anal. Biochem.* **116,** 414–424.

Bienkowski, R. S., Baum, B. J., and Crystal, R. G. (1978a). *Nature* **276,** 413–416.

Bienkowski, R. S., Cowan, M. J., McDonald, J. A., and Crystal, R. G. (1978b). *J. Biol. Chem.* **253,** 4356–4363.

Bigelow, S., Hough, R., and Rechsteiner, M. (1981). *Cell* **25,** 83–93.

Blanck, T. J. J., and Peterkofsky, B. (1975). *Arch. Biochem. Biophys.* **171,** 259–267.

Blobel, G., and Dobberstein, B. (1975). *J. Cell Biol.* **67,** 852–862.

Bornstein, P., and Sage, H. (1980). *Annu. Rev. Biochem.* **49,** 957–1003.

Bornstein, P., and Traub, W. (1979). *In* "The Proteins" (H. Neurath and R. L. Hill. eds.), Vol. 4, pp. 411–632. Academic Press, New York.

Bornstein, P., Horlein, D., McPherson, J., Sandmeyer, S., and Gallis, B. (1982). *In* "New Trends in Basement Membrane Research" (K. Kuehn, H. Schoene, and R. Timpl, eds.) pp. 127–137. Raven, New York.
Bradley, M. O., Hayflick, L., and Schimke, R. T. (1976). *J. Biol. Chem.* **251**, 3521–3529.
Brown, W. J., and Farquhar, M. G. (1984). *Cell* **36**, 295–307.
Burgeson, R. E. (1982). *J. Invest. Dermatol.* **19** (Suppl. 1), 255–305.
Burleigh, M. C. (1977). *In* "Proteinases on Mammalian Cells and Tissues" (A. J. Barrett, ed.), pp. 285–309. North-Holland Publ., New York.
Clark, C. C. (1979). *J. Biol. Chem.* **254**, 10798–10802.
Crawford, S. W., Featherstone, J. A., Holbrook, K., Yong, S. L., Bornstein, P., and Sage, H. (1985). *Biochem. J.* **227**, 491–502.
Curran, S. F., Bienkowski, R. S., and Berg, R. A. (1983). *Fed. Proc.* **42**, 1888.
Dannies, P. S. (1982). *Biochem. Pharmacol.* **31**, 2845–2849.
Davidson, J. M., and Berg, R. A. (1981). *In* "Methods in Cell Biology" (A. R. Hand and C. Oliver, eds.), Vol. 23, pp. 119–133. Academic Press, New York.
Davidson, J. M., McEneany, L. S. G., and Bornstein, P. (1979). *Eur. J. Biochem.* **100**, 551–558.
Dean, R. T. (1977). *Acta Biol. Med. Ger.* **36**, 1815–1820.
Dean, R. T. (1978). "Cellular Degradative Processes", pp. 1–79. Halstead, New York,
Dean, R. T., and Barrett, A. J. (1976). *Biochemistry* **12**, 1–40.
Dean, R. T., and Riley, P. A. (1978). *Biochem. Biophys. Acta* **539**, 230–237.
Dice, J. F., and Walker, C. D. (1980). *Ciba Found. Symp.* **75**, 331–350.
Duchene, M., Wiedebusch, S., Kuhn, K., and Muller, P. K. (1981). *FEBS Lett.* **135**, 119–122.
Duskin, D., and Bornstein, P. (1977). *J. Biol. Chem.* **252**, 955–962.
Duskin, D., Davidson, J. M., and Bornstein, P. (1978). *Arch. Biochem. Biophys.* **185**, 326–332.
Ehrlich, H. P., and Bornstein, P. (1972). *Nature (New Biol.)* **238**, 257–260.
Ehrlich, H. P., Ross, R., and Bornstein, P. (1974). *J. Cell Biol.* **62**, 390–396.
Etlinger, J. D., and Goldberg, A. L. (1977). *Proc. Natl. Acad. Sci. U.S.A.* **74**, 54–58.
Etlinger, J. D., and Goldberg, A. L. (1980). *J. Biol. Chem.* **255**, 4563–4568.
Farquhar, M. G., and Palade, G. E. (1981). *J. Cell Biol.* **91**, 775–1035.
Fessler, J. H., and Fessler, L. I. (1978). *Annu. Rev. Biochem.* **47**, 129–162.
Fessler, L. I., Timpl, R., and Fessler, J. H. (1981). *J. Biol. Chem.* **256**, 2531–2537.
Foster, D. W. (1983). *In* "Diabetes Mellitus" (J. B. Stanbury, J. B. Wyngaardon, D. S. Fredrickson, J. H., Goldstein, and M. S. Brown, eds.), pp. 99–117. McGraw-Hill, New York.
Gibson, G. J., Kielty, C. M., Garner, C., Schor, S. L., and Grant (1983). *Biochem. J.* **211**, 417–426.
Glaumann, H., Sandberg, P. O., and Marzella, L. (1982). *Exp. Cell Res.* **140**, 201–213.
Goldberg, A. L., and St. John, A. C. (1976). *Annu. Rev. Biochem.* **45**, 747–803.
Goldberg, A. L., Baracos, V., Rodemann, P., Waxman, L., and Dinarello, C. (1984). *Fed. Proc.* **43**, 1301–1306.
Grant, M. E., and Jackson, D. S. (1976). *Essays Biochem.* **12**, 77–113.
Graves, P. N., Olsen, B. R., Fietzek, P. P., Prockop, D. J., and Monson, J. M. (1981). *Eur. J. Biochem.* **118**, 363–369.
Habener, J. F., Kronenburg, H. M., Potts, J. T., and Orci, L. (1981). *In* "Methods in Cell Biology" (A. R. Hand and C. Oliver, eds.), Vol. 23, pp. 51–71. Academic Press, New York.
Harwood, R., Grant, M. E., and Jackson, D. S. (1975). *Biochem. J.* **152**, 291–302.

Hay, E. D. (1981). *In* "Cell Biology of Extracellular Matrix" (E. D. Hay, ed.), pp. 379–409. Plenum, New York.

Helseth, D. L., and Veis, A. (1983). *Fed. Proc.* **42,** 1888.

Hendil, K. B. (1981). *FEBS Lett.* **129,** 77–79.

Hentze, M., Hasilik, A., and Von Figura, K. (1984). *Arch. Biochem. Biophys.* **230,** 375–382.

Hershko, A., Ciechanover, A. (1982). *Annu. Rev. Biochem.* **51,** 335–364.

Hershko, A., Heller, H., Ganoth, D., and Ciechanover, A. (1978). *In* "Protein Turnover and Lysosome Function" (H. L. Segal and D. J. Doyle, eds.), pp. 149–170. Academic Press, New York.

Hojima, Y., van der Rest, M., and Prockop, D. J. (1985). *J. Biol. Chem.,* in press.

Housley, T. J., Rowland, F. N., Ledger, D. N., Kaplan, J., and Tanzer, M. L. (1980). *J. Biol. Chem.* **255,** 121–128.

Imberman, M., Oppenheim, F., and Franzblau, C. (1982). *Biochim. Biophys. Acta* **719,** 480–487.

Inouye, K., Sakakibara, S., and Prockop, D. J. (1976). *Biochim. Biophys. Acta* **420,** 133–141.

Jimenez, S. A., Dehm, P., Olsen, B. R., and Prockop, D. J. (1973). *J. Biol. Chem.* **248,** 720–729.

Kao, W. W.-Y., Berg, R. A., and Prockop, D. J. (1977). *J. Biol Chem.* **252,** 8391–8397.

Kao, W. W.-Y., Prockop, D. J., and Berg, R. A. (1979). *J. Biol. Chem.* **254,** 2234–2243.

Karim, A., Cournil, I., and Leblond, L. P. (1979). *J. Histochem. Cytochem.* **27,** 1070–1083.

Kelley, J., Newman, R. A., and Evens, J. N. (1980). *J. Lab. Clin. Med.* **96,** 954–964.

Kivirikko, K. I., and Myllyla, R. (1979). *Int. Rev. Connect. Tissue Res.* **8,** 23–72.

Kivirikko, K. I., and Myllyla, R. (1981). *In* "The Enzymology of Posttranslational Modifications of Proteins" (R. B. Freedman and H. C. Hawkins, eds.) pp. 53–104. Academic Press, New York.

Knowles, S. E., and Ballard, F. J. (1976). *Biochem. J.* **156,** 609–617.

Kruse, N. J., and Bornstein, P. (1975). *J. Biol. Chem.* **250,** 4841–4847.

Laurent, G. J., and McAnulty, R. J. (1983). *Am. Rev. Respir. Dis.* **128,** 82–88.

Ledger, P. W., and Tanzer, M. L. (1984). *Trends Biochem. Sci.* **103,** 313–314.

Leung, M. K. K., Fessler, L. I., Greenberg, D. B., and Fessler, J. H. (1979). *J. Biol. Chem.* **254,** 224–232.

Liau, G., Mudryi, M., de Chrombrughe, B. (1985). *J. Biol. Chem.* **260,** 3773–3777.

Lindenschmidt, R. C., and Witschi, H. P. (1985). *J. Pharmacol. Exp. Ther.* **232,** 346–350.

Lingappa, V. R., Katz, F. N., Lodish, H. F., and Blobel, G. (1978). *J. Biol. Chem.* **253,** 8667–8670.

Livesy, G., Williams, K. E., Knowles, S. E., and Ballard, F. J. (1980). *Biochem. J.* **188,** 895–903.

Morris, N. P., Fessler, L. I., and Fessler, J. H. (1979). *J. Biol. Chem.* **254,** 11024–11032.

Morrisey, J. J., and Cohn, D. (1979). *J. Cell Biol.* **83,** 521–528.

Mortimore, G. E. (1982). *Nutr. Rev.* **40,** 1–12.

Mortimore, G. E., and Mondon, C. E. (1970). *J. Biol. Chem.* **245,** 2375–2383.

Mortimore, G. E., and Pőső, A. R. (1984). *Fed. Proc.* **43,** 1289–1294.

Mortimore, G. E., and Schworer, C. M. (1977). *Nature* **270,** 174–176.

Mortimore, G. E., Neely, A. M., Cox, J., and Guinivan, R. A. (1973). *Biochem. Biophys, Res. Commun.* **54,** 89–95.

Muller, M., Dubiel, W., Rothman, J., and Rapoport, S. (1980). *Eur. J. Biochem.* **109,** 405–410.

Murphy, W. H., von der Mark, K., McEneany, L. S. G., and Bornstein, P. (1975). *Biochemistry* **14**, 3243–3250.

Neblock, D. S. (1984). Ph.D. thesis, Rutgers University.

Neblock, D. S., and Berg, R. A. (1982a). *Biochem. Biophys. Res. Commun.* **105**, 902–908.

Neblock, D. S., and Berg, R. A. (1982b). *Connect. Tissue Res.* **10**, 297–301.

Neblock, D. S., and Berg, R. A. (1984a). *Arch, Biochem. Biophys.* **233**, 338–344.

Neblock, D. S., and Berg, R. A. (1984b). *Fed. Proc.* **43**, 1851.

Neblock. D. S., and Berg, R. A. (1985a). *Ann. N.Y. Acad. Sci.*, in press.

Neblock, D. S., and Berg, R. A. (1985b). Submitted.

Neeley, A. N., Nelson, P. B., and Mortimore, G. E. (1974). *Biochim. Biophys. Acta* **338**, 458–472.

Njieha, F. K., Morikawa, T., Tuderman, L., and Prockop, D. J. (1982). *Biochemistry* **21**, 757–764.

Olsen, B. R., and Berg, R. A. (1979). *Soc. Exp. Biol.* **33**, 57–58.

Olsen. B. R., Guzman, N. A., Engel, J., Condit, C., and Aase, S. (1977). *Biochemistry* **16**, 3030–3037.

Oohira, A., Nogami, H., Ktsukiko, K., Kimata, K., and Suzaki, S. (1979). *J. Biol. Chem.* **254**, 3576–3583.

Orci, L., Halban, P., Amherdt, M., Ravozzola, M., Vassalli, J. D., and Perrelet, A. (1984). *Cell* **39**, 39–47.

Palade, G. (1975). *Science* **189**, 347–358.

Palmiter, R. D., Davidson, J. M., Gagnon, J., Rowe, D. W., and Bornstein, P. (1979). *J. Biol. Chem.* **254**, 1433–1436.

Palotie, A. (1983). *Coll. Rel. Res.* **3**, 105–113.

Peters, T., Jr., Fleischer, B., Fleischer, S. (1971). *J. Biol. Chem.* **246**, 240–244.

Prockop, D. J., and Kivirikko, K. I. (1984). *N. Engl. J. Med.* **311**, 376–386.

Prockop, D. J., Berg, R. A., Kivirikko, K. I., and Uitto, J. (1976). *In* "Biochemistry of Collagen" (G. N. Ramachandran and A. H. Reddi, eds.), pp. 163–273. Plenum, New York.

Quinn, P. S., and Judah, J. D. *Biochem. J.* **172**, 301–309.

Ramirez, F., Sangiorgi, F. O., and Tsipouras, P. (1985). *In* "Human Genes and Diseases" (F. Blasi, ed.). Wiley, New York, in press.

Razooki-Hassan, H. H., White, D. A., and Mayer, R. J. (1982). *Biochem. J.* **202**, 133–138.

Redman, C. M., Banerjee, D., Manning, C., Huang, Y., and Green, K. (1978). *J. Cell Biol.* **77**, 400–416.

Rodemann, H. P., and Goldberg, A. L. (1984). *J. Biol. Chem.* **257**, 1632.

Rosenbloom, J., Endo, R., and Harsch, M. (1976). *J. Biol. Chem.* **251**, 2070–2076.

Sakamoto, M., Sakamoto, S., Brinkley-Parsons, D., and Glimcher, M. J. (1979). *J. Bone Joint Surg.* **61**, 1042–1052.

Sando, H., Borg, J., and Steiner, D. F. (1972). *J. Clin. Invest.* **51**, 1476–1488.

Schmid, T. M., and Linsenmayer, T. F. (1985). *J. Cell Biol.* **100**, 598–605.

Schneir, M., Ramamurthy, N., and Golub, L. (1982). *Diabetes* **31**, 426–431.

Schneir, M., Ramamurthy, N., and Golub, L. (1984). *J. Dent. Res.* **63**, 23–27.

Schuppan, D., Timpl, R., and Glanville, R. S. (1980). *FEBS Lett.* **115**, 297–300.

Sidman, C. L., Potash, M. J., and Kohler, G. (1981). *J. Biol. Chem.* **256**, 13180–13187.

Sly, W. S., Fischer, H. D. *J. Cell. Biochem.* **18**, 67–85.

Snider, G. L., Celli, B. R., Goldstein, R. H., O'Brian, J. J., and Lucey, E. C. (1978). *Am. Rev. Respir. Dis.* **117**, 289–298.

Spencer, C. J., Heaton, J. F., Glehrler, T. D., Richardson, R. I., and Garwin, J. L. (1978). *J. Biol. Chem.* **253**, 7677–7681.

Steiner, D. F., Clark, J. L., Nolan, C., Rubenstein, A. H., Margoliash, E., Melani, F., and Oyer, R. E. (1970). *Nobel Symp., 13th, Stockholm* pp. 123–131.

Steinmann, B., Martin, G., Baum, B., and Crystal, R. G. (1979). *FEBS Lett.* **101**, 269–272.

Steinmann, B., Rao, V. H., and Gitzelmann, R. (1981). *FEBS Lett.* **133**, 142–144.

Tager, H. S., Steiner, D. F., and Patzelt, C. (1981). *In* "Methods in Cell Biology" (A. R. Hand and C. Oliver, eds.), Vol. 23, pp. 73–86. Academic Press, New York.

Tanzawa, K., Berger, J., and Prockop, D. J. (1985). *J. Biol. Chem.* **260**, 1120–1126.

Tartakoff, A. M. (1983). *Cell* **32**, 1026–1028.

Tartakoff, A., and Vassalli, P. (1977). *J. Exp. Med.* **146**, 1332–1345.

Timpl, R., Wiedeman H., von Delden V., Furthmayr, H., and Kuhn, K. (1981). *Eur. J. Biochem.* **120**, 203–211.

Tolstoshev, P., Berg, R. A., Rennard, S. I., Bradley, K. H., Trapnell, B. C., and Crystal, R. G. (1981). *J. Biol. Chem.* **256**, 3135–3140.

Tuderman, L., Kivirikko, K. I., and Prockop, D. J. (1978). *Biochemistry* **17**, 2948–2954.

Uchida, N., Smilowitz, P., Ledger, P. W., and Tanzer, M. L. (1980). *J. Biol. Chem.* **255**, 8638–8644.

Uitto, J., and Prockop, D. J. (1974). *Biochim. Biophys. Acta* **336**, 234–251.

van der Rest, M., Mayne, R., Ninomiya, Y., Seidah, N. G., Chretien, M., and Olsen, B. R. (1985). *J. Cell Biol.* **260**, 220–225.

Walter, P., Gilmore, R., and Blobel, G. (1984). *Cell* **38**, 5–8.

Warburton, M. J., and Poole, B. (1977). *Proc. Natl. Acad. Sci. U.S.A.* **74**, 2427–2431.

Weinstock, M., and Leblond, L. P. (1974). *J. Cell Biol.* **60**, 92–127.

Wilson, M. J., and Hatfield, D. L. (1984). *Biochim. Biophys. Acta* **781**, 205–215.

Woodside, K. H., and Mortimore, G. E. (1972). *J. Biol. Chem.* **247**, 6474–6481.

Yurchenco, P. D., and Furthmayr, H. (1984). *Biochemistry* **23**, 1839–1850.

The Biological Regulation of Collagenase Activity

John J. Jeffrey

Division of Dermatology, Departments of Medicine and Biological Chemistry, Washington University School of Medicine, St. Louis, Missouri

I. Introduction

The development, maintenance, change, and destruction of the architecture of collagenous structures require particularly precise mechanisms to ensure the attainment of the biological end points unique to each of the connective tissues. The fact that the reagents required for these functions must be managed, in biological terms, over vast distances and that many of these reagents exist out of solution, added to the requirement that three-dimensional precision be maintained for long biological times during these processes, imposes singular requirements on the regulatory mechanisms of these tissues. In the vast majority of cases, ordinary homogeneous solution chemistry is inadequate for the tasks at hand; information transfer in the connective tissues

53

requires that data be transmitted which deals with such concepts as "left," "right," "up" and "down," and "how far." This being the case, it comes as no surprise that, for example, the successful regulation of the biosynthesis of collagen requires no fewer than seven enzymatically controlled posttranslational events to ensure both proper quantity and quality of the final product (for review, see Siegel, 1979, Prockop *et al.*, 1979, Prockop and Tuderman, 1982, Kivirikko and Mÿllÿla, 1984). Even after nearly 20 years of intensive study, a number of gaps still exist in our knowledge of the regulation, modulation, and particularly the coordination of most of these enzymatic events.

In the case of the degradation of collagen, an analogously complex picture is beginning to emerge. The past few years have seen the identification and partial analysis of a number of the reagents whose responsibility it is to preside over parts of the process of orderly collagen degradation in vertebrate biology. It needs to be emphasized here that the variety of systems available for the study of various aspects of collagenolysis, while providing a rich tapestry of phenomenology and of apparent biological interactions, has also served to add to the difficulty in making truly appropriate generalizations. Much of the current confusion in the field is the result of a tendency to extrapolate from the findings and their explanation in one system, from a single species, to other systems in other species. Often the phenomena appear similar, but the explanation may well be very different indeed. It will be a major purpose of this article to attempt to identify such extrapolations and to point out cases in which biologically diverse solutions may be employed in the solution of biologically common problems, as well as to identify when possible those instances in which common pathways may exist in diverse systems. It is also the earnest hope of the reviewer that no new unwarranted generalities emerge from this approach.

It should also be mentioned that this article will deal exclusively with the degradation of the so-called interstitial collagens or, for the purpose of this discussion, types I, II, and III. The vast bulk of the information available on the degradation of collagen and its regulation is available only for these genetic types of the substrate. Enzymes have been identified, and in certain cases purified, which degrade types IV and V collagen (Mainardi *et al.*, 1980a,c; Liotta *et al.*, 1979; Salo *et al.*, 1983), but the nature of these molecules and particularly the factors which regulate their activity are largely unknown at this time. It is to be hoped that this area of collagen degradation can itself be the subject of an article such as this in the near future.

This essay will be divided into two broad sections. The first will deal with aspects of the regulation of collagen degradation which derive from the nature of the reagents intrinsic to the process, as they are currently known. Thus, the first section will deal with the nature of the substrate, the enzymes in their various forms, and those molecules produced in normal biology whose specific functions are, wholly or in part, to modify in any way the activity of collagenase. The second part of this review will deal with selected biological systems in which these molecules can be examined with respect to the modulation of their activity by molecules not exclusively designed to interact with the molecules of the collagenolytic system. Into this very broad category falls hormones of various chemical types and a variety of other agents whose primary targets are the cells which produce these molecules.

The fundamental biological and chemical problem of biological collagen degradation has been rather thoroughly treated in a number of previous reviews (Gross, 1976, 1983; Sellers and Murphy, 1980; Woolley, 1984) and will only be briefly discussed here for the purpose of introduction. Collagen, comprising approximately 30% of all the protein of the mammal, displays remarkable resistance to proteolysis. In either soluble or fibrillar form, below its solution denaturation (T_m 40°C) or fibrillar shrinkage (T_s 60°C) temperatures, respectively, type I collagen is essentially undegradable by a wide variety of neutral proteases, even at very high molar ratios. The crucial biological problem presented by this chemical feature of collagen, namely, the removal of collagen from tissues when biologically necessary, is solved by nature by the production of a class of enzymes whose primary purpose appears to be the degradation of collagen.

These enzymes, the collagenases, have now been detected in a wide variety of cells and tissues. As a class they display a neutral pH optimum, require calcium as an activator, and most likely require zinc as an intrinsic metal ion. More remarkably, they also share the property of cleaving the same bond in native collagen molecules (Gly_{775}-X_{776} where X = Leu or Ile), apparently irrespective of the species of origin of either the enzyme or the substrate. This cleavage occurs across all three chains of the collagen molecule, resulting in two cleavage products whose chemical and physical properties are profoundly different from the parent molecule. These products are now soluble and unstable at 37°C, denature rapidly as they are produced, and become suitable substrates for a variety of other tissue proteases. The action of a prototypical collagenase is schematically represented in Fig. 1.

The cleavage of collagen by vertebrate collagenase appears to occur essentially *en bloc,* much as has been observed in the cleavage of procollagen peptides during biosynthetic processing of collagen. Direct evidence for this essentially simultaneous cleavage of all three chains

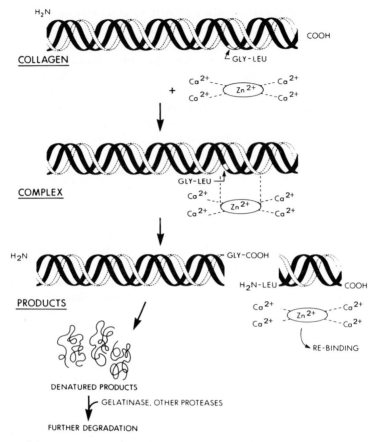

FIG. 1. Schematic representation of the action of collagenase on the native collagen molecule.

is not available, but experience in our own laboratory has shown that at no time do the collagenase cleavage products of type I collagen display anything other than an $\alpha_1^A : \alpha_2^A$ ratio of 2:1 (Welgus *et al.*, 1981, 1983). This is true even when the reaction is performed at high enzyme:substrate ratios, low temperature, and short times (Welgus and Jeffrey, unpublished observations). Thus, there is no perceptible temporal preference of the enzyme for either the α_1 or the α_2 chain of the native substrate.

Considerations such as enzyme preference, coupled with the existence of a highly conserved area of cleavage in the substrate molecule, lead to the first level of regulation of vertebrate collagen degradation:

the nature of the molecules involved and the constraints imposed upon collagenolysis by virtue of these characteristics. In the last several years a number of other macromolecules have been identified which play important, possibly required roles in what are becoming increasingly evident as deserving of the name collagenolytic *system*. In the following sections we shall examine some of the components of the collagenolytic systems of vertebrates, with reference to both their chemistry and their interactions with other components of the system.

II.   REGULATORY ASPECTS OF MOLECULES INTRINSIC TO THE COLLAGENOLYTIC SYSTEM

A.   *The Nature of Latent Collagenase*

The issue of "latent" collagenase has been at the root of possibly the most confusion in the entire field of collagenase research; it has not been fully resolved as of this writing. In 1971, Harper *et al.* first suggested the existence of a proenzyme form for collagenase, from the tadpole. This report was followed by a number of others, most notably those of Vaes (1972) in cultured mouse bone explants, Birkedahl-Hansen *et al.* (1976a) in cultured bovine gingival fibroblasts, and Bauer *et al.* (1975) in cultured human skin fibroblasts, all of which suggested the existence of a collagenase zymogen. This hypothesis was based primarily on the finding, common to all these studies, that limited proteolysis of culture medium with trypsin was necessary for the appearance of active collagenase.

Direct evidence for the existence of a procollagenase was provided by Stricklin *et al.* (1977), who purified and characterized the proenzyme from human skin fibroblasts and showed it to be elaborated as a set of two proteins, of molecular weight 60,000 and 55,000, respectively, each of which could be converted by limited proteolysis with trypsin to an active form, some 10,000 lower in molecular weight. The difference between the two forms of the zymogen appeared to reside in a single peptide, as shown in cyanogen bromide digests (Stricklin *et al.*, 1978), but this difference seemed not to result in a corresponding difference in the catalytic behavior of the active forms against collagen.

It was also shown in these same studies that the zymogen forms of collagenase could undergo an autoactivation process, promoted by repeated freeze-thawing or by prolonged incubation at 37°C, and that the active forms produced by either of these treatments had molecular weights which appeared to be identical to the zymogen forms whence they originated. This finding led these authors to suggest that the autoactivation phenomenon was the result of a conformational change in the procollagenase molecule.

At nearly the same time as the studies of Stricklin *et al.*, Reynolds and co-workers showed that collagenase activity could be elicited from inactive culture medium of a variety of explanted tissues by limited proteolysis, or by the addition of the organomercurial compound, 4-aminophenyl mercuric acetate (APMA) Reynolds *et al.*, 1977; Sellers *et al.*, 1977). On the basis of their studies, these workers concluded that APMA acted by effecting the dissociation of an enzyme–inhibitor complex, releasing active collagenase as a product (Murphy *et al.*, 1977). They were able to isolate inhibitor-containing fractions of culture medium whose inhibitory activity could be blocked by APMA, or which after combining with active collagenase could be again dissociated by the addition of APMA or by trypsin (Murphy *et al.*, 1977; Vater *et al.*, 1978b). The hypothesis advanced by these workers was that, in general, the so-called latency displayed by collagenase was the result of the existence of E–I complexes rather than zymogens (Reynolds *et al.*, 1977). In the years since this suggestion, it has become nearly axiomatic in studies of a variety of impure mixtures that organomercurial-dependent appearance of collagenase activity observed by a number of workers in a variety of systems (Vater *et al.*, 1978b; Harris *et al.*, 1978; Sellers *et al.*, 1980) constituted *prima facie* evidence of such E–I complexes. This unintended consequence of a useful hypothesis has had widespread influence in the literature. In a review of collagenase in 1981, for example (Sellers and Murphy, 1981), the notion of the existence of zymogens as the basis for latent collagenase was not discussed, and the schematic diagram depicting the origin and nature of latent collagenase dealt only with E–I complexes.

Since 1977, however, a number of investigators have demonstrated the existence of zymogen forms of collagenase as primary extracellular products of human skin (Stricklin *et al.*, 1977, 1978; Valle and Bauer, 1979), rabbit synovial (Nagase *et al.*, 1981, 1983), human gingival (Wilhelm *et al.*, 1984), rat (Roswit *et al.*, 1983), and human uterine smooth muscle cells (Roswit, Rifas, and Jeffrey, unpublished) in culture. Birkedahl-Hansen and Taylor (1982) have confirmed, by the use of an ingenious "zymogram" technique (Fig. 2), that the original doublet of Stricklin *et al.* (1977), as well as an analogous set of proteins from gingiva (Wilhelm *et al.*, 1984), display collagenolytic activity when activated by sodium dodecyl sulfate (SDS), which yields active species displaying the molecular weights of the zymogen species as originally reported by Stricklin *et al.* (1977).

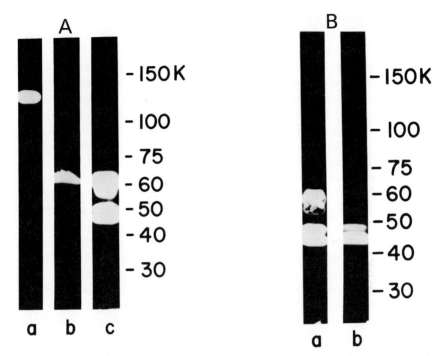

FIG. 2. Collagenase zymograms. Preparations containing collagenase are first sub-jected to SDS–polyacrylamide gel electrophoresis. The SDS is removed with Triton X-100, and the gels incubated 16 hr at 37°C in contact with a film of native reconstituted collagen fibrils. The gel is then removed and the collagen film stained with Coomassie Blue. Clear zones represent areas where collagenolysis has occurred. (A) Activity of *Clostridium histolyticum* collagenase (a), bovine gingival procollagenase (b), and human skin fibroblast collagenase (c). The latter two zymogens have been activated by the SDS in the system but retain the molecular weight characteristic of the proenzymes. (B) Activity of non-trypsin-activated (a) and trypsin-activated (b) human skin fibroblast collagenase. From Birkedahl-Hansen and Taylor (1982), with permission.

Furthermore, Stricklin *et al.* (1983) have shown that organomercuri-als such as APMA (for a more complete discussion of activation, see below) are capable of promoting a conformational change in the proen-zyme of human skin fibroblasts, yielding high molecular weight active forms similar to those originally observed with freeze–thawing or 37°C incubation. These forms then appear to undergo conversion to the lower molecular weight forms of collagenase which are seen after tryp-sin activation. Thus, activation of collagenase by APMA or other organomercurial compounds can, a priori, be as easily due to the activation of a zymogen as to the dissociation of a complex of enzyme and inhibitor, and the two processes cannot be distinguished in impure solutions.

With respect to implications for the regulation of collagenase activity *in vivo,* the existence of zymogens as the primary secretory product of cells clearly indicates the necessity for activation of these inactive species as a necessary step in the initiation of biological collagen degradation. Although only a relatively few cell types have been examined, it appears that secretion of collagenase by the cell of origin as a procollagenase may indeed be a general phenomenon. If so, the activation process assumes major importance in connective tissue biology.

Two further points deserve mention in this discussion. First, most if not all of the organomercurial-dependent latent collagenase activations were observed in organ culture systems as opposed to cell cultures. The former may well represent a biologically more organized system for the study of collagenase metabolism. It may be that in these systems the formation of collagenase–inhibitor complexes of the kind observed by Reynolds *et al.* (1977) is a reflection of mechanisms by which tissues deal with unused, excess activated collagenase to prevent it from acting at unwanted distant sites. Second, in view of the potential importance of these entities, it would be of great interest to be able to critically examine such an adduct in pure form. Indeed, an example may very well exist in the human polymorphonuclear leukocyte, as described by MacCartney and Tschesche (1983a). In this case, the leukocyte collagenase exists as a mixed disulfide complex with an inhibitor (vide infra), and the complex can be dissociated by compounds containing accessible disulfide bonds or by organomercurials such as mersalyl. Thus, at least for the leukocyte, an E–I complex with many of the characteristics described in the organ culture systems described above is put to good biological use.

B.   *Binding of Latent Collagenase to Collagen*

The behavior of latent collagenases in the presence of their native substrate is, at present, somewhat unclear. Harper *et al.* (1971), Stricklin *et al.* (1978), and Halme *et al.* (1980) have reported for tadpole procollagenase, human skin fibroblast zymogen, and rat uterine procollagenase, respectively, that binding to native collagen fibrils does not occur, whereas binding of active enzyme can be observed. On the other hand Vater *et al.* (1978a) have indicated a "partial" binding of rabbit synovial latent collagenase to similar fibrils. In addition, Gillet *et al.* (1976) use collagen coupled to agarose to purify mouse bone procollagenase, and Woessner (1979) has suggested that an inactive form of collagenase is bound to the collagen of rat uterus, together with a serine protease activator. Very recently, studies in this laboratory have shown that human fibroblast procollagenase completely fails to bind to native collagen in solution, whereas the active enzyme binds to the substrate with a K_d of $\sim 10^{-6}$ M and the complex survives gel filtration (Welgus *et al.*, 1985). This may be a case of the biological diversity suggested earlier, and pure reagents in each system will be necessary for the complete resolution of the problem. It would be fascinating if, indeed, biology handled this problem differently either in different species, in different tissues, or for different kinds of processes of collagen degradation. Certainly this question is central to the issue of regulation and one that must be answered in order to fully understand the nature of regulation.

C. Activation of Collagenase

In most respects this extremely important aspect of the regulation of the activity of collagenase is the most poorly defined. A major obstacle to an approach to the problem is a lack of knowledge concerning the end point of the reaction. That is, in no case of biological collagenase action known to this reviewer has the chemical form of the naturally occurring *active* enzyme been shown. This being true, it is difficult to draw firm conclusions about mechanisms of activation. In addition, the several forms of collagenase found in a variety of culture systems may simply be artifacts of culture and more likely to mislead than to edify. That is to say, proteolytic conversion of high molecular weight forms of collagenase may well take place subsequent to diffusion of the latter enzyme into the culture medium from the tissue. Thus, the possibility exists that these forms of the collagenase have no relationship to the form of the enzyme bound to and acting on tissue collagen.

Nevertheless, a wide variety of proteolytic enzymes have been found to activate latent collagenase in a number of tissue and organ culture systems. These include trypsin, which is essentially invariably effective, plasmin (Eeckhout and Vaes, 1977), pancreatic and plasma kallikrein (Eeckhout and Vaes, 1977; Werb *et al.*, 1977), cathepsins B and G (Oronsky *et al.*, 1973), and mast cell proteases (Birkedahl-Hansen *et al.*, 1976b). In addition, rabbit alveolar macrophages contain a protease which activates the latent collagenase contained within these same cells (Horwitz *et al.*, 1976). Similarly, Harper and Gross (1972) earlier reported the production by cultured tadpole skin of a proteolytic activator of the putative zymogen of tadpole collagenase. Vaes and co-workers (1978) suggested the intriguing possibility of a cascade system of activation in a cultured mouse bone system, based primarily upon the observation that full collagenolytic activity in culture medium was not obtained for long periods after a brief activation with trypsin followed by inhibition of the latter protease. The possibility of the existence of such a cascade system for collagenase activation, with its associated multiple control points, would be a most attractive mechanism for regulating the activity of this enzyme.

It should be noted that the above-mentioned studies were all performed in crude preparations, in which it is impossible to monitor specific changes in the chemistry of the collagenase molecule. In the case of the human skin fibroblast procollagenase (Stricklin *et al.*, 1977), which is available in chemically significant amounts as a pure protein preparation, this limitation is absent. Using this molecule as a substrate, it has been possible to isolate, albeit in crude form, activators from two very disparate tissues—human skin itself and involuting rat uterus—which are capable of activating human fibroblast procollagenase by a stoichiometric mechanism (Tyree *et al.*, 1981). That is, activation by these molecules does not require catalysis, such as peptide bond scission, for example, and converts the inactive zymogen to active collagenase by what appears to be a conformational change. These molecules, then, appear to promote the intrinsic ability of the human skin collagenase zymogen to autoactivate in this same fashion and to mimic the effect of organomercurial compounds, such as APMA, on this procollagenase. Thus, Stricklin *et al.* (1983) have shown that these compounds activate human skin procollagenase by inducing a conformational change, which requires the continual presence of the organomercurial, but apparently without alkylating a sulfhydryl group in the collagenase. The mechanism of this unusual process is not known, but the activation process may be related to that observed with the chaotropic ions I^- and SCN^-. The ability of these ions to activate collagenase was first reported by Shinkai and co-workers (1977) in chick skin culture medium. The existence of biological molecules which mimic the effect of these chaotropes is of considerable interest, and may well be significant in the physiological activation of collagenase in some tissues. Interestingly, Vater *et al.* (1983) have reported the existence of an activator molecule from human synovial cell cultures, which extensively purifies with the procollagenase itself and which, these authors report, must be present together with the proenzyme in order for trypsin to activate collagenase. The details of this interesting molecule were not available at this writing; it will be of great interest to see whether this activator acts catalytically (i.e., as an enzyme) or stoichiometrically. Figure 3 schematically depicts the pathways of collagenase activation thus far identified.

It is worth noting at the end of this section, as at the beginning, that the physiologic relevance of none of the pathways of activation described above has been verified, since it is not known in any of the systems what form of collagenase is the physiologically active form. In this regard, as a final indication of the complex nature of this problem, it should be noted that our experience with the human skin fibroblast proenzyme suggests that this species acts as a so-called active zymogen (Kassell and Kay, 1973). Thus, for example, after conformational activation by organomercurials, the zymogen seems to act on itself to yield a number of products (Stricklin *et al.*, 1983), some of which appear identical to those produced by cleavage with trypsin. In view of the existence of this kind of complexity, the task of elucidating the pathways and the participating reagents in the activation of collagenase will be a significant challenge to the collagenase community.

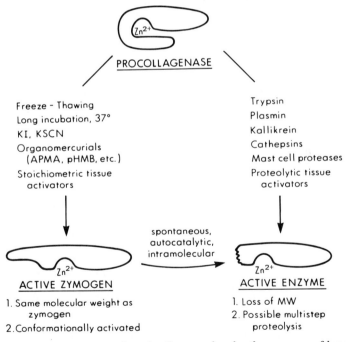

FIG. 3. Schematic representation of pathways whereby the zymogen of human skin fibroblast collagenase can be activated.

D. Nature of Active Collagenase

The collagenases examined to date (Seltzer *et al.*, 1976) appear to require Ca^{2+} as an extrinsic metal, which serves both as an activator and as a thermostabilizer. The K_a for Ca^{2+} is approximately 1 mM, appropriate to the extracellular location of these enzymes. If calcium is removed, collagenase is inactive; readdition of the metal restores activity, but there appears to be a time-dependent irreversible loss of activity in the absence of Ca^{2+}, suggesting that the existence of a initial reversible Ca^{2+}-dependent loss of activity, followed by an irreversible process of denaturation, is occurring under these conditions. Heating Ca^{2+}-free collagenase to 60°C causes a complete loss of activity, while in the presence of 5 mM calcium, the enzyme is stable to temperatures of up to 60°C.

This requirement for freely exchangeable calcium certainly implies the possibility of a pathway for the regulation of the activity of collagenase by varying calcium concentration. To date, however, no system, physiologic or pathologic, has emerged in which this requirement has been implicated in a modulation of collagenase activity or collagen degradation. It may be that, in all but the most desperate pathologies, extracellular calcium concentrations are essentially invariant, and it is for this reason that the enzyme evolved in the way that it did.

The notion that Ca^{2+} acts to preserve a requisite tertiary structure in these enzymes is consistent with the unusual behavior of these enzymes on a variety of ion-exchange matrices. Both human skin fibroblast procollagenase (Stricklin *et al.*, 1977) and rat uterine procollagenase (Roswit *et al.*, 1983), for example, have in common the ability to bind rather strongly to both anion- and cation-exchange resins under essentially the same conditions. Amino acid analyses, however, and pI determination (for the human proenzyme only) indicate that neither of these molecules possesses an unusual charge content. Thus, the calcium may be acting to maintain a three-dimensional structure in which a peculiar spatial *distribution* of charge results, with clustering of positively and negatively charged residues accounting for the unusual chromatographic behavior of these molecules. Changes in environmental Ca^{2+} concentration could result in changes in enzyme conformation and loss of binding or catalytic efficiency.

The collagenases also appear to share a requirement for a second metal, intrinsic Zn^{2+} (Berman and Manabe, 1973; Seltzer *et al.*, 1977; Swann *et al.*, 1981). It is not known at this time whether the requirement is absolute, since no well-characterized apoenzymes of collagenase have as yet been prepared, to allow adding back other metal ions and assessing the resultant activity. Although the regulatory significance of the Zn^{2+} requirement has not been assessed in any well-defined system, an interesting report (Starcher et al., 1980) suggests that nutritional Zn^{2+} deficiency lowers the rate of collagen turnover in chick bone and that this reduction may be due to lowered collagenase levels.

E. Interaction of Collagenase with Substrate

The nature of the active collagenases with their native substrate, collagen, has been only sparsely investigated. A major unresolved question over the years has been whether collagenase alone can complete the degradation of fibrillar collagen as found in vivo. Earlier studies by Leibovitch and Weiss (1971) had suggested that substantially protease-free collagenase was essentially unable to degrade mature, cross-linked collagen fibrils. Added credence was lent to this notion by studies which clearly showed that the introduction of cross-links into reconstituted collagen fibrils markedly slowed the rate of collagenolysis, as measured by release of products from the fibrils (Harris and Farrell, 1972; Vater et al., 1979). On the basis of these findings, the necessity of multienzyme systems for the effective degradation of collagen was hypothesized (Leibovitch and Weiss, 1971; Weiss, 1976). Enzymes in such systems might include gelatinases and proteases which cleaved nonhelical cross-link regions in collagen fibrils, facilitating removal of the products of collagenolytic products from the fibril. On the other hand, Woolley et al. (1975a, 1978b) have shown that highly purified human skin and rheumatoid synovial collagenases are capable of effectively degrading intact, mature collagen fibers. Thus, the issue remains unresolved; clearly the presence of cross-links can be an effective "intrinsic" modifier of collagenolysis. Whether the presence of other proteases do in fact add another layer of regulatory capacity in vivo is not known. No satisfactory system for probing this issue has been developed to date.

In an effort to begin to define some of the aspects of the mechanism of action of collagenase on collagen, Welgus et al. (1980) studied the characteristics of binding of human skin fibroblast collagenase to native, reconstituted guinea pig skin collagen fibrils. The results of this study clearly indicated that collagenase bound tightly ($K_d = 1 \times 10^{-6} M$) to a single affinity class of substrate molecules, which appeared to correspond to those on the outside surface of the roughly 50 nm diameter fibrils present. After binding, the enzyme catalyzed the same cleavage observed when collagen in solution was used as substrate, and at a very slow rate—approximately 25 molecules of collagen per *hour* per molecule of enzyme. This corresponds to approximately one α-chain per minute per enzyme molecule. In addition, and of particular significance from a regulatory standpoint, was the surprising finding that collagenase, once bound, moved from molecule to molecule within a fibril, appearing not to equilibrate with the water of the reaction mixture. That is, activity was essentially dependent only upon the concentration at which the enzyme was originally allowed to bind; subsequent dilution, even by large volumes of buffer, failed to influence either the rate or linearity of the catalysis. Thus collagenase, once bound to fibrillar substrate, brings with it no intimations of its own mortality. Left to itself it appears simply to continue to act until no collagen remains.

The activity of human skin fibroblast collagenase was also examined on native collagen in solution (Welgus *et al.*, 1981), where it was found to behave with normal Michaelis–Menten kinetics, displaying K_m values of 1-2 μM for most collagens examined. Surprisingly, however, values for k_{cat} or V_{max} varied greatly with collagen genetic type. Human type III collagen was degraded 10 times faster than human type I and more than 100 times more rapidly than human type II collagen. The precise reason for these differences remains unknown, but based on this and other studies with human fibroblast collagenase on a variety of collagenous substrates, the following general conclusions can be drawn:

1. Human skin collagenase exhibits slow rates of cleavage of their physiologic substrates, but this is balanced to some extent by high affinities for these substrates (Welgus *et al.*, 1980, 1981). This is not surprising, inasmuch as both enzyme and substrate are macromolecules (Walsh, 1979); catalytic rate in many such cases is sacrificed for avidity of binding. Whether this has any special biological significance for collagenase is not known. Certainly the lack of equilibrium between enzyme and the extrafibrillar water is most unusual. The observation, however, is not entirely new—it was first reported and has been employed as the basis of a useful assay for *in situ* collagenase activity by Ryan and Woessner (1971).

2. Human skin collagenase acts on type II collagen so slowly as to call into question the role of this type of enzyme in cartilage collagen degradation (Welgus *et al.*, 1981). Whether this means that, in spite of its extremely slow catalytic rate of type II collagen, biology nevertheless accepts the limitation or that chondrocytes can synthesize a type II

selective, or possibly specific, collagenase is unknown, but of great interest. Chondrocyte collagenase has been reported (Phadke *et al.,* 1978; Kerwar *et al.,* 1984), but its substrate specificity has not as yet been assessed.

3. Human skin collagenase displays an extraordinary dependence upon temperature, particularly with fibrillar collagen as a substrate (Jeffrey *et al.,* 1983). Whereas "normal" enzymes in general undergo approximately a doubling of their activity for each 10°C increase in temperature, collagenase typically increases its activity some 200-fold over this same temperature span. In terms of more usual temperature changes in homeotherms, this represents a 3-fold change in collagenase activity for every 2 degree change in temperature. This phenomenon was first noted, although not quantitated, by Harris (1974) who suggested its potential importance in inflammatory disease. The assignment of a value to the temperature dependence surely underscores this importance. Simply put, an ongoing process of collagen degradation could be varied approximately 10-fold in either direction by a local or generalized change in temperature of 4°C. This extreme dependence of activity upon temperature could provide a very effective means of regulating the rate of collagenolysis *in vivo.* It will be of great interest to see if this phenomenon is in fact utilized by biological systems in a directive, programmed way.

4. Exclusion of water from collagenous substrates appears to drastically affect the rate of degradation. When human skin collagenase degrades denatured α-chains, which it does slowly (Welgus *et al.,* 1982), it operates as a "normal" enzyme, with normal temperature dependence. When the chains are wound into native molecules, the peptide bonds face into the hydrophobic center of the molecule, water is less available, and collagenolysis becomes a more energy-requiring process. When the monomers are aggregated into fibrils, water is further excluded and the exquisite temperature dependence noted above, the result of an extremely high energy of activation, is observed. In the case of type III collagens (Welgus *et al.,* 1984), it appears that the packing of monomers into fibrils is tighter, the consequent exclusion of water greater, and the energy dependence of collagenolysis even greater. It is this, latter finding—so far observed only under *in vitro* conditions—that may offer a basis for biology to offset the far greater susceptibility of type III collagen than type I in solution. Under laboratory conditions, the type III collagens appear to pack more tightly than type I collagens, with the result that, as fibrils, the rate of their degradation by collagenase is not vastly different from that of type I collagen

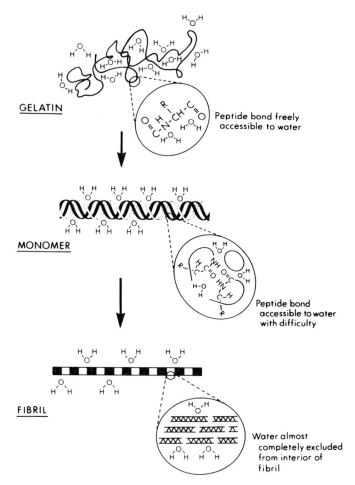

GELATIN

Peptide bond freely
accessible to water

MONOMER

Peptide bond
accessible to water
with difficulty

FIBRIL

Water almost
completely excluded
from interior of
fibril

FIG. 4. Schematic illustration of the progressive inaccessibility of water to the site of
catalysis of collagenous substrates by collagenase as the level of molecular organization
increases.

fibrils under the same conditions (Welgus *et al.*, 1984). Figure 4 summarizes this progressive exclusion of water as a function of the molecular organization of collagen, and the enzymologic consequences of this
process.

In any event, it should be emphasized that the extent of hydration of
collagen fibrils—the amount of water available for hydrolysis—can
drastically affect the rate of collagenolysis, and could be a major intrinsic regulatory factor in any number of processes of collagen breakdown. In fact, it is not inconceivable that mature collagen fibrils, hav-

ing expressed water over a period of time as packing perfection increases, may be essentially protected from collagenolysis solely on this basis. Under laboratory conditions, for example, maintaining reconstituted guinea pig type I fibrils in a humidified atmosphere at 37°C for 5 days lowers their susceptibility to a constant concentration of collagenase to one-third that of 1-day-old fibrils (Welgus and Jeffrey, unpublished observations).

5. Many type III collagens contain a "weak" helix in the region of the collagenase cleavage site. Based on studies on the action of human skin fibroblast collagenase on a number of type III collagens, it is clear that, in some species, a weak region in the helix, at or surrounding to cleavage site, exists and appears to persist to some extent in fibrillar form (Welgus et al., 1984). Thus, type collagen from human, dog, and cat all display distinct breaks in Arrhenius plots relating catalytic activity to temperature. All these collagens are susceptible to trypsin, as originally reported by Miller et al. (1976), which cleaves an X-Arg bond eight residues C-terminal to the collagenase cleavage site. They are also susceptible to elastase, originally found by Mainardi et al. (1980b) to cleave human type III collagen. This susceptibility to non-collagenolytic proteases can be observed even after aggregation of these collagens into fibrils (Welgus et al., 1984). Very high concentrations of trypsin, for example, are required, but complete dissolution of typical collagen substrate gels can be achieved by this enzyme. Thus, the possibility cannot be excluded that proteases other than collagenase, if present in sufficiently high concentrations, can degrade type III collagen in vivo.

Interestingly, not all species of type III collagen display the same degree of helix lability. Guinea pig type III displays only a barely perceptible nonlinearity in its Arrhenius plot, and chick type III collagen invariably yields completely linear plots. Concomitantly, these collagens display markedly lower rates of catalysis by collagenase and markedly higher resistance to trypsin. In fact, chick type III collagen is as resistant to trypsin as is type I collagen. The reasons for these differences are unknown, but clearly the helical integrity of type III collagen is variable between species, and is strongly correlated with the susceptibility of these molecules to collagenase as well as other proteases.

Gross and co-workers have attempted to identify features in the collagen molecule at or near the cleavage site which would suggest a basis for the susceptibility to collagenase (Highberger et al., 1979). The results have been inconclusive, for the most part because of our lack of knowledge concerning precisely what forces contribute to the stability of the collagen helix. Interestingly, a 36-residue peptide from $\alpha_1(I)$ containing the collagenase cleavage site fails to renature under precisely identical conditions in which a peptide of identical length from another region of the chain renatures extensively (Gross *et al.*, 1980). This result suggests the possibility of helix lability in the region of the cleavage site. Unfortunately, it is not completely clear that the inability of a given peptide to renature is identical with the stability of that same peptide, were it in triple helical configuration. More information bearing on this question would be invaluable to our understanding of how collagen can contribute to its own susceptibility to degradation.

Similar, but not yet as extensive, studies have been performed using another pure enzyme available in chemical amounts, that from postpartum rat uterine cells in culture (Roswit *et al.*, 1983). Interestingly, this enzyme, which is elaborated for the purpose of a massive and rapid removal of collagen, fails to display the selectivity against collagen types observed with the human skin collagenase. Thus, types I, II, and III collagens are degraded at approximately the same rates (Welgus *et al.*, 1983). In this case, the biological purpose for which a given collagenolytic enzyme is intended may confer upon it an intrinsic specifier of its activity. In this regard, it would be extremely interesting to have this kind of information for human leukocyte collagenase, which has been reported to have a marked preference for type I collagen as opposed to type III (Horwitz *et al.*, 1977).

It should also be noted that studies similar to those employing human skin collagenase have been performed with pure tadpole collagenase by Hayashi *et al.* (1980a), using bovine types I, II, and III collagens in solution. No departure from linearity was noted in the Arrhenius plots with any of these substrates. Values of activation energy for the tadpole collagenase (40–60 kcal/mol) acting on bovine collagens are similar to those obtained with the human enzyme. Interestingly these authors also found that the degradation of either types III or II collagen is anomalously affected by the presence of the opposite type collagen in the same solution (Hayashi *et al.*, 1980b). They speculate that the tadpole enzyme may not obey classical Michaelis–Menten kinetics. On the other hand, Bicsak and Harper (1984) report that the tadpole collagenase does, in fact, display normal kinetic behavior. The tadpole enzyme is the only pure collagenase to date which is known to be produced by an epithelial cell (Eisen and Gross, 1965), and it will be extremely interesting to see if this enzyme is indeed qualitatively different in its interaction with collagen than collagenase of mesenchymal origin. In any event, from the foregoing examples it can be seen that the biological diversity stressed in the introduction to this review manifests itself rather dramatically in the nature of both the collagen substrate and in the chemical and kinetic properties of the various collagenases studied to date.

Before leaving this subject, it is worth briefly touching on the question of the biological necessity for enzymes other than collagenase in the process of total collagen degradation. Instinctively, most workers in the field would most probably agree that collagen degradation does not end with the action of collagenase. There is, however, much less known about other proteases that might be involved in the degradation of the products of the initial cleavage by collagenase. A number of gelatinolytic proteases have been described, most notably from tadpole tissues (Harper and Gross, 1970) and from human synovium (Harris and Krane, 1972), skin (Seltzer et al., 1981), and leukocytes (Sopata and Dancewicz, 1974). These gelatinases all seem to be metalloproteases, and are capable of effectively degrading denatured collagen to small peptides. Very little is known regarding the regulation of the production or activity of these enzymes. Very probably they are essential for the removal of the products of initial collagenase activity from the fiber, especially when extensive intramolecular cross-linking is present. It should be mentioned as well that at least some collagenases appear to have gelatinolytic as well as collagenolytic activity. Nagai et al. originally noted this property of tadpole collagenase (1964), and reported that, in addition to Gly-Ile and Gly-Leu bonds, the hydrolysis of Gly-Ala, Gly-Phe, and Gly-Val appeared to be catalyzed by the enzyme as well. Woolley et al. (1978b) originally reported that human skin collagenase possesses gelatinolytic activity, and Welgus et al. (1982) have confirmed and extended this observation, showing that denatured α_2-chains are degraded much faster by this enzyme than are α_1-chains. The rate of gelatinolysis by human skin collagenase, based on α-chain disappearance is considerably lower than the rate of collagenolysis. Additionally, it was found that only NH_2-terminal Leu and Ile were produced during the process. Recently, Welgus et al. have examined pure rat uterine collagenase for gelatinolytic activity and have found that this enzyme attacks denatured collagen chains approximately 10 times more rapidly than it does native collagen (Welgus and Jeffrey, unpublished). Interestingly, although Gly-Leu and Gly-Ile are the predominant NH_2-terminal amino acids produced by this activity, significant amounts of NH_2-Phe, -Ala, and -Val were also observed, much as originally observed by Nagai et al. (1964). Considerable care was taken to ensure purity of the enzyme preparation, and the gelatinolytic activity does appear to be a property of the collagenase itself. This raises the intriguing possibility that, in the rapidly involuting uterus, a single molecule is used both as a collagenase and a gelatinase, a case of intrinsic co-regulation. Finally, during the examination of the rat uterine collagenase for its gelatinolytic activity, it was found that human skin fibroblast collagenase, acting as a gelatinase, can also cleave the denatured chains at Gly-Ala and Gly-Val loci, as well as the previously observed Gly-Leu and Gly-Ile bonds. These cleavages are apparently not as easily catalyzed by the human skin as by the rat uterine collagenase, but they do occur. Here, again, is a possible example of biological diversity superimposed on underlying similarity; the three enzymes may be able to cleave a similar set of Gly-X bonds, where X is generally a nonpolar amino acid, but each enzyme may do so at very different rates for as yet unknown biological advantage.

F. Interaction of Collagenase with Inhibitors

The nature of the interaction of collagenases with biologically occurring inhibitors has, as suggested in an earlier section, been somewhat confusing due in great measure to the existence of a number of different molecules able to inhibit collagenase. The subject of collagenase inhibitors was reviewed recently in this series (Sellers and Murphy, 1980), and the reader is referred to that review for an extensive catolog of collagenase inhibitors from various sources. Since the appearance of that review, it has become clear that inhibitors are not always (and in cell culture systems perhaps seldom) the cause of collagenase latency. Rather, there is now documentation in a number of systems for the existence of zymogen forms of collagenase, which can be activated by organomercurials. Hence, previous reports attributing the phenomenon of organomercurial activation of latent collagenase to E–I complex dissociation must be reevaluated in this light. On the other hand, the inhibitors isolated by a number of laboratories, and purified by at least two (Cawston et al., 1981; Stricklin and Welgus, 1983), most probably represent a class of metalloprotease inhibitors present in a wide variety of connective tissues (Welgus and Stricklin, 1983). This class of inhibitors, referred to by many as "TIMP" (tissue inhibitor of metallo proteinase) (Murphy and Sellers, 1980) is characterized by molecular weights of approximately 30,000, stability to heat, and inactivation by reductive alkylation. They do not appear to be inactivated or prevented from acting by organomercurials. These inhibitors, as a class, appear to form tight complexes with collagenase with a 1:1 stoichiometry. In general, they fail to inhibit the collagenase from Clostridium histolyti-

cum or nonmetalloproteinases, although other metalloproteinases of connective tissue origin do appear to be inhibited by these molecules.

Until recently, sufficient differences appeared to exist between a number of the inhibitors such that including them in a single class appeared unwarranted. Recent work on two of them, however, has suggested that they are very similar entities. For example, preliminary studies on the inhibitor from human skin fibroblasts suggested that this molecule did not form a stable E–I complex in the absence of substrate, although the kinetics of its inhibition of collagenase suggested the formation of such a complex (Welgus *et al.*, 1977). Similarly, the inhibitor from rabbit bone was reported to be inactivated by organomercurials (Sellers *et al.*, 1977), whereas that from skin fibroblasts was not (Stricklin and Welgus, 1983). Recently, however, with the use of different methodology, a complex between human skin fibroblast collagenase and its cosynthesized inhibitor has been demonstrated (Welgus *et al.*, 1985). The complex is sufficiently stable to survive gel-filtration on both conventional and high-performance liquid chromatography (HPLC) matrices. Furthermore, a recent report (Cawston *et al.*, 1983) indicates that the purified inhibitor from rabbit bone, which similarly forms a complex with purified collagenase, is not inactivated by APMA. It appears then that the two inhibitors are very similar in all major respects. It is similarly likely that a variety of other inhibitors reported in the past few years will, when fully characterized, share these properties.

In addition, Welgus, and Stricklin (1983) have recently shown that a molecule functionally and immunologically identical to the inhibitor produced by human skin fibroblasts is also produced by every human mesodermal cell line they examined. This finding implies very wide distribution for this molecule in humans, and the existence of virtually identical molecules in rabbit (Murphy and Sellers, 1980), porcine (Nolan *et al.*, 1978; Kerwar *et al.*, 1980), bovine (Nolan *et al.*, 1980), and human tissues (Stricklin and Welgus, 1983; Welgus and Stricklin, 1983; Welgus *et al.*, 1977; Vater *et al.*, 1979) suggests a wide distribution for a molecule of this type in nature.

Of interest with respect to its implication in the regulation of collagenolysis is the finding that the human skin fibroblast inhibitor is unable to bind either to collagen or, most importantly, to procollagenase. This lack of interaction between inhibitor and zymogen was first indicated from kinetic studies (Welgus *et al.*, 1977) and, more recently, by direct demonstration of a complex between inhibitor and active collagenase and by the failure of such a complex to form between zymogen and inhibitor (Welgus *et al.*, 1985). Thus, in the case of the human skin fibroblast collagenolytic system, in which the zymogen appears unable to interact with either its substrate or its inhibitor, the process of zymogen activation assumes new importance in the modulation of collagenase activity in physiology.

The nature of the interaction between these inhibitors and active collagenase is of considerable interest with respect to the regulation of enzyme activity by these entities. All the inhibitors of this class examined to date have been reported to have very high affinities for collagenase. Thus, Vater *et al.* (1979) estimated a K_d of ~10^{-8} M for the human tendon inhibitor, Cawson *et al.* (1983) report a K_d of 1.4×10^{-10} M for the rabbit bone molecule, and Welgus *et al.* (1985) observed that the K_d is <10^{-9} M for the human skin fibroblast inhibitor. It should be emphasized that the measurements of such constants for tight enzyme–inhibitor complexes is difficult and subject to considerable imprecision (Bieth, 1974); nevertheless, two points should be made. First, in every case, the dissociation constant for the E–I complex is 2–4 orders of magnitude lower than the K_d of the E–S complex of ~1 μM measured for human skin collagenase, both in solution and in fibrillar form. The crucial point is that the affinity of inhibitor for enzyme is very much greater than that of enzyme for substrate, arguing to the potential effectiveness of the inhibitor not only in binding free inhibitor, but in competing for collagenase already bound to collagen during ongoing processes of degradation *in vivo*. Certainly under laboratory conditions, the human fibroblast inhibitor is effective in inhibiting collagenase which has been prebound to reconstituted fibrils (Welgus and Jeffrey, unpublished observations).

Second, the binding of these inhibitors to collagenase is so tight, and the affinity so high, that the process is essentially a stoichiometric one, very much akin to the titration of a strong acid with a strong base. The regulatory implications of such a steeply sloped titration is that a relatively small change in inhibitor concentration results in a very large change in enzyme activity. By constructing the system this way, nature provides an extremely sensitive mechanism for regulating the rate of collagenase activity. Thus, biology makes use of the principle of stoichiometry, rather than of catalysis (such as, for example, a proteolytic inactivation of collagenase) to regulate collagenolytic activity for the purposes of achieving temporal and spatial specificity at the tissue level. This is illustrated in Fig. 5. It will be of considerable interest, as research continues in this important area, to determine whether the interrelationships that exist between inhibitor, collagenase, and substrate will be found to exist when the other metallopro-

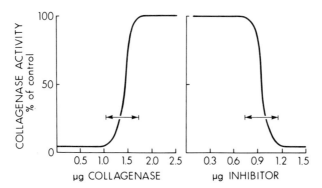

FIG. 5. Illustration of the consequences of the very tight binding of collagenase and its mesenchymal cell-produced inhibitor. Whether a given amount of inhibitor is titrated with collagenase (left panel), or a given amount of collagenase is titrated with inhibitor (right panel), massive changes in enzyme activity occur upon relatively small changes in the amounts of either reagent.

teinases which are inhibited by these inhibitors can be subjected to the same kind of analysis. In addition, specific information on the chemical and physical properties, and the regulatory pathways, of the members of this important class of connective tissue molecules should provide major insight into the way nature manages the turnover of connective tissue.

For a number of years considerable attention has been focused on ability of serum to inhibit collagenases of tissue origin (see Sellers and Murphy, 1980, for review). The exact identity and number of different inhibitors of collagenase in serum has been unclear, but recent studies by MacCartney and Tschesche (1983a,b) and by Stricklin and Welgus (1983; Welgus and Stricklin, 1983) have shed new light on this question. There has been universal agreement for some time that α_2-macroglobulin is an effective inhibitor of collagenase, as it is for so many other proteases (Abe and Nagai, 1973; Werb et al., 1974). On the other hand, α_1-antitrypsin, at first thought to have inhibitory activity (Bauer et al., 1972), is now agreed to be essentially ineffective as an anticollagenase (Werb et al., 1974; Berman et al., 1973a; Woolley et al., 1975b; Eisen et al., 1977). Woolley (1976, 1978a) reported the existence of a protein in the β_1 fraction of serum that inhibited collagenase and termed it β_1-anticollagenase. Its characteristics remained undefined until MacCartney and Tschesche (1983b), as part of their investigation of human leukocyte collagenase and its inhibitor, purified β_1-anticollagenase from serine and reported its amino acid composition and characteristics. Pure β_1-anticollagenase, MW 31,000, inhibited active leukocyte collagenase by formation of a tight 1:1 stoichiometric complex. The inhibition appears to proceed via a free sulfhydryl group in the inhibitor, since alkylation with iodoacetamide inactivates the inhibitor. In addition, the inhibitor–enzyme complex could be reactivated by the addition of disulfide-containing molecules such as oxidized glutathione or by organomercurials such as mersalyl. In these latter respects, the mechanism of inhibition appears to be very similar to that exhibited by the leukocyte collagenase inhibitor (MacCartney and Tschesche, 1983a). Here again, addition of compounds which could participate in disulfide exchange reactions reversed the inhibitor. Despite the apparent similarity of mechanism, however, the two molecules appear not to be the same, as assessed by amino acid composition. Clear differences were present in a number of amino acid residues. Of even greater interest was the fact that neither of these molecules was identical to the inhibitor produced by cultured human skin fibroblasts, and which is also present in significant amounts in human serum (Stricklin and Welgus, 1983; Welgus and Stricklin, 1983). In the case of the latter inhibitor, neither its mechanism of action, nor its amino acid composition resembled those of either β_1-anticollagenase or the leukocyte inhibitor.

As of this writing, there appear to be at least three identifiable collagenase inhibitors, other than α_2-macroglobulin, in human blood—either intra- or extracellularly. All have similar molecular weights and form tight complexes with collagenase but appear to be distinct molecules. The leukocyte inhibitor most probably serves to maintain that cell's collagenase in an inactive form until its release is needed. MacCartney and Tschesche (1983b) have shown that the oxidative burst accompanying the release of a number of granular components of leukocytes effectively dissociates the leukocyte collagenase from its inhibitor. The function of the two other inhibitors, however, is unknown. Woolley (1975b) has suggested that β_1-anticollagenase functions as a scavenger of collagenase, after which it transfers the latter to α_2-macroglobulin for clearance to the liver. In view of the fact that significant concentrations of human skin fibroblast inhibitor appear in serum, there is, conversely, no reason to suppose *a priori* that β_1-anticollagenase does not exist in significant quantity in human connective tissues.

The preceding sections have dealt with the components of the collagenolytic system itself and have attempted to present our current knowledge of the ways in which each of these components interact with others of the system. The use of the term collagenolytic system appears warranted by the number of components now identified which are explicitly produced by cells for the purpose of directly affecting the rate and/or the extent of collagen degradation in mammalian tissues. A schematic representation of a composite collagenolytic system is contained in Fig. 6. In it is indicated pathways in which, to the extent we now know, interaction is allowed as well as those that appear not to occur. Again, it should be emphasized that all the relationships depicted in this figure may not exist in all systems, or may exist in altered form, either qualitatively or quantitatively. It will be the exciting task of the next few years to further explore these interactions with a view to better defining their exact nature.

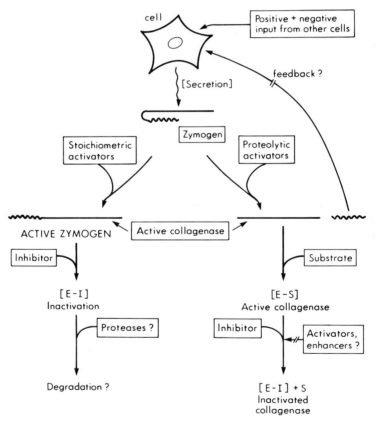

FIG. 6. Schematic representation of a collagenolytic system, with the reagents known to date indicated as acting at their appropriate loci.

III. Extrinsic Regulation of Collagenase Activity: A
Selective Survey of Collagenolytic Systems and Their
Regulation

The following section of this review will present the salient features
of the regulation of collagenase activity in a number of individual
tissue or organ systems. A narrative approach will be taken; no attempt will be made to exhaustively discuss specific aspects of any system. The reader is referred to the papers cited for details and precise
data. The purpose of this section is, therefore, to provide an overview of
the range and variety of mechanisms which have been identified or
suggested to be operative in the processes by which collagenase activity can be modulated in various vertebrate systems. As noted at the
beginning of this article, this section will deal primarily with the regulation of collagenase by those biological agents *extrinsic* to the collagenolytic systems discussed above. That is, by entities whose physiological role is not solely intended to be as a regulator of collagenase.
Lastly, it should be emphasized that the systems discussed below do
not comprise, by any means, an exhaustive list of those systems which
have been examined over the years. Rather, they have been selected to
provide the reader with a feeling for the variety of approaches that
biology adopts in the control of the degradation of collagen.

A. Uterus

The postpartum involution of the mammalian uterus represents the
most massive and rapid process of collagen degradation in normal
physiology. In the human uterus, for example, some 30 g of collagen is
degraded over a period of approximately 10 days (Woessner and
Brewer, 1963), or roughly one-twentieth the time required for the synthesis of the same collagen during gestation. The overall subject of
uterine collagen and its degradation has been reviewed by Woessner
(1982); this section will deal only with the regulation of the process of
collagenolysis in the postpartum uterus.

The majority of the experimental work dealing with uterine collagen
degradation has been performed in the rat. Gestation in this animal is
22 days, with the bulk of the collagen synthesized in the last 12 days of
pregnancy. After delivery, all of the accumulated collagen, and more,
is resorbed in approximately 3 days, resulting in a uterus which contains less collagen than before implantation. An indication that most
mammals effect the process of uterine collagen involution in an analogous, if not an identical, manner has been suggested by Koob and Ryan

(1980). They point out that, as a fraction of gestation time, the curves representing the rates of collagen accumulation and degradation are superimposable for a wide range of mammalian species.

In the rat, the postpartum involution of the uterus is accompanied by the appearance of collagenase, either in the medium of explant cultures (Jeffrey and Gross, 1970; Jeffrey et al., 1971a) or bound tightly to the collagen of the tissue itself (Ryan and Woessner, 1971). By either method, the uterus can be shown to synthesize the enzyme only during the period of active involution; none is observed either in late pregnancy or after degradation is complete (Eisen et al., 1970). Clearly, the uterus possesses effective pathways for the initiation of the production of collagenase as well as for the termination of its synthesis. The nature of these pathways has been a matter of some uncertainty.

Woessner and co-workers, working with the in vivo rat, have found that estradiol, when administered to postpartum animals, retards the involution of the uterus in general, with collagen degradation somewhat more inhibited than overall wet weight (Woessner, 1969). When the uterine tissue from estradiol-treated animals is examined for endogenous, tightly bound collagenase, it was found that the levels of the enzyme are diminished in the steroid-injected animals (Ryan and Woessner, 1972; Woessner, 1979). On the other hand, Jeffrey and Koob (1974) have found that progesterone is also capable of inhibiting the degradation of collagen in the in vivo rat. In this case the inhibition was quite selective for collagen, with virtually no effect observed on overall uterine weight; however, the effect could only be maintained for roughly 24 hr, after which time collagen degradation proceeded at the normal rate. Almost identical results had been earlier reported by Goodall (1966) in the involuting rabbit uterus. On the other hand, Halme and Woessner (1975) were able to observe inhibition of in vivo collagen degradation in the rat only with very high concentrations of progesterone. The reason for the quantitative disparity remains unknown, but it is clear that in the whole animal both estradiol and progesterone can affect the catabolism of collagen in the postpartum uterus.

Data from in vitro systems, on the other hand, paint a somewhat different picture. In the explant culture system first described by Jeffrey and Gross (1970), progesterone but not estradiol or testosterone effectively and selectively prevents the appearance of collagenase (Jeffrey et al., 1971b). This inhibition of the appearance of collagenase by the principal steroid of pregnancy is accompanied by a complete cessation of the degradation of collagen which occurs in the cultured explants (Jeffrey et al., 1971a,b). Similar observations have been made in organ cultures of the involuting uterine deciduoma in rats (Jeffrey, 1981). Again, in this interesting system, estradiol is without effect. In both culture systems the effect of progesterone is synergistic with dibutyryl cyclic AMP (Jeffrey, 1981; Koob and Jeffrey, 1974); concentrations of steroid or cyclic nucleotide which by themselves have no inhibitory effect can be shown to completely prevent collagenase production when added to cultures together. The nature and the physiologic significance of this interaction are, at present, unknown. The existence of this synergism, however, indicates the complexity of the overall system for regulation of the metabolism of collagen in the all-important process of mammalian reproduction.

Further evidence of the complexity of the regulation of collagenase in this tissue was provided by the study of Tyree *et al.* (1980), who showed that addition of progesterone to cultured postpartum uterine explants resulted first in the production of control levels of collagenase, but in an inactive form. At the same time, it was found that the steroid reduced the amount of an activator of these inactive forms which is normally produced by the cultured tissue. Thus, the initial effect of the steroid was to prevent activation of collagenase by inhibiting the production of activator. Prolonged incubation with progesterone then resulted in a lowered amount of total (active + inactive) collagenase. The tentative conclusion from this study was that progesterone acts by way of a dual mechanism to control collagenolysis in the uterus. First, it lowers activator levels rapidly enough to prevent conversion of inactive collagenase to its active form, providing for a rapid cessation of active collagenase production. Second, the steroid lowers the production of collagenase itself in a slower process. Of particular interest in the rapid process is the potential advantage to biology of utilizing a stoichiometric, rather than a catalytic, mechanism of collagenase activation. In the stoichometric mechanism, a modest reduction in an activator level can have a profound effect on activation, if the affinity of activator for proenzyme is high. This is very similar to the effect of small changes in collagenase inhibitor on the activity of the enzyme (Welgus *et al.*, 1977) and suggests the possibility that such stoichiometric interactions are particularly important in a variety of regulatory processes in connective tissue metabolism.

In cultured postpartum uterine explants, Koob *et al.* (1981) found that the glucocorticoids hydrocortisone and dexamethasone were also effective in preventing the appearance of collagenase. On a molar basis, hydrocortisone was approximately one order of magnitude less effective than progesterone in producing a 50% inhibition in collagenase production. Whether the mechanism of inhibition by these steroids is the same as that of the progestational steroids is not known at this time. In very recent work, Jeffrey *et al.* (unpublished), utilizing a cell culture system derived from postpartum uterus, have found that progesterone and medroxyprogesterone acetate, but not estradiol or testosterone, effectively and selectively inhibit the production of procollagenase by these cells, as assayed both by enzymatic activity and by immunoreactivity, measured by a sensitive ELISA for rat collagenase. The time course of disappearance of enzyme is consistent with a mechanism whereby the steroids inhibit the production of a messenger RNA. Definitive assignment of this pathway, however, must await further documentation.

B.   Rheumatoid Synovium

Rheumatoid arthritis is a chronic destructive disease of the connective tissue, characterized by extensive erosion and inappropriate remodeling of cartilage and bone in the joints of affected individuals. The involvement of collagenase in this disease was first implicated when it was found that explant cultures of rheumatoid synovium produce relatively large quantities of collagenase in culture (Evanson *et al.*, 1967, 1968). In the intervening years, a great deal of elegant work has appeared which indicates that a complex set of interactions exists in the rheumatoid joint which acts to modulate the production of collagenase in the disease. Involved in the process are resident cells of the synovium, inflammatory cells, and their products, as well as immune cells and a variety of hormones. As a result of these extensive investigations, the pathways involved in the regulation of collagenase in this pathologic state are probably the best documented of any such process to date.

A major key to the understanding of the regulatory aspects of collagenase production in this disease process has come from the work of Krane and co-workers, who first showed that cells derived from rheumatoid synovium could be grown in culture and produce collagenase (Dayer *et al.*, 1976). The enzyme-producing cell originally appeared not to be the fibroblast, as it is in the skin, but rather a stellate, or dendritic, cell (Woolley *et al.*, 1978c, 1979) of unknown lineage. Interestingly, however, these cells can be induced to change their shape to a more fibroblast-like cell by the inhibition of prostaglandin synthesis in the cultures by indomethacin (Baker *et al.*, 1983). Stellate morphology can then be restored by the addition of prostaglandin E_2 (PGE$_2$), itself a major cellular product of the stellate cell in culture (Dayer *et al.*, 1976). It may be that the major collagenase producing cell in the synovium is, in fact, the fibroblast.

The production of both collagenase and PGE_2 has been shown to be the result of the action of a protein factor obtained from human peripheral blood monocytes and called mononuclear cell factor (MCF) by Dayer *et al.* (1977a,b). This molecule displays functional similarity with interleukin I (Dayer *et al.*, 1981), but identity with the latter molecule has not been definitively established. Nevertheless, the identification of monocytes–macrophages (cells associated with the inflammatory process in rheumatoid arthritis) as the source of MCF, and as playing a major role in the onset of collagenolysis in the disease, seems clearly established. It should be noted that prostaglandin production is neither required, nor apparently associated with, the production of collagenase by these cells (Baker *et al.*, 1983; Krane and Amento, 1983). Addition of indomethacin at concentrations sufficient to block PGE_2 production had no effect on the appearance of collagenase in the medium.

More recently, evidence for further complexity in the pathways of collagenase regulation in the rheumatoid synovium has been provided by the finding that the activated T lymphocyte appears to play a critical role in the mediation of the monocyte–macrophage induction of collagenase by the synovial cells (Dayer *et al.*, 1979a; Amento *et al.*, 1982). Thus, for example, co-cultures of lectin-stimulated T cells and monocytes produce high levels of MCF. Unstimulated T cells fail to induce MCF production. Thus, another cell type intrinsic to the inflammatory process appears to be at least capable of exerting a major regulatory role for collagenase in rheumatoid arthritis.

Other factors of potential importance in the pathology of rheumatoid arthritis have been reported in recent years. They include agents that can influence the maturation of the blood-borne monocyte to the mature macrophage. Such agents may be typified by 1,25-dihydroxyvitamin D_3, which promotes the differentiation of the monocytic cell line U937 to the macrophage phenotype with an attendant production of MCF by these cells (Dayer *et al.*, 1979b; Krane and Amento, 1983). In addition, it has been shown that incubation of monocyte–macrophages with purified IgG molecules can markedly increase the capacity of these cells to produce MCF (Dayer *et al.*, 1980). In this regard, it has recently been shown that the IgG rheumatoid factor complexes shown to exist in the human rheumatoid joint are themselves capable of stimulating MCF synthesis by monocytes (Nardella *et al.*, 1983). Thus, arthritis-associated immune complexes may contribute to the continuation and severity of the connective tissue damage characteristic of the disease.

In addition to these modulators, there is the finding that bacterially produced endotoxin also exerts a stimulatory effect on monocyte MCF production (Dayer *et al.*, 1979b). Thus, infection of the joint can be envisioned as a potential contributor to disease-associated damage. Of considerable interest also is the finding that at least two genetic types of collagen, including type II, are capable of stimulating MCF production by the monocyte–macrophage (Dayer *et al.*, 1982). This raises the possibility that collagen synthesis in response to inflammatory signals or in an effort to repair the damaged structures of the joint may contribute additional impetus for the destruction of the joint.

With regard to the existence of mechanisms by which collagenase production in the rheumatoid synovium can be inhibited, the literature is considerably more scanty. Early studies in explant cultures indicated that glucocorticoids are effective in blocking the appearance of the enzyme (Koob *et al.*, 1974). Recently, certain retinoids have been shown to decrease the level of collagenase production in rabbit synovial fibroblasts (Brinckerhoff *et al.*, 1980b). Perhaps the best hope for ultimate control of collagenolysis in this disease process may be the rational manipulation of the naturally produced protein inhibitor of the enzyme in the synovial tissues themselves (Welgus *et al.*, 1977; Murphy *et al.*, 1981).

The resident cell of the articular cartilage, the chondrocyte, has also been implicated in the pathogenesis of rheumatoid arthritis; at least two studies have shown that cultures of these cells can be induced to synthesize collagenase by a factor or factors produced by stimulated macrophages (Phadke *et al.*, 1978; Kerwar *et al.*, 1984). In studies by Kerwar *et al.*, in which the nature of the factor was explored (1984), it is suggested on the basis of molecular weight and indomethacin-independent production, that the chondrocyte stimulating factor is not MCF as described by Dayer *et al.* (1981). Further exploration of this potential participation of the resident cells of the cartilage in the destructive process would be of considerable use.

Clearly, the modulation of the collagenolysis associated with rheumatoid arthritis is very complex, with an extraordinary number of pathways available to exacerbate the process of connective tissue destruction. Some of these stimuli act in ways which may promote a self-perpetuation of the disease process, such that at some point in the progress of the disease, joint destruction becomes self-sustaining.

C. Skin

The mammalian skin undergoes architecturally specific remodeling of its collagen during such processes as wound healing, fetal development, and adolescent growth. The ability of the skin of normal mammals, including the human, to produce collagenase has been amply documented (for review, see Bauer *et al.*, 1972). Pathologically, collagenase has been documented to be increased in the skin of patients afflicted with the severe, blistering disease, recessive dystrophic epidermolysis bullosa (RDEB) (Bauer and Eisen, 1978). In addition, there have been persistent suggestions that impairment in collagen degradation plays a role in hypertrophic scar and keloid formation (Cohen *et al.*, 1975), as well as at least a permissive role in the mechanism of tumor invasion (Dresden *et al.*, 1972; Bauer *et al.*, 1977). In view of its potential importance in both normal physiology and in pathology, the pathways of regulation of collagenase in this tissue are of great interest.

Production of collagenase by human skin, and that of several other species, has been documented in both explant and cell culture systems (Bauer *et al.*, 1972; Stricklin *et al.*, 1977). Indeed, the collagenase from human skin fibroblasts is perhaps the best characterized of the collagenases from the standpoint of its mechanism of action. As discussed in a previous section, the enzyme appears to be secreted as a zymogen, whose physiologic mechanism of activation is as yet unknown (Stricklin *et al.*, 1977, 1978, 1983). In the explant system, production of collagenase can be prevented by the addition of glucocorticoids to the culture medium (Koob *et al.*, 1974). Both hydrocortisone and its potent synthetic analog dexamethasone completely prevent the appearance of the enzyme at concentrations in the physiologic range. The inhibition is manifested in losses of both enzymatic activity and immunoreactive protein. Preliminary studies in the cell culture system suggest that the steroids act at the level of messenger RNA transcription and not at the level of translation (Kronberger *et al.*, 1985). Steroid hormones of other classes—estrogens, progestogens, and androgens—are without effect in this system. Thus, the effect appears to be quite glucocorticoid specific.

The ability of physiologic concentrations of the glucocorticoids to completely block the production of collagenase brings into question the notion that glucocorticoids produce atrophy in the skin *in vivo* by inducing the production of collagenase (Houck *et al.*, 1968). Certainly the *in vitro* results stand in sharp contrast to this view. Recent studies by

Cutroneo and co-workers (Rokowski *et al.,* 1981; Sterling *et al.,* 1983) now strongly suggest that the primary effect these hormones have in both skin and lung is on collagen synthesis. This view is supported by the study of Jeffrey *et al.* (1985) who found that, in the actively growing neonatal rat skin, collagenase activity is essentially absent and that treatment of these young animals with steroids results in complete cessation of collagen accumulation in the skin. Thus, at this point the exact biological time or states in which the glucocorticoids do, in fact, exert their effect on collagenase production is not clear; it may not be unreasonable to postulate that these hormones function primarily in regulating the day-to-day basal catabolic rate of collagen in mammalian skin.

Evidence that the epidermis may participate in the regulation of collagenase production by dermal cells has been provided by the studies of Johnson-Wint and Bauer (1984), who showed that an 18 kDa cytokine derived from rabbit corneal epithelial cells can significantly increase the production of collagenase by human skin fibroblasts in culture. Although an *in vivo* role for such a factor is lacking at this time, its existence would provide an attractive basis for explaining previous observations that the epidermis plays an important role in the regulation of collagenase production in healing wounds (Grillo and Gross, 1967).

Other agents that have been shown to modulate collagenase production by human skin in either explant or cell culture systems include dibutyryl cyclic AMP, which is a potent inhibitor of the production of the enzyme in organ culture (Koob *et al.,* 1974, 1981). Thus, in the skin, as in the uterus (Koob and Jeffrey, 1974) and in the cornea (Berman *et al.,* 1976), the cyclic nucleotide appears to exert an analogous, if not identical, inhibitory effect on collagenase production. Interestingly, this effect of cyclic AMP on resident tissue cells is opposite from that exerted by the cyclic nucleotide upon peritoneal macrophages (vide infra), as well as from that reported on collagenase production in tadpole skin (Harper and Toole, 1973).

It has also been shown that certain derivatives of vitamin A, the retinoids, are capable of lowering the production of collagenase by human skin fibroblasts in culture (Bauer *et al.,* 1982). The inhibition is selective; general protein synthesis is essentially unaffected. The mechanism of action of these pharmacologic agents is unknown, but their action on collagenase production takes on added significance in view of the clinical effectiveness of these same compounds in the treatment of severe acne. It should also be mentioned that the action of the retinoids on collagenase production has also been observed in cultures of rabbit synovial fibroblasts (Brinckerhoff *et al.*, 1980a), suggesting that a wide range of cells respond to these compounds.

D. Cornea

The cornea of the eye has been the subject of considerable study with respect to collagen degradation over the past several years. In large measure because of the therapeutic considerations in such pathologic conditions as corneal ulceration and scarring, a number of investigators have examined both explant and cell culture systems for their ability to produce the enzyme and for pathways of regulation of collagenase. Thus, several have reported that collagenolytic activity in explant cultures of alkali-burned rabbit cornea was correlated with the ulceration caused by the alkali insult (Brown *et al.*, 1970b; Anderson *et al.*, 1971; Berman *et al.*, 1971). The enzyme has been partially characterized (Berman *et al.*, 1973b, 1977) and bears numerous similarities to those collagenases now more extensively purified. The metalloproteinase nature of the enzyme (Berman and Manabe, 1973) gave rise to extensive study of the usefulness of classical collagenase inhibitors in reversing the damage produced by these agents (Brown *et al.*, 1969; Berman, 1975).

The biological regulation of collagenase activity in the cornea has been examined in a number of studies over the years. Thus, for example, there is a report that high concentrations of dexamethasone can induce collagenase activity in corneal fibroblasts (Brown *et al.*, 1970a). This intriguing finding has not, as yet, been confirmed. Standing as it does in opposition to the inhibitory effect of glucocorticoids on a number of collagenase-producing cells and tissues, the documentation and definition of such a pathway would be of considerable interest. In another study (Berman *et al.*, 1976), dibutyryl cyclic AMP has been found to inhibit the production of collagenase by corneal explants. This activity of the cyclic nucleotide is similar to that observed in both skin and uterine culture systems, and suggests the possibility of a more universal mechanism of regulation in fibroblasts.

Studies of particular interest, not only with respect to the regulation of collagenase in the cornea itself but also in terms of the importance of epithelial–mesenchymal interactions in the regulation of collagen remodeling, have come from Johnson-Muller and Gross (1978). These studies (Gross *et al.*, 1980) evolved from the early observations of Newsome and Gross that the epithelium from alkali-burned rabbit cornea could stimulate corneal fibroblasts to make collagenase. Further studies of this initial phenomenon led Johnson-Wint and Gross (1984) to the finding that cytochalasin B-treated corneal epithelium could induce inactive corneal fibroblasts to produce collagenase. It was found that the epithelial cells, treated with cytochalasin, released factors into the medium which stimulated the fibroblasts. The phenomenon appeared quite complex, and conceivably all the more important for ultimate biological usefulness in that, depending upon the density of epithelial cells in the cultures, factors which either stimulated or inhibited collagenase production were produced by cytochalasin B treatment. Such a biphasic response, although in need of considerable further study, raises the possibility that the epithelium can regulate the production of collagenase in both a positive and negative direction. Such a capability could easily be critically important in a process such as wound healing, in which, for example, collagenase activity can be observed at the leading margin of the wound but not at geographically more distant sites (Grillo and Gross, 1967).

The stimulatory and inhibitory factors have been partially characterized, and it has been found that the principal form of either factor has a molecular weight of approximately 19,000 (Gross and Highberger, 1980; Johnson-Wint and Gross, 1984). Interestingly, the stimulating factor, or cytokine, has also been shown to have stimulatory activity upon human skin fibroblasts in culture (Johnson-Wint and Bauer, 1984), raising the possibility that the cytokine, or an analogous molecule, is produced by the epithelium of several tissues. Such a possibility would have wide-ranging biological consequences. Epithelial–mesenchymal interactions as regulators of collagenase production are among the earliest reported phenomena to be described in the field. Thus, tadpole tailfin resorption (Eisen and Gross, 1965), mammalian wound healing (Grillo and Gross, 1967), and tumor cell–host cell interactions (Bauer *et al.*, 1977) all have been described in terms of one cell type inducing the production of collagenase in another. Yet these phenomena have remained largely unexplored in specific terms.

E. Macrophages

Macrophages are ubiquitous members of the cast of cells present during most, if not all, processes of tissue inflammation. Derived from the monocytes of the peripheral circulation, their participation in the induction of the collagenolytic process in rheumatoid arthritis has been discussed previously. The macrophage, however, in addition to its ability to elicit collagenase production by a variety of cell types, is itself capable of producing collagenase. Peritoneal macrophages from mouse (Werb and Gordon, 1975), rabbit (Horwitz and Crystal, 1976), and guinea pig (Wahl *et al.*, 1974, 1975) have been shown to elaborate the enzyme. Furthermore, the regulation of collagenase production by these cells appears to be complex and may vary with species of origin.

Probably the best characterized macrophage system at the present time is that from the guinea pig peritoneum, as described primarily by Wahl and co-workers (Wahl *et al.*, 1977; McCarthy *et al.*, 1980) these cells, elicited from the peritoneum by mineral oil injection and cultured in serum-free medium, fail to produce collagenase in the resting state. The enzyme can be induced by treatment of the cells with bacterial lipopolysaccharide (LPS) or with secreted products of lectin-stimulated lymphocytes. Interestingly, the production of collagenase by these cells appears to be secondary to the synthesis of prostaglandin E_2 by the induced cells. This is in contrast to the cells of the human synovial system, in which prostaglandin synthesis can be dissociated from collagenase production. In the macrophage, the PGE_2 response in turn appears to result in a rise in intracellular cyclic AMP, which may yet be a more direct mediator of collagenase production.

The production of collagenase by the guinea pig macrophage can be prevented by the addition of dexamethasone at reasonably physiological concentrations (Wahl and Winter, 1984). Of interest was the finding that the glucorticoid exerted parallel effects on the production of prostaglandins. Moreover, the effect of the steroid on both PGE_2 and collagenase production could be reversed by the addition of exogenous dibutyryl cyclic AMP, PGE_2, arachidonic acid, or phospholipase A_2. Thus, the primary effect of the glucocorticoid appears to be on the pathway whereby prostaglandins are produced from arachidonic acid, rather than a more direct effect upon the production of collagenase message as indicated in the case of human fibroblasts. It should be mentioned that macrophages from other species also display glucocorticoid inhibition of collagenase (Werb, 1978); at this time, however, it is not known whether a prostaglandin-mediated pathway is operative in these cells. Interestingly, Bhatnagar *et al.* (1982) have reported that endotoxin stimulates, and that prostaglandin and cyclic AMP mediate, the production of collagenase in rat liver Kupffer cells in culture.

Of further interest in the guinea pig macrophage system is the response of these cells to the microtubule active compound colchicine. Colchicine, when added to cultures of macrophages together with LPS, prevents the production of collagenase, whereas the prostaglandin response is unaffected. If, however, the compound is added 24 hr after LPS, collagenase synthesis is unaffected. Wahl and Winter suggest that the effect of colchicine is upon the activation of the macrophage by agents such as LPS, resulting in the failure of the cell to produce a variety of normal products associated with the inflammatory response. Again, it should be noted that mouse macrophages have been reported to be *stimulated* by colchicine (Gordon and Werb, 1976), suggesting the possibility of significant species differences in the behavior of these cells. It will be of considerable interest to have a more thorough comparison of macrophages from a variety of species in view of the importance of the responses of these cells to pharmacological and physiological modifiers of the inflammatory response.

F. Bone

The specific nature of the resorption of the organic matrix of bone—made up of over 90% type I collagen fibers—is a question still unresolved despite nearly 20 years of intensive investigation by a number of workers. The mechanism, and the regulation, of this process of collagen degradation remains one of the most intriguing problems currently under study in the field of collagenolysis. The general topic of bone resorption has been well reviewed by Vaes (1980). The purpose of this section will be only to provide a perspective on the current status of knowledge concerning collagen degradation in bone.

The pivotal issue in bone collagen degradation, and the issue that makes this tissue particularly intriguing, is whether a specific neutral collagenase is involved in the process of normal bone turnover. Uncertainty with regard to this point is, in part, a consequence of the fact that the cell associated with, and generally agreed to preside over, bone resorption, the osteoclast, produces a zone of low pH at the surface of the bone being resorbed. This fact raised questions as to whether a neutral collagenase could act in this region. This uncertainty has been intensified by the elegant series of studies of Vaes and co-workers, who have been unable to correlate the presence of collagenase with parathyroid hormone-dependent bone resorption.

The studies of this group have made use of organ cultures of embryonic mouse bone (Vaes, 1965) which resorb when parathyroid hormone (PTH) is added to the culture medium. When the rudiments are undergoing hormone induced resorption, no collagenase, either in active or latent form, can be detected in the culture medium. Instead, a wide variety of lysosomal enzymes are released from the tissue into the medium (Vaes, 1967, 1968). This is in contrast to the observation that readily detectable collagenase activity—essentially all latent—can be detected in these same cultures in the presence of heparin (Shimizu *et al.*, 1963; Sakamoto *et al.*, 1972; Vaes, 1972). Under this latter condition the increase in collagenase production by the explants is not accompanied by resorption of the tissue. When both heparin and PTH are added to the cultures simultaneously (Lenaers-Claeys et al., 1979; Francois-Gillet et al., 1981), the resorption expected from the added PTH and the level of collagenase associated with the addition of heparin are both observed, but neither additional resorption nor collagenase production is seen when both agents are present. Thus the production of collagenase and the resorption of matrix appear to be essentially completely dissociable.

On the basis of these results, coupled with the finding by Vaes' group and those of others that PTH-induced resorption is invariably associated with the appearance of lysosomal enzymes (Vaes, 1967, 1968; Eilon and Raisz, 1978), Vaes concludes that the mechanism of PTH-stimulated bone resorption at least is not mediated by a neutral collagenase. This group hypothesizes that, at the lowered pH in the microenvironment near the osteoclast, lysosomal proteases are capable of degrading a collagen which, compromised by the acidic environment, is now susceptible to enzymes not normally associated with collagen degradation. Direct proof for this hypothesis has not, as yet, been forthcoming, and this notion must still be considered speculative. Nevertheless, the accumulation of circumstantial evidence is impressive in suggesting that the normal parathyroid-mediated resorption of bone, one of the most massive processes of collagen degradation in vertebrate physiology, may in fact not employ a specific collagenase.

Of interest with regard to this general problem, it has recently been shown that osteoblasts or "osteoblast-like" cells (Sakamoto and Sakamoto, 1984; Otsuka et al., 1984), are capable of producing collagenase in culture, a finding which would be consistent with Vaes' hypothesis. The question of the function of the osteoblast collagenase has not been answered; an attractive possibility is that the bone uses this capability of the osteoblast in a wound healing process, as in the healing of fractures. More trivially, it could be that, under certain circumstances, the expression of collagenase in culture may be a fortuitous consequence of placing a mesenchymal cell in tissue culture. This problem is not unique to bone, however. It must be borne in mind in all these systems discussed here that the expression of collagenase in culture does not imply that the enzyme is similarly expressed in vivo.

IV. SUMMARY AND FUTURE PERSPECTIVE

To end this essay, the author would return the beginning paragraphs and reemphasize the complexity of systems required to be in place in order to produce rational changes in the shape of an organ or tissue. In terms of explaining organized processes of collagen degradation, a great deal of progress has been made in the last few years in at least identifying many—although not by any means necessarily all—of the molecules which can be envisioned as participating in such a process. Thus, collagenase zymogens have been described in numerous tissues, and protein inhibitors of collagenase seem to be ubiquitous as well. It appears, and anthropomorphically attractively so, that the inhibitors interact only with the active form of the enzyme, emphasizing that the activation of the zymogen as a watershed event in collagen degradation. The question of the activation of inactive primary secretory forms of collagenase is one which will need to be more aggressively addressed in the future. The problem is a difficult one since, as noted, the physiologically active form of the enzyme has not been conclusively identified in a single tissue, whereas *in vitro* activation can be effected by so many pathways. Nevertheless, it is to be hoped that this singularly crucial event in collagen metabolism can be described with some precision in the near future.

Another area which should provide very substantial new information in the near future will come from studies on the naturally synthesized collagenase inhibitors now being identified and purified from a wide variety of sources. The potential for these molecules to delimit the biological activity of collagenase in time and space makes further knowledge of their regulation and tissue distribution of enormous importance. Such studies on a number of these inhibitors should be forthcoming.

Additionally, the potential for these inhibitors as therapeutic agents can not be minimized; since they are naturally occurring and possess extremely high affinity constants they could make ideal agents for the prevention of untimely collagenolysis in any number of pathologies. Their eventual use in diseases such as rheumatoid arthritis or recessive dystrophic epidermolysis bullosa could represent major therapeutic triumphs. Still to be assessed, however, is the problem of whether such inhibitors can be confined to the area of interest and not equilibrate with the entire organism. Furthermore, the apparent ability of these inhibitors to interact with enzymes other than collagenase leaves open the question as to whether they will be of sufficient specificity to be of truly significant clinical use. Nevertheless, it will be exciting to follow developments in this area.

Another area certain to be explored rigorously in the future is that of the role of cell–cell interaction in the regulation of collagen remodeling. The most obvious example to date of the importance of those interactions has been in the area of rheumatoid arthritis, a pathologic process. There are, however, strong indications that such interactions are of similar importance in normal physiology as well. Thus, further analysis of the interactions between mesenchymal cells and other cell types with a view toward producing or modulating physiologically important processes of collagen degradation are almost certain to produce useful information in the future.

In the area of more fundamental biology, the current availability of molecular biological technology should ultimately enable qualitative advances to be made in the mechanisms by which any of the relevant tissue macromolecules of a collagenolytic system are regulated by a given agent, and the precise biological sequelae of such a regulatory mechanism. The availability of the gene for a collagenase whose production is known to be regulated by one or more factors, whether biological or pharmacological, will eventually allow the definition of exactly how such modulations are effected in the tissue. At the moment no such gene is available, but given the state of the art in molecular biology, its appearance can hardly be far away in time.

The most basic questions of all with respect to collagen remodeling and its control, namely the total description of the exact mechanisms by which the three-dimensional architecture of a tissue (much less right- and left-handed versions of certain tissues) is specified, must still be viewed as distant, dimly perceived goals. Nevertheless, as unattainable as they may appear at this time, one must have a certain faith that, as the molecules involved in these processes continue to be identified, purified, and described in precise chemical terms, we are *ipso facto* approaching these ultimate answers. Twenty-five years ago workers in this field despaired of even finding a true collagenolytic enzyme; the breadth and depth of developments since that time should encourage us to think that today's insoluble problems will bring a set of solutions as exciting as those that have appeared since that time.

ACKNOWLEDGMENTS

Support during the preparation of this review and for some of the studies described herein was provided by USPHS Grants HD05291, AM12129, and AM02784.

REFERENCES

Abe, S., and Nagai, Y. (1973). *J. Biochem.* **73,** 897–900.
Amento, E. P., Kurmick, J. J., Epstein, A., and Krane, S. M. (1982). *Proc. Natl. Acad. Sci. U.S.A.* **79,** 5307–5311.
Anderson, R. E., Kuns, M. E., and Dresden, M. H. (1971). *Ann. Ophthalmol.* **3,** 619–621.
Baker, D. G., Dayer, J.-M., and Roelke, M. (1983). *Arthritis Rheum.* **26,** 8–13.
Bauer, E. A., and Eisen, A. Z. (1978). *J. Exp. Med.* **148,** 1378–1387.
Bauer, E. A., Eisen, A. Z., and Jeffrey, J. J. (1972). *J. Invest. Dermatol.* **59,** 50–55.

Bauer, E. A., Stricklin, G. P., Jeffrey, J. J., and Eisen, A. Z. (1975). *Biochem. Biophys. Res. Commun.* **64**, 232–240.

Bauer, E. A., Gordon, J. M., Reddick, M. E., and Eisen, A. Z. (1977). *J. Invest. Dermatol.* **69**, 363–367.

Bauer, E. A., Seltzer, J. L., and Eisen, A. Z. (1982). *J. Am. Acad. Dermatol.* **6**, 603–607.

Berman, M. B. (1975). *In* "International Ophthalmology Clinics" (D. Pavan-Langston, ed.), Vol. 15, no. 4, pp. 49–66. Little, Brown, Boston.

Berman, M., and Manabe, R. (1973). *Ann. Ophthalmol.* **5**, 1193–1209.

Berman, M., Dohlman, C. H., Gnadinger, M., and Davison, P. F. (1971). *Exp. Eye Res.* **12**, 255–257.

Berman, M. B., Barber, J. C., and Talamo, R. C. (1973a). *Invest. Ophthalmol.* **12**, 759.

Berman, M. B., Kerza-Kwiatecki, A., and Davison, P. F. (1973b). *Exp. Eye Res.* **15**, 367–373.

Berman, M. B., Cavanagh, H. D., and Gage, J. (1976). *Exp. Eye Res.* **22**, 209–218.

Berman, M. B., Leary, R., and Gage, J. (1977). *Exp. Eye Res.* **25**, 435–445.

Bhatnagar, R., Schade, U., Rietschel, E. T., and Decker, K. (1982). *Eur. J. Biochem.* **125**, 125–130.

Bicsak, T. A., and Harper, E. (1984). *J. Biol. Chem.* **259**, 13145–13150.

Bieth, J. (1974). *Bayer Symp.* **V**, 463–469.

Birkedahl-Hansen, H., and Taylor, R. E. (1982). *Biochem. Biophys. Res. Commun.* **107**, 1173–1178.

Birkedahl-Hansen, H., Cobb, C. M., Taylor, R. E., and Fullmer, H. (1976a). *Biochim. Biophys. Acta* **429**, 229–238.

Birkedahl-Hansen, H., Cobb, C. M., Taylor, R. E., and Fullmer, H. M. (1976b). *Biochim. Biophys. Acta* **438**, 273–286.

Brinckerhoff, C. E., Gross, R. H., Nagase, H., Sheldon, L., Jackson, R. C., and Harris, E. D., Jr. (1980a). *N. Engl. J. Med.* **303**, 432–436.

Brinckerhoff, C. E., McMillan, R. M., Dayer, J.-M., and Harris, E. D., Jr. (1980b). *N. Engl. J. Med.* **303**, 432–436.

Brown, S. I., Akiya, S., and Weller, C. A. (1969). *Arch. Ophthalmol.* **82**, 95–97.

Brown, S. I., Weller, C. A., and Vidrich, A. M. (1970a). *Am. J. Ophthalmol.* **70**, 744–747.

Brown, S. I., Weller, C. A., and Wasserman, H. E. (1970b). *Arch. Ophthalmol.* **83**, 370–373.

Cawston, T. E., Galloway, W. A., Mercer, E., Murphy, G., and Reynolds, J. J. (1981). *Biochem. J.* **195**, 159–165.

Cawston, T. E., Murphy, G., Mercer, E., Galloway, W. A., Hazleman, B. L., and Reynolds, J. J. (1983). *Biochem. J.* **211**, 313–318.

Cohen, T. K., Diegelmann, R. F., and Bryant, C. P. (1975). *Surg. Forum* **26**, 61–62.

Cooper, T. W., Welgus, H. G., Stricklin, G. P., and Eisen, A. Z. (1985). *Proc. Natl. Acad. Sci. U.S.A.* **82**, 2779–2783.

Dayer, J.-M., Krane, S. M., and Russell, R. G. G. (1976). *Proc. Natl. Acad. Sci. U.S.A.* **73**, 945–949.

Dayer, J.-M., Robinson, D. R., and Krane, S. M. (1977a). *J. Exp. Med.* **145**, 1399–1404.

Dayer, J.-M., Russell, R. G. G., and Krane, S. M. (1977b). *Science* **195**, 181–183.

Dayer, J.-M., Breard, J., Chess, L., and Krane, S. M. (1979a). *J. Clin. Invest.* **64**, 1386–1392.

Dayer, J.-M., Passwell, J. H., Schneeburger, E. E., and Krane, S. M. (1979b). *J. Clin. Invest.* **64**, 1386–1392.

Dayer, J.-M., Passwell, J. H., Schneeburger, E. E., and Krane, S. M. (1980). *J. Immunol.* **124**, 1712–1720.

Dayer, J.-M., Stephenson, M. L., and Schmidt, E. (1981). *FEBS Lett.* **124,** 253–256.
Dayer, J.-M., Trentham, D. E., and Krane, S. M. (1982). *Collagen Rel. Res.* **2,** 523–540.
Dresden, M. H., Heilman, S. A., and Schmidt, J. D. (1972). *Cancer Res.* **32,** 993–996.
Eeckhout, Y., and Vaes, G. (1977). *Biochem. J.* **166,** 21–31.
Eilon, G., and Raisz, L. G. (1978). *Endocrinology* **103,** 1969–1975.
Eisen, A. Z., and Gross, J. (1965). *Dev. Biol.* **12,** 408–418.
Eisen, A. Z., Bauer, E. A., and Jeffrey, J. J. (1970). *J. Invest. Dermatol.* **55,** 359–373.
Eisen, A. Z., Bauer, E. A., Stricklin, G. P., Seltzer, J. L., Koob, T. J., and Jeffrey, J. J. (1977). *Cholesteatoma Int. Conf., 1st.* pp. 115–123.
Evanson, J. M., Jeffrey, J. J., and Krane, S. M. (1967). *Science* **158,** 499–502.
Evanson, J. M., Jeffrey, J. J., and Krane, S. M. (1968). *J. Clin. Invest.* **47,** 2639–2681.
Francois-Gillet, C., Delaisse, J.-M., Eeckhout, Y., and Vaes, G. (1981). *Biochim. Biophys. Acta* **673,** 1–9.
Gillet, C., Eeckhout, Y., and Vaes, G. (1977). *FEBS Lett.* **74,** 126–128.
Goodall, F. R. (1966). *Science* **152,** 356–358.
Gordon, S., and Werb, Z. (1976). *Proc. Natl. Acad. Sci. U.S.A.* **73,** 872–876.
Grillo, H. C., and Gross, J. (1967). *Dev. Biol.* **15,** 300–317.
Gross, J. (1976). *In* "Biochemistry of Collagen" (G. N. Ramachandran and A. H. Reddi, eds.), pp. 275–310. Plenum, New York.
Gross, J. (1983). *In* "Cell Biology of Extracellular Matrix" (E. Hay, ed.), pp. 217–253. Plenum, New York.
Gross, J., Highberger, J. H., Johnson-Wint, B., and Biswas, C. (1980). *In* "Collagenase in Normal and Pathological Connective Tissues" (D. E. Woolley and J. M. Evanson, eds.), pp. 11–35. Wiley, New York.
Halme, J., and Woessner, J. F. (1975). *J. Endocrinol.* **66,** 357–362.
Halme, J., Tyree, B., and Jeffrey, J. J. (1980). *Arch. Biochem. Biophys.* **199,** 51–60.
Harper, E., and Gross, J. (1970). *Biochim. Biophys. Acta* **198,** 286–292.
Harper, E., and Gross, J. (1972). *Biochem. Biophys. Res. Commun.* **48,** 1147–1152.
Harper, E., and Toole, B. P. (1973). *J. Biol. Chem.* **248,** 2625–2626.
Harper, E., Bloch, K. J., and Gross, J. (1971). *Biochemistry* **10,** 3035–3041.
Harris, E. D., Jr., and Farrell, M. E. (1972). *Biochim. Biophys. Acta* **278,** 133–141.
Harris, E. D., Jr., and Krane, S. M. (1972). *Biochim. Biophys. Acta* **258,** 566–576.
Harris, E. D., Jr., and McCroskery, P. A. (1974). *N. Engl. J. Med.* **290,** 1–6.
Harris, E. D., Jr., Mainardi, C. L., and Vater, C. A. (1978). *Clin. Res.* **26,** 515A.
Hayashi, T., Nakamura, T., Hori, H., and Nagai, Y. (1980a). *J. Biochem.* **87,** 809–815.
Hayashi, T., Nakamura, T., Hori, H., and Nagai, Y. (1980b). *J. Biochem.* **87,** 993–995.
Highberger, J. H., Corbett, C., and Gross, J. (1979). *Biochem. Biophys. Res. Commun.* **89,** 202–208.
Horwitz, A. L., and Crystal, R. G. (1976). *Biochem. Biophys. Res. Commun.* **69,** 296–303.
Horwitz, A. L., Kelman, J. A., and Crystal, R. G. (1976). *Nature* **264,** 772–774.
Horwitz, A. L., Hance, A. J., and Crystal, R. G. (1977). *Proc. Natl. Acad. Sci. U.S.A.* **74,** 897–901.
Houck, J. C., Sharma, V. K., Patel, J. M., and Gladner, J. A. (1968). *Biochem. Pharmacol.* **17,** 2081–2090.
Jeffrey, J. J. (1981). *Collagen Rel. Res.* **1,** 257–268.
Jeffrey, J. J., and Gross, J. (1970). *Biochemistry* **9,** 269–278.
Jeffrey, J. J., and Koob, T. J. (1974). *Excerpta Med. Int. Congr. Ser.* **273,** 1115–1121.
Jeffrey, J. J., Coffey, R. J., and Eisen, A. Z. (1971a). *Biochim. Biophys. Acta* **252,** 136–142.

Jeffrey, J. J., Coffey, R. J., and Eisen, A. Z. (1971b). *Biochim. Biophys. Acta* **252,** 143–149.

Jeffrey, J. J., Welgus, H. G., Burgeson, R. E., and Eisen, A. Z. (1983). *J. Biol. Chem.* **258,** 11123–11127.

Jeffrey, J. J., Di Petrillo, T. L., Counts, D. F., and Cutroneo, K. R. (1985). *Collagen Rel. Res.* **5,** 157–165.

Johnson-Muller, B., and Gross, J. (1978). *Proc. Natl. Acad. Sci. U.S.A.* **75,** 4417–4421.

Johnson-Wint, B., and Bauer, E. A. (1985). *J. Biol. Chem.* **260,** 2080–2085.

Johnson-Wint, B., and Gross, J. (1984). *J. Cell. Biol.* **98,** 90–96.

Kassell, B., and Kay, J. (1973). *Science* **180,** 1022–1027.

Kerwar, S. S., Nolan, J. C., Ridge, S. C., Oronsky, A. L., and Slakey, L. (1980). *Biochim. Biophys. Acta* **632,** 183–191.

Kerwar, S. S., Ridge, S. C., Landes, M. J., and Nolan, J. C. (1984). *Agent Action* **14,** 54–57.

Kivirikko, K. I., and Myllyla, R. (1984). *In* "Extracellular Matrix Biochemistry" (K. A. Piez and A. H. Reddi, eds.), pp. 83–118. Elsevier, Amsterdam.

Koob, T. J., and Jeffrey, J. J. (1974). *Biochim. Biophys. Acta* **354,** 61–70.

Koob, T. J., and Ryan, K. (1980). *In* "Dilatation of the Uterine Cervix" (P. Stubblefield and F. Naftolin, eds.), pp. 135–145. Raven, New York.

Koob, T. J., Jeffrey, J. J., and Eisen, A. Z. (1974). *Biochem. Biophys. Res. Commun.* **61,** 1083–1088.

Koob, T. J., Eisen, A. Z., and Jeffrey, J. J. (1981). *Biochim. Biophys. Acta* **629,** 13–23.

Krane, S. M., and Amento, E. P. (1983). *J. Rheumatol.* **115,** 7–12.

Kronberger, A., Valle, K. J., Eisen, A. Z., Jeffrey, J. J., and Bauer, E. A. (1985). *Biochim. Biophys. Acta* **825,** 227–235.

Leibovitch, S. J., and Weiss, J. (1971). *Biochim. Biophys. Acta* **25,** 109–121.

Lenaers-Claeys, G., and Vaes, G. (1979). *Biochim. Biophys. Acta* **584,** 375–388.

Liotta, L. A., Abe, S., Robey, P. G., and Martin, G. R. (1979). *Proc. Natl. Acad. Sci. U.S.A.* **76,** 2268–2272.

McCarthy, J. B., Wahl, S. M., Rees, J. C., Olsen, C. E., Sandberg, A. L., and Wahl, L. M. (1980). *J. Immunol.* **124,** 2405–2409.

MacCartney, H. W., and Tschesche, H. (1983a). *Eur. J. Biochem.* **130,** 79–83.

MacCartney, H. W., and Tschesche, H. (1983b). *Eur. J. Biochem.* **130,** 85–92.

Mainardi, C. L., Dixit, S. N., and Kang, A. H. (1980a). *J. Biol. Chem.* **255,** 5435–5441.

Mainardi, C. L., Hasty, D. L., Seyer, J. M., and Kang, A. H. (1980b). *J. Biol. Chem.* **255,** 12006–12010.

Mainardi, C. L., Seyer, J. M., and Kang, A. H. (1980c). *Biochem. Biophys. Res. Commun.* **97,** 1108–1115.

Miller, E. J., Finch, E. D., Chung, E., and Butler, W. (1976). *Arch. Biochem. Biophys.* **173,** 631–637.

Murphy, G., and Sellers, A. (1980). *In* "Collagenase in Normal and Pathological Connective Tissues" (D. E. Woolley and J. M. Evanson, eds.), pp. 65–81. Wiley, New York.

Murphy, G., Cartwright, E. C., Sellers, A., and Reynolds, J. J. (1977). *Biochim. Biophys. Acta* **483,** 493–498.

Murphy, G., McGuire, M. B. G., and Russell, R. G. G. (1981). *Clin. Sci.* **61,** 711–716.

Nagai, Y., Lapiere, C. M., and Gross, J. (1964). *Sixth Int. Congr. Biochem.* **II,** 135.

Nagase, H., Jackson, R. C., Brinckerhoff, C. E., Vater, C. A., and Harris, E. D., Jr. (1981). *J. Biol. Chem.* **256,** 11951–11954.

Nagase, H., Brinckerhoff, C. E., Vater, C. A., and Harris, E. D., Jr. (1983). *Biochem. J.* **214,** 281–288.

Nardella, F. A., Dayer, J.-M., Roelke, M., Krane, S. M., and Mannik, M. (1983). *Rheumatol. Int.* **3,** 183–186.

Nolan, J. C., Ridge, S. C., Oronsky, A. L., Slakey, L. L., and Kerwar, S. S. (1978). *Biochem. Biophys. Res. Commun.* **83,** 1183–1190.

Nolan, J. C., Ridge, S. C., Oronsky, A. L., and Kerwar, S. S. (1980). *Artherosclerosis* **35,** 93–102.

Oronsky, A. L., Perper, R. J., and Schroder, H. C. (1973). *Nature* **246,** 417–419.

Otsuka, K., Sodek, J., and Limeback, H. (1984). *Eur. J. Biochem.* **145,** 123–129.

Phadke, K. D., Lawrence, M., and Nanda, S. (1978). *Biochem. Biophys. Res. Commun.* **85,** 490–496.

Postlethwaite, A. E., Lackman, L. B., Mainardi, C. L., and Kang, A. H. (1983). *J. Exp. Med.* **157,** 801–806.

Prockop, D. J., and Tuderman, L. (1982). *In* "Methods in Enzymology" (L. W. Cunningham and D. W. Fredeoiksen, eds.), Vol. 82, Part A, pp. 305–319. Academic Press, New York.

Prockop, D. J., Kivirikko, K. I., Tuderman, L., and Guzman, N. A. (1979). *N. Engl. J. Med.* **301,** 13–23.

Reynolds, J. J., Muraphy, G., Sellers, A., and Cartwright, E. (1977). *Lancet* ii, 333–335.

Rokowski, R. J., Sheehy, J., and Cutroneo, K. R. (1981). *Arch. Biochem. Biophys.* **210,** 73–81.

Roswit, W. T., Halme, J. H., and Jeffrey, J. J. (1983). *Arch. Biochem. Biophys.* **225,** 285–295.

Ryan, J. N., and Woessner, J. F. (1971). *Biochem. Biophys. Res. Commun.* **44,** 144–149.

Ryan, J. N., and Woessner, J. F. (1972). *Biochem. J.* **127,** 705–715.

Sakamoto, S., and Sakamoto, M. (1984). *Biochem. Int.* **9,** 51–58.

Sakamoto, S., Goldhaber, P., and Glimcher, M. J. (1972). *Calcium Tissue Res.* **10,** 142–151.

Salo, T., Liotta, L., and Tryggvason, K. (1983). *J. Biol. Chem.* **258,** 3058–3063.

Sellers, A., and Murphy, G. (1981). *Int. Rev. Connect. Tissue Res.* **9,** 151–182.

Sellers, A., Cartwright, E., Murphy, G., and Reynolds, J. J. (1977). *Biochem. J.* **163,** 303–307.

Sellers, A., Meikle, M. C., and Reynolds, J. J. (1980). *Calcium Tissue Int.* **31,** 35–43.

Seltzer, J. L., Welgus, H. G., Jeffrey, J. J., and Eisen, A. Z. (1976). *Arch. Biochem. Biophys.* **173,** 355–361.

Seltzer, J. L., Jeffrey, J. J., and Eisen, A. Z. (1977). *Biochim. Biophys. Acta* **484,** 179–187.

Seltzer, J. L., Adams, S. A., Grant, G. A., and Eisen, A. Z. (1981). *J. Biol. Chem.* **256,** 4662–4668.

Shimizu, M., Glimcher, M. J., Travis, D., and Goldhaber, P. (1963). *Biochem. Biophys. Res. Commun.* **130,** 1175–1180.

Shinkai, H., Kawamoto, T., Hori, H., and Nagai, Y. (1977). *J. Biochem.* **81,** 261–263.

Siegel, R. C. (1979). *Int. Rev. Connect. Tissue Res.* **8,** 73–118.

Sopata, I., and Dancewicz, A. M. (1974). *Biochim. Biophys. Acta* **370,** 510–523.

Starcher, B. C., Hill, C. H., and Madaras, J. G. (1980). *J. Nutr.* **110,** 2095–2102.

Sterling, K. M., Harris, M. J., Mitchell, J. J., De Petrillo, T. L., Delaney, G. L., and Cutroneo, K. R. (1983). *J. Biol. Chem.* **258,** 7644–7647.

Stricklin, G. P., and Welgus, H. G. (1983). *J. Biol. Chem.* **258,** 12252–12258.

Stricklin, G. P., Bauer, E. A., Jeffrey, J. J., and Eisen, A. Z. (1977). *Biochemistry* **16,** 1607–1615.

Stricklin, G. P., Eisen, A. Z., Bauer, E. A., and Jeffrey, J. J. (1978). *Biochemistry* **17,** 2331–2337.

Stricklin, G. P., Jeffrey, J. J., Roswit, W. T., and Eisen, A. Z. (1983). *Biochemistry* **22,** 61–68.

Swann, J. C., Reynolds, J. J., and Galloway, W. A. (1981). *Biochem. J.* **195,** 41–49.

Tschesche, H., and Macartney, H. W. (1981). *Eur. J. Biochem.* **120,** 183–190.

Tyree, B., Halme, J., and Jeffrey, J. J. (1980). *Arch. Biochem. Biophys.* **202,** 314–317.

Tyree, B., Seltzer, J. L., Halme, J., Jeffrey, J., and Eisen, A. Z. (1981). *Arch. Biochem. Biophys.* **208,** 440–443.

Vaes, G. (1965). *Exp. Cell Res.* **39,** 470–474.

Vaes, G. (1967). *Biochem. J.* **103,** 802–804.

Vaes, G. (1968). *J. Cell Biol.* **39,** 676–697.

Vaes, G. (1972). *Biochem. J.* **126,** 275–289.

Vaes, G. (1980). *In* "Collagenase in Normal and Pathological Connective Tissues" (D. E. Woolley and J. M. Evanson, eds.), pp. 185–207. Wiley, New York.

Vaes, G., Eeckhout, Y., Lenaers-Claeys, G., Francois-Gillet, C., and Druetz, J. E. (1978). *Biochem. J.* **172,** 261–264.

Valle, K.-J., and Bauer, E. A. (1979). *J. Biol. Chem.* **254,** 10115–10122.

Vater, C. A., Mainardi, C. L., and Harris, E. D., Jr. (1978a). *Biochim. Biophys. Acta* **539,** 238–247.

Vater, C. A., Mainardi, C. L., and Harris, E. D., Jr. (1978b). *J. Clin. Invest.* **62,** 987–992.

Vater, C. A., Harris, E. D., Jr., and Siegel, R. C. (1979a). *Biochem. J.* **181,** 639–645.

Vater, C. A., Mainardi, C. L., and Harris, E. D., Jr. (1979b). *J. Biol. Chem.* **254,** 3045–3053.

Vater, C. A., Nagase, H., and Harris, E. D., Jr. (1983). *J. Biol. Chem.* **258,** 9374–9382.

Wahl, L. M., and Winter, C. C. (1984). *Arch. Biochem. Biophys.* **230,** 661–667.

Wahl, L. M., Wahl, S. M., Martin, G. R., and Mergenhagen, S. E. (1974). *Proc. Natl. Acad. Sci. U.S.A.* **71,** 3598–3601.

Wahl, L. M., Wahl, S. M., Martin, G. R., and Mergenhagen, S. E. (1975). *Science* **187,** 261–263.

Wahl, L. M., Olsen, C. E., Sandberg, A. L., and Mergenhagen, S. E. (1977). *Proc. Natl. Acad. Sci. U.S.A.* **74,** 4955–4958.

Walsh, C. (1979). "Enzymatic Reaction Mechanisms," pp. 34–35. Freeman, San Francisco.

Weiss, J. B. (1976). *Int. Rev. Connect. Tissue Res.* **7,** 101–157.

Welgus, H. G., and Stricklin, G. P. (1983). *J. Biol. Chem.* **258,** 12259–12264.

Welgus, H. G., Stricklin, G. P., Eisen, A. Z., Bauer, E. A., Cooney, R. V., and Jeffrey, J. J. (1979). *J. Biol. Chem.* **254,** 1938–1943.

Welgus, H. G., Jeffrey, J. J., Stricklin, G. P., Roswit, W. T., and Eisen, A. Z. (1980). *J. Biol. Chem.* **255,** 6806–6813.

Welgus, H. G., Jeffrey, J. J., and Eisen, A. Z. (1981). *J. Biol. Chem.* **256,** 9511–9515.

Welgus, H. G., Jeffrey, J. J., Stricklin, G. P., and Eisen, A. Z. (1982). *J. Biol. Chem.* **257,** 11534–11539.

Welgus, H. G., Kobayashi, G. K., and Jeffrey, J. J. (1983). *J. Biol. Chem.* **258,** 14162–14165.

Welgus, H. G., Wootten, J. M., Fliszar, K., Minor, R. E., Burgeson, R. E., and Jeffrey, J. J. (1984). *J. Biol. Chem.*, in press.

Welgus, H. G., Stricklin, G. P., Eisen, A. Z., and Jeffrey, J. J. (1985). *Collagen Rel. Res.*, in press.

Werb, Z. (1978). *J. Exp. Med.* **147,** 1695–1712.

Werb, Z., and Gordon, S. (1975). *J. Exp. Med.* **142,** 346–360.

Werb, Z., Burleigh, P. M. C., Barrett, A. J., and Starkey, P. M. (1974). *Biochem. J.* **139**, 359–368.

Werb, Z., Mainardi, C. L., Vater, C. A., and Harris, E. D., Jr. (1977). *N. Engl. J. Med.* **296**, 1017–1023.

Wilhelm, S. M., Javed, T., and Miller, R. L. (1984). *Collagen Rel. Res.* **4**, 129–152.

Woessner, J. F. (1969). *Biochem. J.* **112**, 637–646.

Woessner, J. F. (1979). *Biochem. J.* **180**, 95–102.

Woessner, J. F. (1982). *In* "Collagen in Health and Disease" (J. B. Weiss and M. I. V. Jayson, eds.), pp. 506–527. Churchill-Livingstone, London.

Woessner, J. F., and Brewer, T. H. (1963). *Biochem. J.* **89**, 75–82.

Woolley, D. E. (1984). *In* "Extracellular Matrix Biochemistry" (K. A. Piez and A. H. Reddi, eds.), pp. 119–151. Elsevier, Amsterdam.

Woolley, D. E., Glanville, R. W., Crossley, M. J., and Evanson, J. M. (1975a). *Eur. J. Biochem.* **54**, 611–622.

Woolley, D. E., Roberts, D. R., and Evanson, J. M. (1975b). *Biochem. Biophys. Res. Commun.* **66**, 747–754.

Woolley, D. E., Roberts, D. R., and Evanson, J. M. (1976). *Nature* **261**, 325–327.

Woolley, D. E., Akroyd, C., Evanson, J. M., Soames, J. V., and Davies, R. M. (1978a). *Biochim. Biophys. Acta* **522**, 205–217.

Woolley, D. E., Glanville, R. W., Roberts, D. R., and Evanson, J. M. (1978b). *Biochem. J.* **169**, 265–276.

Woolley, D. E., Harris, E. D., Jr., Mainardi, C. L., and Brinckerhoff, C. E. (1978c). *Science* **200**, 773–775.

Woolley, D. E., Brinckerhoff, C. E., Mainardi, C. L., Vater, C. A., Evanson, J. M., and Harris, E. D., Jr. (1979). *Ann. Rheum. Dis.* **38**, 262–270.

Feedback Regulation of Collagen Synthesis

Peter K. Müller, Andreas G. Nerlich,
Joachim Böhm, Luu Phan-Than

Max-Planck-Institut für Biochemie, Martinsried, Federal Republic of Germany

and

Thomas Krieg

Dermatologische Klinik Ludwig-Maximilians-Universität, München, Federal Republic of Germany

REGULATION OF MATRIX ACCUMULATION

I. Introduction

A. *Clinical Aspects of Collagen Regulation*

Collagen is the most abundant connective tissue protein, with a predominant localization in bone, cartilage, tendon, muscle, and skin as well as in the septal parts of all parenchymal organs. A concise regulation of the metabolism of collagen is essential for the normal function of connective tissue. The disturbance of normal collagen production, secretion, or degradation therefore causes malfunction, resulting in a variety of pathological symptoms. Thus, a lack of collagen coincides with a reduction in tissue stability, as seen for example in osteogenesis imperfecta (Hollister, 1981), while an overproduction and accumulation of collagen leads to an enhanced tissue rigidity, as seen for example in scleroderma (Leroy, 1974) or pulmonary fibrosis (Rennard and Crystal, 1982), or to a displacement of parenchymal cells with subsequent malfunction of the organ, as in liver cirrhosis (Rojkind, 1970). The most important clinical conditions which are related to a disturbed regulation of collagen synthesis are summarized in Table I and represent a variety of different diseases which affect different organ systems. An enhanced collagen production also occurs under physiological conditions in all reparative processes, like wound or fracture healing. In these instances, however, the synthesis of collagen declines when tissue repair is completed.

B. *Biochemistry of Collagen*

Collagens are a family of proteins whose common feature is a triple helical domain formed by three tightly coiled polypeptide chains (Fig. 1). The ability to form this helix and its stability and length are determined by the amino acid sequence of the individual chains (for review see Piez, 1984). The typical collagen sequence Gly-X-Y is repeated many times, with type I collagen, e.g., containing more than 330 of these subunits. A glycine in every third position is essential for triple helix formation, and positions X and Y often are proline and hydroxyproline, respectively. Hydroxyproline is synthesized from proline after translation of the chains and is characteristic for collagen.

Up to now 10 genetically different types of collagen have been described, each of them composed of one to three different chains (see Bornstein and Sage, 1980; Martin *et al.*, 1985). The interstitial collagen types include types I–III. Type I, the most abundant collagen in mammals, is a heterotrimer composed of two different chains, while

TABLE I

SELECTED EXAMPLES OF CLINICALLY IMPORTANT
FIBROTIC PROCESSES

Hepatic cirrhosis
Pulmonary fibrosis
Atherosclerosis
Systemic (progressive) sclerosis (scleroderma)
Hypertrophic scars/keloid
Myelofibrosis
Endomyocardial fibrosis
Pancreatic fibrosis
Retroperitoneal fibrosis
Thickened basement membranes in diabetic kidney and
    blood vessels

both type II and III are homotrimers. Type II is specific for cartilage
and the vitrous body and is synthesized by chondrocytes, whereas fibroblasts produce types I and III simultaneously.

C. Regulation of Collagen Synthesis

During biosynthesis of collagen (Fig. 2) several modifications of the
peptide chains occur which are essential for a functionally intact collagen molecule (for review see Kivirikko and Myllylä, 1984). After transcription of the distinct collagen gene(s) the high molecular weight
RNA is processed to functional mRNA. The collagen chains are then
synthesized on membrane-bound ribosomes. After several intra- and

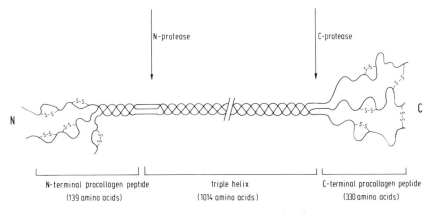

FIG. 1. The type I procollagen molecule.

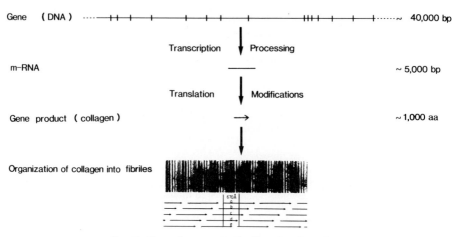

F_{IG}. 2. From the gene to the functional product.

extracellular posttranslational modifications including, e.g., hydroxyl-ation of proline and lysine and cleavage of N- and C-terminal procolla-gen peptides, the collagen molecules then are deposited in the extracel-lular space. At all the steps mentioned a modulation and regulation of collagen production is possible.

Regulation of collagen synthesis at the level of transcription is evi-dent. The expression of the various genes coding for different collagen types is specific for a given tissue. Changes in the normal cell-specific pattern have been described for chondrocytes cultured *in vitro* for ex-tended times. These cells "dedifferentiate", and the morphological change from round chondrocytes to the flattened shape of fibroblasts is accompanied by a switch from type II to type I collagen (Müller *et al.*, 1979; Bornstein and Sage, 1980). Several groups have shown that fi-broblasts transformed by viruses specifically reduce the transcription of collagen genes (Adams *et al.*, 1979; Sandmeyer *et al.*, 1981; Sobel *et al.*, 1981; Avvedimento *et al.*, 1981). Ascorbate, an important cofactor of several enzymes of collagen biosynthesis, seems to act both on tran-scription and translation of collagen mRNAs (Pinell, 1982).

Translational control of collagen mRNA has attracted much inter-est. The first reports suggesting translational control came from an experimental liver fibrosis model. Rojkind and Deleon (1970) found that the intracellular pool of free amino acids such as proline appears to regulate collagen production. 6-Diazo-5-oxonorleucine, an analog of glutamine, which inhibits the synthesis of nucleic acids, stimulates protein synthesis in chick embryo tibiae in general and specifically increases translation of collagen mRNA. This was interpreted as being due to an altered posttranscriptional control (Bhatnagar and Rapaka, 1971). It is also obvious that there exist some further regulatory sites during the posttranslational processing of the collagen molecule. One particular site is represented by the hydroxylation of proline which is crucially important for the stability of the triple helix formation (Baum *et al.*, 1980). The experimental inhibition of prolyl hydroxylation with $\alpha\alpha'$- dipyridyl therefore leads to a decreased stability of the collagen chain and an increase in the intra- and extracellular degradation of the molecules (Prockop *et al.*, 1979). Finally, the degradation of the collagen chains represents a further site for the regulation of extra- and intracellular accumulation of this molecule (Krane, 1982; see Berg, this volume).

The feedback control mechanism of collagen production exerted by aminopropeptides was first suggested following the discovery of procollagen as the precursor form of collagen and its accumulation in a disorder that coincides with enhanced collagen synthesis (Bornstein *et al.*, 1972; Prockop *et al.*, 1973; Lenaers *et al.*, 1971; Fjolstadt and Helle, 1974; Lichtenstein *et al.*, 1973).

II. THE AMINOPROPEPTIDES

A. *Structure of Aminopropeptides*

Procollagen, the precursor form of interstitial collagen, consists of the mature collagen triple helix and additional peptides at the amino- and carboxy-terminal ends of the helix (Fessler and Fessler, 1978; Martin *et al.*, 1975; Prockop *et al.*, 1979). The procollagen peptides account for approximately 10% (aminopeptide) and 20% (carboxypeptide) of the mass of procollagen. These are specifically cleaved off by certain neutral proteases during the metabolic processing of the collagen molecule.

An intermediate form in the process of conversion from procollagen to collagen which still contains the amino-terminal peptide extension but not the carboxypropeptide, is named pN-collagen (Smith *et al.*, 1977; Martin *et al.*, 1975). These pN-collagens were first identified in dermatosparactic skin of calves. Examination of these molecules extracted from skins by electron microscopy showed 13–25 nm long extensions which consist of about 139 amino acid residues (Becker *et al.*, 1976; Rhode *et al.*, 1979b).

The aminopropeptide was originally isolated as a fragment which did not show the characteristic composition of collagen (Furthmayr *et al.*, 1972). In later studies a longer form of the aminopropeptide was found that contained both noncollagenous and collagenous sequences (Becker *et al.*, 1976; Nowack *et al.*, 1976a; Pesciotta *et al.*, 1980). This led to the two-domain model of the aminopropeptide for the proα1(I) chain of type I procollagen and the proα1(III) chain of type III procollagen (see Timpl and Glanville, 1982). At the amino end there is a globular noncollagenous segment, termed Col 1, containing five intrachain disulfide bridges. A schematic diagram of the aminopropeptides is depicted in Fig. 3. The remainder of the aminopropeptide is a collagenous tripel helical segment of about 14 Gly-X-Y triplets (Kühn *et al.*, 1982). Between this collagenous region and the telopeptide of the collagen α chain, occurs another short region of nonhelical sequence, the Col 2 fragment.

There are two major differences between the aminopropeptides of type I and type III collagens. The latter contain three interchain disulfide bridges between three identical chains. This enables the aminopropeptide of type III procollagen to withstand both denaturation and cleavage by bacterial collagenase (Fessler and Fessler, 1979). The

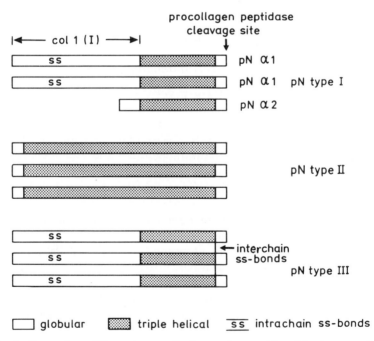

FIG. 3. Comparison of the amino-terminal extension peptides of the interstitial collagens.

aminopropeptides of type I collagen are susceptible to collagenase digestion (Becker *et al.*, 1976) and are made up of two extension peptides from proα1(I) chains and one from the proα2(I) chain. Compared with the aminopropeptide of proα1(I) chain, the propeptide of proα2(I) is approximately half the size and consists mainly of the collagenous region plus a short noncollagenous sequence linked to the α2(I) telopeptide. The aminopropeptide of the proα2(I) chain seems not to contain intrachain disulfide bridges and is readily degraded by collagenase (Harwood *et al.*, 1977; Morris *et al.*, 1979). Type II procollagen has a similar extension peptide which has an intermediate size. The amino acid sequence of the type II aminopropeptide was recently deduced from the nucleotide sequence of a cDNA clone for this portion of procollagen (Khono *et al.*, 1984). The propeptide synthesized as preproα chain is mainly triple helical and contains 25 Gly-X-Y repeats. It has a total length of approximately 92 amino acids.

Proline and hydroxyproline residues are found in the triple helical part of the aminopropeptide in even higher amounts than in the major collagen helix of the molecule. This indicates that the collagenous sequence of the aminopropeptide is very stable. The melting point of the type III collagen propeptide triple helix is at 53°C (Bruckner *et al.*, 1978), while the melting range of the type I procollagen peptides occurs between 35 and 45°C (Engel *et al.*, 1977).

The sequence of the aminopropeptide has some special properties. About one-fourth of the amino acids are Asp and Glu residues, while Hyl is not present. The cystein content is especially high in α1(I) aminopropeptides (Hörlein *et al.*, 1978).

B. *Metabolism of the Aminopropeptides*

Aminopropeptides are synthesized as segments of intact procollagen chains. The first biosynthetic product of collagen metabolism, however, is not the procollagen chain, but a preproduct with an additional extension connected to the N-terminus of the aminopropeptides (prepropeptide). This sequence is characterized by containing several hydrophobic amino acid residues, as found for many other polypeptides secreted into the rough endoplasmic reticulum of the cells. The amino acid sequence has been partially elucidated for the chick proα1(I) chain (Palmiter *et al.*, 1970) and consists of 19 amino acid residues as found also for preproα1(II) (Khono *et al.*, 1984). At the time of secretion or afterwards the aminopropeptides are cleaved from the procollagen molecules by specific proteases. There presumably exist not only different proteases for N- and C-propeptides, but also for different collagen types (see Fessler and Fessler, 1978). The removal of the propeptides occurs *en bloc,* presumably by cleaving a single peptide bond (Fessler and Fessler, 1979; Leung *et al.,* 1979; Tuderman *et al.,* 1978). The cleavage site for the N-protease is a Pro-Glu bond in the nonhelical part of the aminopropeptide. The procollagen N-protease or peptidase, has been shown to be essential for normal collagen deposition since in dermatosparactic sheep and calves, which lack the enzyme (Lapiere *et al.,* 1971), this seems to be responsible for the tissue fragility.

C. *Stability of the Propeptides in Vivo and Its Distribution in Body Fluids and Tissues*

First evidence for a relatively high stability of the aminopropeptides arose from the experimental investigations of Layman *et al.* (1971) and Pontz *et al.* (1973), who reported a persistance of the aminopropeptides in the medium of cultured cells. Metabolism of propeptides was suggested by the identification of smaller forms of the peptides in tissues, serum, and urine (Niemela *et al.,* 1982; Rohde *et al.,* 1983). The portion that is excreted into the urine is the noncollagenous domain (Col 1) (Raedsch *et al.,* 1983; Rohde *et al.,* 1979a). The proteolytic separation of the noncollagenous and the collagenous fragment may be a physiologic process preceeding their elimination from the body.

Rhode *et al.* (1979a) found by immunoassay that the aminopropeptide in human serum is quite stable. This observation is consistent with the physical data that show a high stability of the type III aminopropeptides towards denaturation and enzymatic attack.

Additionally, there exists evidence that under certain conditions some aminopropeptides are not processed at all and persist as structural elements in the collagen fibrils. Persistence of aminopropeptides seems to be related to the thickness of the fibril. Thus, fibrils with small diameters appear to contain a high proportion of aminopropeptides. This observation led to the hypothesis that the aminopropeptides are involved in the regulation of fibril diameter (Fleischmajer *et al.,* 1981).

Aminopropeptides have been isolated not only from tissues, but also from various body fluids. Thus, these peptides were detected in calf serum and amniotic fluid (Nowack *et al.,* 1976b), human serum and ascitic fluid (Rhode *et al.,* 1979a), lung lymph fluid of sheep (Nerlich *et al.,* 1984), as well as in the fluid of bronchoalveolar lavage of humans. (Low *et al.,* 1983). Similarly, aminopropeptides have also been isolated from the medium of cells in culture, including fibroblasts (Pontz *et al.,* 1973) and epithelial cells (Alitalio *et al.,* 1980).

D. Preparation of Aminopropeptides

The main sources for the preparation of aminopropeptides are the skin of dermatosparactic animals, which contains pN-collagen (Hörlein *et al.*, 1978) due to defective cleavage, and fetal skin, which has a relatively high content of aminopropeptides (particularly of type III collagen) presumably due to a high rate of synthesis. The preparation of aminopropeptides of type I collagen from dermatosparactic calf skin involves cleavage of the triple helical part of type I collagen by bacterial collagenase and isolation of the aminopropeptide fraction by chromatography on DEAE–cellulose, agarose molecular sieve, and phosphocellulose (Wiestner *et al.*, 1979). Aminopropeptides from type III collagen are preferentially obtained by extraction of fetal calf skin, which is followed by cleavage with collagenase, chromatographic purification on DEAE–cellulose and molecular sieve chromatography (Nowack *et al.*, 1976b). The precursor form of type II collagen has not been isolated in quantity.

III. Experiments on Feedback Inhibition of Aminopropeptides on Collagen Biosynthesis

A. Translational Control

In eukaryotes the sites of transcription and translation are located in different compartments of the cell. An RNA copy of a transcription unit is made in the nucleus and processed. The functional mRNA is transported into the cytoplasm where it may be translated. In contrast to prokaryotes, where transcription and translation occur simultaneously, both processes are separated in eukaryotes. This offers additional possibilities to modulate gene expression. A general increase in translation of mature mRNA in cytoplasm was shown for the early development in sea urchin. Unfertilized eggs increase translation at least 50-fold from the same number of mRNAs after fertilization (Brandhorst, 1976). Translational control also is evident in virus-infected cells, where synthesis of host proteins is reduced although the mRNA is still present (Fernandez-Munoz and Darnell, 1976; Skup *et al.*, 1981). During mitosis cells decrease the level of translation by one-third without degrading mRNA (Fan and Penman, 1970). Translational control of collagen synthesis was shown by Focht and Adams (1984). In their studies, hybridization with specific probes revealed that chick chondrocytes contain type I and type III mRNA, but that they were not translated either in the cells or in cell-free systems.

These findings indicate that there are specific mechanisms to regulate which mRNAs present are translated. Rhagow *et al.* (1984) isolated a factor from fibrotic rat liver which enhances translation of type I mRNA 4- to 6-fold without affecting other proteins suggesting that positive regulators also are present.

B. *Dermatosparaxis*

In this inborn error of collagen metabolism the affected animals show extremely enhanced bruisability of skin that tears even under slight trauma (Lenaers *et al.*, 1971; Fjolstadt and Helle, 1972). Electron microscopic examination of the skin reveals an irregular organization of collagen (Fig. 4) that shows no large bundles of fibers as in normal skin. Extraction of the skin collagen and analysis of SLS crystalites additionally shows the presence of collagen molecules retaining the aminoterminal propeptide (Becker *et al.*, 1976; Rhode *et al.*, 1979b). Soon after the description of the molecular abnormality in dermatosparactic animals, Lichtenstein *et al.* (1973) found a similar defect in collagen in the skin of patients with a severe form of Ehlers–Danlos syndrome type VII (arthrochalasis multiplex congenita). The underlying molecular defects in EDS type VII and dermatosparaxis appear to differ, since in the first case there is a mutation in the proα2(I) chain (Steinmann *et al.*, 1980) preventing the peptides from cleavage, whereas in the animal disease there is a defect in the procollagen peptidase (Lapiere *et al.*, 1971). In addition, Lichtenstein *et al.* (1973) noticed that cells from patients with a low removal of aminopropeptides showed an elevated rate of collagen synthesis. Therefore they raised the hypothesis that cleavage of amino-terminal extension peptides may regulate synthesis of collagen by feedback inhibition. This was corroborated by Wiestner *et al.* (1982a) who showed that the slow rate of procollagen conversion was accompanied by a higher rate of collagen synthesis in dermatosparactic sheep fibroblasts. In this study, the low rate of procollagen conversion coincided with an increased synthesis of both type I and type III collagen. However measurement of the levels of mRNA for the proα2(I) chain showed that the levels of mRNA were only marginally different between dermatosparactic and normal fibroblast strains (Lozano *et al.*, 1983).

C. *The Biological Activity of Aminopropeptides in Cell Culture*

In a set of experiments, feedback inhibition of collagen synthesis by aminopropeptides was directly verified (Wiestner *et al.*, 1979, 1982b;

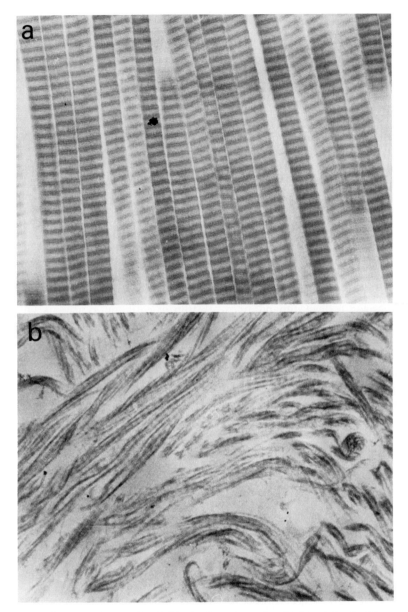

FIG. 4. Electron micrographs of thin sections through calf skin stained with uranyl acetate. (a) Skin of normal calf, (b) skin of dermatosparactic calf. (Pictures taken by H. Wiedemann.)

TABLE II

INHIBITION OF COLLAGEN SYNTHESIS BY AMINO-TERMINAL
EXTENSION PEPTIDE OF PROCOLLAGEN TYPE I
ON CELLS IN CULTURE

Cell culture	Species	Tissue	Collagen type	Inhi-bition
Fibroblast	Calf	Skin	I, III	+
Fibroblast	Human	Skin	I, III	+
Chondrocyte	Calf	Cartilage	II	−
Chondrocyte	Calf	Cartilage	I	−
Fibroblast	Chick	Tendon	I	−
Chondrocyte	Chick	Sterna	II	−
Chondrocyte	Chick	Sterna	I	−

Paglia *et al.*, 1981; Kühn *et al.*, 1982). These authors analyzed the effect of aminopropeptides from type I and III collagen on collagen production in various types of cells from different species (Table II). These studies showed that the propeptides from type I and III procollagen caused a dose dependent inhibition of collagen synthesis with a 50% inhibition of synthesis at 6 μM of either peptide. Peptides derived from other portions of the collagen molecule showed no inhibitory activity. Furthermore, synthesis of noncollagenous proteins was not altered. The synthesis of both proα1(I) and proα2(I) chains showed an equal inhibition (Fig. 5), and there was no change in the level of hydroxyproline in the collagen chains or in the level of intracellular

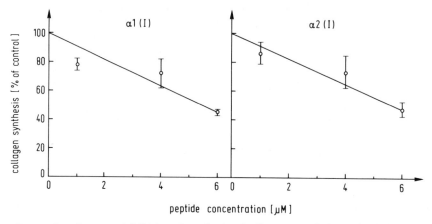

FIG. 5. Simultaneous inhibition of synthesis of collagen type I chains by Col 1(I) in cultured fibroblasts.

degradation. Additional experiments showed that aminopropeptides obtained from procollagen type I and III inhibited collagen synthesis in fibroblast strains, which produce collagen type I and III, but did not alter the synthesis of type II collagen by chondrocytes. Also, the propeptides failed to inhibit collagen production in chondrocytes which had switched to type I synthesis after extended culture.

In the various experiments described above aminopropeptides isolated from calf skin collagen were used. No evidence for interspecies differences were noted. Both human and calf fibroblasts respond to the same extent. In general, these studies showed specificity for fibroblasts over other cells. Whether this reflects a difference in the uptake of peptides by the different cell types has not been determined. Due to the low level of collagen type III synthesis in cultured fibroblasts it was not possible to obtain definitive data on the relative sensitivity of type I to type III collagen synthesis. However preliminary results suggest that both are affected in a similar fashion (Phan-Than *et al.*, 1982).

D. Action of Propeptides on the Cell-Free Synthesis of Procollagen Chains

Previous studies have established that it is possible to obtain rather efficient translation of collagen mRNAs in a cell-free lysate of reticulocytes and that full length chains including even the signal peptide at the amino-terminal end of the proα chains are produced (Monson and Goodman, 1978). No posttranslational modifications of the chains occur in this system. To study the possible intracellular site and mechanism of collagen synthesis inhibition, Paglia *et al.* (1979) examined the effect of the propeptides on the translation of proα1(I) and proα2(I) mRNA by a cell-free lysate. Addition of the amino-terminal propeptide from either type I or type III procollagen caused a marked inhibition of translation of the proα1(I) and proα2(I) collagen mRNA. The translation of other mRNAs like that for globin was not inhibited by the propeptides (Hörlein *et al.*, 1981). Translation of type III mRNA isolated from a rhabdomyosarcoma cell strain, where type III accounts for approximately 90% of total collagen (Krieg *et al.*, 1979), also was reduced by Col 1(I) (Phan-Than *et al.*, 1982) (Fig. 6). Interestingly, the translation of proα1(II) mRNA was also inhibited by the addition of Col 1(I) to the lysate while, as discussed above, no inhibition was observed in whole cells. Furthermore, translation of α1(II) mRNA was, in contrast to type I mRNAs, not reduced by Col 1(III) (Paglia *et al.*, 1981). Comparing structural features of collagen mRNAs, Yamada *et al.* (1983) showed that the mRNAs coding for α1(I), α2(I), and α1(III)

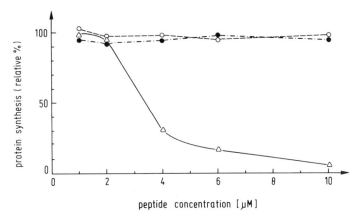

FIG. 6. Specific inhibition of translation of procollagen type III mRNA in a cell-free system. △, Procollagen mRNA + Col 1(I); ●, globin mRNA + Col 1(I); ○, procollagen mRNA + triple helical peptide α1CB3.

collagen contain inverted repeats at their 5′ ends and are able to form a hairpin structure in which the initiation codon AUG is contained. In the α1(II) mRNA this hairpin cannot be formed (E. Pöschl, personal communication). Whether this observation has implications for the mechanism of feedback inhibition remains to be established.

Structural studies on fragments of the propeptides showed that the inhibitory activity resided in the Col 1 fragment. Peptides from the helical portion of collagen had no inhibitory action (Paglia *et al.,* 1979). Hörlein and co-workers (1981) confirmed the findings of Paglia *et al.* (1981) and further analyzed the active domain of the propeptides. They showed that reduction and alkylation destroyed the specific activity. These modified peptides caused a nonspecific inhibition of the translation of all mRNAs examined. Enzymatic cleavage of the type I aminopropeptide with trypsin and *Staphylococcus aureus* V8 protease produced a tetrapeptide (Pro-Thr-Asp-Glu) which still retained the inhibiting activity. Whereas the intact Col 1(I) aminopropeptide interferes with elongation and/or termination of translation, the tetrapeptide is a general inhibitor of translation and prevents the initiation. In a later study they report that this inhibition of protein synthesis is associated with changes in protein phosphorylation and suggest that the active inhibitory peptide itself is phosphorylated (McPherson *et al.,* 1982). These studies thus demonstrate that aminopropeptides specifically are able to inhibit the translation of collagen mRNAs and also suggest that the observed cell type specificity is not due to differencies in the translational control of procollagen chains but more by cellular features such as different kinds of or levels of receptors for propeptides on the cell surface.

IV. CLINICAL IMPORTANCE OF COLLAGEN FEEDBACK REGULATION

Disorders associated with an enhanced collagen production and deposition could be due to defects of control mechanisms such as that described for the aminopropeptides. Beyond fibrotic diseases which are summarized in Table III, there are several physiological conditions in which an organism responds to injuries and triggers regeneration by a stimulated collagen production. Similarly, marked changes occur in the rate of collagen synthesis during development.

In conclusion, the rate of collagen synthesis is strictly regulated under physiological conditions, while this regulation could be lost in fibrotic diseases. Two main types of observation on pathological conditions are related to the regulation by aminopropeptides: (1) the levels of free aminopropeptides in various pathological conditions and different body fluids and (2) the effects of the propeptides on fibroblasts with an elevated rate of collagen synthesis, such as seen in scleroderma skin fibroblasts. The amount of free aminopropeptides of type III and, to a lesser extent, type I collagen in various body fluids correlates well with a beginning fibrotic process. An especially positive correlation was established between the type III aminopropeptide level and histological signs of inflammatory reactions and cell necrosis in liver biopsies, but not with other laboratory parameters (Rhode et al., 1979a) (Table III).

In in vitro experiments with scleroderma fibroblasts which produce excessive amounts of collagen (Krieg et al., 1978) demonstrated an inhibitory effect of the Col 1(I) peptide, similar to that observed by Wiestner et al. (1979). Thus collagen synthesis was reduced by about 30% while the production of noncollagenous proteins was not affected. These findings were recently confirmed by Perlish et al. (1983). Defective procollagen conversion and therefore increased production in dermatosparaxis might resemble a lost control of collagen synthesis in acquired fibrotic diseases.

Major problems are still unresolved and not all the data obtained are conclusive. The clinical importance of fibrotic processes requires an intensive investigation of the mechanisms underlying the feedback inhibition of collagen synthesis by aminopropeptides before any thera-

TABLE III

LIST OF ALTERED LEVELS OF AMINOPROPEPTIDES IN VARIOUS PATHOLOGICAL CONDITIONS

Disease (reference)	Source	Peptide[a]	Increase
Alcoholic liver disease (Rhode *et al.,* 1978)	Serum	NP III NP I	+ + +
Alcoholic liver disease, chronic hepatitis, schistosomiasis (Koda *et al.,* 1982)	Serum	NP I	+/+ +
Alcoholic liver cirrhosis (Niemela *et al.,* 1983)	Serum	NP III	+ +
Alcoholic liver cirrhosis (Raedsch *et al.,* 1983)	Bile	NP III	+ +
Chronic liver disease (Hahn *et al.,* 1982; Pencev *et al.,* 1982; Pierard *et al.,* 1982)	Serum	NP III	+ +
Chronic liver disease (Rhode *et al.,* 1979a)	Serum, ascites	NP III	+
Chronic active liver disease (Ackermann *et al.,* 1981)	Serum	NP III	+ +
Hepatic cirrhosis, acute viral hepatitis, amoebic liver abscess, schistosomiasis (Bolarin *et al.,* 1984)	Serum	NP III	+/+ +
Primary biliary cirrhosis (Savolainen *et al.,* 1983)	Serum	NP III	+ +
Chronic endomyocardial fibrosis (Bolarin *et al.,* 1983)	Serum	NP III	+/+ +
Hepatocellular carcinoma, other malignant diseases (Bolarin *et al.,* 1982)	Serum	NP III	+ +
Myelofibrosis (Hochweiss *et al.,* 1982)	Serum	NP III	+ +
Paget's disease of bone (Simon *et al.,* 1981)	Serum	NP III CP I	+ +
Pulmonary fibrosis, sarcoidosis (Low *et al.,* 1983)	Bronchoalveolar lavage	NP III	+ +
Acute pulmonary fibrosis (sheep) (Nerlich *et al.,* 1984)	Lymph fluid	NP III	+ +
Scleroderma (Fleischmajer *et al.,* 1981)	Skin fibroblasts	NP III	+ +

[a] CP I, carboxypropeptide from type I collagen; NP I, aminopropeptide from type I collagen; NP III, aminopropeptide from type III collagen.

peutical applications can be conceived. The radioimmunoassays for quantitation of free aminopropeptides that are available at present represent a valuable tool for the diagnostic detection of an increased collagen turnover, as seems to be the basic cause of pathological symptoms in fibrosis, a widespread diagnosis in human pathology. This clinical importance implies that further intensive investigations in regard to a therapeutical application must coincide with the detailed elucidation of the molecular mechanisms enabling the aminopropeptides to regulate collagen synthesis.

ACKNOWLEDGMENTS

We thank G. Martin for critical reading of the manuscript. The studies of our group were supported by grants from the Deutsche Forschungsgemeinschaft (Mu 378/13 and Kr 558/4-2/3). A. Nerlich was a fellow of the Wilhelm-Sander-Stiftung; T. Krieg was a recipient of a Heisenberg fellowship.

REFERENCES

Ackermann, W., Pott, G., Voss, B., Müller, K. M., and Gerlach, U. *Clin. Chim. Acta* **112,** 365–369 (1981).
Adams, S. L., Alwine, J. C., de Crombrugghe, B., and Pastan, I. *J. Biol. Chem.* **254,** 4935–4838 (1979).
Alitalo, K., Kurkinen, M., Vaheri, A., Krieg, T., and Timpl, R. *Cell* **19,** 1053–1062 (1980).
Avvedimento, E., Yamada, Y., Lovelace, E., Vogeli, G., de Crombrugghe, B., and Pastan, I. *Nucleic Acids Res.* **9,** 1123–1131 (1981).
Baum, S. J., Moss, J., Breul, S. D., Berg, R. A., and Crystal, R. G. *J. Biol. Chem.* **255,** 2843–2847 (1980).
Becker, U., Timpl, R., Helle, O., and Prockop, D. J. *Biochemistry* **15,** 2853–2862 (1976).
Bhatnagar, R. S., and Rapaka, S. S. R. *Nature New Biol.* **234,** 92–93 (1971).
Bolarin, D. M., and Andy, J. J. *Ann. Clin. Res.* **15,** 123–127 (1983).
Bolarin, D. M., Savolainen, E. R., and Kivirikko, K. I. *Int. J. Cancer* **29,** 401–405 (1982).
Bolarin, D. M., Savolainen, E. R., and Kivirikko, K. I. *Eur. J. Clin. Invest.* **14,** 90–95 (1984).
Bornstein, P., and Sage, H. *Annu. Rev. Biochem.* **49,** 957–1003 (1980).
Bornstein, P., Ehrlich, H. P., and Wyke, A. W. *Science* **175,** 544–546 (1972).
Brandhorst, B. P. *Dev. Biol.* **52,** 310–317 (1976).
Bruckner, P., Bächinger, H. P., Timpl, R., and Engel, J. *Eur. J. Biochem.* **90,** 596–603 (1978).
Engel, J., Bruckner, P., Becker, U., Timpl, R., and Rutschmann, B. *Biochemistry* **16,** 4026–4033 (1977).
Fan, H., and Penman, S. *J. Mol. Biol.* **50,** 655–670 (1970).
Fernandez-Munoz, R., and Darnell, J. E. *J. Virol.* **126,** 719–726 (1976).
Fessler, J. H., and Fessler, L. I. *Annu. Rev. Biochem.* **47,** 129–162 (1978).
Fessler, L. I., and Fessler, J. H. *J. Biol. Chem.* **254,** 233–239 (1979).
Fjolstadt, M., and Helle, O. *J. Pathol.* **112,** 183–188 (1974).
Fleischmajer, R., Perlish, J. S., Krieg, T., and Timpl, R. *J. Invest. Dermatol.* **76,** 400–403 (1981).
Fleischmajer, R., Olsen, B. R., Timpl, R., Perlish, J., and Lovelace, O. *Proc. Natl. Acad. Sci. U.S.A.* **80,** 3354–3358 (1983).
Focht, R. J., and Adams, S. L. *Mol. Cell. Biol.* **4,** 1843–1852 (1984).
Furthmayer, H., Timpl, R., Stark, M., Lapiere, Ch. M., and Kühn, K. *FEBS Lett.* **28,** 247–250 (1972).
Hahn, E. G., Pencev, D., Pittner, P., Kalbfleisch, H., Bruguera, M., and Timpl, R. *In* "Connective Tissue of the Normal and Fibrotic Human Liver" (U. Gerlach, G. Polt, J. Rauterberg, and B. Voss, eds.), pp. 205–206. Thieme, Stuttgart (1982).

116   PETER K. MÜLLER *ET AL.*

Harwood, R., Merry, A. H., Woolley, D. E., Grant, M. E., and Jackson, D. S. *Biochem. J.* **161**, 405–418 (1977).
Hochweiss, S., Hahn, E. G., Gilbert, H., Donovan, P. B., and Berk, P. D. *Clin. Res.* **30**, A 403 (1982).
Hollister, D. W. *Coll. Rel. Res.* **1**, 227–234 (1981).
Hörlein, D., Fietzek, P. P., and Kühn, K. *FEBS Lett.* **89**, 279–282 (1978).
Hörlein, D., McPherson, J., Han Goh, S., and Bornstein, P. *Proc. Natl. Acad. Sci. U.S.A.* **78**, 6163–6167 (1981).
Khono, K., Martin, G. R., and Yamada, Y. *J. Biol. Chem.* **259**, 13668–13673 (1984).
Kivirikko, K. I., and Myllylä, R. *In* "Extracellular Matrix Biochemistry" (K. A. Piez, and A. H. Reddi, eds.), pp. 83–118. Elsevier, Amsterdam (1984).
Koda, K., Wu, G. Y., Hait, P., and Seifter, S. *Hepatology* **2**, 720 (1982).
Krane, S. *Connect. Tissue Res.* **10**, 51–59 (1982).
Krieg, T., Hörlein, D., Wiestner, M., and Müller, P. K. *Arch. Dermatol. Res.* **263**, 171–180 (1978).
Krieg, T., Timpl, R., Alitalo, K., Kurkinen, M., and Vaheri, A. *FEBS Lett.* **104**, 405–409 (1979).
Kühn, K., Wiestner, M., Krieg, T., and Müller, P. K. *Connect. Tissue Res.* **10**, 43–50 (1982).
Lapiere, Ch. M., Lenaers, A., and Kohn, L. D. *Proc. Natl. Acad. Sci. U.S.A.* **68**, 3054–3058 (1971).
Layman, D. L., McGoodwin, E. B., and Martin, G. R. *Proc. Natl. Acad. Sci. U.S.A.* **68**, 454–458 (1971).
Lenaers, A., Ansay, M., Nusgens, B. V., and Lapiere, Ch. M. *Eur. J. Biochem.* **23**, 533–543 (1971).
Leroy, E. C. *J. Clin. Invest.* **54**, 880–889 (1974).
Leung, M. K. K., Fessler, L. I., Greenberg, D. B., and Fessler, J. H. *J. Biol. Chem.* **254**, 224–232 (1979).
Lichtenstein, J. R., Martin, G. R., Kohn, L. D., Byers, P. H., and McKusick, L. A. *Science* **182**, 298–300 (1973).
Low, R. B., Cutroneo, K. R., Davis, G. S., and Giancola, M. S. *Lab. Invest.* **48**, 755–759 (1983).
Lozano, G., Helle, O., and Miler, P. K. *EMBO J.* **2**, 1223–1227 (1983).
Martin, G. R., Byers, P. H., and Piez, K. A. *Adv. Enzymol.* **42**, 167–191 (1975).
Martin, G. R., Müller, P. K., Timpl, R., and Kühn, K. *TIBS* **10**, 285–287 (1985).
McPherson, J. M., Hörlein, D., Abbott-Brown, D., and Bornstein, P. *J. Biol. Chem.* **257**, 8557–8560 (1982).
Monson, J. M., and Goodman, H. M. *Biochemistry* **17**, 5122–5128 (1978).
Morris, N. P., Fessler, L. I., and Fessler, J. H. *J. Biol. Chem.* **254**, 11024–11032 (1979).
Müller, P. K., Lemmen, C., Gay, S., Gauss, V., and Kühn, K. *Exp. Cell Res.* **108**, 47–55 (1977).
Müller, P. K., Kirsch, E., Gauss-Müller, V., and Krieg, T. *Mol. Cell. Biochem.* **34**, 73–85 (1981).
Nerlich, A. G., Nerlich, M. L., Langer, I., and Demling, R. H. *Exp. Mol. Pathol.* **40**, 311–319 (1984).
Niemela, O., Risteli, L., Sotaniemi, E. A., and Risteli, J. *Clin. Chim. Acta* **124**, 39–44 (1982).
Niemela, O., Risteli, L., Sotaniemi, E. A., and Risteli, J. *Gastroenterology* **85**, 254–259 (1983).
Nowack, H., Olsen, B. R., and Timpl, R. *Eur. J. Biochem.* **70**, 205–216 (1976a).

Nowack, H., Rhode, H., and Timpl, R. *Hoppe Seyler's Z. Physiol. Chem.* **357**, 601–604 (1976b).

Nowack, H., Olsen, B. R., and Timpl, R. *Eur. J. Biochem.* **70**, 205–216 (1976c).

Paglia, L., Wilczek, J., Diaz de Leon, L., Martin, G. R., Hörlein, D., and Müller, P. K. *Biochemistry* **18**, 5030–5034 (1979).

Paglia, L. M., Wiestner, M., Duchene, M., Ouellette, L. A., Hörlein, D., Martin, G. R., and Müller, P. K. *Biochemistry* **20**, 3523–3527 (1981).

Palmiter, R. D., Davidson, J. M., Gagnon, J., Rowe, D. W., and Bornstein, P. *J. Biol. Chem.* **254**, 1433–1436 (1979).

Pencev, D., Pittner, P., Hahn, E. G., Timpl, R., and Martini, G. A. *In* "Connective Tissue of the Normal and Fibrotic Human Liver" (U. Gerlach, G. Pott, J. Rauterberg, and B. Voss, eds.), pp. 212–214. Thieme, Stuttgart (1982).

Perlish, J. S., Fleischmajer, R., Timpl, R., and Carter, V. *Arthritis Rheum.* **26**, S30 (1983).

Pesciotta, D. M., Silkowitz, M. H., Fietzek, P. P., Graves, P. N., Berg, R. A., and Olsen, B. R. *Biochemistry* **19**, 2447–2454 (1980).

Phan-Than, L., Timpl, R., Müller, P. K., and Krieg, T. *J. Invest. Dermatol.* **78**, 330 (1982).

Pierard, D., Plomteux, G., Amrani, N., Robin, M., Gielen, J., and Lapiere, Ch. M. *In* "Connective Tissue of the Normal and Fibrotic Human Liver" (U. Gerlach, G. Pott, J. Rauterberg, and B. Voss, eds.), pp. 217–218. Thieme, Stuttgart (1982).

Piez, K. A. *In* "Extracellular Matrix Biochemistry" (K. A. Piez and A. H. Reddi, eds.), pp. 1–39. Elsevier, Amsterdam (1984).

Pinell, S. R. *J. Invest. Dermatol.* **79**, 735–765 (1982).

Pontz, B. F., Müller, P. K., and Meigel, W. N. *J. Biol. Chem.* **248**, 7558–7564 (1973).

Prockop, D. J., Dehm, P., Olsen, B. R., Berg, R. A., Grant, M. E., Uitto, J., and Kivirikko, K. I. *In* "Biology of Fibroblast" (E. Kulonen and J. Pikkarainen, eds.), pp. 311–320. Academic Press, New York (1973).

Prockop, D. J., Kivirikko, K. I., Tuderman, L., and Guzman, N. A. *N. Engl. J. Med.* **301**, 13–23, 77–85 (1979).

Raedsch, R., Stiehl, A., Sieg, A., Walker, S., and Kommerell, B. *Gastroenterology* **85**, 1265–1270 (1983).

Rennard, S. I., and Crystal, R. G. *In* "Collagen in Health and Disease" (J. B. Weiss and M. I. V. Jayson, eds.), pp. 424–444. Churchill, Edinburgh (1982).

Rhagow, R., Gossage, D., Seyer, J. M., and Kang, A. H. *J. Biol. Chem.* **259**, 12718–12723 (1984).

Rhode, H., Hahn, E., and Timpl, R. *Fresenius Z. Anal. Chem.* **290**, 151–152 (1978).

Rhode, H., Vargas, L., Hahn, E., Kalbfleisch, H., Bruguera, M., and Timpl, R. *Eur. J. Clin. Invest.* **9**, 451–459 (1979a).

Rhode, H., Wachter, E., Richter, W. J., Bruckner, P., Helle, O., and Timpl, R. *Biochem. J.* **179**, 631–642 (1979b).

Rhode, H., Langer, I., Krieg, T., and Timpl, R. *Coll. Rel. Res.* **3**, 371–379 (1983).

Rojkind, M., and Deleon, D. L. *Biochim. Biophys. Acta* **217**, 512–522 (1970).

Rojkind, M., and Perez-Tamayo, R. *Int. Rev. Connect. Tissue Res.* **10**, 333–393 (1983).

Sandmeyer, S., Smith, R., Kiehn, D., and Bornstein, P. *Cancer Res.* **41**, 830–838 (1981).

Savolainen, E. R., Miettinen, T. A., Pikkarainen, P., Salaspuro, M. P., and Kivirikko, K. I. *Gut* **24**, 136–142 (1983).

Simon, L. S., Kovitz, K. L., Krane, I. M., and Krane, S. M. *Arthritis Rheum.* **24**, S58 (1981).

Skup, D., Zarbl, H., Millward, S. *J. Mol. Biol.* **151**, 35–55 (1981).

Smith, B. D., McKenney, K. H., and Lustberg, T. J. *Biochemistry* **16**, 2980–2985 (1977).

Sobel, M. E., Yamamoto, T., de Crombrugghe, B., and Pastan, I. *Biochemistry* **20,** 2678–2684 (1981).

Steinmann, B., Tuderman, L., Peltonen, L., and Martin, G. R. *J. Biol. Chem.* **255,** 8887–8893 (1980).

Timpl, R., and Glanville, R. W. *Clin. Orthop.* **158,** 224–242 (1981).

Tuderman, L., Kivirikko, K. I., and Prockop, D. J. *Biochemistry* **17,** 2948–2954 (1978).

Wiestner, M., Krieg, T., Hörlein, D., Glanville, R. W., Fietzek, P., and Müller, P. K. *J. Biol. Chem.* **254,** 7016–7023 (1979).

Wiestner, M., Rhode, H., Helle, O., Krieg, T., Timpl, R., and Müller, P. K. *EMBO J.* **1,** 513–516 (1982a).

Wiestner, M., Rhode, H., Helle, O., Krieg, T., Timpl, R., and Müller, P. K. *In* "New Trends in Basement Membrane Research" (K. Kühn, H. Schöne, and R. Timpl, eds.), pp. 139–143. Raven, New York (1982b).

Yamada, Y., Mudryj, M., and de Crombrugghe, B. *J. Biol. Chem.* **258,** 14914–14919 (1983).

Steroid Hormone Regulation of Extracellular Matrix Proteins

Kenneth R. Cutroneo, Kenneth M. Sterling Jr.,* and Susan Shull

Department of Biochemistry, College of Medicine, University of Vermont, Burlington, Vermont

* Present address: Division of Pediatric Gastroenterology, Mount Sinai School of Medicine, New York, New York, 10029.

REGULATION OF MATRIX ACCUMULATION

I. Introduction

The extracellular matrix is a defined structural entity in tissues acting as a scaffold to which cells attach (for review, Hay, 1981). We now know that the extracellular matrix may also influence the biochemical function of cells in both connective and soft tissues. Studies involving communication between cells and the extracellular matrix should provide exciting information for cell biologists in the future.

The three major proteinaceous components of the extracellular matrix are collagen, elastin, and glycoproteins. Collagen, although it is a glycoprotein, has very short carbohydrate extensions. This fibrous protein is comprised of a heterogeneous family of proteins including types I through X. Collagen types I through V are better characterized than VI through X. The biosynthesis of the collagen component of the extracellular matrix has recently been reviewed by Olsen (1981). The relationship and interactions between collagen synthesis and degradation have been reviewed by Tanzer (1982). A wealth of information has also been gained concerning the pathology of connective tissues in various acquired and heritable disorders (for review, Gay and Miller, 1978; Hollister *et al.*, 1982; Prockop and Kivirikko, 1984). In a number of these disease states, changes in the ratio of certain collagen types have been documented. Furthermore, alterations in the rates of collagen synthesis and degradation have also been noted in various diseased tissue.

Elastin, another functional component of the extracellular matrix, is present in practically every organ of the body. The structure and biosynthesis of elastin in normal and diseased tissues have recently been reviewed (Sandberg *et al.*, 1981). In addition, two recent articles have focused on the control of elastin synthesis and the regulation of elastin gene expression (Burnett *et al.*, 1982; Davidson and Crystal, 1982). The studies of diseases characterized by abnormal elastin metabolism will provide the basis for investigating and defining the molecular defects in the regulation of elastin gene expression.

Fibronectin belongs to a class of glycoproteins which make up the extracellular matrix. This proteinaceous component of the extracellular matrix is found in blood as well as in tissues. A striking characteristic of fibronectin is that it is insoluble in tissues while being soluble in plasma and other body fluids. The function of this cell-surface protein is to attach cells to the extracellular matrix. A recent review has appeared in the literature concerned with the structure and function of fibronectin (Ruoslahti *et al.*, 1981).

The primary objective of this article is to present and evaluate the literature regarding steroid hormone regulation of the synthesis of the three major proteinaceous components of the extracellular matrix: collagen, elastin, and fibronectin. Steroid-hormone-induced inhibitory and stimulatory effects on the synthesis of one or all of these proteins may lead to an alteration of the composition and architecture of the extracellular matrix. Furthermore, since the extracellular matrix is tightly associated with cells, steroid-hormone-induced changes of these matrix proteins may result in abnormal biochemical functions of cells.

II.   GLUCOCORTICOID REGULATION OF COLLAGEN METABOLISM
IN TISSUES

A. Skin

Natural and synthetic glucocorticoids have profound effects on collagen metabolism in skin. A review of the effects of glucocorticoids on collagen synthesis appeared previously (Cutroneo *et al.*, 1981).

Topical glucocorticoids are used in the treatment of various dermatological diseases (Miller and Munro, 1980). The development of potent fluorinated topical glucocorticoids has resulted in marked beneficial effects in many dermatoses. The major therapeutic effects of topical corticosteroids result from their marked antiinflammatory activity. However, repeated and prolonged treatment with corticosteroids results in skin atrophy which is associated with telangiectasia

(Stevanovic, 1972; Asboe-Hansen, 1976; Jablonska *et al.*, 1979; Bondi and Kligman, 1980). Topical glucocorticoids inhibit growth, prevent regeneration of the connective tissue matrix, and decrease epidermal thickness. These adverse changes in structure result in altered skin function. The degree of changes in skin induced by these steroids varies markedly with the different corticosteroid preparations. To test the ability of different corticosteroid preparations to affect skin atrophy, an excellent rat model was established which has been well characterized by Smith *et al.* (1976). Rats are treated topically for 28 days with corticosteroids and double skin thickness is determined.

Glucocorticoids also influence skin wound healing (for review see Goforth and Gudas, 1980). Cortisol treatment results in reduced extensibility and increased stiffness of wounds (Oxlund *et al.*, 1979). This makes the skin more vulnerable to rupturing forces. Prednisolone also decreases wound tensile strength during corneal wound healing (Phillips *et al.*, 1983). After thermal burns, deep ulceration and perforation developed in control animals but not in the prednisolone-treated group. Following glucocorticoid treatment of rats, Oxlund *et al.* (1982) observed a biphasic effect. Skin strength and stability at first increased due to an increase in collagen cross-links. Second, collagen synthesis decreased resulting in skin thinning and an ultimate decrease in collagen content. No change was observed in the ratio of type I to type III collagen. A similar biphasic effect of hydrocortisone on skin mechanical properties and skin thickness was observed by Vogel (1974). In another study, glucocorticoids decreased the mechanical strength and total collagen content in healing wounds of the stomach and duodenum (Gottrup and Oxlund, 1981).

Glucocorticoids selectively decrease collagen synthesis and therefore produce an antianabolic effect on skin collagen metabolism. In weanling rats, glucocorticoid treatment resulted in a decrease of urinary hydroxyproline as a measure of collagen metabolism (Kivirikko and Laitinen, 1965; Kivirikko *et al.*, 1965; Smith and Allison, 1965; Smith, 1967). Furthermore, Kivirikko *et al.* (1965) reported that after an injection of radioactive proline the specific activity of urinary radioactive hydroxyproline was lower in cortisone-treated rats than in control rats. In this same study glucocorticoids decreased the specific and total activity of radioactive hydroxyproline in soluble collagen of skin. Smith and Allison (1965) demonstrated that radioactive glycine incorporation into skin and femur collagen was decreased in cortisone-treated rats. This antianabolic effect of glucocorticoids on skin collagen metabolism was also observed by Uitto *et al.* (1972). These investigators found that a variety of glucocorticoids decreased collagen synthesis in explants of human skin. The inhibitory effect of glucocorticoids on proteinaceous hydroxyproline in skin was most pronounced with the fluorinated antiinflammatory steroids. This study concluded that the degree of inhibition of collagen synthesis by different corticosteroids may relate to the atrophic skin effects of these steroids. However, all these early studies suggested that glucocorticoids decreased both collagen and noncollagen protein synthesis in a nonselective manner. These workers concluded that the inhibitory effect of glucocorticoids on skin collagen synthesis resulted from a general inhibition of protein synthesis.

A genetic study was carried out to determine the degree of inhibition of collagen synthesis by dexamethasone in populations in mice exhibiting a high frequency (A/J) and low frequency (NIH Swiss Webster) of spontaneous or stress-induced facial malformation (Robey, 1979). The ratio of collagen to noncollagen protein in the skin of the dexamethasone-treated A/J mice increased slightly, probably due to a greater loss of noncollagen proteins. However, dexamethasone inhibited skin collagen synthesis in both mouse strains. Analogously, glucocorticoid treatment of rats results in a decrease of salt-soluble collagen in skin (Smith, 1967).

Glucocorticoid administration to neonatal rats resulted in a selective decrease of collagen synthesis (Cutroneo and Counts, 1975). Rats were treated for 3 consecutive days with triamcinolone diacetate. Radioactive proline was administered, and the degree of inhibition of formation of radioactive proteinaceous hydroxyproline was compared to total skin proline incorporation. Collagen synthesis was decreased to a greater extent than total skin protein synthesis. This was the first demonstration of a selective effect of glucocorticoids on collagen synthesis in skin. DNA synthesis was also reduced in the skin of glucocorticoid-treated neonatal rats. This inhibitory effect on DNA synthesis in skin paralleled the degree of inhibition of collagen synthesis (Newman and Cutroneo, 1978). Whether a relationship exists between the inhibition of DNA synthesis and collagen synthesis by glucocorticoids in skin remains to be seen.

To rule out a possible catabolic effect of glucocorticoids on skin collagen, rats were treated with triamcinolone diacetate for 3 consecutive days and were pulse labeled with radioactive proline. Polysomes were isolated from the skins of control and glucocorticoid-treated rats and were translated in a wheat germ lysate system in the presence of puromycin to release peptidyl nascent chains. The incorporation of radioactive proline in collagen nascent chains was decreased to a greater extent than proline incorporation in noncollagen nascent chains in the glucocorticoid-treated neonatal rats. Furthermore, the degree of inhibition of nascent chain synthesis for both collagen and noncollagen proteins was the same as the degree of inhibition for total skin collagen and noncollagen protein synthesis in both dose and temporal response studies. Although collagen synthesis is decreased to a greater extent than noncollagen protein synthesis, fibronectin synthesis is increased. Procollagen type I and procollagen type III syntheses are decreased to the same extent (Fig. 1). The inhibitory effect of glucocorticoids on type I procollagen and type III procollagen synthesis was the same at various doses and times following glucocorticoid administration (Shull and Cutroneo, 1983). Furthermore, the inhibition of type I and type III procollagen synthesis was reversed 72 hr after glucocorticoid administration.

Associated with the selective inhibition of collagen synthesis in skin is a decrease in the activities of the intracellular posttranslation modification enzymes. Prolyl hydroxylase activity is decreased in the skin of neonatal rats following glucocorticoid administration (Cutroneo and Counts, 1975; Cutroneo *et al.*, 1975; Risteli, 1977; Newman and Cutroneo, 1978; Benson and LuValle, 1981). The decrease of prolyl hydroxylase activity represents a decrease of total skin antigenic enzyme (Cutroneo *et al.*, 1975). Beside prolyl hydroxylase, lysyl hydroxylase, collagen galactosyltransferase, and collagen glucosyltransferase are

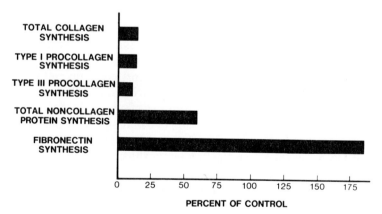

FIG. 1. Neonatal rats were treated at 12 mg/kg of triamcinolone diacetate, intraperitoneally, for 3 consecutive days. Twenty-four hours after the last treatment, the rats were injected intraperitoneally with radioactive proline when measuring collagen synthesis. Rats were injected with radioactive leucine when measuring fibronectin synthesis. Total collagen and noncollagen protein synthesis was determined using the purified bacterial collagenase assay. The syntheses of type I procollagen, type III procollagen, and fibronectin were determined using monospecific antibodies to these proteins.

decreased in skin following glucocorticoid treatment (Risteli, 1977). Glucocorticoids have also been shown to decrease the induction of galactosylhydroxylysine glucosyltransferase in suction blisters in human abdominal skin (Oikarinen *et al.*, 1983a). The activity of the extracellular enzyme lysyl oxidase is also decreased in skin by glucocorticoid treatment (Benson and LuValle, 1981). However, these results are rather tenuous since collagen cross-linking is increased in the skin of glucocorticoid treated rats (Oxlund *et al.*, 1982; Counts *et al.*, 1985). Although the posttranslational modification enzymes of collagen synthesis are decreased in skin following glucocorticoid treatment, glucose-6-phosphate dehydrogenase and aspartate aminotransferase activities are not (Newman and Cutroneo, 1978).

The decreased prolyl hydroxylase in skin does not result in the production of hydroxyproline deficient collagen. The degree of prolyl hydroxylation of procollagen nascent chains in the skin of rats treated with triamcinolone diacetate is the same as that of the nascent chains isolated from control rats (Newman and Cutroneo, 1978). The nascent chain data definitively indicate that although skin prolyl hydroxylase is decreased by glucocorticoid treatment, prolyl hydroxylation of procollagen is not affected. Since the majority of prolyl hydroxylation occurs on nascent procollagen peptides (Miller and Udenfriend, 1970), determination of the degree of prolyl hydroxylation of total cellular procollagen is not a definitive index that the procollagen synthesized is underhydroxylated since the newly synthesized random coil procollagen is rapidly catabolized intracellularly.

Glucocorticoid effects on cellular metabolism are mediated by specific proteinaceous receptors in target tissues. Glucocorticoid receptors have been located and characterized in skin (Eppenberger and Hsia, 1972; Epstein and Munderloh, 1981; Epstein, 1983; Smith *et al.*, 1983). The receptors resemble those of other tissues in their chromatographic properties, binding affinities, the specific steroid to which they bind, quantities, molybdate stabilization, heat lability, and protease susceptibility (Epstein and Munderloh, 1981; Smith *et al.*, 1983). The results of these glucocorticoid receptor studies in skin are consistent with the binding protein being the skin glucocorticoid receptor. A glucocorticoid-receptor-mediated decrease of collagen synthesis through a selective decrease of procollagen mRNA may explain the inhibitory effect of glucocorticoids on procollagen synthesis.

The glucocorticoid-mediated selective inhibition of type I collagen synthesis in skin is controlled by a decrease in the functional and total amount of proα1(I) and proα2(I) mRNAs. Polysomes were isolated from control and glucocorticoid-treated neonatal rats and translated in a

wheat germ lysate system (McNelis and Cutroneo, 1978). The polysomes isolated from glucocorticoid-treated rats synthesized less collagen and noncollagen protein than control polysomes. Furthermore,
collagen synthesis was decreased to a greater extent than noncollagen
protein synthesis. However, in another study from this laboratory,
Rokowski et al. (1981b) separated the membrane-bound and free polysomes before translating them in the wheat germ lysate system. Noncollagen protein synthesis directed by the dermal free polysomes was
decreased to the same extent as collagen synthesis directed by the
membrane-bound polysomes. However, the inhibitory effects of glucocorticoids on collagen synthesis was selective since noncollagen protein synthesis directed by membrane-bound polysomes was decreased
to a lesser extent than collagen synthesis. In addition, the synthesis of
prolyl hydroxylase directed by total dermal polysomes was not effected
by glucocorticoid treatment (Rokowski et al., 1981a,b). A selective effect of glucocorticoids on collagen synthesis was also observed when
polysomal poly(A) RNA isolated from the dermis of control and glucocorticoid-treated neonatal rats was translated in the nuclease-treated
reticulocyte lysate system (Rokowski et al., 1981b). To determine if
glucocorticoids decrease the concentrations of proα1(I) and proα2(I)
mRNAs, pCg54 proα1(I) and the pCg45 proα2(I), cloned cDNAs, were
used. Dot hybridization analysis of total chick skin RNA indicated a
dose-dependent decrease of proα1(I) and proα2(I) mRNAs in neonatal
chicks treated with dexamethasone (Sterling et al., 1983a) (Fig. 2).
Based on the data above it is unlikely that the glucocorticoid-mediated
inhibition of procollagen synthesis in skin results from an alteration of
the specific activity of the prolyl-tRNA pool(s) in skin.

The dermal atrophy caused by topical application of corticosteroids,
and to a greater extent the fluorinated corticosteroids, results from an
inhibitory effect of these steroids on normal skin collagen synthesis.
We have attempted for the past 14 years to block the inhibitory effect
of glucocorticoids on skin collagen synthesis while maintaining the
antiinflammatory activity of these steroids. The approaches which we
have used are (1) coadministration of anabolic steroids, (2) coadministration of retinoic acid derivatives, and (3) the discovery of new antiinflammatory steroids which might not inhibit normal skin collagen synthesis. The first two ventures have proven futile. The last has been
encouraging. We have identified two new antiinflammatory steroids,
methyl prednisolonate and methyl 20-dihydroprednisolonate. These
corticosteroids are antiinflammatory because they protect against rat
hind paw edema (Lee and Trottier, 1980), inhibit granuloma formation
(Soliman and Lee, 1981), and stabilize lysosomes (Heiman et al., 1982).

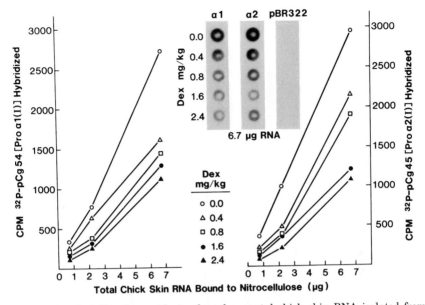

FIG. 2. Dot hybridization analysis of total neonatal chick skin RNA isolated from chicks receiving no steroid or dexamethasone at the doses indicated. The chicks were sacrificed 18 hr after intraperitoneal steroid administration. Since the cDNAs were in pBR322, nick-translated pBR322 was also used to insure that there was no hybridization of total skin RNA to pBR322 sequences. (From Sterling *et al.*, 1983a.)

However, compared to the parent compound, prednisolone, these corticosteroids produce less of a decrease in thymus weight and no decrease in liver glycogen, plasma corticosterone, plasma ACTH, adrenal weight, or growth (Lee and Soliman, 1982). Methylprednisolonate and methyl 20-dihydroprednisolonate have lower affinities for hepatic cytosol receptors than prednisolone (Lee *et al.*, 1981). Although methylprednisolonate and methyl 20-dihydroprednisolonate are antiinflammatory steroids, they do not inhibit skin collagen synthesis (DiPetrillo *et al.*, 1984; Fig. 3). Furthermore, methylprednisolonate and methyl 20-dihydroprednisolonate do not cause skin atrophy when applied topically to rats for 30 consecutive days (Fig. 4).

The net effect of glucocorticoids on skin collagen production and accumulation depends on not only the inhibitory effect of these steroids on collagen synthesis but also possible effects of these steroids on collagen degradation. Evidence in the literature indicates that glucocorticoids decrease collagen degradation in skin. Koob *et al.* (1974) demonstrated that hydrocortisone and dexamethasone decreased both

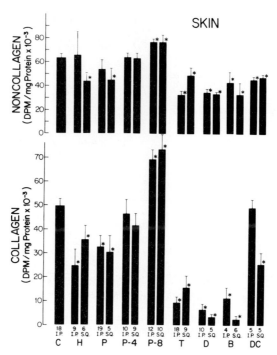

FIG. 3. Equivalent doses of antiinflammatory steroids based on 60 mg/kg of hydrocortisone were administered either intraperitoneally or subcutaneously for 3 consecutive days to neonatal rats. The amount of collagen and noncollagen synthesis was determined by the purified bacterial collagenase assay after labeling animals with radioactive proline. The numbers on the abscissa are sample sizes. The asterisks indicate significance as compared to control (C) at $p \leq 0.05$. Hydrocortisone (H), prednisolone (P), methyl 20-dihydroprednisolonate (P-4), methyl prednisolonate (P-8), triamcinolone (T), dexamethasone (D), betamethasone (B), and dichlorisone (DC). (From DiPetrillo *et al.*, 1984.)

collagen degradation and the appearance of collagenase in the media of normal human skin explants. In neonatal rats, triamcinolone decreased the degradation of noncollagen protein in skin (Cutroneo and Clarke, 1979). In addition, collagen degradation and collagenase activity remained unchanged in neonatal rat skin following triamcinolone treatment *in vivo* (Jeffrey *et al.*, 1985).

B. *Granuloma*

The initial observation that endogenous glucocorticoids in guinea pigs regulate collagen formation in granuloma tissue was made by Robertson and Sanborn (1958). These workers found that adrenalec-

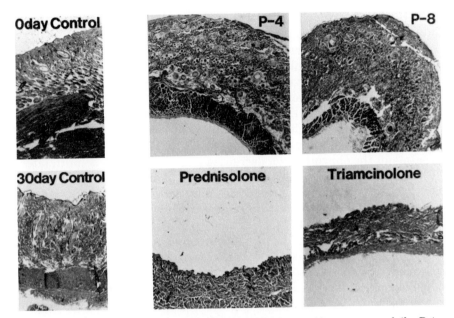

FIG. 4. Rats (100 g) were topically treated with 0.5% steroid creams once daily. P-4, Methyl 20-dihydroprednisolonate; P-8, methyl prednisolonate. (From DiPetrillo et al., 1984.)

tomy resulted in an increase of collagen in carrageenan-induced granuloma. Glucocorticoids were later shown to decrease granuloma growth (Nocenti et al., 1964; Tsurufuji et al., 1974; Wehr et al., 1976; Freeman et al., 1979; Salmela, 1981), DNA (Tsurufuji et al., 1974; Wehr et al., 1976; Freeman et al., 1979; Salmela, 1981), RNA (Tsurufuji et al., 1974; Salmela, 1981), collagen (Wehr et al., 1976; Salmela, 1981), noncollagen protein (Tsurufuji et al., 1974; Wehr et al., 1976), mucopolysaccharides (Tsurufuji et al., 1974), the release of lysosomal hydrolases (Freeman et al., 1979), cell proliferation (Freeman et al., 1979), and the development of vascularity (Wehr et al., 1976; Salmela, 1981). It would appear that glucocorticoids inhibit a spectrum of biochemical and cellular parameters which are elevated during sponge-induced and carrageenan-induced granuloma formation. However, the inhibitory effects of glucocorticoids on granuloma formation and the involution of existing granuloma remain unexplained in molecular terms. Ohno et al. (1972) demonstrated that DNA synthesis in glucocorticoid-treated granuloma is markedly inhibited while DNA degradation was not significantly affected. Whether the inhibitory actions of glucocorticoids on DNA synthesis and procollagen synthesis are related in this model remains to be seen.

During granuloma formation prolyl hydroxylase activity is markedly decreased in granuloma tissue by various glucocorticoids (Cutroneo *et al.*, 1971; Wehr *et al.*, 1976; Kruse *et al.*, 1978; Counts and Cutroneo, 1979). Furthermore, the decrease of prolyl hydroxylase activity in granuloma is directly related to the glucocorticoid inhibition of granuloma growth (Cutroneo *et al.*, 1971). Unlike in liver, in which the enzyme is significantly decreased after 12 hr of glucocorticoid treatment, the enzyme is not decreased in granuloma tissue until later (Counts and Cutroneo, 1979). This may explain the findings of other investigators who demonstrated that glucocorticoid treatment did not result in a decrease of prolyl hydroxylase activity (Nakagawa *et al.*, 1971; Tsurufuji *et al.*, 1974). Although granuloma prolyl hydroxylase activity is decreased following glucocorticoid treatment, hydroxyproline-deficient collagen is not synthesized in granuloma tissue (Nakagawa *et al.*, 1971; Kruse *et al.*, 1978).

Glucocorticoids decrease granuloma collagen content by decreasing fibroblast number as well as the synthesis and secretion of collagen molecules per cell. Nocenti *et al.* (1964) demonstrated that hydrocortisone decreased the formation of radioactive proteinaceous hydroxyproline concomitant with a decrease in the hydroxyproline content in experimental granulomas. In another study, betamethasone markedly inhibited the incorporation of radioactive proline into collagen and noncollagen protein (Fukuhara and Tsurufuji, 1969). The inhibitory effect of betamethasone on the synthesis of both collagen and noncollagen protein was significant as early as 1 hr after the administration of the glucocorticoid (Nakagawa *et al.*, 1971). Furthermore, the inhibition of granuloma collagen synthesis was significantly greater than the inhibition of total granuloma protein synthesis (Nakagawa *et al.*, 1971; Tsurufuji *et al.*, 1974; Kruse *et al.*, 1978). In addition, Nakagawa and colleagues demonstrated that glucocorticoids decrease the synthesis of procollagen, the immediate precursor of collagen (Nakagawa and Tsurufuji, 1972b; Tsurufuji *et al.*, 1974). Although it is well established that glucocorticoids decrease granuloma growth, much remains to be known about the molecular mechanisms by which corticosteroids decrease granuloma growth and collagen synthesis.

Glucocorticoid regulation of the net amount of collagen in granulomas may result from the control of protein degradation. Ohno and Tsurufuji (1970) demonstrated that hydrocortisone increased the degradation of total granuloma protein while the incorporation of radioactive tyrosine into granuloma protein was reduced. However, Nakagawa and Tsurufuji (1972a) demonstrated that betamethasone specifically inhibited collagen degradation in granuloma *in vivo* and reduced the amount of dialyzable hydroxyproline in a granuloma mince system. These last two studies suggest that glucocorticoids increase the catabolism of noncollagen granuloma protein while decreasing collagen degradation. Studying physiological parameters of the granuloma tissue, Vogel (1971) demonstrated that granuloma tensile strength increased after treatment with prednisolone acetate. This finding is in accord with a glucocorticoid-mediated inhibition of collagen degradation.

The inhibitory effects of corticosteroids on granuloma growth and macromolecular syntheses are reversible by discontinuation of steroid treatment or coadministration of vitamin A. After steroid withdrawal, granulomatous inflammation is followed by recovery of granuloma weight, DNA, and noncollagen protein (Shin *et al.*, 1974). Recovery of the incorporation of radioactive thymidine into DNA and radioactive proline into noncollagen protein of granuloma also occurs. Recovery of collagen synthesis in this "rebound" granuloma model is not complete until 4 days after cessation of corticosteroid treatment.

The inhibitory effect of corticosteroids on granuloma growth and collagen accumulation may be reversed or retarded by coadministration of vitamin A (Ehrlich and Tarver, 1971; Ehrlich *et al.*, 1973; Wehr *et al.*, 1976). In addition, coadministration of vitamin A in animals treated with glucocorticoids totally blocks the inhibitory effect of the corticosteroid on DNA and total granuloma protein (Wehr *et al.*, 1976). One must be cautious as to the clinical relevance of these findings since simultaneous treatment of vitamin A to patients taking corticosteroids as well as other antiinflammatory agents may result in exacerbation of the inflammatory process.

C. Bone

Glucocorticoids have dramatic inhibitory effects on the composition, growth, structural integrity, and collagen synthesis of the skeleton. In particular, high pharmacological doses given either locally or systemically produce toxicological effects on bone. Physiological concentrations of both naturally occurring and synthetic corticosteroids produce anabolic effects on bone metabolism, particularly on collagen synthesis.

Corticosteroid administration to rabbits results in a marked decrease of bone mass (Thompson and Urist, 1973). Ribs, femur, and vertebral body mass are significantly decreased by pharmacological doses of cortisone. This loss of bone mass after prolonged treatment with corticosteroids results in the development of osteoporesis (Saville and Kharmosh, 1967; Gallagher *et al.,* 1973; Hahn *et al.,* 1974). Adrenalectomy results in increased collagen synthesis in both the metaphysis and diaphysis of the bone matrix (Cruess and Sakai, 1972).

Naturally occurring and synthetic corticosteroids were injected into the chorioallantoic membrane of chick embryos (Uitto and Mustakallio, 1971). Radioactive proline was administered, and the formation of radioactive proteinaceous hydroxyproline was determined as an index of collagen synthesis in tibiae. Collagen synthesis was markedly decreased by all corticosteroids tested. Although there was no difference in the degree of inhibition, prolyl hydroxylase activity was not affected. In this study, glucocorticoid treatment was administered for only 12 hr which is not enough time to affect this enzyme in bone, as indicated previously. In an analogous *in vitro* experiment, betamethasone inhibited hydroxyproline formation to a greater extent than did other corticosteroids. In both the *in vivo* and *in vitro* studies, total proline incorporation was decreased to the same extent as hydroxyproline formation indicating that glucocorticoids are general inhibitors of bone protein synthesis. Blumenkrantz and Asboe-Hansen (1976) also demonstrated a glucocorticoid-mediated decrease of radioactive proteinaceous hydroxyproline in chick embryo tibia explants. These workers also demonstrated decreased collagen secretion into the medium. It should be noted that this latter study employed high doses of corticosteroids as did the *in vitro* studies of Uitto and Mustakallio (1971). These latter bone studies and others in the literature indicate that there is no specificity of the effect of glucocorticoids on collagen synthesis. This is in marked contrast to many more recent studies which indicate that glucocorticoids selectively decrease collagen synthesis in many different connective tissues and cells. Rokowski *et al.* (1981b) demonstrated that treatment of neonatal rats with triamcinolone results in a greater decrease of calvaria collagen synthesis as compared to the inhibition of noncollagen protein synthesis. This selective inhibition of bone collagen synthesis may explain the induction of osteoporosis by pharmacological doses of corticosteroids. Osteoporosis may result from both increased bone resorption and decreased bone formation.

The effect of glucocorticoids on collagen synthesis in fetal rat calvaria cultures is biphasic (Canalis, 1983a,b). After 24 hr dexamethasone and hydrocortisone increased the incorporation of radioactive proline into collagen to a greater extent than into noncollagen protein.

Physiological concentrations of corticosteroids administered for a short term maintain the differentiated function of osteoblasts. This increased collagen synthesis is not associated with either increased DNA or RNA synthesis. The inactive glucocorticoid analogs epicortisol and deoxycorticosterone do not effect collagen synthesis.

Hydrocortisone does not affect collagen synthesis of calvaria dissected prior to culture into the periosteum and nonpercosteal central bone (Canalis, 1984). The stimulatory effect on collagen synthesis was seen only if the two bone sections were cultured in the same vial and were in contact with each other. These data suggest the participation of specific bone factors in cortisol stimulation of collagen synthesis. This anabolic effect of glucocorticoids on bone collagen synthesis agrees with the ability of physiological doses of hydrocortisone to inhibit bone resorption (Stern, 1969; Raisz et al., 1972; Yasumura, 1976) and may result from the glucocorticoid-induced decreased proliferation of osteoclast precursor cells. However, in our laboratory we have never observed in vivo a stimulatory effect of any glucocorticoid on bone collagen synthesis regardless how small a dose of corticosteroid was used. The biological significance of the stimulatory effect of glucocorticoids on collagen synthesis in the calvaria explants still remains questionable.

In cultures treated for longer periods of time bone collagen synthesis is markedly depressed. This may result from an inhibition of osteoblast proliferation and/or decreased collagen synthesis per cell. Dexamethasone and hydrocortisone treatment of the calvaria explants for 96 hr results in a decrease of collagen synthesis, noncollagen protein synthesis, and DNA and RNA synthesis (Dietrich et al., 1979). Glucocorticoid-mediated inhibition of collagen synthesis in the calvaria explants is associated with decreased number of osteoblasts (Canalis, 1983a). In addition, hydrocortisone, corticosterone, and dexamethasone significantly decrease DNA content after 96 hr of treatment. These inhibitory effects are not observed after 24 hr of glucocorticoid treatment. Thus corticosteroids have a biphasic effect on collagen synthesis in fetal rat calvaria cultures in vitro. Since cortexolone also increased and decreased collagen synthesis in the calvaria explants at 24 and 96 hr of treatment, respectively (Dietrich et al., 1979), the biological significance of these results may be questionable since this steroid is a glucocorticoid antagonist, although it is possible that this antagonist may have some inherent glucocorticoid agonist activity. The significance of these studies on corticosteroid-induced modulation of collagen synthesis in fetal rat calvaria awaits more definitive in vivo investigations.

Similar stimulatory and inhibitory effects of glucocorticoids were also noted for alkaline phosphatase activity.

Another interesting finding of this same research group is that conditioned medium prepared from fetal rat calvaria organ cultures and cell cultures stimulates DNA and collagen synthesis in fetal rat calvaria organ cultures (Canalis *et al.*, 1980). Hydrocortisone treatment enhanced the collagen-stimulating effect of this nondialyzable and heat-stable growth factor(s) in the conditioned medium. Other studies have demonstrated that physiological doses of glucocorticoids sensitize bone cells to parathyroid hormone (Chen and Feldman, 1978; Wong, 1979). A recent comprehensive review summarizes the effects of steroid hormones, polypeptides and other hormones, vitamins, growth factors, and local factors on the regulation of collagen synthesis, noncollagen protein synthesis, DNA content, DNA synthesis, and alkaline phosphatase activity in bone (Canalis, 1983b).

Little is known about the molecular mechanisms by which glucocorticoids regulate bone cell collagen metabolism. The convincing evidence that bone cells may be target cells for glucocorticoid action rests on the findings that bone cells have high affinity cytoplasmic receptors (Feldman *et al.*, 1975; Chen *et al.*, 1977; Choe *et al.*, 1978; Chen and Feldman, 1979). Oikarinen and Ryhanen (1981) determined the ability of mRNA isolated from the calvaria of chick embryos treated with hydrocortisone to direct the synthesis of type I procollagen in the nuclease-treated reticulocyte lysate. Glucocorticoid treatment resulted in a decrease of translatable type I procollagen mRNAs in calvaria. Interestingly, there was a 12-hr lag before this response occurred. Since type I procollagen mRNAs were quantified by a translation assay, one can not say that glucocorticoid treatment results in decreases of type I procollagen mRNAs in calvaria. Hybridization studies using recombinant cDNAs to $\text{pro}\alpha1(\text{I})$ mRNA and $\text{pro}\alpha2(\text{I})$ mRNA should be done.

The results above on the inhibitory and stimulatory effects of glucocorticoids on collagen synthesis in bone should be contrasted to studies on bone collagen degradation. Prednisolone suppresses the development of arthritis and decreases the increased collagenase activity in bone, other tissues, and in the serum of the arthritic rat (Kuberasampath and Bose, 1980). Furthermore, this corticosteroid inhibits the enhanced collagen catabolism in these arthritic rats (Kuberasampath and Bose, 1979, 1980). Smith (1967) reported that glucocorticoids have an anticatabolic effect on femur collagen. In addition, Cruess and Hong (1975) demonstrated that cortisone decreased collagenase activity in metaphyseal bone.

D. Normal Lung and Fibrotic Lung

Lung has a defined extracellular matrix composed of various proteinaceous components including multiple collagen types, elastin, and glycoproteins. There are many different cell types which originate from various embryonic origins (Gail and Lenfant, 1983). The biochemical profile of many of these cells is altered during chronic inflammation of the lower respiratory tract (Crystal et al., 1984a). In idiopathic pulmonary fibrosis, a fatal disorder which starts as an alveolitis and advances to interstitial fibrosis, collagen metabolic processes in lung become abnormal which results in distinct changes in lung collagen content and in the ratio of different collagen types. Zapol et al. (1979) demonstrated that morphological evidence of lung fibrosis in humans is correlated with a significant increase of lung collagen content in patients with diffuse interstitial lung fibrosis following severe acute respiratory failure. In still another study, Last et al. (1983) found a specific increase of type I collagen content in the lungs of patients with adult respiratory distress syndrome. There remains a problem in determining the significance of the above findings of increased collagen content in human biopsy specimens. It is extremely important to obtain biopsy specimens which are to be compared from the same section of the lung lobe of each patient. Furthermore, many investigators feel that fibrotic lung disease, at least in humans, results from collagen rearrangement rather than an increase of lung collagen content (Crystal et al., 1976). Changes in the arrangement of collagen types have been found in biopsy specimens of patients with lung fibrosis (Madri and Furthmayr, 1980). These morphological findings agree with the findings of the biochemical studies of Seyer et al. (1976). These workers demonstrated that the ratio of type I to type III collagen is increased in fibrotic lung.

Corticosteroids are used in a variety of pulmonary diseases. These drugs have been prescribed in the treatment of respiratory distress syndrome with certain precautions (Ballard and Ballard, 1979). Glucocorticoids are also used to treat diffuse interstitial pulmonary disease (Winterbauer et al., 1978; Crystal et al., 1984b). Patients with less than 1 year of duration have a more favorable response to corticosteroid therapy than patients who have had the disease for more than 2 years. A favorable progress is indicated by the fact that responders to therapy have improved lung volumes and gas exchange. Some patients treated with corticosteroids fall into the good responder group, while others are resistant to therapy and constitute the moderate and low responding groups (Turner-Warwick *et al.*, 1980). A possible explanation for the different groups of responders to corticosteroid therapy is variation in the quantity of glucocorticoid receptors in lung cells between control and idiopathic pulmonary fibrosis patients. Indeed, cytoplasmic glucocorticoid receptors are present in lung (Ballard and Ballard, 1974). In an interesting study, Ozaki *et al.* (1982) found that patients with idiopathic pulmonary fibrosis who were good responders to glucocorticoid therapy had more glucocorticoid receptors in bronchoalveolar cells than normal volunteers.

In experimental animals glucocorticoids selectively decrease collagen synthesis in normal lung. As has been previously shown for skin, glucocorticoid receptors are also present in fetal lung (Ballard and Ballard, 1972; Giannapoulos *et al.*, 1973; Giannopoulos, 1975a,b). Cytoplasmic glucocorticoid receptors in lung exist in nonactivated and activated forms (Giannopoulos, 1975a). These glucocorticoid receptors bind and are taken up by lung nuclei (Giannopoulos, 1975b). In addition, these steroid receptors have been shown to bind nuclear components of lung.

Glucocorticoids administered to neonatal rats coordinately decrease type I and type III procollagen synthesis of lung (Shull and Cutroneo, 1983). Collagen synthesis *in vitro* directed by total lung polysomes and polysomal poly(A) RNA isolated from glucocorticoid-treated rats is selectively decreased (Rokowski *et al.*, 1981b). Noncollagen protein synthesis is decreased to a lesser extent than collagen synthesis. This selective action of corticosteroids on lung collagen synthesis is further indicated since collagen synthesis by membrane-bound polysomes is decreased while noncollagen protein synthesis is increased. However, noncollagen protein synthesis by free polysomes isolated from glucocorticoid-treated rats is decreased to the same extent as collagen synthesis. The polysomal or polysomal poly(A) RNA directed synthesis of at least one noncollagen lung protein, prolyl hydroxylase, is not affected by glucocorticoid treatment. Therefore the inhibitory effect of glucocorticoids on procollagen synthesis in lung does not result from a steroid-induced alteration of the specific activity of the prolyl-tRNA precursor pools.

Bleomycin, a glycopeptide antineoplastic agent, is used in the treatment of several types of malignancies. This drug causes DNA damage (Muller *et al.*, 1972; Sausville *et al.*, 1978a,b) and inhibits DNA synthesis (Suzuki *et al.*, 1968; Muller *et al.*, 1975). The interaction of bleomycin with purified DNA results in single- and double-stranded DNA breaks in addition to release of free bases (Muller *et al.*, 1972; Kuo and Haidle, 1973; Takeshita *et al.*, 1974; Haidle and Lloyd, 1978). The major limiting toxicity of this antineoplastic agent is pulmonary fibrosis which can be induced in animals by intratracheal or intraperitoneal injection of bleomycin (Adamson and Bowden, 1974; Adamson, 1976; Snider et al., 1978; Giri et al., 1980; Tom and Montgomery, 1980; Fasske and Morgenroth, 1983). This bleomycin model of lung fibrosis is characterized by fibrotic morphological changes in lung structure and architecture and an alteration in the biochemical profile of lung cells. These morphological observations support the time-related changes in lung collagen content and metabolism induced by bleomycin treatment.

A very comprehensive description of the general changes of collagen structure, function, and metabolism in fibrotic tissue has recently appeared (Nimni, 1983). In animals treated with bleomycin, the collagen content of lung is increased (McCullough et al., 1978; Sikic et al., 1978; Starcher et al., 1978; Goldstein et al., 1979; Giri et al., 1983). This increased collagen content results from increased collagen synthesis (Clark et al., 1980; Phan et al., 1980; Zuckerman et al., 1980; Laurent and McAnulty, 1983) and decreased degradation of newly synthesized collagen (Laurent and McAnulty, 1983). However, there is another report in the literature that the degradation of newly synthesized collagen is markedly increased (Clark et al., 1980). There has also been reported a change in the ratio of collagen types in bleomycin-induced lung fibrosis (Reiser and Last, 1983). Type I collagen is increased relative to types III and V collagens. The latter two collagen types remained at control values. Two recent studies reported the presence of factors in bleomycin-treated fibrotic tissues which were able to modulate both fibroblast proliferation and collagen synthesis in either lung minces or in human lung fibroblasts (Phan and Thrall, 1981; Clark et al., 1982). Pulmonary tissue is selectively susceptible to fibrosis induced by bleomycin since there is a lack of metabolism of this antineoplastic agent in lung tissue of rodents (Lazo and Humphreys, 1983).

The bleomycin model has been used to determine the ameliorative properties of corticosteroids in lung fibrosis. Several groups have been successful in preventing or partially blocking the bleomycin-induced increase of lung collagen content and lung collagen synthesis by concomitant corticosteroid treatment. Using methylprednisolone after intratracheal administration of bleomycin, Phan et al. (1981) demonstrated that this glucocorticoid prevented an increase in lung collagen content but only partially suppressed total lung collagen synthesis. This corticosteroid was injected intramuscularly at 18 mg/kg daily for 2 weeks after bleomycin instillation. Our laboratory was able to suppress totally the bleomycin-induced increases in lung collagen content and collagen synthesis by alternate day therapy with triamcinolone starting 24 hr after a single intratracheal dose of bleomycin (Sterling *et al.*, 1982a). A total response to steroid treatment was obtained with 8 mg/kg when given intraperitoneally. These total inhibitory effects were not seen using a dose of 4 mg/kg (Fig. 5).

Other models have been used to investigate the effects of glucocorticoids on lung injury and the fibrotic process. The antioxidant butylated hydroxytoluene produces lung damage which is potentiated by hyperoxia to produce lung fibrosis (Kehrer and Witschi, 1981). Prednisolone treatment decreased mortality but had no effect on lung collagen accumulation. However, when prednisolone was given for 12 successive days, the increase in collagen accumulation in lung was prevented (Hakkinen *et al.*, 1983). Using the ozone model, Hesterberg and Last (1981) demonstrated that concurrent administration of methylprednisolone during the exposure to ozone prevented the increased rate of

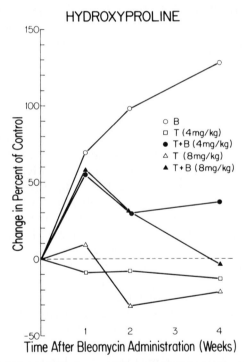

FIG. 5. Fischer 344 rats (125 g) were given a single intratracheal injection of bleomycin (0.6 units/100 g rat) or saline. Twenty-four hours after bleomycin administration, groups of rats were injected every other day with triamcinolone (4 or 8 mg/kg ip) or saline. (From Sterling *et al.*, 1982a.)

lung collagen synthesis. Glucocorticoid treatment appears to prevent pulmonary fibrosis by suppressing cellular recruitment to the site of injury, reducing cell proliferation, and decreasing collagen synthesis (Koenig et al., 1983). The biological significance of all the above findings that glucocorticoids prevent, retard, or partially block increased collagen content and synthesis in experimental pulmonary fibrosis models rests on demonstrating the morphological reversal of pulmonary fibrosis and the amelioration of the abnormal mechanical properties of the diseased lung.

E. Normal Liver and Fibrotic Liver

Liver is composed of a limited number of different cell types which adhere to a defined extracellular matrix (Rojkind and Ponce-Noyola, 1982). Approximately 80% of the liver is composed of cellular elements. The major proteinaceous components of the extracellular matrix of the liver are the cell-connecting glycoprotein fibronectin and types I, III, IV, and V collagens. The extracellular matrix of liver is also composed of laminin, a component of basement membranes, and possibly other glycoproteins which as yet remain to be purified and characterized.

During physical insult, the liver progresses through the various phases of inflammation including the destructive, reparative, and chronic inflammatory phases. During the inflammatory process in liver, various components of the extracellular matrix undergo changes in composition and metabolism (Rojkind and Dunn, 1979; Rojkind and Perez-Tamayo, 1983). We will focus on changes of collagen components of the extracellular matrix during the process of liver fibrosis and subsequent treatment with corticosteroids.

In human and rat fibrotic liver disease, total liver collagen content is elevated (Rojkind and Perez-Tamayo, 1983). This increase in collagen content is most likely related to the distortion of the architecture of fibrotic livers. In particular the amounts of type I, type I trimer, type III, type IV, and type V are markedly elevated. In alcoholic liver fibrosis, prolyl hydroxylase activity is increased in proportion to the increase of the percentages of collagen synthesis in fibrotic liver (Mann et al., 1979). Beside increases in the amounts of the various collagen types in fibrotic liver disease which probably result from increased collagen synthesis, there are also unexplained functional changes in tissue collagen polymorphism. These changes may have defined pathological implications in the onset and progression of fibrotic liver disease. Seyer et al. (1977) found that although normal human liver contains 47% type III collagen, cirrhotic liver contains less type III collagen, which ranged in liver biopsy specimens from 18 to 34%. In this latter study the collagen types were analyzed by cyanogen bromide peptide analysis. However, Rojkind and colleagues have found an increase in the ratio of type III to type I collagen in human alccholic liver cirrhosis (Rojkind and Martinez-Palomo, 1976). In another study, this same group found that in cirrhotic livers with greater than 20 mg of collagen per gram of liver, type I collagen was predominant and that the ratio of type I to type III collagens was significantly increased (Rojkind *et al.,* 1979).

Corticosteroids have been used in a variety of liver diseases (Tanner and Powell, 1979; Sherlock, 1981). However, the clinical usefulness of the glucocorticoids in treating hepatic fibrotic disease is at best questionable. Although the currently marketed corticosteroids may not ameliorate fibrotic liver disease, the development of new glucocorticoids showing increased efficacy for liver disease may progress to the point of producing clinically useful corticosteroids for treatment of fibrotic liver disease.

One of the most popular experimental systems of liver fibrosis is the CCl_4 model. After induction of cirrhosis in rat liver by administration of CCl_4 to rats, liver collagen content increases significantly (Ehrinpreis *et al.,* 1980; Seyer, 1980; Rojkind *et al.,* 1983). This increase in collagen content is associated with increased liver collagen synthesis (Galligani *et al.,* 1979; Ehrinpreis *et al.,* 1980; Seyer, 1980). In primary liver organ cultures, the relative rate of collagen synthesis was significantly higher in CCl_4-damaged liver (Galligani *et al.,* 1979). The activity of prolyl hydroxylase was also increased in CCl_4-induced fibrotic liver tissue. Type I and type III interstitial collagens are increased to the same extent, with the type III collagen constituting 35–40% of the total of type I and type III collagens (Seyer, 1980). Alternately, Rojkind *et al.* (1983) found that type I collagen is the predominant collagen type in the extracellular matrix of cirrhotic rat liver. The CCl_4 experimental model should be extremely useful in the future in determining the possible beneficial effects of corticosteroids on collagen metabolism in cirrhotic rat liver.

Glucocorticoid administration to rats results in changes in collagen metabolism in normal liver. Following glucocorticoid treatment, total liver collagen is decreased (Hirayama *et al.,* 1971). Liver prolyl hydroxylase is markedly decreased by glucocorticoid treatment of rats in a time-dependent manner (Cutroneo *et al.,* 1971). Glucocorticoid treatment of hypoxic animals results in the prevention of hypoxia-induced liver damage (Galvin and Lefer, 1979). In another liver injury system, rats were treated with dimethylnitrosamine with and without medroxyprogesterone (Saarni *et al.*, 1983). This steroid caused an inhibitory effect on the accumulation of liver collagen and the increase of prolyl hydroxylase activity. From the above-mentioned studies of the effects of glucocorticoids on collagen metabolism of both normal and cirrhotic liver, it appears that more controlled studies need to be done. Only after such studies are completed will we be able to draw conclusions as to the potential usefulness of marketed and new corticosteroids in the treatment of fibrotic liver diseases.

F. Other Tissues

There are several other model systems in which glucocorticoids alter tissue collagen metabolism. Glucocorticoid treatment of certain inbred strains of mice at certain phases of their development induces cleft palate formation (Greene and Kochhar, 1975; Salomon and Pratt, 1979; Gasser and Goldman, 1983). The degree of incidence of cleft palate induction in mice is genetically determined. Glucocorticoid treatment of the developing inbred mice, A/J, a highly susceptible mouse strain, results in marked inhibition of craniofacial growth and an increased incidence of cleft palate production. One possible genetic basis for this increased susceptibility to cleft palate formation is a higher mesenchymal cellular concentration of glucocorticoid receptors. Dexamethasone inhibition of human embryonic palatal mesenchymal cell growth is closely related to the specific binding of radiolabeled dexamethasone to cells (Yoneda and Pratt, 1981). Glucocorticoid inhibition of both mesenchymal cell growth and collagen synthesis may at least in part be responsible for abnormal palate development.

There is indirect evidence that altered collagen metabolism is involved in cleft palate formation. Administration of the lathrogen β-aminopropionitrile to pregnant rats results in a high incidence of cleft palate in the offspring (Steffek *et al.*, 1972). In another study, Pratt and King (1972) demonstrated that 98% cleft palate rat fetuses were produced after a single injection of β-aminopropionitrile when administered on day 15 of gestation. Cleft palate formation in the rat fetuses treated with β-aminopropionitrile was correlated with an inhibition of collagen cross-linking although collagen synthesis was not affected. More direct evidence of changes in collagen metabolism during secondary palate formation exists. Palatal mouse explants from mice of low and high incidence of cleft palate formation were incubated with radioactive proline (Uitto and Thesleff, 1979). The formation of radioactive hydroxyproline, the activity of prolyl hydroxylase, and the various collagen types produced were characterized. Parameters of collagen synthesis increased during the closure of the palatal shelves. The predominant collagen was type I while lesser amounts of type II and type III collagen were synthesized. Hydrocortisone at a physiological dose increased collagen formation in the palatal explants of both mouse strains. However, pharmacological doses of corticosteroids were shown to inhibit the proliferation of neonatal chondrocytes and significantly reduce the DNA, RNA, and protein contents in chondylar cartilage of neonatal mice (Silbermann and Maor, 1979).

In dental pulp, collagen synthesis is selectively decreased following corticosteroid treatment of rabbits (Uitto and Manthorpe, 1983). Proline incorporation into collagen was determined in both molar and incisor pulps following glucocorticoid administration. A similar selective inhibitory effect on collagen synthesis in these pulps was demonstrated during starvation.

Glucocorticoids have also been shown to affect vascular collagen metabolism (Manthorpe *et al.*, 1980; Manthorpe, 1983). Prednisolone inhibits intimal thickening of injured aortas. Collagen synthesis of vascular connective tissue during inflammation and tissue repair is more sensitive to corticosteroid treatment than the connective tissues of the undamaged vascular wall. However, the effects on collagen synthesis of long-term treatment with prednisolone are more pronounced in normal skin as compared to either damaged or undamaged vascular wall. In developing chick aorta of embryos treated with hydrocortisone, the percentage of collagen synthesis of total aortic protein synthesis is decreased (Eichner and Rosenbloom, 1979). However, this inhibitory effect varied between different experiments. The most striking effect of corticosteroid in this experiment was a significant increase in the rate of tropoelastin synthesis, which will be discussed later.

III. GLUCOCORTICOID REGULATION OF COLLAGEN METABOLISM IN CELLS

A. *Fibroblasts*

Rodent fibroblasts are susceptible to glucocorticoid-induced inhibition of growth and collagen synthesis. Mouse fibroblasts have been shown to contain functional glucocorticoid receptors (Hackney *et al.*, 1970; Pratt *et al.*, 1975; Aronow, 1978). Furthermore, glucocorticoid-sensitive cells bind more glucocosteroid action.

Glucocorticoids inhibit cell proliferation, DNA synthesis, and protein synthesis in mouse fibroblasts (Ruhmann and Berliner, 1965;

Verbruggen *et al.*, 1981, 1983). In the latter studies, glucocorticoids selectively inhibited collagen synthesis. Inhibition of collagen synthesis was greater than the inhibition of total protein synthesis. Mouse fibroblasts obtained from the more glucocorticoid-susceptible A/J mice had a greater response to corticosteroid treatment than fibroblasts obtained from the less susceptible C57BC6/J mice. Glucocorticoid treatment of mouse fibroblasts also results in a decrease of the ratio of newly synthesized type III to type I procollagens (Verbruggen and Abe, 1982). Type I procollagen remains unchanged while type III procollagen is significantly decreased following glucocorticoid treatment.

In neonatal rat dermal fibroblasts obtained from glucocorticoid-treated rats, collagen synthesis is selectively decreased (Counts *et al.*, 1979). Although prolyl hydroxylase is decreased in these cells, under-hydroxylated collagen is not produced. This enzyme is apparently not rate limiting for the hydroxylation of certain prolyl residues in collagen nascent chains synthesized in the glucocorticoid-treated fibroblasts. Since glucocorticoids selectively decrease the synthesis of collagen peptides, the enyzme to nascent chain ratio is apparently in the normal range to allow complete hydroxylation of the susceptible prolyl residues in pro α chains. Similarly, in granuloma-derived fibroblasts hydrocortisone decreased prolyl hydroxylase activity while collagen prolyl hydroxylation was not affected (Kruse *et al.*, 1978). In addition, in a cloned fibroblast line derived from a rat carrageenan granuloma, glucocorticoids decreased both collagen synthesis and amino acid uptake (Murota, 1976).

To determine the molecular mechanism by which glucocorticoids decrease type I procollagen synthesis, the total cellular content of proα1(I) and proα2(I) mRNAs were determined in embryonic chick skin and chick lung fibroblasts (Sterling *et al.*, 1983a). As shown in Fig. 6, a correlation is observed between the inhibitory effects of glucocorticoids on collagen synthesis and the proα1(I) and proα2(I) mRNA content. These data indicate that glucocorticoids truly decrease procollagen synthesis. The glucocorticoid-mediated inhibition of procollagen synthesis does not result from an alteration of the prolyl-tRNA pool(s) in chick skin and chick lung fibroblasts.

Glucocorticoids are readily taken up by human skin fibroblasts (Ponec and Kempenaar, 1983). These corticosteroids readily inhibit the proliferation of these fibroblasts in culture (Ponec *et al.*, 1977a; McCoy *et al.*, 1980). The inhibitory effect of glucocorticoids on human skin fibroblast cell growth is also observed with anabolic steroids (Ponec *et al.*, 1979a). Therefore this growth-inhibitory effect is not limited to only antianabolic steroids. The degree of inhibition of fibro-

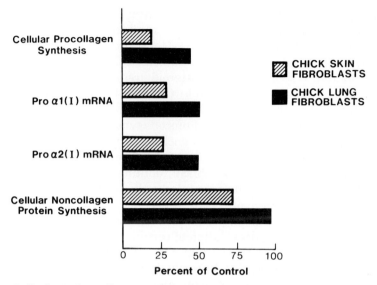

FIG. 6. To determine collagen synthetic rates, embryonic chick skin fibroblasts and chick lung fibroblasts were treated with dexamethasone for 22 hr. Radioactive proline was then added to the medium and the cultures were incubated for another 2 hr. Cellular collagen synthesis was determined by using the collagenase digestion assay. The contents of cellular proα1(I) and proα2(I) mRNAs were determined by using cloned cDNA probes in the dot hybridization assay.

blast proliferation is dependent on the growth phase of the cultures (Ponec *et al.*, 1979b). Fibroblasts at early growth phases are more susceptible than cells at late growth phases. Furthermore, glucocorticoids elicit different responses in normal and diseased fibroblasts (Russell *et al.*, 1978; Priestley and Brown, 1980). Russell *et al.* (1978) demonstrated that hydrocortisone decreased collagen synthesis in normal human fibroblasts but was not effective in decreasing collagen synthesis in keloid-derived fibroblasts. However, a later study by this group showed a strain-to-strain variation of the degree of inhibition of collagen synthesis in keloid-derived fibroblasts to hydrocortisone treatment. McCoy *et al.* (1980), using triamcinolone, demonstrated a decrease of collagen synthesis in both normal and keloid-derived fibroblasts. The differences in response of normal and keloid-derived fibroblasts by Russell *et al.* (1978) to glucocorticoid treatment are not the result of cellular differences of glucocorticoid receptors with respect to the total number of binding sites, the dissociation constants, steroid specificity, or nuclear receptor binding (Gadson *et al.*, 1984). However, a differential effect of glucocorticoids on normal and keloid-derived fibroblasts was observed for system A amino acid transport (Russell *et al.,* 1984c). Glucocorticoids increase the V_{max} of system A amino acid transport one- to twofold in normal fibroblasts and five-to tenfold in keloid-derived fibroblasts.

One study, which needs substantiation, suggests that other factors beside glucocorticoid receptor binding are responsible for glucocorticoid regulation of cell growth (Ponec *et al.,* 1980). Although pharmacological doses of glucocorticoids decrease human skin fibroblast cell growth, selected glucocorticoids at physiological concentrations increase the growth rate of human skin fibroblasts (Priestley, 1978; Runikis *et al.,* 1978).

As has been shown in other tissues and cell lines, glucocorticoid treatment of human skin fibroblasts results in a selective inhibition of collagen synthesis (Ponec *et al.,* 1977b; Priestley, 1978; McCoy *et al.,* 1980; Saarni *et al.,* 1980, Russell *et al.,* 1981). The glucocorticoid-mediated inhibition of collagen synthesis in human skin fibroblasts is observed only in the presence of ascorbate (Russell *et al.,* 1981). This inhibition of collagen synthesis in human skin fibroblasts is mediated by a decrease in the total cellular translatable procollagen mRNAs (Oikarinen *et al.,* 1983b).

Glucocorticoids, as has been observed in many tissues and other cell lines, markedly decrease prolyl hydroxylase activity in human skin fibroblasts (Trupin *et al.,* 1983). Although corticosteroids selectively decrease collagen synthesis, there is no inhibitory effect on collagen prolyl hydroxylation in human skin fibroblasts (Ponec *et al.,* 1979c).

The effect of glucocorticoids on collagen synthesis observed in human skin fibroblasts is not always inhibitory. A review has been published on the variability of glucocorticoid effects on collagen synthesis (Booth *et al.,* 1982). In fact, corticosteroids have been shown to increase collagen synthesis in some human skin fibroblast cultures (Harvey *et al.,* 1974; Doherty and Saarni, 1976). There are several possible explanations for the apparent variability of these results. First, many investigators have used ethanol as a glucocorticoid vehicle. Ethanol nonspecifically inhibits collagen and noncollagen protein synthesis at a dose greater than 0.05% (Thanassi *et al.,* 1980). In addition, Saarni and Tammi (1978) demonstrated that glucocorticoids increased collagen synthesis when the preincubation time was 0–24 hr. However, with a preincubation time of 84 hr, glucocorticoids inhibited collagen synthesis. Another variable in studying the effects of glucocorticoids on collagen synthesis in human skin fibroblasts is that hydrocortisone affects proline uptake in these cells (Russell *et al.,* 1982a). In addition cultured human skin fibroblasts are heterogeneous, which may result in heterosensitivity for collagen synthesis to glucocorticoid administration.

Human lung fibroblasts contain glucocorticoid receptors (Cristofalo and Rosner, 1979; Rosner and Cristofalo, 1981). Hydrocortisone treatment of human lung fibroblasts results in increased cell proliferation (Cristofalo and Rosner, 1979; Rosner and Cristofalo, 1979, 1981). Recently it has been shown that in embryonic lung fibroblasts hydrocortisone decreases the interdivision time independently for a given cell (Absher and Cristofalo, 1984). The hydrocortisone stimulation of fibroblast growth is observed using physiological doses. It would be of interest to see if synthetic glucocorticoids also increase lung fibroblast cell growth when using either physiological and/or pharmacological doses of glucocorticoid. The significance of these findings will not be realized until other biochemical parameters of fibroblast metabolism beside cell growth are determined. In addition, human lung fibroblasts may have to be grown on extracellular matrix components and then challenged with hydrocortisone to test the physiological significance of these findings.

Glucocorticoid administration to rats following an intratracheal injection of bleomycin blocks the accumulation of collagen in lung as previously shown (Fig. 5). Bleomycin-induced pulmonary fibrosis involves the participation of many cell types, cell–cell interactions, stimulatory and inhibitory factors, morphological changes, immunological changes, and alterations of lung biochemical processes. An interesting observation was made by Otsuka *et al.* (1976). These investigators demonstrated that bleomycin increased collagen synthesis in cultured rat granuloma fibroblasts. Both Clark *et al.* (1980b) and Sterling *et al.* (1982b) later investigated the direct effects of bleomycin on collagen metabolism in human lung fibroblasts. Clark's group found that total procollagen synthesis increased while the proportion of newly synthesized type III decreased. Procollagen synthesis was predominantly that of type I procollagen. We found (Sterling *et al.*, 1982b) that although cellular collagen synthesis is increased by bleomycin, both intracellular and extracellular collagen degradation are increased. This may have significance in light of the proposed restructuring model of pulmonary fibrosis *in vivo*.

The bleomycin-induced increase of cellular collagen synthesis in embryonic chick lung and chick skin fibroblasts is blocked by dexamethasone treatment (Sterling *et al.*, 1983b) (Fig. 7). The bleomycin-induced increase of cellular collagen synthesis has been shown to result from a partitioning of procollagen type I mRNAs into polysomes. As seen in Fig. 7, dexamethasone treatment of bleomycin treated chick lung and

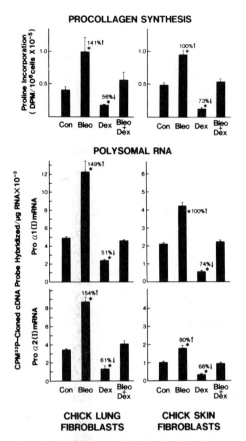

FIG. 7. Primary embryonic chick lung and chick skin fibroblasts were treated for 24 hr with bleomycin and for the next 24 hr with dexamethasone. Prior to cell collection radioactive proline was added to the cultures. Cell layer collagen and noncollagen protein synthesis was determined by the collagenase digestion assay. Cellular levels of proα1(I) and proα2(I) mRNAs were determined using cloned cDNA probes by dot blot hybridization analysis. The asterisks indicate significance as compared to control (Con) at $p \leq 0.05$.

chick skin fibroblasts results in a blocking of the increase in polysomal type I procollagen mRNAs.

B. Hepatocytes

Parenchymal cells derived from liver have been shown to synthesize collagen. Epithelial cell lines in culture have been shown to synthesize collagen (Sakakibara *et al.*, 1976). This group has also cloned liver epithelial cells which have been shown to synthesize collagen in culture (Sakakibara *et al.,* 1978, 1982; Hata *et al.,* 1980). These investigators demonstrated that cloned liver cell lines synthesize type I, type I trimer, and type III collagens (Hata *et al.,* 1980). They also showed the distribution within the liver of type I and type IV collagen, laminin, and fibronectin using the unlabeled peroxidase–antiperoxidase technique (Sakakibara *et al.,* 1982).

Other investigators have shown that nonproliferating primary hepatocytes synthesize collagen (Guzelian *et al.,* 1981; Hatahara and Seyer, 1982; Tseng *et al.,* 1982; Diegelmann *et al.,* 1983; Guzelian *et al.,* 1984). In an interesting study, Diegelmann and colleagues, using indirect immunofluorescence, demonstrated that primary hepatocyte systems synthesized types I, III, and IV collagens at different times during cell incubation (Diegelmann *et al.,* 1983). These workers also showed that glucocorticoids markedly decrease hepatocyte collagen synthesis (Guzelian *et al.,* 1984). This system of glucocorticoid regulation of epithelial collagen synthesis has several advantages. The inhibition of collagen synthesis is selective since this corticosteroid has no effect on noncollagen protein synthesis. The steroid-mediated inhibitory effect on collagen synthesis is observed at physiological glucocorticoid concentrations (i.e., 10^{-8} and 10^{-9} M). Finally, the inhibitory effect is also persistent after the cell cultures are briefly exposed to glucocorticoid.

The partial mechanism by which glucocorticoids decrease hepatocyte procollagen synthesis has been elucidated by Jefferson *et al.* (1984). These workers demonstrated that glucocorticoids decrease the cytoplasmic concentration of type I procollagen mRNAs. These findings may be of importance in light of a therapeutic effect of corticosteroids in cirrhosis. These results are exciting since collagen synthesis by the hepatocyte may be an important biochemical process during the development of hepatic fibrosis and its subsequent treatment with corticosteroids.

C.   *Other Cells*

Glucocorticoids also regulate collagen synthesis in other cell types. When added to chick embryo tendon cells, betamethasone selectively decreased collagen synthesis with no effect on prolyl hydroxylase activity (Oikarinen, 1977a). In other studies, only selected corticosteroids decreased collagen synthesis in isolated chick embryo tendon cells (Saarni and Hopsu-Havu, 1976; Saarni, 1977). Betamethasone produced the most potent inhibition of collagen synthesis. Collagen synthesis and the activities of prolyl hydroxylase, lysyl oxidase, collagen galactosyltransferase, and collagen glucosyltransferase were all decreased in chick embryo tendon cells after four daily injections of hydrocortisone (Oikarinen, 1977b).

Glucocorticoids selectively decrease collagen synthesis in chondrocytes isolated from articular cartilage (Guenther et al., 1984). Although this effect is not seen in primary cultures, significant inhibition of collagen synthesis by corticosteroids is observed in secondary cultures. The glucocorticoid-mediated inhibitory effect on collagen synthesis is apparently specific since noncollagen protein synthesis is not affected by steroid treatment. These data agree with the detection of glucocorticoid receptors in cultured articular chondrocytes (Blondelon et al., 1980).

Glucocorticoids are potent regulators of collagen metabolism in synovial fibroblasts. Corticosteroid treatment suppresses collagenase synthesis in these cells (Brinckerhoff et al., 1980; Brinckerhoff and Harris, 1981). Beside suppressing collagenase production these steroids also increase a collagenase inhibitor (McGuire et al., 1981).

Hydrocortisone treatment of human aortic smooth muscle cells resulted in decreased cell growth as measured by thymidine incorporation into DNA and DNA content (Jarvelainen et al., 1982). Glucocorticoid treatment increased collagen and noncollagen protein synthesis and lysyl oxidase activity. Glucocorticoids also inhibit bovine aortic smooth muscle cell proliferation (Longenecker et al., 1984). This corticosteroid-mediated inhibition of aortic smooth muscle cell growth is associated with an increase of collagen and noncollagen protein synthesis in both primary cultures and cloned cells during log-phase growth (Leitman et al., 1984). Although the specific activity of the intracellular proline pool in dexamethasone-treated aortic smooth muscle cells is increased, normalization for this change resulted in a greater than twofold increase of the rates of collagen and noncollagen protein synthesis. The ratio of type I and type III collagen in aortic smooth muscle cells did not change following dexamethasone treatment.

Glucocorticoids regulate the production of collagen in transformed fibroblasts. Dexamethasone treatment of transformed cells causes the accumulation of collagen and other extracellular matrix components (Furcht et al., 1979a,b). These investigators concluded that if the presence of collagen represents the differentiated state of fibroblasts, then dexamethasone treatment of transformed fibroblasts provides at least in part a drug-induced reversion back to the "normal" differentiated state.

Beside having direct effects on collagen metabolism in fibroblasts, glucocorticoids also alter collagen degradation by affecting other cell types. Corticosteroids have profound effects on macrophages associated with wound repair (Leibovich and Ross, 1975). Physiological concentrations of antiinflammatory steroids selectively and reversibly inhibit the secretion of collagenase by macrophanges (Werb, 1978; Werb *et al.,* 1978a). These effects of glucocorticoids on macrophages are mediated by specific glucocorticoid receptors (Werb *et al.,* 1978a,b). In addition Wahl and Winter (1984) demonstrated that dexamethasone and lipopolysaccharide treatment of macrophages results in an inhibition of prostaglandin E_2 and collagenase production. This effect is reversed by phospholipase A_2, arachidonic acid, prostaglandin E_2, and dibutyryl-cAMP. The phospholipase inhibitor mepacrine inhibits prostaglandin E_2 and collagenase production.

IV. Sex Hormone Regulation of Collagen Metabolism in Tissues

A. Bone

Sex hormones affect collagen metabolism in a variety of tissues and cells. Sex steroids are known to affect skeletal metabolism. The effect of estrogen on bone collagen during immobilization osteoporosis was studied by analyzing femur and tibia hydroxyproline content and determining femur cortical thickness (Orimo *et al.,* 1971). The decreased hydroxyproline content of bone during osteoporesis was significantly blocked by estrogen administration. This was correlated with inhibition of decreased femur density and cortical thickness. Collagen formation is enhanced by medullary bone induced by estradiol in male quail (Turner and Schraer, 1977). This anabolic effect of estrogen on bone collagen metabolism appears to result from the differentiation of osteogenic precursor cells to osteoblasts.

In fractured bones of castrated female rats, high doses of estradiol resulted in a reduction of collagen synthesis (Langeland, 1975). In normal bone of estradiol-treated castrated female rats, collagen synthesis decreased in a dose-dependent manner (Langeland and Teig, 1975a). Bone pieces incubated with this sex hormone synthesized less collagen than control bone pieces, although the doses of estradiol were nonphysiological (Langeland, 1977). In these studies, the inhibitory effect of estrogen on collagen synthesis was correlated with bone collagen resorption.

Oophorectomy results in increases in the collagen content of bone and incorporation of radioactive proline into collagen (Cruess and

Hong, 1979). Bone collagen content is decreased to normal by estrogen administration while the increased collagen synthesis is only partially reversed. Another spectrum of biochemical changes was noted in intact and castrated male rats treated with estrogen (Cruess and Hong, (1978). In other endocrine ablation studies, estrogen administration to thyro-parathyroidectomized/castrated female rats resulted in a reduced rate of bone collagen resorption with no effect of this sex hormone on bone collagen metabolism in hypophysectomized/castrated rats (Langeland and Teig, 1975b).

Estrogen treatment inhibits the lathyritic effect of β-aminopropionitrile not only in bone but also in skin (Henneman, 1972). Lysyl oxidase activity is increased in both bone and skin by estrogen treatment (Sanada et al., 1978). Pyridinoline, a nonreducible collagen cross-link, is increased in bone of testectomized mice after estrogen treatment while the reducible cross-links are not (Shimizu et al., 1982). Therefore, estrogen treatment may accelerate bone collagen maturation in the extracellular matrix.

The reported effects of sex hormones on bone collagen content and collagen synthesis are complemented by bone collagen degradation. When methaphyseal bone of rats treated with estradiol are placed in culture, there is a decrease of collagenase secreted into the culture medium (Cruess and Hong, 1976).

Bone collagen metabolism is also affected by other sex hormones. Estrogen and to a greater extent testosterone has an anabolic effect on bone collagen metabolism in young gonadectomized rats (Kowalewski et al., 1971). Progesterone treatment of fetal rat calvaria explants results in a selective inhibition of collagen synthesis (Canalis and Raisz, 1978). This inhibitory effect on collagen synthesis was correlated with the inhibition of DNA and RNA synthesis. By testing a series of other sex hormones in the fetal rat calvaria explant system, these investigators concluded that estrogens and androgens do not significantly regulate bone formation in vitro. However, many future studies of bone explant and bone cell culture systems will have to be carried out before definitive conclusions can be drawn.

B.   Granuloma

Progesterone alone as well as progesterone plus estrogen decrease collagen content and tensile strength of granulation tissue in oophorectomized rats (Pallin et al., 1975). In another study it was noted that in guinea pigs bearing carrageenan-induced granulomas and treated with estrogen, total collagen content of both skin and granuloma was reduced (Henneman, 1968). Estrogen treatment decreases granuloma soluble collagen which mainly represents newly synthesized collagen. In addition, estrogen and progesterone have been shown to retard collagen accumulation while selectively decreasing collagen synthesis during experimental granulation tissue formation (Hagberg *et al.,* 1980). The synthesis of different collagen types in granulation tissue is not differentially affected by sex hormone treatment.

C. *Uterus*

In the immature rat, estrogen administration results in increases of both collagen and noncollagen protein content of the uterus (Salvador and Tsai, 1973a). This effect is also observed with estrone, diethylstilbestrol, and ethynylestradiol-3-methyl ether. During hormone treatment the percentage of total protein that is collagen remains unchanged. Collagen and noncollagen proteins are significantly lost from the uterus of adult rats after ovariectomy. After 4 days of administration of estradiol to ovarectomized rats, noncollagen protein is partially restored while the collagen content of the uterus is not increased. Sex hormones have also been shown to regulate collagen content in uterine endometrium but not in the myometrium of the rat (Yochim and Blahna, 1976).

Prolyl hydroxylase activity of the uterus of normal rats is markedly increased as compared to ovariectomized rats (Salvador and Tsai, 1973b). Estradiol administration to either normal or ovariectomized animals results in an increase of uterine prolyl hydroxylase activity. This increase of enzyme activity was also observed in rats treated with estriol, estrone, diethylstilbestrol, and ethynylestradiol-3-methyl ether. In contrast to the estrogen-induced elevation of prolyl hydroxylase activity in the uterus, enzyme activity is decreased in heart, kidney, and lung (Salvador *et al.,* 1976). In uterus, the increase of prolyl hydroxylase activity is associated with an increase of total antigenic enzyme protein.

Estrogen treatment has potent effects on uterine collagen metabolism. Estradiol administration to ovariectomized rats results in an increase of collagen synthesis in the uterus (Dyer *et al.,* 1980). Estradiol treatment stimulates the synthesis of both type I and type III collagens with adequate conversion of procollagens to collagens (Mandell and Sodek, 1982). In addition, increases in the synthesis of noncollagen proteins are observed.

The effects of sex hormones on uterine collagen content and collagen synthesis may also be related to the effects of these steroid hormones on collagen catabolism. Estradiol administration to rats inhibits collagen loss from the involuting uterus (Ryan and Woessner, 1972). This results from an inhibition of collagen degradation and not from an effect of this steroid hormone on collagen synthesis. During postpartum involution of the uterus, collagen breakdown is correlated with collagenase activity, both of which are inhibited by estradiol treatment (Ryan and Woessner, 1974; Woessner, 1979). CI-628, an estrogen antagonist, decreased the inhibitory effect of estrogen on collagen breakdown in the involuting uterus (Woessner, 1976). These data suggest that the effect of estradiol on postpartum involuting uterus is receptor mediated. Progesterone also retards uterine involution and collagen breakdown (Halme and Woessner, 1975). This sex hormone has been reported to reduce uterine collagenase activity. Subsequently, both estradiol and progesterone were shown to reduce collagen breakdown in explants of human cervix (Wallis and Hillier, 1981). A more complete discussion of the effect of sex hormones on uterus collagenase activity appears in another chapter of this volume (Jeffrey).

D. Vascular Tissue

Contraceptive and sex steroids have potent effects on vascular collagen metabolism. Wolinsky (1973a) demonstrated that the accumulation of both collagen and elastin in the rat aortic wall is regulated by endogenous estrogen. Estrogen replacement inhibits the accumulation of these connective tissue matrix components in aorta. Estradiol and mestranol–norethynodrel administration to castrated male and female rats result in decreased aortic collagen and collagen synthesis (Fischer and Swain, 1977, 1980). These investigators also demonstrated that estradiol treatment increases the degradation of aortic collagen in ovariectomized rats (Fischer, 1972). From studies in intact and castrated male rats treated with estradiol and testosterone, it was concluded that estradiol and to a lesser extent testosterone increases aortic collagen degradation (Fischer and Swain, 1978). With the ablation of sex hormones, aortic collagen remains relatively inert. In a very intriguing study, these same investigators demonstrated that in rabbits fed an atherogenic diet and treated with the contraceptive hormone mestranol–norethynodrel a decreased rate of collagen synthesis and a decreased deposition of cholesterol in the aorta (Fischer et al., 1981). This treatment protocol may retard the progression of atherosclerosis.

Androgen treatment of male rats also elicits changes in collagen of the aortic wall (Wolinsky, 1972a). The amount of collagen is significantly increased by androgen treatment while noncollagen protein remains unchanged. It is apparent from the above discussion that sex hormones may have profound effects on the vascular wall structure and functions. Indeed, these effects may be mediated by sex hormone regulation of collagen metabolism at the level of gene expression.

E. Other Tissues

Collagen synthesis is decreased by estradiol in the tendons of castrated female rats. Fascia collagen degradation is increased similar to the degradation evidenced in aortic tissue (Fischer, 1973). Estradiol treatment results in decreased collagen synthesis and an increase of collagen degradation in the skin of guinea pigs (Henneman, 1971). However, estradiol treatment of rats results in a decreased skin collagen degradation (Skosey and Damgaard, 1973).

Estrogen treatment results in a selective increase of collagen synthesis in the sex skin of monkeys (Bentley *et al.*, 1971). In an in-depth study, testosterone was found to have no effect on collagen synthesis and wound healing in both normal and castrated rats (Shamberger *et al.*, 1982).

Androgens markedly affect collagen in the male accessory sex organs (Mariotti *et al.*, 1981). The collagen content of the ventral prostate and seminal vesicles increases during puberty and is prevented by prepubertal castration. Dihydrotestosterone treatment of these castrated animals restored the collagen content of these sex organs to normal. Estrogen treatment did not have the same restorative effect. In addition epithelial collagen of the sex organs of adult animals is reduced by castration (Mariotti and Mawhinney, 1981). This reduction is prevented by dihydrotestosterone treatment.

The effects of sex hormones on connective tissue metabolism were analyzed biochemically and morphologically in the capsular ligament (Hama *et al.*, 1976). Ovariectomy resulted in an increase of collagen content and fibril diameter. These parameters were decreased by estrogen administration as well as estrogen in combination with progesterone. Testosterone administration to orchiectomized male rats increased collagen parameters.

Wahl *et al.* (1977) demonstrated that postpartum pubic symphysis ligaments in culture undergo a reduction of collagen content. This loss of collagen is partially inhibited by estrogen while progesterone significantly impaired ligament resorption. Progesterone was shown to markedly decrease collagenase activity while estrogen was less effective.

V. SEX HORMONE REGULATION OF COLLAGEN METABOLISM IN CELLS

A. Fibroblasts

Differential effects of estradiol are seen in skin and lung fibroblasts of the AKR strain mouse embryos (Hosokawa *et al.*, 1981). Collagen synthesis is increased by estrogen to a greater extent in skin fibroblasts that in lung fibroblasts. This effect is selective since total protein synthesis is increased in skin fibroblasts to a lesser degree than collagen synthesis. In lung fibroblasts treated with estrogen, total protein synthesis is increased to a greater extent than collagen synthesis.

B. Aortic Smooth Muscle Cells

The aortic smooth cell system provides an excellent model to study the effects of estrogen on collagen metabolism. Estrogen has no effect on aortic smooth muscle cell growth which is a distinct advantage in studying the effects of any hormone on collagen metabolic parameters (Beldekas *et al.*, 1981). In aortic smooth muscle cells estradiol slightly reduces prolyl hydroxylation of collagen while prolyl hydroxylase activity is not affected. Although total protein synthesis is not affected, collagen synthesis was decreased as a function of estradiol concentration. Estradiol reduces the syntheses of type I and type II procollagens. The ratio of these procollagen types is also altered by estradiol treatment. In a later study these investigators demonstrated that estradiol treatment results in increased processing of type I procollagen as compared to type III procollagen during a 1-hr pulse period (Beldekas *et al.*, 1982).

C. Macrophages

The steady-state concentration of collagen may also be regulated by degradation. Sex hormones regulate the production of collagenase by peritoneal macrophages which in turn may regulate collagen degradation in tissues (Wahl, 1977). Macrophages obtained from nonpregnant guinea pigs were stimulated by endotoxin to secrete collagenase in culture. Progesterone or estrogen treatment of guinea pigs resulted in an inhibition of endotoxin stimulation of collagenase production. The addition of these two sex hormones to macrophages in culture resulted in a marked inhibition of collagenase activity at lower doses than was necessary for each hormone alone to elicit an inhibitory effect.

VI. GLUCOCORTICOID REGULATION OF ELASTIN METABOLISM IN TISSUES

Reports on the effect of glucocorticoids on elastin synthesis and degradation in tissues and cells are less abundant than reports concerned with steroid hormone regulation of collagen metabolism. However, interesting as well as significant information is available.

A. *Vascular Tissue*

Differential regulation of elastin genes has been observed in the aorta during chick embryogenesis (Barrineau *et al.*, 1981). This differential expression of elastin genes during development may be under hormonal control.

Glucocorticoid treatment of chick embryos and embryonic chick aortas incubated *in vitro* markedly alters tropoelastin synthesis in aortic tissue (Eichner and Rosenbloom, 1979; Burnett *et al.*, 1980). A significant increase in the rate of tropoelastin synthesis was observed in the aorta of hydrocortisone treated 8-day chick embryos and 8-day chick embryo aorta treated *in vitro* with hydrocortisone. The level of tropoelastin synthesis was similar to that found in aortas isolated from 14- to 18-day embryos. Furthermore, the increase of tropoelastin synthesis was selective with respect to procollagen synthesis and general protein synthesis. These data indicate that the regulation of tropoelastin synthesis in the developing chick embryo aorta may be intimately related to glucocorticoid levels during embryogenesis. Subsequent studies from the same laboratory using cell-free translation indicated that the hydrocortisone-induced increase of tropoelastin synthesis in the chick embryo aorta results from an increase in the amount of functional tropoelastin mRNA (Burnett *et al.*, 1980).

The administration of the synthetic glucocorticoid dexamethasone to chick aorta in organ culture also elicits an increased rate of tropoelastin synthesis (Foster *et al.*, 1983). In addition, the proportion of tropoelastin a with respect to tropoelastin b is greater after dexamethasone treatment. The opposite is true in untreated aorta. Thus, the evidence suggests that not only can glucocorticoids mediate an increase in tropoelastin synthesis in the chick aorta via increased tropoelastin mRNA levels, but glucocorticoids can also differentially modulate the proportional amounts of tropoelastin a and b.

An earlier study indicated that pharmacologic doses of glucocorticoids did not effect the amount of aortic insoluble elastin (Manthorpe *et al.*, 1974, 1980). The difference observed between embryonic chick aorta and 5-month-old rabbit aorta in response to glucocorticoids may be due to species difference and/or may be an age-related phenomenon.

Experimentally induced hypertension in the rat causes a significant increase in the total amount of elastin as well as collagen in the aorta (Wolinsky *et al.*, 1974). Administration of methylprednisolone to these hypertensive rats inhibits the accumulation of elastin in aortic tissue. Inhibition of elastin accumulation in the aorta of hypertensive rats appears to be contradictory to the findings in normal embryonic chick aorta in which glucocorticoid administration caused an increase in elastin synthesis as described above. However, these conflicting results may be due to species-dependent, dose-related, and/or age-related differences. In addition, the increased amount of elastin in the aorta in response to hypertension is probably a result of increased synthesis and turnover in response to vascular injury. Thus, glucocorticoids may only inhibit the amount of elastin being synthesized as a result of hypertension. Glucocorticoid treatment does not effect elastin accumulation in the aorta of normotensive rats.

Glucocorticoid regulation of aortic elastin synthesis *in ovo* or in organ culture can provide useful information in elucidating the molecular mechanism(s) of this specific tissue response. However, whole tissue studies, while important for understanding biological phenomenon *in vivo*, limit one's ability to ascertain which cell type(s) respond to the steroid hormone.

B. Skin and Lung

Glucocorticoids decrease the amounts of collagen synthesis and glycosaminoglycan synthesis in rabbit skin (Manthorpe *et al.*, 1974, 1980). The connective tissue parameters studied, including elastin, are more sensitive to changes induced by glucocorticoids in skin.

Glucocorticoid treatment of pregnant rhesus monkeys does not significantly alter the elastin content of fetal monkey lung (Beck *et al.*, 1981). However, the ratio of collagen to elastin is significantly increased in the lungs of the treated group. In addition, dexamethasone treatment of chick embryos does not alter the rate of elastin synthesis or the ratio of tropoelastin a to b in lung (Foster *et al.*, 1983). Thus, significant modifications of elastin metabolic parameters in response to glucocorticoid appear to be confined to the vascular tissue and skin.

VII. GLUCOCORTICOID REGULATION OF ELASTIN METABOLISM IN CELLS

A. *Ligamentum Nuchae Fibroblasts*

A well-characterized cell system has appeared in the literature to study the effects of steroid hormones on the synthesis and degradation of elastin (Mecham *et al.*, 1981, 1984a,b). The process of elastogenic differentiation in bovine ligamentum nuchae fibroblasts may be useful to elucidate the mechanism(s) of regulation of elastin gene expression during development. In this model, the undifferentiated ligament fibroblasts from early gestation animals initiate elastin synthesis when grown on extracellular matrix isolated from late gestation ligamentum nuchae. After such differentiation, the early gestation fibroblasts show a positive chemotactic response to elastin. This positive response persists after the removal of the extracellular matrix.

Mecham *et al.* (1984c) have also demonstrated that bovine ligamentum nuchae fibroblasts are stimulated by glucocorticoids to synthesize two to three times more tropoelastin than nontreated cells. Glucocorticoid enhancement of tropoelastin synthesis is selective and is time and dose dependent. The synthesis of tropoelastin a and b is coordinately elevated following glucocorticoid treatment. This is in contrast to the differential sitmulation of tropoelastin a and b synthesis in glucocorticoid treatment embryonic chick aorta (Foster *et al.*, 1983). The glucocorticoid-induced synthesis of tropoelastin occurs only in differentiated cells from late gestation animals and is consistent with a glucocorticoid-receptor-mediated process. However, undifferentiated cells which are not induced by glucocorticoid to synthesize elastin also have glucocorticoid receptors.

It will be of great interest to see what factor(s) is (are) responsible for the ability of differentiated ligament fibroblasts to increase tropoelastin production in response to glucocorticoid treatment. Furthermore, the bovine ligament fibroblast model may provide a worthwhile system to determine the mechanism of action of the glucocorticoid-receptor complex upon the DNA sequences which are possibly involved in the regulation of tropoelastin gene expression by glucocorticoids.

B. Polymorphonuclear Leukocytes and Macrophages

The steady-state concentration of elastin in tissue is dependent not only on elastin synthesis but also on the regulation of elastin degradation. Glucocorticoids inhibit the secretion of elastase by activated polymorphonuclear leukocytes (Hart, 1984) and macrophages (Werb, 1978; Werb et al., 1978; Dahlgren et al., 1980; Ackerman et al., 1981). This process in macrophages is apparently glucocorticoid-receptor mediated (Werb et al., 1978). The inhibition of secretion of elastase by macrophages and polymorphonuclear leukocytes may be one of the mechanisms by which glucocorticoids can ameliorate the symptoms of pulmonary disease in which there is a degeneration of the interstitial connective tissue components including elastin.

VIII. Sex Hormone Regulation of Elastin Metabolism in Vascular Tissue

The sex steroid hormones have been reported to have notable effects on the aortic elastin content in rats (Wolinsky, 1972a,b; Fischer, 1972; Wolinsky, 1973a,b; Fischer and Swain, 1977, 1978, 1980). Estradiol administration to ovariectomized female rats results in a decrease of elastin content in the aorta (Fischer, 1972). It was concluded that the decreased amount of elastin results from an increased degradation of newly synthesized elastin. Although aortic elastin is decreased, the net result is a higher proportion of elastin with respect to collagen and decreased stiffness of the vessel wall. Estradiol administration to intact male rats causes a significantly lower amount of total elastin in the aorta, indicating that the effect of estradiol overrides that of endogenous testosterone (Fischer and Swain, 1977).

Aortic elastin content in ovariectomized and intact female rats is differentially affected by administration of various sex steroids and also the contraceptive steroids (Fischer and Swain, 1980). Progesterone administration to castrated female rats results in an increased percentage of aortic elastin but no change in total aortic elastin. Testosterone treatment of ovariectomized rats did not change the total content of elastin in the aorta but did result in a slightly increased percentage of aortic elastin. Testosterone treatment of intact female rats showed a slight depression in total aortic elastin as well as a marked decrease in the percentage of elastin. The combination of mestranol–norethynodrel administered to ovariectomized rats resulted in a significant decrease in aortic elastin without changing the percentage of aortic elastin. The differential effect of the individual sex steroids on female rat aortic elastin content may indicate different molecular mechanisms for affecting such changes.

Estrogen or antiandrogen treatment of hypertensive intact male rats results in an inhibition of the hypertension induced accumulation of aortic elastin (Wolinsky, 1972b, 1973b). Alternatively, progesterone treatment of hypertensive male rats failed to inhibit the increase in aortic elastin. Cyproterone acetate, an antiandrogen, inhibits the increase in aortic elastin due to hypertension but does not significantly alter the amount of elastin in the aorta of rapidly growing normotensive rats. Thus, estrogen and antiandrogens appear to be specific inhibitors of hypertension-induced elastin accumulation in the aorta. Aortic elastin synthesis is increased in female rabbits fed an atherogenic diet (Fischer *et al.,* 1981). However, combination therapy of the contraceptive steroids mestranol and norethynodrel partially inhibits this increase of aortic elastin synthesis.

From the studies mentioned above, it is apparent that the female sex hormone estrogen, the contraceptives mestranol and norethynodrel, and the antiandrogen cyproterone can protect against the pathological accumulation of elastin which occurs in cardiovascular diseases. It remains to be seen whether or not these sex steroids as well as glucocorticoids regulate elastin synthesis and content in other elastin containing tissues. Sex steroid hormones may have a physiological role in determining connective tissue composition and mediating sexual induced differentiation of connective tissues.

IX. STEROID HORMONE REGULATION OF FIBRONECTIN METABOLISM IN LIVER AND CELLS

Owens and Cimino (1982), using isolated perfused rat liver, demonstrated that a significant proportion of plasma fibronectin is synthesized by the liver. Addition of puromycin to the liver perfusate diminished but did not totally block fibronectin production during 10 hr of perfusion. The basal level of fibronectin synthesis was also unaffected by this protein synthesis inhibitor. When liver perfusate solutions were supplemented with insulin and cortisol, the net synthesis of fibronectin increased after 6 hr of perfusion.

Fibronectin is associated with cellular adhesiveness and cell shape. Transformed and neoplastic cells generally lose their capacity to express and to bind to fibronectin in cell culture. These cells exhibit altered morphology, are frequently less differentiated than their parent cells, and are less adhesive in cell-to-cell interactions (for reviews see Yamada and Olden, 1978; Pearlstein *et al.,* 1980; Hynes and

Yamada, 1982). The major producers of fibronectin are fibroblasts and endothelial cells. Glucocorticoid regulation of fibronectin synthesis has been demonstrated in both normal and neoplastic cells.

A. Hepatocytes

Glucocorticoid regulation of fibronectin synthesis has been demonstrated in normal untransformed hepatocytes. Using indirect immunofluorescence microscopy, Marceau *et al.* (1980) examined the effects of dexamethasone on hepatocytes from newborn rats. Primary cell cultures grown in serum-free medium exhibited a defined fibronectin extracellular matrix as early as 24 hr after glucocorticoid treatment. Hepatocytes not treated with glucocorticoid exhibited little immunofluorescence staining for fibronectin. Phase contrast microscopy of the glucocorticoid-treated hepatocytes revealed epithelial cell morphology. In this primary cell culture system of liver, fibroblast growth was inhibited by glucocorticoid treatment.

B. Fibroblasts

Oliver *et al.* (1983) demonstrated that fibronectin synthesis by normal human foreskin fibroblasts is increased twofold following glucocorticoid treatment. These cells were grown in the presence of 10% serum-supplemented medium and dexamethasone for 5 days. Fibronectin synthesis was assessed by immunoprecipitation of radiolabeled proteins. This glucocorticoid-mediated increase of fibronectin synthesis, but not the basal level of fibronectin synthesis, was blocked by the glucocorticoid antagonist RU-486. This suggests that this glucocorticoid mediated response is receptor mediated.

C. Endothelial Cells

Hydrocortisone treatment of primary cultures of human umbilical endothelial vein cells in a defined serum-free medium did not alter fibronectin production (Berliner, 1981). However, dexamethasone treatment of umbilical vein endothelial cells in medium containing 20% serum caused an increase in fibronectin production (Piovella *et al.*, 1982). In these studies, it is important to distinguish the effects of glucocorticoids on cells binding to fibronectin from the cellular synthesis of fibronectin. Cells grown under serum-rich conditions may accumulate bovine plasma fibronectin on their surfaces when exposed to exogenous glucocorticoids.

D. Transformed Cells

The phenotypic switch evidenced by increased fibronectin production following glucocorticoid treatment of transformed cells has been interpreted as a step toward a more normal expression and a more differentiated state. Baumann and Eldredge (1982) demonstrated that fibronectin is induced by glucocorticoids in rat hepatoma cells. Fibronectin synthesis in dexamethasone-treated cells was increased two- to fourfold. The fibronectin synthesized by these glucocorticoid-treated cells was capable of binding gelatin and was only partially active in cell binding ability to either normal fibroblasts or neoplastic cells.

Furcht *et al.* (1979a,b) observed an accumulation of extracellular matrix in human skin fibroblasts transformed *in vitro* with SV40 and treated with the synthetic glucocorticoid dexamethasone. Immunocytochemical analysis of these cells revealed an extracellular matrix composed of fibronectin and procollagen type I. An attempt was made to stimulate fibronectin accumulation in these transformed cells by addition of other steroid hormones. Progesterone and testosterone elicited no changes in fibronectin production.

Mouse 3T3 fibroblasts grown under serum starved conditions lose most of their cell-associated fibronectin (Chen *et al.*, 1977) and become synchronized (Brooks, 1976). Cell-surface-associated fibronectin was lowest during mitosis (Stenman *et al.*, 1977). However, during mitosis these cells did not have reduced amounts of intracellular fibronectin. Hydrocortisone did not increase fibronectin synthesis when these cells were cultured under low serum conditions. Of the 13 serum components and hormones tested, only epidermal growth factor induced fibronectin accumulation on the cell surface (Chen *et al.*, 1977).

Dexamethasone treatment of human fibrosarcoma cells results in a 10-fold increase of fibronectin synthesis over untreated cells (Oliver *et al.*, 1983). Newly synthesized radiolabeled fibronectins were immunoprecipitated and subjected to SDS–PAGE resolution and fluorographic analysis. As was observed in normal human foreskin fibroblasts, the dexamethasone-mediated increase in fibronectin synthesis was blocked by the glucocorticoid antagonist RU-486. However, the basal level of fibronectin synthesis was not affected.

Glucocorticoid treatment of rat glioma cells also increases the production of cell-surface-associated fibronectin as determined by immunofluorescent staining (Armelin and Armelin, 1983). These fully transformed cells do not normally accumulate fibronectin on their cell surfaces. Varients of this cell line were also shown to respond to hydrocortisone treatment by an increased extracellular deposition of fibronectin.

A great deal of work still remains to be done in this area of research before the mechanisms of glucocorticoid regulation of fibronectin synthesis are more fully understood. Studies using recombinant DNA technology should yield exciting information on the molecular regulation mechanisms of fibronectin gene expression by steroid hormones.

X. FUTURE PROSPECTIVES OF STEROID HORMONE REGULATION OF THE SYNTHESIS OF THE PROTEINACEOUS COMPONENTS OF THE EXTRACELLULAR MATRIX

A. Fibroblast Heterogeneity and Glucocorticoid Heterosensitivity

The effects of glucocorticoids on cellular collagen synthesis are cell specific. Vascular smooth muscle cells increase collagen synthesis while fibroblasts decrease collagen synthesis in response to glucocorticoids. More importantly, there may be variability in the response of certain cells to glucocorticoid administration. The heterogeneity of fibroblasts in culture may result in heterosensitivity of glucocorticoid regulation of collagen synthesis as well as the synthesis of other proteinaceous components of the extracellular matrix.

Human fibroblasts in culture are a heterogeneous population of cells (Smith and Hayflick, 1974; Kaufman et al., 1975; Bowman and Daniel, 1975; Ko et al., 1977; Zavala et al., 1978; Harper and Grove, 1979; Kelley et al., 1983). Various studies have indicated heterogeneity in proliferation potential, biochemical synthetic activities, and morphology. In a recent study, subsets of human diploid fibroblasts have been separated using a fluorescence-activated cell sorter (Brodin et al., 1984). A subset of fibroblasts with a high affinity for C1q was isolated which synthesized DNA, grew faster than parent cultures, and synthesized increased amounts of type III and type V collagens. This functional heterogeneity of fibroblasts in culture may result in differences in response to steroid-hormone-mediated regulation of the synthesis of the extracellular matrix protein components. For example, in human cloned keloid skin fibroblasts, glucocorticoids decreased collagen synthesis to different extents among different clones (Russell et al., 1982b). These data suggest functional heterogeneity of the cloned fibroblast population. However, this variation among clones may reflect either differences in clonal growth or changes in phenotypic expression as a result of cell culturing, which may reflect differences in population density. There is also other evidence in the literature of varied responses of collagen synthesis to glucocorticoid treatment in human skin fibroblasts (Booth *et al.*, 1982). In addition, rat calvaria bone cells were divided into subpopulations which have different rates of collagen synthesis (Guenther *et al.*, 1984). While glucocorticoids selectively decreased collagen synthesis in one of these cell populations, no response to corticosteroid treatment was noted in another subpopulation.

B. In Vitro Transcription Systems

Differential regulation of protein synthesis by glucocorticoids in fibroblasts has been well established in this review. Glucocorticoid regulation of collagen synthesis in fibroblasts appears to be a receptor-mediated process (Fig. 8). The glucocorticoid antagonists progesterone and RU-486 (Chobert *et al.*, 1983; Jung-Testas and Baulieu, 1983; Oliver *et al.*, 1983) blocked the glucocorticoid-mediated inhibition of collagen synthesis. The agonist 5β-dihydrocortisol (Weinstein *et al.*, 1983)

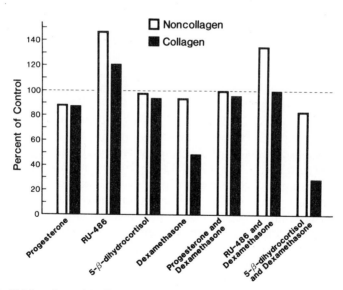

FIG. 8. Chick embryo skin fibroblasts were pretreated with either progesterone, RU-486, or 5β-dihydrocortisol for 24 hr. The cells were then treated for the next 24 hr with dexamethasone both with or without the agonist and antagonist. After labeling the cells with radioactive proline, collagen and noncollagen syntheses were determined by the collagenase digestion assay.

potentiated the inhibitory effect of glucocorticoid on collagen synthesis.

Much work remains to be done to reveal the molecular mechanism(s) by which steroid hormones regulate extracellular protein gene expression. Several transcriptional systems are available to elucidate these mechanisms. Nuclei can be isolated from control and steroid-treated cells and transcribed *in vitro*. Cloned cDNA probes can be used to monitor the synthesis of protein-specific hnRNAs *in vitro*. Alternatively, purified steroid–receptor complexes can be added to untreated nuclei and the up and downs of the synthesis of specific hnRNAs can be determined. However, isolated nuclei systems may be complicated by possible rapid metabolism of newly synthesized hnRNA.

In vitro transcription of recombinant genomic probes provides another method for investiagting the regulation of eukaryotic protein gene expression by steroid hormones. However, the *in vitro* transcription systems developed by Manley *et al.* (1980) and Weil *et al.* (1979) do not respond to regulatory signals. The development of totally purified *in vitro* transcription systems, including recombinant genomic DNA with promoter and structural gene regions, purified transcription factors, and purified steroid–receptor complexes will probably surmount the less well-defined transcriptional lysate systems presently available.

C. Transfection Systems

Recently, a recombinant gene system which expresses chloramphenicol acetyltransferase in mammalian cells has been developed (Groman *et al.*, 1982). This model system has been applied to the study of the procollagen $\alpha2(I)$ promoter in transfected mouse 3T3 cells (Schmidt *et al.*, 1984). The procollagen $\alpha2(I)$ promoter is fused to the chloramphenicol acetyltransferase gene which then comes under the regulatory control of the procollagen $\alpha2(I)$ promoter. When the transfected clones are transformed with Maloney mouse sarcoma virus, endogenous procollagen type I mRNAs and chloramphenicol acetyltransferase activity were diminished. The procollagen $\alpha2(I)$ promoter activity may be modulated by specific regulatory signals. This genetically engineered model may be used in the future to test the procollagen $\alpha2(I)$ promoter response to added steroid hormones. However, successful modulation of chloramphenicol acetyltransferase activity by an exogenous steroid hormone would only indicate that the procollagen $\alpha2(I)$ promoter is somehow involved. Addition of an inhibitor of protein synthesis such as cycloheximide would determine whether or not newly synthesized cellular proteins, in response to steroid hormone administration, may play a role in affecting the procollagen $\alpha2(I)$ promoter activity. Although this system may faithfully reflect alterations in procollagen $\alpha2(I)$ promoter activity upon addition of a steroid hormone, one has no control over the character of flanking host genomic DNA within which the recombinant genomic DNA is inserted. It must be remembered that in transfection experiments, the inserted recombinant DNA may be modified. This modification may alter steroid-hormone-induced regulation of procollagen gene expression. Factors such as the degree of DNA methylation or chromatin organization of the inserted recombinant DNA and flanking DNA cannot be readily assessed. These factors which are referred to as epigenetic structures could be critical for the variable response of the procollagen $\alpha2(I)$ promoter in transfected cells to steroid hormone administration.

To circumvent these complexities in the study of procollagen $\alpha2(I)$ promoter regulation, one can employ genomic fusion plasmids containing a transforming fragment of the bovine papilloma virus (BPV) type I (Lowy *et al.*, 1980; Law *et al.*, 1981, 1982; Ostrowski *et al.*, 1983). Recombinant plasmid vectors of this type offer several advantages including extrachromosomal replication and amplification and maintenance in the episomal state during propagation (Ostrowski *et al.*, 1983). Recombinant genomic plasmids containing the procollagen $\alpha2(I)$ promoter fused to an appropriate coding sequence offer a well-defined model system for the investigation of steroid-hormone-induced regulation of extracellular matrix protein gene expression. Steady-state RNA levels can be determined after glucocorticoid administration as well as *in vitro* transcription of subnuclear fractions containing the recombinant minichromosomes (Ostrowski *et al.*, 1983). The experimental analysis of secondary differences in the inserted DNA and flanking DNA is facilitated by the readily obtained purified minichromosomes. Future studies employing these model systems should definitively elucidate the molecular mechanism(s) by which glucocorticoids and other steroid hormones regulate the synthesis of procollagen as well as other extracellular matrix proteins.

Acknowledgments

We thank Dr. Helga Boedtker for the cDNA plasmid probes for type I procollagen. We also thank Dr. George J. Cardinale for the prolyl hydroxylase antibody and Dr. R. Hynes for the fibronectin antibody. We thank Mr. Robert A. Shaw, Ms. Sara W. Andrews, and Carol F. Cutroneo, who helped in the preparation of this manuscript, and our other colleagues who have collaborated on the studies described in this review: Thomas A.

DiPetrillo, Mike J. Harris, John Mitchell, Debra Cockayne, Grace Delaney, and Sharon Illeyne. These studies were supported by NIH Grants AM 19808 and HL 14212. K. M. Sterling was supported by the Cancer Biology Training Grant CA 09826.

REFERENCES

Absher, M., and Cristofalo, V. J. (1984). *J. Cell. Physiol.* **119**, 315–319.

Ackerman, N. R., Jubb, S. N., and Marlowe, S. L. (1981). *Biochem. Pharmacol.* **30**, 2147–2155.

Adamson, I. Y. R. (1976). *Environ. Health Perspect.* **16**, 119–126.

Adamson, I. Y. R., and Bowden, D. H. (1974). *Am. J. Pathol.* **77**, 185–198.

Armelin, M. C. S., and Armelin, H. A. (1983). *J. Cell Biol.* **97**, 459–465.

Aronow, L. (1978). *Fed. Proc.* **37**, 162–166.

Asboe-Hansen, G. (1976). *Dermatologica* **152**, 127–132.

Ballard, P. L., and Ballard, R. A. (1972). *Proc. Natl. Acad. Sci. U.S.A.* **69**, 2668–2672.

Ballard, P. L., and Ballard, R. A. (1974). *J. Clin. Invest.* **53**, 477–486.

Ballard, P. L., and Ballard, R. A. (1979). *Pediatrics* **63**, 163–165.

Barrineau, L. L., Rich, C. B., Przybyla, A., and Foster, J. A. (1981). *Dev. Biol.* **87**, 46–51.

Baumann, H., and Eldredge, D. (1982). *J. Cell Biol.* **95**, 29–40.

Beck, J. C., Mitzner, W., Johnson, J. W. C., Hutchins, G. M., Foidart, J. M., London, W. T., Palmer, A. E., and Scott, R. (1981). *Pediatr. Res.* **15**, 235–240.

Beldekas, J. C., Smith, B., Gerstenfeld, L. C., Sonenshein, G. E., and Franzblau, C. (1981). *Biochemistry* **20**, 2162–2167.

Beldekas, J. C., Gerstenfeld, L., Sonenshein, G. E., and Franzblau, C. (1982). *J. Biol. Chem.* **257**, 12252–12256.

Benson, S. C., and LuValle, P. A. (1981). *Biochem. Biophys. Res. Commun.* **99**, 557–562.

Bentley, J. P., Nakagawa, H., and Davies, G. H. (1971). *Biochim. Biophys. Acta* **244**, 35–46.

Berliner, J. A. (1981). *In Vitro* **17**, 985–992.

Blondelon, D., Adolphe, M., Zizine, L., and Lechat, P. (1980). *FEBS Lett.* **117**, 195–198.

Blumenkrantz, N., and Asboe-Hansen, G. (1976). *Acta Endocinol.* **83**, 665–672.

Bondi, E. E., and Kligman, A. M. (1980). *Prog. Dermatol.* **14**, 1–4.

Booth, B. A., Tan, E. M. L., Oikarinen, A., and Uitto, J. (1982). *Int. J. Dermatol.* **21**, 333–337.

Bordin, S., Page, R. C., and Narayanan, A. S. (1984). *Science* **223**, 171–173.

Bowman, P. D., and Daniel, C. W. (1975). *Adv. Exp. Med. Biol.* **53**, 107–122.

Brinckerhoff, C. E., and Harris, E. D., Jr. (1981). *Biochim. Biophys. Acta* **677**, 424–432.

Brinckerhoff, C. E., McMillan, R. M., Dayer, J-M., and Harris, E. D., Jr. (1980). *N. Engl. J. Med.* **303**, 432–436.

Brooks, R. F. (1976). *Nature* **260**, 248–250.

Burnett, W., Eichner, R., and Rosenbloom, J. (1980). *Biochemistry* **19**, 1106–1111.

Burnett, W., Yoon, K., Finnigan-Bunick, A., and Rosenbloom, J. (1982). *Invest. Dermatol.* **79**, 138s–145s.

Canalis, E. (1983a). *Endocrinology* **112**, 931–939.

Canalis, E. (1983b). *Endocr. Rev.* **4**, 62–77.

Canalis, E. (1984). *Calcif. Tissue Int.* **36**, 158–166.

Canalis, E., and Raisz, L. G. (1978). *Calcif. Tissue Res.* **25**, 105–110.

Canalis, E., Peck, W. A., and Raisz, L. G. (1980). *Science* **210**, 1021–1023.

Chen, L. B., Gudor, R. C., Sun, T. T., Chen, A. B., and Mosesson, M. W. (1977). *Science* **197**, 776–778.

Chen, T. L., Aronow, L., and Feldman, D. (1977). *Endocrinology* **100**, 619–628.
Chen, T. L., and Feldman, D. (1978). *Endocrinology* **102**, 589–596.
Chen, T. L., and Feldman, D. (1979). *J. Clin. Invest.* **63**, 750–758.
Chobert, M. N., Barouki, R., Finidori, J., Aggerbeck, M., Hanoune, J., Philibert, D., and Deraedt, R. (1983). *Biochem. Pharmacol.* **32**, 3481–3483.
Choe, J., Stern, P., and Feldman, D. (1978). *J. Steroid Biochem.* **9**, 265–271.
Clark, J. G., Overton, J. E., Marino, B. A., Uitto, J., and Starcher, B. C. (1980a). *J. Lab. Clin. Med.* **96**, 943–953.
Clark, J. G., Starcher, B. C., and Uitto, J. (1980b). *Biochim. Biophys. Acta* **631**, 359–370.
Clark, J. G., Kostal, K. M., and Marino, B. A. (1982). *J. Biol. Chem.* **257**, 8098–8105.
Counts, D. F., and Cutroneo, K. R. (1979). *J. Pharm. Pharmacol.* **31**, 780–782.
Counts, D. F., Rojas, F. J., and Cutroneo, K. R. (1979). *Mol. Pharmacol.* **15**, 99–107.
Counts, D. F., Shull, S., and Cutroneo, K. R. *Connect. Tissue Res.,* in press.
Cristofalo, V. J., and Rosner, B. A. (1979). *Fed. Proc.* **38**, 1851–1856.
Cruess, R. L., and Hong, K. C. (1975). *Proc. Soc. Exp. Biol. Med.* **148**, 887–890.
Cruess, R. L., and Hong, K. C. (1976). *Calcif. Tissue Res.* **20**, 317–320.
Cruess, R. L., and Hong, K. C. (1978). *Proc. Soc. Exp. Biol. Med.* **159**, 368–373.
Cruess, R. L., and Hong, K. C. (1979). *Endocrinology* **104**, 1188–1193.
Cruess, R. L., and Sakai, T. (1972). *Clin. Orthop. Relat. Res.* **86**, 253–259.
Crystal, R. G., Fulmer, J. D., Roberts, W. C., Moss, M. L., Line, B. R., and Reynolds, H. Y. (1976). *Ann. Intern. Med.* **85**, 769–788.
Crystal, R. G., Bitterman, P. B., Rennard, S. I., Hance, A. J., and Keogh, B. A. (1984a). *N. Engl. J. Med.* **310**, 154–166.
Crystal, R. G., Bitterman, P. B., Rennard, S. I., Hance, A. J., and Keogh, B. A. (1984b). *N. Engl. J. Med.* **310**, 235–244.
Cutroneo, K. R., and Clarke, D. H. (1979). *Biochem. Pharmacol.* **28**, 3229–3231.
Cutroneo, K. R., and Counts, D. F. (1975). *Mol. Pharmacol.* **11**, 632–639.
Cutroneo, K. R., Costello, D., and Fuller, G. C. (1971). *Biochem. Pharmacol.* **20**, 2797–2804.
Cutroneo, K. R., Stassen, F. L. H., and Cardinale, G. J. (1975). *Mol. Pharmacol.* **11**, 44–51.
Cutroneo, K. R., Rokowski, R., and Counts, D. F. (1981). *Coll. and Relat. Res.* **1**, 557–568.
Dahlgren, M. E., Davies, P., and Bonney, R. J. (1980). *Biochim. Biophys. Acta* **630**, 338–351.
Davidson, J. M., and Crystal, R. G. (1982). *J. Invest. Dermatol.* **79**, 133s–137s.
Diegelmann, R. F., Guzelian, P. S., Gay, R., and Gay, S. (1983). *Science* **219**, 1343–1345.
Dietrich, J. W., Canalis, E. M., Maina, D. M., and Raisz, L. G. (1979). *Endocrinology* **104**, 715–721.
DiPetrillo, T., Lee, H., and Cutroneo, K. R. (1984). *Arch. Dermatol.* **120**, 878–883.
Doherty, N. S., and Saarni, H. (1976). *J. Pharm. Pharmacol.* **28**, 656–657.
Dyer, R. F., Sodek, J., and Heersche, J. N. M. (1980). *Endocrinology* **107**, 1014–1021.
Ehrinpreis, M. N., Giambrone, M. A., and Rojkind, M. (1980). *Biochim. Biophys. Acta* **629**, 184–193.
Ehrlich, H. P., and Tarver, H. (1971). *Proc. Soc. Exp. Biol. Med.* **137**, 936–938.
Ehrlich, H. P., Tarver, H., and Hunt, T. K. (1973). *Ann. Surg.* **177**, 222–227.
Eichner, R., and Rosenbloom, J. (1979). *Arch. Biochem. Biophys.* **198**, 414–423.
Eppenberger, U., and Hsia, S. L. (1972). *J. Biol. Chem.* **247**, 5463–5469.
Epstein, E. H., Jr. (1983). *In* "Biochemistry and Physiology of the Skin" (L. A. Goldsmith, ed.), Vol II, pp. 1200–1209. Oxford Univ. Press, New York.

Epstein, E. H., Jr., and Munderloh, N. H. (1981). *Endocrinology* **108**, 703–711.

Fasske, E., and Morgenroth, K. (1983). *Lung* **161**, 133–146.

Feldman, D., Dziak, R., Koehler, R., and Stern, P. (1975). *Endocrinology* **96**, 29–36.

Fischer, G. M. (1972). *Endocrinology* **91**, 1227–1232.

Fischer, G. M. (1973). *Endocrinology* **93**, 1216–1218.

Fischer, G. M., and Swain, M. L. (1977). *Am. J. Physiol.* **232**, H617–H621.

Fischer, G. M., and Swain, M. L. (1978). *Endocrinology* **102**, 92–97.

Fischer, G. M., and Swain, M. L. (1980). *Exp. Mol. Pathol.* **33**, 15–24.

Fischer, G. M., Cherian, K., and Swain, M. L. (1981). *Atherosclerosis* **39**, 463–467.

Foster, J. A., Rich, C. B., and Karr, S. R. (1983). *Int. Rev. Connect. Tissue Res.* **10**, 65–95.

Freeman, P. C., Mangan, F. R., and Watkins, D. K. (1979). *Biochem. Pharmacol.* **28**, 573–578.

Fukuhara, M., and Tsurufuji, S. (1969). *Biochem. Pharmacol.* **18**, 2409–2414.

Furcht, L. T., Mosher, D. F., Wendelschafer-Crabb, G., Woodbridge, P. A., and Foidart, J. M. (1979a). *Nature* **277**, 393–395.

Furcht, L. T., Mosher, D. F., Wendelschafer-Crabb, G., Woodbridge, P. A., and Foidart, J. M. (1979b). *Cancer Res.* **39**, 2077–2083.

Gadson, P. F., Russell, J. D., and Russell, S. B. (1984). *J. Biol. Chem.* **259**, 11236–11241.

Gail, D. B., and Lenfant, C. J. M. (1983). *Am. Rev. Respir. Dis.* **127**, 366–387.

Gallagher, J. C., Aaron, J., Horsman, A., Wilkinson, R., and Nordin, B. E. C. (1973). *Clin. Endocrinol. Metab.* **2**, 355–368.

Galligani, L., Lonati-Galligani, M., and Fuller, G. C. (1979). *Toxicol. Appl. Pharmacol.* **48**, 131–137.

Galvin, M. J., and Lefer, A. M. (1979). *J. Reticuloendothel. Soc.* **25**, 61–72.

Gasser, D. L., and Goldman, A. S. (1983). *Biochem. Actions Horm.* **10**, 357–382.

Gay, S., and Miller, E. J. (1978). *In* "Collagen in the Physiology and Pathology of Connective Tissue" (E. J. Miller and S. Gay, eds.), pp. 1–110. Fischer, Stuttgart.

Giannopoulos, G. (1975a). *J. Biol. Chem.* **250**, 2904–2910.

Giannopoulos, G. (1975b). *J. Biol. Chem.* **250**, 2896–2903.

Giannopoulos, G., Mulay, S., and Solomon, S. (1973). *J. Biol. Chem.* **248**, 5016–5023.

Giri, S. N., Schwartz, L. W., Hollinger, M. A., Freywald, M. E., Schiedt, M. J., and Zuckerman, J. E. (1980). *Exp. Mol. Pathol.* **33**, 1–14.

Giri, S. N., Chen, Z. L., Younker, W. R., and Schiedt, M. J. (1983). *Toxicol. Appl. Pharmacol.* **71**, 132–141.

Goforth, P., and Gudas, C. J. (1980). *J. Foot Surg.* **19**, 22–28.

Goldstein, R. H., Lucey, E. C., Franzblau, C., and Snider, G. L. (1979). *Am. Rev. Respir. Dis.* **120**, 67–73.

Gorman, C. M., Moffat, L. F., and Howard, B. H. (1982). *Mol. Cell. Biol.* **2**, 1044–1051.

Gottrup, F., and Oxlund, H. (1981). *J. Surg. Res.* **31**, 165–171.

Greene, R. M., and Kochhar, D. M. (1975). *Teratology* **11**, 47–56.

Guenther, H. L., Felix, R., and Fleisch, H. (1984). *Calcif. Tissue Int.* **36**, 145–152.

Guzelian, P. S., Qureshi, G. D., and Diegelmann, R. F. (1981). *Coll. Relat. Res.* **1**, 83–93.

Guzelian, P. S., Lindblad, W. J., and Diegelmann, R. F. (1984). *Gastroenterology* **86**, 897–904.

Hackney, J. F., Gross, S. R., Aronow, L., and Pratt, W. B. (1970). *Mol. Pharmacol.* **6**, 500–512.

Hagberg, L., Pallin, B., Ahonen, J., Penttinen, R., and Zederfeldt, B. (1980). *Surg. Gynecol. Obstet.* **151**, 740–746.

Hahn, T. J., Boisseau, V. C., and Avioli, L. V. (1974). *J. Clin. Endocrinol. Metab.* **39**, 274–282.

Haidle, C. W., and Lloyd, R. S. (1978). *In* "Bleomycin: Current Status and New Development" (S. K. Carter, S. T. Crooke, and H. Umezawa, eds.), pp. 21–33. Academic Press, New York.

Hakkinen, P. J., Schmoyer, R. L., and Witschi, H. P. (1983). *Am. Rev. Respir. Dis.* **128**, 648–651.

Halme, J., and Woessner, J. F., Jr. (1975). *J. Endocrinol.* **66**, 357–362.

Hama, H., Yamamuro, T., and Takeda, T. (1976). *Acta Orthop. Scand.* **47**, 473–479.

Harper, R. A., and Grove, G. (1979). *Science* **204**, 526–527.

Hart, D. H. L. (1984). *Blood* **63**, 421–426.

Harvey, W., Grahame, R., and Panayi, G. S. (1974). *Ann. Rheum. Dis.* **33**, 437–441.

Hata, R-I., Ninomiya, Y., Nagai, Y., and Tsukada, Y. (1980). *Biochemistry* **19**, 169–176.

Hatahara, T., and Seyer, J. M. (1982). *Biochim. Biophys. Acta* **716**, 431–438.

Hay, E. D. (1981). *J. Cell Biol.* **91**, 205s–223s.

Heiman, A. S., Nathoo, Z. N., and Lee, H. J. (1982). *Drug Dev. Res.* **2**, 377–382.

Henneman, D. H. (1968). *Endocrinology* **83**, 678–690.

Henneman, D. H. (1971). *Biochem. Biophys. Res. Commun.* **44**, 326–332.

Henneman, D. H. (1972). *Clin. Orthop.* **83**, 245–254.

Hesterberg, T. W., and Last, J. A. (1981). *Am. Rev. Respir. Dis.* **123**, 47–52.

Hirayama, C., Morotomi, I., and Hiroshige, K. (1971). *Experientia* **27**, 893–894.

Hollister, D. W., Byers, P. H., and Holbrook, K. A. (1982). *Adv. Hum. Genet.* **12**, 1–87.

Hosokawa, M., Ishii, M., Inoue, K., Yao, C. S., and Takeda, T. (1981). *Connect. Tissue Res.* **9**, 115–120.

Hynes, R. O., and Yamada, K. M. (1982). *J. Cell Biol.* **95**, 369–377.

Jablonska, S., Groniowska, M., and Dabroswki, J. (1979). *Br. J. Dermatol.* **100**, 193–206.

Jarvelainen, H., Halme, T., and Ronnemaa, T. (1982). *Acta Med. Scand. (Suppl.)* **660**, 114–122.

Jefferson, D. M., Reid, L. M., Gianbrone, M. A., Shafritz, D. A., and Zern, M. A. (1984). *East Coast Connect. Tissue Soc. 4th Annu. Meet.*

Jeffrey, J. J., Di Petrillo, T., Counts, D. F., and Cutroneo, K. R. (1985). *Coll. Relat. Res.* **5**, 157–165.

Jung-Testas, I., and Baulieu, E. E. (1983). *Exp. Cell Res.* **147**, 177–182.

Kaufman, M., Pinsky, L., Straisfeld, C., Shanfield, B., and Zilahi, B. (1975). *Exp. Cell Res.* **96**, 31–36.

Kehrer, J. P., and Witschi, H. (1981). *Toxicology* **20**, 281–288.

Kelley, R. O., Perdue, B. D., and Uruchurtu-Valdivia, R. A. (1983). *Anat. Rec.* **206**, 329–339.

Kivirikko, K. I., and Laitinen, O. (1965). *Acta Physiol. Scand.* **64**, 356–360.

Kivirikko, K. I., Laitinen, O., Aer, J., and Halme, J. (1965). *Biochem. Pharmacol.* **14**, 1445–1451.

Ko, S. D., Page, R. C., and Narayanan, A. S. (1977). *Proc. Natl. Acad. Sci. U.S.A.* **74**, 3429–3432.

Koenig, W. J., Cross, C. E., Hesterberg, T. W., and Last, J. A. (1983). *Chest* **83**, 5S–7S.

Koob, T. J., Jeffrey, J. J., and Eisen, A. Z. (1974). *Biochem. Biophys. Res. Commun.* **61**, 1083–1088.

Kowalewski, K., Heron, F., and Russell, J. C. (1971). *Acta Endocrinol.* **67**, 740–755.

Kruse, N. J., Rowe, D. W., Fujimoto, Y., and Bornstein, P. (1978). *Biochim. Biophys. Acta* **540**, 101–116.

Kuberasampath, T., and Bose, S. M. (1979). *Agents Actions* **9**, 502–509.

Kuberasampath, T., and Bose, S. M. (1980). *Agents Actions* **10**, 78–84.

Kuo, M. T., and Haidle, C. W. (1973). *Biochim. Biophys. Acta* **335,** 109–114.

Langeland, N. (1975). *Acta Endocrinol.* **80,** 603–612.

Langeland, N. (1977). *Acta Orthop. Scand.* **48,** 266–272.

Langeland, N., and Teig, V. (1975a). *Acta Endocrinol.* **80,** 784–794.

Langeland, N., and Teig, V. (1975b). *Acta Endocrinol.* **80,** 795–800.

Last, J. A., Siefkin, A. D., and Reiser, K. M. (1983). *Thorax* **38,** 364–368.

Laurent, G. J., and McAnulty, R. J. (1983). *Am. Rev. Respir. Dis.* **128,** 82–88.

Law, M.-F., Lowy, D. R., Dvoretzky, I., and Howley, P. M. (1981). *Proc. Natl. Acad. Sci. U.S.A.* **78,** 2727–2731.

Law, M. F., Howard, B., Sarver, N., and Howley, P. M. (1982). *In* "Eukaryotic Viral Vectors" (Y. Glusman, ed.), pp. 79–85. Cold Spring Harbor Laboratory, Cold Spring Harbor, New York.

Lazo, J. S., and Humphreys, C. J. (1983). *Proc. Natl. Acad. Sci. U.S.A.* **80,** 3064–3068.

Lee, H. J., and Soliman, M. R. I. (1982). *Science* **215,** 989–991.

Lee, H. J., and Trottier, R. (1980). *Res. Commun. Chem. Pathol. Pharmacol.* **27,** 611–614.

Lee, H. J., Bradlow, H. L., Moran, M. C., and Sherman, M. R. (1981). *J. Steroid Biochem.* **14,** 1325–1335.

Leibovich, S. J., and Ross, R. (1975). *Am. J. Pathol.* **78,** 71–100.

Leitman, D. C., Benson, S. C., and Johnson, L. K. (1984). *J. Cell Biol.* **98,** 541–549.

Longenecker, J. P., Kilty, L. A., and Johnson, L. K. (1984). *J. Cell Biol.* **98,** 534–540.

Lowy, D. R., Dvoretzky, I., Shober, R., Law, M. F., Engel, L., and Howley, P. M. (1980). *Nature* **287,** 72–74.

McCoy, B., Diegelmann, R. F., and Cohen, I. K. (1980). *Proc. Soc. Exp. Biol. Med.* **163,** 216–222.

McCullough, B., Collins, J. F., Johanson, W. G., Jr., and Grover, F. L. (1978). *J. Clin. Invest.* **61,** 79–88.

McGuire, M. B., Murphy, G., Reynolds, J. J., and Russell, R. G. G. (1981). *Clin. Sci.* **61,** 703–710.

McNelis, B., and Cutroneo, K. R. (1978). *Mol. Pharmacol.* **14,** 1167–1175.

Madri, J. A., and Furthmayr, H. (1980). *Hum. Pathol.* **11,** 353–363.

Mandell, M. S., and Sodek, J. (1982). *J. Biol. Chem.* **257,** 5268–5273.

Manley, J. L., Fire, A., Cano, A., Sharp, P. A., and Gefter, M. L. (1980). *Proc. Natl. Acad. Sci. U.S.A.* **77,** 3855–3859.

Mann, S. W., Fuller, G. C., Rodil, J. V., and Vidins, E. I. (1979). *Gut* **20,** 825–832.

Manthorpe, R. (1983). *Acta Endocrinol. (Suppl.)* **259,** 1–40.

Manthorpe, R., Helin, G., Kofod, B., and Lorenzen, I. (1974). *Acta Endocrinol.* **77,** 310–324.

Manthorpe, R., Garbarsch, C., and Lorenzen, I. (1980). *Acta Endocrinol.* **95,** 271–281.

Marceau, N., Goyette, R., Valet, J. P., and Deschenes, J. (1980). *Exp. Cell Res.* **125,** 497–502.

Mariotti, A., and Mawhinney, M. (1981). *Prostate* **2,** 397–408.

Mariotti, A., Thornton, M., and Mawhinney, M. (1981). *Endocrinology* **109,** 837–843.

Mecham, R. P., Lange, G., Madaras, J., and Starcher, B. (1981). *J. Cell Biol.* **90,** 332–338.

Mecham, R. P., Griffin, G. L., Madaras, J. G., and Senior, R. M. (1984a). *J. Cell Biol.* **98,** 1813–1816.

Mecham, R. P., Madaras, J. G., and Senior, R. M. (1984b). *J. Cell Biol.* **98,** 1804–1812.

Mecham, R. P., Morris, S. L., Levy, B. D., and Wrenn, D. S. (1984c). *J. Biol. Chem.* **259,** 12414–12418.

Miller, J. A., and Munro, D. D. (1980). *Drugs* **19,** 119–134.

Miller, R. L., and Udenfriend, S. (1970). *Arch. Biochem. Biophys.* **139**, 104–113.

Muller, W. E. G., Yamazaki, Z. I., Breter, H. J., and Zahn, R. K. (1972). *Eur. J. Biochem.* **31**, 518–525.

Muller, W. E. G., Totsuka, A., Nusser, I., Zahn, R. K., and Umezawa, H. (1975). *Biochem. Pharmacol.* **24**, 911–915.

Murota, S. I., Koshihara, Y., and Tsurufuji, S. (1976). *Biochem. Pharmacol.* **25**, 1107–1113.

Nakagawa, H., and Tsurufuji, S. (1972a). *Biochem. Pharmacol.* **21**, 839–846.

Nakagawa, H., and Tsurufuji, S. (1972b). *Biochem. Pharmacol.* **21**, 1884–1886.

Nakagawa, H., Fukuhara, M., and Tsurufuji, S. (1971). *Biochem. Pharmacol.* **20**, 2253–2261.

Newman, R. A., and Cutroneo, K. R. (1978). *Mol. Pharmacol.* **14**, 185–198.

Nimni, M. E. (1983). *Semin. Arthritis Rheum.* **13**, 1–86.

Nocenti, M. R., Lederman, G. E., Furey, C. A., and Lopano, A. J. (1964). *Proc. Soc. Exp. Biol. Med.* **117**, 215–218.

Ohno, T., and Tsurufuji, S. (1970). *Biochem. Pharmacol.* **19**, 1–8.

Ohno, T., Ishibashi, S., and Tsurufuji, S. (1972). *Biochem. Pharmacol.* **21**, 1057–1062.

Oikarinen, A. (1977a). *Biochem. Pharmacol.* **26**, 875–879.

Oikarinen, A. (1977b). *Biochem. J.* **164**, 533–539.

Oikarinen, A., Peltonen, L., Hintikka, J., Foidart, J. M., and Kiistala, U. (1983a). *Br. J. Dermatol.* **108**, 171–178.

Oikarinen, J., and Ryhanen, L. (1981). *Biochem. J.* **198**, 519–524.

Oikarinen, J., Pihlajaniemi, T., Hamalainen, L., and Kivirikko, K. I. (1983b). *Biochim. Biophys. Acta* **741**, 297–302.

Oliver, N., Newby, R. F., Furcht, L. T., and Bourgeois, S. (1983). *Cell* **33**, 287–296.

Olsen, B. R. (1981). *In* "Cell Biology of Extracellular Matrix" (E. D. Hay, ed.), Chap. 6, pp. 139–177. Plenum, New York.

Orimo, H., Fujita, T., Yoshikawa, M., Hayano, K., and Sakurada, T. (1971). *Endocrinology* **88**, 102–105.

Ostrowski, M. C., Richard-Foy, H., Wolford, R. G., Berard, D. S., and Hager, G. L. (1983). *Mol. Cell. Biol.* **3**, 2045–2057.

Otsuka, K., Murota, S. I., and Mori, Y. (1976). *Biochim. Biophys. Acta* **444**, 359–368.

Owens, M. R., and Cimino, C. D. (1982). *Blood* **59**, 1305–1309.

Oxlund, H., Fogdestam, I., and Viidik, A. (1979). *Surg. Gynecol. Obstet.* **148**, 876–880.

Oxlund, H., Sims, T., and Light, N. D. (1982). *Acta Endocrinol.* **101**, 312–320.

Ozaki, T., Nakayama, T., Ishimi, H., Kawano, T., Yasuoka, S., and Tsubura, E. (1982). *Am. Rev. Respir. Dis.* **126**, 968–971.

Pallin, B., Ahonen, J., and Zederfeldt, B. (1975). *Acta Chir. Scand.* **141**, 710–714.

Pearlstein, E., Gold, L. I., and Garcia-Pardo, A. (1980). *Mol. Cell. Biochem.* **29**, 103–128.

Phan, S. H., and Thrall, R. S. (1981). *Am. J. Pathol.* **106**, 156–164.

Phan, S. H., Thrall, R. S., and Ward, P. A. (1980). *Am. Rev. Respir. Dis.* **121**, 501–506.

Phan, S. H., Thrall, R. S., and Williams, C. (1981). *Am. Rev. Respir. Dis.* **124**, 428–434.

Phillips, K., Arffa, R., Cintron, C., Rose, J., Miller, D., Kublin, C. L., and Kenyon, K. R. (1983). *Arch. Ophthalmol.* **101**, 640–643.

Piovella, F., Giddings, J. C., Ricetti, M. M., Almasio, P., and Ascari, E. (1982). *Haematologica* **67**, 58–63.

Ponec, M., and Kempenaar, J. A. (1983). *Arch. Dermatol. Res.* **275**, 334–344.

Ponec, M., de Haas, C., Bachra, B. N., and Polano, M. K. (1977a). *Arch. Dermatol. Res.* **259**, 117–123.

Ponec, M., Hasper, I., Vianden, G. D. N. E., and Bachra, B. N. (1977b). *Arch. Dermatol. Res.* **259**, 125–134.

Ponec, M., de Haas, C., Kempenaar, J. A., and Bachra, B. N. (1979a). *Arch. Dermatol. Res.* **266**, 75–82.

Ponec, M., de Haas, C., Bachra, B. N., and Polano, M. K. (1979b). *Arch. Dermatol. Res.* **265**, 219–227.

Ponec, M., Kempenaar, J. A., Van Der Meulen-Van Harskamp, G. A., and Bachra, B. N. (1979c). *Biochem. Pharmacol.* **28**, 2777–2783.

Ponec, M., DeKloet, E. R., and Kempenaar, J. A. (1980). *J. Invest. Dermatol.* **75**, 293–296.

Pratt, R. M., Jr., and King, T. G. (1972). *Dev. Biol.* **27**, 322–328.

Pratt, W. B., Kaine, J. L., and Pratt, D. V. (1975). *J. Biol. Chem.* **250**, 4584–4591.

Priestley, G. C. (1978). *Br. J. Dermatol.* **99**, 253–261.

Priestley, G. C., and Brown, J. C. (1980). *Br. J. Dermatol.* **102**, 35–41.

Prockop, D. J., and Kivirikko, K. I. (1984). *N. Engl. J. Med.* **311**, 376–386.

Raisz, L. G., Trummel, C. L., Wener, J. A., and Simmons, H. (1972). *Endocrinology* **90**, 961–967.

Reiser, K. M., and Last, J. A. (1983). *J. Biol. Chem.* **258**, 269–275.

Risteli, J. (1977). *Biochem. Pharmacol.* **26**, 1295–1298.

Robertson, W. van B., and Sanborn, E. C. (1958). *Endocrinology* **63**, 250–252.

Robey, P. G. (1979). *Biochem. Pharmacol.* **28**, 2261–2266.

Rojkind, M., and Dunn, M. A. (1979). *Gastroenterology* **76**, 849–863.

Rojkind, M., and Martinez-Palomo, A. (1976). *Proc. Natl. Acad. Sci. U.S.A.* **73**, 539–543.

Rojkind, M., and Perez-Tamayo, R. (1983). *Int. Rev. Connect. Tissue Res.* **10**, 333–393.

Rojkind, M., and Ponce-Noyola, P. (1982). *Coll. Relat. Res.* **2**, 151–175.

Rojkind, M., Giambrone, M. A., and Biempica, L. (1979). *Gastroenterology* **76**, 710–719.

Rojkind, M., Rojkind, M. H., and Cordero-Hernandez, J. (1983). *Coll. Relat. Res.* **3**, 335–347.

Rokowski, R., Cutroneo, K. R., Guzman, N. A., Fallon, A., and Cardinale, G. J. (1981a). *J. Biol. Chem.* **256**, 1340–1345.

Rokowski, R. J., Sheehy, J., and Cutroneo, K. R. (1981b). *Arch. Biochem. Biophys.* **210**, 74–81.

Rosner, B. A., and Cristofalo, V. J. (1979). *Mech. Ageing Dev.* **9**, 485–496.

Rosner, B. A., and Cristofalo, V. J. (1981). *Endocrinology* **108**, 1965–1971.

Ruhmann, A. G., and Berliner, D. L. (1965). *Endocrinology* **76**, 916–927.

Runikis, J. O., McLean, D. I., and Stewart, W. D. (1978). *J. Invest. Dermatol.* **70**, 348–351.

Ruoslahti, E., Engvall, E., and Hayman, E. G. (1981). *Coll. Relat. Res.* **1**, 95–128.

Russell, J. D., Russell, S. B., and Trupin, K. M. (1978). *J. Cell. Physiol.* **97**, 221–230.

Russell, S. B., Russell, J. D., and Trupin, K. M. (1981). *J. Cell. Physiol.* **109**, 121–131.

Russell, S. B., Russell, J. D., and Trupin, J. S. (1982a). *J. Biol. Chem.* **257**, 9525–9531.

Russell, J. D., Russell, S. B., and Trupin, K. M. (1982b). *In Vitro* **18**, 557–564.

Russell, S. B., Russell, J. D., and Trupin, J. S. (1984c). *J. Biol. Chem.* **259**, 11464–11469.

Ryan, J. N., and Woessner, J. F. (1972). *Biochem. J.* **127**, 705–713.

Ryan, J. N., and Woessner, J. F., Jr. (1974). *Nature* **248**, 526–528.

Saarni, H. (1977). *Biochem. Pharmacol.* **26**, 1961–1966.

Saarni, H., and Hopsu-Havu, V. K. (1976). *Br. J. Dermatol.* **95**, 566–567.

Saarni, H., and Tammi, M. (1978). *Biochim. Biophys. Acta* **540**, 117–126.

Saarni, H., Jalkanen, M., and Hopsu-Havu, V. K. (1980). *Br. J. Dermatol.* **103**, 167–173.

174 KENNETH R. CUTRONEO *ET AL.*

Saarni, H. U., Savolainen, E. R., and Sotaniemi, E. A. (1983). *Res. Commun. Chem.* *Pathol. Pharmacol.* **42,** 61–69.
Sakakibara, K., Saito, M., Umeda, M., Enaka, K., and Tsukada, Y. (1976). *Nature* **262,** 316–318.
Sakakibara, K., Takaoka, T., Katsuta, H., Umeda, M., and Tsukada, Y. (1978). *Exp. Cell* *Res.* **111,** 63–71.
Sakakibara, K., Suzuki, T., Tsukada, Y., and Nagai, Y. (1982). *Cell Struct. Funct.* **7,** 213–228.
Salmela, K. (1981). *Scand. J. Plast. Reconstr. Surg.* **15,** 87–91.
Salomon, D. S., and Pratt, R. M. (1979). *Differentiation* **13,** 141–154.
Salvador, R. A., and Tsai, I. (1973a). *Biochem. Pharmacol.* **22,** 37–46.
Salvador, R. A., and Tsai, I. (1973b). *Arch. Biochem. Biophys.* **154,** 583–592.
Salvador, R. A., Tsai, I., and Stassen, F. L. H. (1976). *Biochem. Pharmacol.* **25,** 907–912.
Sanada, H., Shikata, J., Hamamoto, H., Ueba, Y., Yamamuro, T., and Takeda, T. (1978).
Biochim. Biophys. Acta **541,** 408–413.
Sandberg, L. B., Soskel, N. T., and Leslie, J. G. (1981). *N. Engl. J. Med.* **304,** 566–579.
Sausville, E. A., Peisach, J., and Horwitz, S. B. (1978a). *Biochemistry* **17,** 2740–2746.
Sausville, E. A., Stein, R. W., Peisach, J., and Horwitz, S. B. (1978b). *Biochemistry* **17,** 2746–2754.
Saville, P. D., and Kharmosh, O. (1967). *Arthritis Rheum.* **10,** 423–430.
Schimdt, A., Pastan, I., and de Crombrugghe, B. (1984). *East Coast Connect. Tissue Soc.* *4th Annu. Meet.*
Seyer, J. M. (1980). *Biochim. Biophys. Acta* **629,** 490–498.
Seyer, J. M., Hutcheson, E. T., and Kang, A. H. (1976). *J. Clin. Invest.* **57,** 1498–1507.
Seyer, J. M., Hutcheson, E. T., and Kang, A. H. (1977). *J. Clin. Invest.* **59,** 241–248.
Shamberger, R. C., Thistlethwaite, P. A., Thibault, L. E., Talbot, T. L., and Brennan, M. F. (1982). *J. Surg. Res.* **33,** 58–68.
Sherlock, S. (1981). *Semin. Liver Dis.* **1,** 354–364.
Shimizu, K., Higuchi, K., Yamamuro, T., Ohtsuji, T., and Takeda, T. (1982). *Experientia* **38,** 864–866.
Shin, K. H., Nakagawa, H., and Tsurufuji, S. (1974). *Biochem. Pharmacol.* **23,** 381–387.
Shull, S., and Cutroneo, K. R. (1983). *J. Biol. Chem.* **258,** 3364–3369.
Sikic, B. I., Young, D. M., Mimnaugh, E. G., and Gram, T. E. (1978). *Cancer Res.* **38,** 787–792.
Silbermann, M., and Maor, G. (1979). *Growth* **43,** 273–287.
Skosey, J. L., and Damgaard, E. (1973). *Endocrinology* **93,** 311–315.
Smith, J. R., and Hayflick, L. (1974). *J. Cell Biol.* **62,** 48–53.
Smith, J. G., Jr., Wehr, R. F., and Chalker, D. K. (1976). *Arch. Dermatol.* **112,** 1115–
1117.
Smith, K., Shuster, S., and Rawlins, M. (1983). *Endocrinology* **96,** 229–239.
Smith, Q. T. (1967). *Biochem. Pharmacol.* **16,** 2171–2179.
Smith, Q. T., and Allison, D. J. (1965). *Endocrinology* **77,** 785–791.
Snider, G. L., Hayes, J. A., and Korthy, A. L. (1978). *Am. Rev. Respir. Dis.* **117,** 1099–
1108.
Soliman, M. R. I., and Lee, H. J. (1981). *Res. Commun. Chem. Pathol. Pharmacol.* **33,**
357–360.
Starcher, B. C., Kuhn, C., and Overton, J. E. (1978). *Am. Rev. Respir. Dis.* **117,** 299–305.
Steffek, A. J., Verrusio, A. C., and Watkins, C. A. (1972). *Teratology* **5,** 33–40.
Stenman, S., Wartiovaara, J., and Vaheri, A. (1977). *J. Cell Biol.* **74,** 453–467.

Sterling, K. M., Jr., DiPetrillo, T., Cutroneo, K. R., and Prestayko, A. (1982a). *Cancer Res.* **42**, 405–408.

Sterling, K. M., Jr., DiPetrillo, T. A., Kotch, J. P., and Cutroneo, K. R. (1982b). *Cancer Res.* **42**, 3502–3506.

Sterling, K. M., Jr., Harris, M. J., Mitchell, J. J., DiPetrillo, T. A., Delaney, G. L., and Cutroneo, K. R. (1983a). *J. Biol. Chem.* **258**, 7644–7647.

Sterling, K. M., Jr., Harris, M. J., Mitchell, J. J., and Cutroneo, K. R. (1983b). *J. Biol. Chem.* **258**, 14438–14444.

Stern, P. H. (1969). *J. Pharmacol. Exp. Ther.* **168**, 211–217.

Stevanovic, D. V. (1972). *Br. J. Dermatol.* **87**, 548–556.

Suzuki, H., Nagai, K., Yamaki, H., Tanaka, N., and Umezawa, H. (1968). *J. Antibiot.* **21**, 379–386.

Takeshita, M., Horwitz, S. B., and Grollman, A. P. (1974). *Virology* **60**, 455–465.

Tanner, A. R., and Powell, L. W. (1979). *Gut* **20**, 1109–1124.

Tanzer, M. L. (1982). *In* "Disorders of Mineral Metabolism" (C. L. Comar and F. Bronner, eds.), Vol. II, pp. 237–269. Academic Press, New York.

Thanassi, N. M., Rokowski, R. J., Sheehy, J., Hart, B., Absher, M., and Cutroneo, K. R. (1980). *Biochem. Pharmacol.* **29**, 2417–2424.

Thompson, J. S., and Urist, M. R. (1973). *Calcif. Tissue Res.* **13**, 197–215.

Tom, W.-M., and Montgomery, M. R. (1980). *Toxicol. Appl. Pharmacol.* **53**, 64–74.

Trupin, J. S., Russell, S. B., and Russell, J. D. (1983). *Coll. Relat. Res.* **3**, 13–23.

Tseng, S. C. G., Lee, P. C., Ells, P. F., Bissell, D. M., Smuckler, E. A., and Stern, R. (1982). *Hepatology* **2**, 13–18.

Tsurufuji, S., Nakagawa, H., Ohno, T., and Fukuhara, M. (1974). *In* "Biochemistry and Pathology of Connective Tissue" (Y. Otaka, ed.), pp. 139–151. Igaku Shoin, Tokyo.

Turner, R. T., and Schraer, H. (1977). *Calcif. Tissue Res.* **24**, 157–162.

Turner-Warwick, M., Burrows, B., and Johnson, A. (1980). *Thorax* **35**, 593–599.

Uitto, J., and Mustakallio, K. K. (1971). *Biochem. Pharmacol.* **20**, 2495–2503.

Uitto, J., Teir, H., and Mustakallio, K. K. (1972). *Biochem. Pharmacol.* **21**, 2161–2167.

Uitto, V. J., and Thesleff, I. (1979). *Arch. Oral Biol.* **24**, 575–583.

Uitto, V. J., and Manthorpe, R. (1983). *Arch. Oral Biol.* **28**, 241–246.

Verbruggen, L. A., and Abe, S. (1982). *Biochem. Pharmacol.* **31**, 1711–1715.

Verbruggen, L. A., Salomon, D. S., and Greene, R. M. (1981). *Biochem. Pharmacol.* **30**, 3285–3289.

Verbruggen, L. A., Orloff, S., Rao, V. H., and Salomon, D. S. (1983). *Scand. J. Rheumatol.* **12**, 360–366.

Vogel, H. G. (1971). *Arzneimittelforschung* **21**, 2039–2044.

Vogel, H. G. (1974). *Connect. Tissue Res.* **2**, 177–182.

Wahl, L. M. (1977). *Biochem. Biophys. Res. Commun.* **74**, 838–845.

Wahl, L. M., and Winter, C. C. (1984). *Arch. Biochem. Biophys.* **230**, 661–667.

Wahl, L. M., Blandau, R. J., and Page, R. C. (1977). *Endocrinology* **100**, 571–579.

Wallis, R. M., and Hillier, K. (1981). *J. Reprod. Fertil.* **62**, 55–61.

Wehr, R. F., Smith, J. G., Jr., Counts, D. F., and Cutroneo, K. R. (1976). *Proc. Soc. Exp. Biol. Med.* **152**, 411–414.

Weil, P. A., Luse, D. S., Segall, J., and Roeder, R. G. (1979). *Cell* **18**, 469–484.

Weinstein, B. I., Gordon, G. G., and Southern, A. L. (1983). *Science* **222**, 172–173.

Werb, Z. (1978). *J. Exp. Med.* **147**, 1695–1712.

Werb, Z., Foley, R., and Munck, A. (1978a). *J. Immunol.* **121**, 115–121.

Werb, Z., Foley, R., and Munck, A. (1978b). *J. Exp. Med.* **147**, 1684–1694.

Winterbauer, R. H., Hammar, S. P., Hallman, K. O., Hays, J. E., Pardee, N. E., Morgan, E. H., Allen, J. D., Moores, K. D., Bush, W., and Walker, J. H. (1978). *Am. J. Med.* **65,** 661–672.

Woessner, J. F., Jr. (1976). *J. Endocrinol.* **70,** 157–158.

Woessner, J. F., Jr. (1979). *Biochem. J.* **180,** 95–102.

Wolinsky, H. (1972a). *J. Clin. Invest.* **51,** 2552–2555.

Wolinsky, H. (1972b). *Circ. Res.* **30,** 341–349.

Wolinsky, H. (1973a). *Proc. Soc. Exp. Biol. Med.* **144,** 864–867.

Wolinsky, H. (1973b). *Circ. Res.* **33,** 183–189.

Wolinsky, H., Goldfischer, S., Schiller, B., and Kasak, L. E. (1974). *Circ. Res.* **34,** 233–241.

Wong, G. L. (1979). *J. Biol. Chem.* **254,** 6337–6340.

Yamada, K. M., and Olden, K. (1978). *Nature* **275,** 179–184.

Yasumura, S. (1976). *Am. J. Physiol.* **230,** 90–93.

Yochim, J. M., and Blahna, D. G. (1976). *J. Reprod. Fertil.* **47,** 79–82.

Yoneda, T., and Pratt, R. M. (1981). *J. Craniofacial Genet. Dev. Biol.* **1,** 411–423.

Zapol, W. M., Trelstad, R. L., Coffey, J. W., Tsai, I., and Salvador, R. A. (1979). *Am. Rev. Respir Dis.* **119,** 547–554.

Zavala, C., Herner, G., and Fialkow, P. J. (1978). *Exp. Cell Res.* **117,** 137–144.

Zuckerman, J. E., Hollinger, M. A., and Giri, S. N. (1980). *J. Pharmacol. Exp. Ther.* **213,** 425–431.

Control of Elastin Synthesis: Molecular and Cellular Aspects

Jeffrey M. Davidson* and M. Gabriella Giro†

Department of Pathology, University of Utah School of Medicine, and Research Service, Veterans Administration Medical Center, Salt Lake City, Utah

* Present address: Department of Pathology, Vanderbilt University School of Medicine and Research Service, Veterans Administration Medical Center, Nashville, Tennessee 37203.

† Permanent address: Istituto di Istologia–Embriologia, Università di Padova, 35100 Padova, Italy.

177

I. Introduction

Elastin is an unusual biological substance. It is the least soluble protein in the body, one of the most hydrophobic polypeptides, and extremely durable, perhaps lasting the lifetime of the organism. These properties have made the study of elastin biosynthesis both important and difficult, since many of the conventional ways to analyze control of synthesis have had to be adapted to an unconventional system. Elastin also has an unique physiologic role: it is the biological rubber used by vertebrates to absorb mechanical stress with perfect recoil, most significantly in the integumentary, pulmonary, and vascular systems, but also in a variety of specialized elastic ligaments.

This article will attempt to describe our present understanding of the known and potential control mechanisms involved in production and destruction of elastin, with particular attention to experimental approaches. The reader is referred to other contemporary articles for details of elastin structure (Sandberg and Davidson, 1984), cross-linking (Rucker and Tinker, 1977; Eyre *et al.*, 1984; Kagan, this volume), cell-free translation of elastin mRNA (Foster *et al.*, 1983), association with nutritional and disease states (Sandberg *et al.*, 1981b; Rÿhanen and Uitto, 1982; Rosenbloom, 1984; Tinker and Rucker, 1985; Davidson, 1985), and the nature of elastin-associated proteins (Cleary and Gibson, 1983).

A. General Aspects of Elastin Structure

The elastic properties of the most specialized elastic tissue, the ligamentum nuchae of grazing ungulates, were appreciated by crossbow fabricators more than 700 years ago. The elastic fiber has been recognized as a morphologic entity for over a century, and it was readily assigned as the structural basis for the elasticity of lung, skin, and blood vessels. Several characteristic histologic stains (Frances and Robert, 1984; Gomori, 1950; Brury and Wallington, 1976) reveal elastic fibers in good contrast.

1. Elastic Fiber Morpholology

When elastic tissue is stained with Verhoef–Van Gieson (Verhoef, 1908) or similar agents, a characteristic wavy fibrous network is revealed, which represents the elastic fiber in its retracted state. If tissues are fixed under tension or stress, elastic fibers lose their wavy appearance and exhibit weak birefringence with polarized optics, suggesting reorientation of their substructure into a more ordered array.

At the ultrastructural level, most preparations of elastic tissue appear highly amorphous and stain poorly with conventional techniques. Tannic acid has been the most successful mordant for ultrastructural analysis.

In many tissues, elastic fibers consist of two entities, the amorphous elastin component and a microfibrillar component. This latter structure, a 8- to 15-nm microfibril, has been thought to provide a developmental framework for the deposition of elastin (Greenlee et al., 1966; Ross and Bornstein, 1969; Fahrenbach et al., 1966; Gibson and Cleary, 1983), but elastin can occur in its apparent absence (e.g., in elastic cartilage; Quintarelli et al., 1979). An extremely comprehensive and detailed review of this component is available (Clearly and Gibson, 1983). Recent data may suggest that some of the preparations of so-called microfibrillar protein (Ross and Bornstein, 1969) are extremely similar if not identical to type VI collagen (Knight et al., 1984), although immunohistochemical evidence suggests that there are other proteins unique to elastic fibers whose staining does not codistribute with that of type VI collagen. Type VI collagen is not uniquely associated with elastic fibers (von der Mark et al., 1984) and is unlikely to be the microfibrillar protein.

2. ELASTIN COMPOSITION AND STRUCTURE

There are many unusual features of elastin chemistry. One of the original methods used to isolate the protein was extraction in 0.1 N NaOH at 98°C for 45 min (Lansing et al., 1952). Despite the numerous published studies which have claimed greater purification or less contamination (see Davidson, 1985, for review), from the point of view of establishing the nature and composition of elastin there has been no definitive improvement in the isolation technique. Elastin is a highly cross-linked polymer of a soluble subunit, tropoelastin. Early studies had shown that base-insoluble elastin was cleaved by oxalic acid hydrolysis to generate peptides, the larger of which was called α-elastin, sharing with the tropoelastin monomer the property of *coacervation,* i.e., the formation of aggregates at higher (>20°C) temperatures (Partridge et al., 1955).

Elastin is extremely rich in glycine, valine, alanine, and proline. It is very low in charged residues. Although elastin contains some hydroxyproline, apparently produced by the same enzymatic process as in collagen, the proteins are quite unrelated in primary structure with one possible exception (Smith et al., 1981). The amino acid composition of elastins from higher vertebrates appears highly conserved. Elastin hydrolysates are characteristically devoid of histidine, tryptophan, and methionine, but may contain a small amount (two residues) of cysteine (Yoon *et al.*, 1985). A very important characteristic of elastin is the presence of two kinds of tetrafunctional cross-links, desmosine and its isomer isodesmosine, which are the ultimate products of the oxidative deamination of three adjacent lysyl residues and their condensation with a fourth lysyl ε-amino group to form a pyridinium ring structure stable to acid hydrolysis (see Kagan, this volume). Cross-link formation is a critical step in elastin synthesis. In most tissues, the amount of desmosine plus isodesmosine is proportional to the amount of insoluble elastin (Starcher, 1977). The production of reactive aldehydes from the lysyl ε-amino groups is catalyzed by lysyl oxidase, a copper-dependent amine oxidase (see Kagan, this volume, for an extensive review).

Copper-deficient pigs were known to have severe connective tissue abnormalities, including aortic aneurysms (Shields *et al.*, 1962; Kadar *et al.*, 1977). Carnes and co-workers were able to isolate from copper-deficient aortas a soluble protein which had the amino acid composition of elastin but a much higher lysine content and no desmosines (Sandberg *et al.*, 1969; Smith *et al.*, 1972). This molecule, with an apparent molecular weight of 72,000, was named tropoelastin by analogy with the collagen nomenclature of the time.

To date, the primary structure of tropoelastin has been largely deduced from tryptic peptides which intrinsically lack the overlapping sequences needed to order the fragments. The structure of these peptides has been recently reviewed (Sandberg and Davidson, 1984). Several characteristic sequences are prominent, including a pentapeptide repeat (PGVGV), a hexapeptide repeat (PGVGVA), and a putative cross-link-site sequence (AAAKAAKF). The pentapeptide repeat is proposed to have the potential to form a "β-spiral" structure consisting of β-turn elements (Urry *et al.*, 1978, 1982), and the cross-link regions are proposed to be in a more rigid α-helical conformation (Gray *et al.*, 1973). However, other physical–chemical data (Torchia and Piez, 1973; Aaron and Gosline, 1981) argue for a highly anisotropic or random arrangement for the polypeptide chains in the relaxed state.

   a. Solubility Properties. Elastin is insoluble in 8 M urea, 6 M guanidinium hydrochloride plus dithiothreitol, hot alkali, and weak organic acids (Franzblau, 1971; Anwar, 1982). Elastin can be partially hydrolyzed by hot oxalic acid to produce soluble peptides of similar amino acid composition: α-elastin (>50,000 M_r) and β-elastin (10,000–50,000 M_r), the former having the property of coacervation upon warming (Partridge *et al.*, 1955). Elastin is readily hydrolyzed by pancreatic and leukocyte elastases and by pepsin, but many other enzymes apparently cut the molecule infrequently enough to leave the cross-linked network intact. Insoluble elastin is resistant to bacterial and vertebrate collagenases.

Tropoelastin is soluble in physiologic solutions and dilute acetic acid but coacervates upon warming. At pH 5 in ammonium formate buffer, tropoelastin partitions into the organic phase of a buffer–butanol–propanol mixture, indicating its extremely hydrophobic nature. Tropoelastin contains many lysyl residues before it is cross-linked, and it is readily cleaved by many proteases, including trypsin. Thus, protease inhibitors are necessary during the purification of the protein.

b. Cross-Links. Recent analysis of tropoelastin cDNA sequences (see below) tends to confirm the hypotheses put forward by Gray *et al.* (1973) and Anwar and associates (1977) that four lysyl residues from two tropoelastin chains condense to form the desmosine structure, although only one report of a multimeric intermediate has been published (Abraham and Carnes, 1978). Many cross-link intermediates, however, have been described, and desmosine formation can occur in tissue over several days (Kagan, this volume). Interestingly, desmosines have recently been found in eggshell membrane proteins of birds and lizards (Leach *et al.*, 1981; Cox *et al.*, 1982); moreover, the avian oviduct is enriched in the enzyme lysyl oxidase (Harris *et al.*, 1980). There are numerous structural intermediates which have been isolated from elastic tissue. Presumably some of these are involved in the biosynthetic pathway of cross-link formation, but others may be artifacts of the hydrolysis process (Eyre *et al.*, 1984).

B. Biological Significance of Elastin

1. TISSUE DISTRIBUTION

Elastin is widely distributed in connective tissues, but it is most abundant in the thoracic aorta of warm-blooded vertebrates and the ligamentum nuchae of ungulates, where it comprises 40 to >60% of the dry mass of adult tissue. Elastin is prominent in the walls of all the major arteries and arterioles in the form of elastic lamellae: concentric, fenestrated cylinders of elastic tissue which surround the vessel lumen. Elastic fibers appear to be intimately associated with the vascular smooth muscle cell periphery (Clark and Glagov, 1985). Elastin is less prominent in venous structures. It is also an important constituent of lung tissue, both in alveolar septa and in visceral pleura (Horowitz *et al.*, 1976), as well as the deeper layers of the skin. Elastin is a constituent of the true vocal cords, the interspinous ligamenta flava of humans, elastic cartilage such as in the ear, and the digital flexor tendons of rodents (Sandberg *et al.*, 1981b). Elastin is also found in Bruch's membrane of the eye and the interstitium of the cervix. The relative proportions of amorphous elastin and the microfibrillar component vary as a function of the developmental maturity of these tissues (Greenlee *et al.*, 1966) and anatomic location (Cleary and Gibson, 1983).

2. Physiologic Role

Elastin appears to be uniquely designed to serve one function: the storage and return of mechanical energy. During systole, a considerable fraction of the hydraulic output of the heart is absorbed by distention of the thoracic aorta, which in turn provides elastic recoil during diastole. Lesser arteries complement this role. In pulmonary respiration, inhalation distends the elastic elements, which then provide the primary energy for emptying the air spaces of the lung. The nuchal ligament of grazing animals supports a large head, even during sleep, with little muscular exertion. Elastin in the skin serves to keep the tissue taut yet able to withstand considerable distortion. Elastin is almost always codistributed with collagen, a protein providing tensile strength, and the relative proportions of elastin and collagen, as well as their physical arrangement, determine the mechanical properties of most connective tissues.

3. Association with Pathologic States

Much of our understanding of the role of elastin comes from the pathologies associated with its absence or overabundance (Rÿhanen and Uitto, 1982; Rosenbloom, 1984; Davidson, 1985). In particular, pulmonary emphysema, the loss of elastic recoil in lung parenchyma, has come to attention as a disease involving the destruction of elastin. This destruction is thought to be mediated by the unregulated or stimulated activity of leukocyte elastases (Janoff and Carp, 1983). Humans genetically deficient in α1-antiprotease activity and many smokers are thus at high risk for the disease.

Cutis laxa is a genetic syndrome which frequently involves the loss of elastic tissue and is manifested as loose, sagging skin, joint hypermobility, and, in severe forms of the disease, pulmonary emphysema. The mode of inheritance is usually autosomal recessive. One case is reported with X-linkage, but it has been shown to result from a lysine oxidase deficiency (Byers *et al.*, 1980) which is secondary to defective copper metabolism (Peltonen *et al.*, 1983). Another rare elastic tissue disorder, pseudoxanthoma elasticum, results in abnormal accumulations of elastin in the frequently stretched areas of the skin, calcification of elastic fibers, rupture of Bruch's membrane (behind the retina), and occasional rupture of the visceral arteries (Rÿhanen and Uitto, 1982; Uitto, 1984).

Accumulations of elastin are noted in several rare skin disorders, such as Buschke–Ollendorf syndrome and elastosis perforans serpiginosa (Rÿhanen and Uitto, 1982; Uitto, 1984; Volpin *et al.*, 1978). Elastosis (the overaccumulation of elastic tissue) is characteristic of chronically sun-exposed skin (Smith *et al.*, 1962; Danielsen and Kobayasi, 1972; Johnston *et al.*, 1984) and perhaps older skin in humans. Elastic fibers are one of the constituents of the atherosclerotic plaque, probably being synthesized by the neointimal smooth muscle cells associated with the lesion. Elastosis is also reported in periductal regions of breast tumors (Adnet *et al.*, 1981; Reyes *et al.*, 1982) and some forms of liver fibrosis (Thung and Gerber, 1982). In animal models of emphysema, instillation of proteases destroys elastin (Kuhn *et al.*, 1976) but also stimulates nonfunctional resynthesis of the protein (reviewed in Clark *et al.*, 1983). Bleomycin treatment also appears transiently to stimulate lung elastin accumulation (Starcher *et al.*, 1978; Cantor *et al.*, 1984).

II. Molecular Biology

Elastin has only recently been accessible to the molecular biologist, and our present understanding of the overall organization of the gene is limited. Figure 1 depicts the current status of our information on the structural arrangement of the elastin gene, based on studies of the sheep (Davidson and Crystal, 1982; Davidson *et al.*, 1984a) and bovine (Cicila *et al.*, 1984; Rosenbloom, 1984) genes and a sheep cDNA clone (Yoon *et al.*, 1984, 1985).

A. *Organization of the Elastin Gene*

1. Size

Segments of the elastin gene have been isolated from sheep (Davidson *et al.*, 1984a), cow (Cicilia *et al.*, 1984), and human (Goldstein *et al.*,

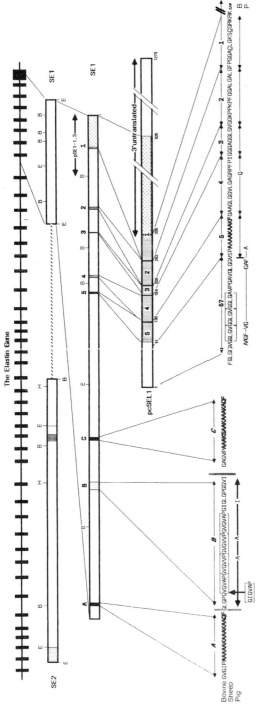

Fig. 1. Current concept of the elastin gene. The top line illustrates the probable dispersity of a hypothetical intact elastin gene, having < 7% coding sequence (solid vertical bars). Line 2 indicates the overall arrangement of two sheep genomic isolates, SE1 and SE2. Letters represent restriction enzyme sites (B = BamHI; E = EcoRI; H = HindIII). The dashed line represents an undetermined amount of genomic DNA separating the two clones, which are provisionally assigned to the same gene. Gray areas in SE2 represent the actual limits of the cloned DNA. 3′ sites were deduced by genomic mapping experiments. Line 3 shows the exon–intron map of the bovine gene (Rosenbloom, 1984). Exons 1–5 have been unambiguously identified at the 3′-terminus of SE1, and exon 1 largely consists of 3′-untranslated sequence (hatched area). Exons A–C are a synthesis of information from the bovine and sheep genes. Dark bars represent exons with potential cross-link sites, and dotted bars represent hydrophobic exons. The extent of the subclone used in most of the hybridization reactions in this laboratory (pSS1) is indicated as subclone pSE1–1.3. Below is shown the organization of a cDNA transcript derived from SE1, clone pcSEL1 (Yoon et al., 1984, 1985). The hatched area indicates the extent of correspondence of genomic and cDNA sequence. Line 5 indicates the conceptual translation of bovine (B) and sheep (S) DNA sequences derived from these exons, along with their relationship to the known porcine (P) tropoelastin amino acid sequences. Regions of homology are shown as horizontal lines with amino acid substitutions shown. In exon B, there appears to be an additional hexapeptide repeat unit present in the pig sequence. Peptide repeat units are indicated by brackets, and potential cross-link sites are shown in bold lettering.

1985) genomic libraries. Using purified elastin mRNA as a probe, an extensive region of the sheep genome was isolated from a genomic library (Davidson *et al.*, 1984a). Although the complete elastin gene has not been isolated, the sheep gene probably spans >40 kb (kilobases) of DNA, yet encodes a 3.5-kb mRNA product. The bovine elastin gene appears to have an extremely homologous structure to the sheep gene, even at the level of restriction enzyme sites (Rosenbloom, 1984); however, a recently reported human clone shows somewhat greater variation at the level of restriction enzyme patterns. Preliminary evidence, based on genomic Southern blot hybridization and quantitative dot hybridization with cloned elastin sequences, suggests that there is a single elastin gene in the sheep (Olliver *et al.*, 1986). The human elastin gene has recently been localized to chromosome 2 (Emanuel *et al.*, 1985).

2. INTRON–EXON RELATIONSHIPS

Initial evidence of the dilution of coding sequences in the elastin gene came from R-loop analysis of a 9.9-kb fragment of the sheep gene (SE1). These studies (Davidson *et al.*, 1984a) showed the presence of at least seven large R-loops corresponding to intervening sequences, interspersed with small regions (≤120 bp) of mRNA–DNA homology.

a. Sequence Analysis. DNA sequence analysis of the sheep and bovine genomic clones is incomplete, but a large amount of the 3'-terminus of the bovine gene has been sequenced as well as selected portions of the sheep gene. Figure 1 illustrates the current status of primary structural information. These studies, largely carried out by Rosenbloom and co-workers in collaboration with this laboratory (Rosenbloom, 1984), quantify the extremely dilute nature of the gene, which contains several small exons interrupted by enormous intervening sequence segments. Sequence analysis has also begun to align the protein sequences generated by Sandberg and co-workers (Sandberg and Davidson, 1984).

In contrast to the protein-coding portion of the gene, the 3'-untranslated region of the sheep elastin gene is found in a large uninterrupted sequence which, based upon cDNA sequence analysis, extends beyond the 3'-terminus of the clone SE1 (Yoon *et al.*, 1985). This exon contains at least 664 bases (973 in the bovine gene), and the 44 nucleotides at its 5'-terminus comprise the newly deduced carboxy-terminus of tropoelastin. The most intriguing aspect of the conceptual translation of this segment is the presence of two cysteine residues within an unusually basic, hydrophilic "tail" on the protein. Molecular hybridization analyses with the 3'-terminus of SE1 (pSE1–1.3 or pSS1) suggest considerable interspecific homology among the sheep (Davidson *et al.,* 1984b), cow (J. M. Davidson and R. P. Mecham, unpublished results), pig (Davidson *et al.,* 1985), human (Giro *et al.,* 1985), hamster (Raghow *et al.,* 1985), and rat (Frisch *et al.,* 1985) elastin genes. Since this subclone (pSS1) contains largely untranslated coding sequences (Yoon *et al.,* 1985), it likely represents a conserved area of the expressed portion of the elastin gene. Recent sequence analysis of bovine and human DNA indicates a very high degree (>90%) of nucleotide extent and sequence homology, which may suggest a significant role for unexpressed, 3' mRNA sequence (Ornstein *et al.,* 1985).

   b. Splice Sites. According to present information, splicing in the elastin gene follows conventional rules for acceptor and donor sequences (Breathnach and Chambon, 1981). Rosenbloom (1984) has reported that splicing sites appear to occur most frequently within glycine codons. Multiple translation products have been reported from elastin mRNA (mRNA$_e$) as differentially migrating protein bands on acrylamide–SDS gels (Davidson *et al.,* 1982a; Foster *et al.,* 1980a, 1982, 1983), and the possibility exists that these forms arise from differential splicing of a single pre-mRNA$_e$ transcript. Raju *et al.* (1985) recently reported the isolation of two bovine cDNA clones which retain enough sequence homology to suggest either alternative splicing or multiple gene products.

3. Exons as Domains

   The nature of the exons in the bovine elastin gene has been deduced by comparison of genomic DNA sequences (Cicila *et al.,* 1984) with the sequence of a 1.2-kb sheep elastin cDNA clone (Yoon *et al.,* 1984; Rosenbloom, 1984) and the known protein sequence of porcine tropoelastin (Sandberg *et al.,* 1980; Sandberg and Davidson, 1984). Interestingly, the exons derived from the translated region of the gene are representative of the two domains of the elastin molecule: cross-link sites and hydrophobic regions of elastin genes (Fig. 1). Cross-link sites are interspersed between hydrophobic sequences including some of the well-known peptide repeat regions, consistent with the concept that intervening sequences serve to isolate and preserve functional protein domains by reducing the frequency of genetic recombination (Gilbert, 1978). As discussed above, the final, hydrophilic domain of the translated portion of the mRNA is continuous with a large exon encoding the 3'-untranslated region of elastin mRNA, contains two cysteine residues, and is highly homologous in deduced sequences from sheep, bovine, and human DNA.

a. *Evidence for Multiple Genes.* Several investigators have put forward the hypothesis that distinct genetic types of elastin are present in cartilage (Keith *et al.,* 1978; Field *et al.,* 1978) or during aortic development (Foster *et al.,* 1980a; Barrineau *et al.,* 1981). In addition, studies of the compositional changes in aortic elastin have also prompted speculation that different elastin genes might be expressed during the aging of the vasculature (John and Thomas, 1972; Spina *et al.,* 1983). Biosynthetic studies, however, have largely ruled out the presence of a cartilage-specific elastin (Heeger and Rosenbloom, 1980; Foster *et al.,* 1980b). In the chicken aorta, an elastin-like protein, called "tropoelastin a," is described (Foster *et al.,* 1980a; Karr and Foster, 1984; Rich and Foster, 1984), but its relationship to the two forms of authentic tropoelastin is unclear. While amino acid microsequencing of the signal peptide sequence of sheep tropoelastin has shown microheterogeneity at two positions (Davidson *et al.,* 1982b), and a number of investigators have shown newly synthesized tropoelastin to run as a doublet on SDS–polyacrylamide gels (Davidson *et al.,* 1982a,b; Foster *et al.,* 1984; Mecham *et al.,* 1984b), the relationship between the upper band of these doublets and tropoelastin a from the chick is not certain. Structurally distinct bovine cDNA clones have been reported (Raju *et al.,* 1985).

b. *Evidence for a Single Gene.* A number of lines of evidence argue for a unique elastin gene. Genomic blot experiments have qualitatively identified unique fragments of the sheep and human genome which respond as single-copy genes (P. A. LuValle and J. M. Davidson, unpublished results). Preliminary gene-copy-number experiments in the sheep suggest the same conclusion (Olliver *et al.,* 1985). Thus, if other forms of the elastin gene are present, they must lack significant homology to the 3'-genomic and cDNA probes used to detect elastin DNA sequences. In addition, the role of allelic variation or polymorphism within the elastin gene is unresolved. Although the two large fragments of the sheep elastin gene (SE1 and SE2; Davidson and Crystal, 1982) are not contiguous, cross-hybridization of the two recombinant clones has not identified any closely homologous regions as might be expected if SE1 and SE2 were different elastin genes (P. A. Luvalle and J. M. Davidson, unpublished results). Definitive isolation and sequence analysis of tropoelastin a, its gene, or its mRNA will be required to clarify the issue of multiple genes.

B.   Structure of Elastin mRNA

Because elastin is highly expressed in certain tissues during development, isolation and characterization of elastin mRNA and the cloning of cDNAs has been possible.

1.   Size

Tropoelastin contains about 850 amino acid residues, yet elastin mRNA from several species is at least 3500 nucleotides long (Davidson and Crystal, 1982; Burnett et al., 1981; Giro et al., 1985; Frisch et al., 1985; Davidson et al., 1985a), implying a large amount of untranslated mRNA sequence. Sequence analysis of a sheep elastin cDNA clone has confirmed the presence of a 974-nucleotide 3'-untranslated region, about half of which is present in the 3'-terminal genomic clone, pSE1-1.3 (pSS1; Yoon et al., 1985). Thus much of the additional mass of mRNA$_e$ is accounted for in this region. Human and bovine genomic clones appear to contain the entire 3'-untranslated region in a single exon (Cicila et al., 1984; Rosenbloom, 1984; Ornstein et al., 1985). In the rat, an additional mRNA species about 4.2 kb in length has been observed (Frisch et al., 1985).

2.   Sequence Content

Two cDNA clones of elastin mRNA have been isolated and characterized to date. The first cDNA to be described was a short (200 nucleotides) segment from the 3'-untranslated region of chick aortic mRNA$_e$ (Burnett et al., 1981), and more recently results have appeared describing the complete sequence of a 1.3-kb cDNA clone derived from sheep mRNA$_e$ (Yoon et al., 1984, 1985). A number of interesting features of the protein were revealed (Fig. 1): (1) the carboxy-terminus of the protein contains two cysteinyl residues within a very basic peptide sequence; (2) at least one potential cross-link site with the predicted arrangement of paired lysyl residues within a cluster of alanyl residues (. . . AAAAKAAKFGAA . . .) was confirmed; (3) DNA sequencing identified 58 previously unreported amino acid residues at the carboxy-terminus of ovine tropoelastin which overlap convincingly with known porcine sequence; (4) alignment and assignment of some of the carboxy-terminal, porcine tryptic peptides was made.

Full-length cDNA clones of mRNA$_e$ may be exceedingly difficult to obtain because of the high G + C content of the molecule, which likely promotes formation of secondary structures resistant to reverse transcription. Thus, despite the low exon:intron ratio (<0.1), considerable effort is being directed toward sequence analysis of the elastin gene. It may take some time before the primary structure of tropoelastin is determined.

3. UNTRANSLATED TERMINI

Although several other mRNAs are known to contain large 3'-untranslated regions, their role in RNA processing or utilization is unknown. This area of mRNAs is often highly divergent among isotypes and species; however, homology has been reported among α-actin 3'-termini as well (Ponte *et al.*, 1984), and it can only be speculated that the striking conservation of sequence in this region may contribute in some way to the function of the mRNA. Specific sequences near the polyadenylation site seem to be generally important for addition of poly(A), but the length of the 3'-terminus in elastin mRNA is much greater than needed for adenylation signals. It is known that the entire 3'-terminal segment is contained in one exon in bovine and human genes (Cicila *et al.*, 1984; Rosenbloom, 1984; Ornstein *et al.*, 1985), and this is likely to be true of the sheep gene as well. The 5'-terminus of neither the mRNA nor the gene has yet been isolated.

4. ALTERNATIVE SPLICING—EVIDENCE FOR MULTIPLE RNAS

One intriguing explanation for the multiple forms of elastin proposed by several laboratories would be differential splicing of primary gene transcripts in either a tissue-specific or developmentally regulated fashion. Such processes are known to occur with many other proteins including fibronectin (Tamkun *et al.*, 1984; Kornblihtt *et al.*, 1984; Schwarzbauer *et al.*, 1983). Two species of elastin mRNA have been clearly resolved in Northern blots from rat smooth muscle cells (Frisch *et al.*, 1985), but their relationship to the translation products is not known. Two different bovine cDNA clones have been reported (Raju *et al.*, 1985). The protein mass difference most investigators have reported for the tropoelastin doublets seen by SDS–PAGE is about 1000–2000 Da (Karr *et al.*, 1981; Foster *et al.*, 1983; Rich and Foster, 1984; Davidson *et al.*, 1982b), which would correspond to about 60 nucleotides in the mRNA$_e$, a rather small difference to be resolved in a 3500-nucleotide molecule. Since the doublets are seen in translation products, posttranslational modification is also an unlikely explanation for their differential electrophoretic mobility. Alternative splicing would be unlikely to explain the significant compositional differences reported for tropoelastin "a" (e.g., a high cysteine and histidine content).

III.   Biosynthesis and Secretion

Much of the biosynthetic machinery for elastin production is quite conventional with respect to other secretory proteins. Thus, only the unique or critical aspects of elastin biosynthesis need be discussed in this section. Figure 2 schematically illustrates our current concept of cellular elastin synthesis.

A.   Transcription, Translation, and Translocation

The details of elastin gene transcription have not been described. The diagram shown suggests the likelihood that $mRNA_e$ is capped. Based on current understanding of elastin gene structure (Davidson *et al.*, 1984a; Rosenbloom, 1984), a prodigious amount of splicing occurs after transcription, which may serve as a means of regulating $mRNA_e$ levels. Capped, spliced, and polyadenylated $mRNA_e$ is probably transported to the site of translation as a messenger ribonucleoprotein particle.

Elastin mRNA is translated on membrane-bound polysomes (Ry̆hanen *et al.*, 1978) and in the reticulocyte lysate (Burnett *et al.*, 1980; Foster *et al.*, 1981; Davidson *et al.*, 1982a) as an M_r 72,000–74,000 polypeptide. A 26-residue signal peptide is present in the cell-free translation product of $mRNA_e$ from both chick aorta (Karr *et al.*, 1981) and sheep nuchal ligament (Davidson *et al.*, 1982b), and the secreted form of tropoelastin is therefore about M_r 2000 smaller based on electrophoretic mobility. The 26-residue signal sequence in sheep tropoelastin is analogous to that of other secreted proteins; however, sequence microheterogeneity may indicate allelic variation in elastin structure.

Based on the foregoing information, the higher molecular weight forms of tropoelastin ("proelastin") that have been described in the literature (Foster *et al.*, 1978; Heng-Khoo *et al.*, 1979; Rucker *et al.*, 1979), are likely artifacts of isolation; however, tropoelastin may in fact be tightly associated with proteases or other peptides under certain circumstances (Mecham *et al.*, 1976; Mecham and Foster, 1977; Romero *et al.*, 1985). Evidence has recently been presented to suggest that rat smooth muscle cells secrete a larger (M_r 77,000) form of tropoelastin which is processed to an M_r 71,000 product (Chipman *et al.*,

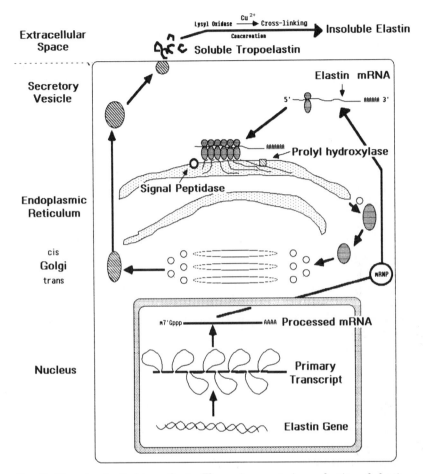

FIG. 2. Steps in elastin biosynthesis. The major events in production of elastin are indicated in this scheme. Potential regulation may occur at each point, and various pathological processes may also affect each stage. Not shown are the equally or more complex pathways by which elastin may be degraded, nor are indicated the nature or location of possible interactions with other matrix components.

1985). Interestingly, rat and hamster mRNA$_e$ is larger than that of other species (Frisch *et al.*, 1985; Raghow *et al.*, 1985).

As yet, no evidence of translational control of elastin synthesis has been found. Pretranslational control has thus far been the predominant mechanism (Davidson and Crystal, 1982; Burnett *et al.*, 1982); however, it has been observed that elastin-synthesizing tissues appear to have intrinsically different translational efficiencies. In the sheep, lung tissue appeared to produce far more elastin molecules per $mRNA_e$ molecule than did nuchal ligament cells (Davidson *et al.*, 1981, 1984b). Detailed studies of transit time, elongation rates, and initiation rates are now required to establish this potential level of control. Stability of $mRNA_e$ may also play a role in regulation of expression. For example, recent evidence suggests that glucocorticoids may act on collagen synthesis at a posttranscriptional level, apparently by affecting mRNA half-lives (Hamalainen *et al.*, 1985).

B.   Hydroxylation

Although hydroxyproline was described in elastin some time ago, its role in elastin biology is unknown. Elastin polypeptidyl proline is cotranslationally hydroxylated by the membrane-bound, endoplasmic reticulum enzyme, proline hydroxylase. This enzyme, whose function is critical to collagen synthesis and triple-helix thermostability, may act adventitiously on elastin prolyl residues within appropriate primary sequences in elastin-synthesizing cells that are simultaneously producing collagen. Hydroxyproline seems unnecessary for tropoelastin secretion or stability, since several triple-helix-disrupting proline analogs (Rosenbloom and Cywinsky, 1976b) and the iron chelator α,α'-dipyridyl (Uitto *et al.*, 1976) have no effect on tropoelastin secretion.

As elaborated below, ascorbic acid, the vitamin necessary for prolyl hydroxylation, exerts a negative effect on elastin accumulation in cell culture (Dunn and Franzblau, 1982; Faris *et al.*, 1984) and also appears to suppress elastin production (J. Alford, P. A. LuValle, and J. M. Davidson, unpublished observations). It has been proposed that hydroxyprolyl residues may destabilize the conformation of tropoelastin molecules (Bhatnagar *et al.*, 1978).

C.   Transport and Exocytosis

The kinetics of secretion of tropoelastin have been evaluated in suspension cultures cells from the 17-day embryonic chick aorta (Kao *et al.*, 1982). These authors concluded that secretion was a first-order process with a secretion time of about 1 hr. Since the time for synthesis of nascent elastin chains is estimated at 8–15 min, these molecules appear to move through a complex secretory pathway.

Elastin leaves the cell via the classical pathway for protein secretion. After signal peptide cleavage, completed chains traverse the endoplasmic reticulum (Saunders and Grant, 1984) to the Golgi apparatus (Damiano *et al.*, 1984) and reach the cell surface in spinous secretory vesicles ("acanthosomes," Fahrenbach *et al.*, 1966). The fact that tropoelastin was detected in the trans Golgi apparatus was somewhat surprising, since there is no evidence of processing, i.e., glycosylation, of the molecule before secretion. Elastic fibers show an intimate association of amorphous elastin with a microfibrillar glycoprotein component, which might explain the need to traverse the Golgi region.

Secretion of elastin is perturbed by anticytoskeletal drugs (Uitto *et al.*, 1976). Recently, the sodium ionophore monensin has also been shown to block tropoelastin secretion in smooth muscle cells (Frisch *et al.*, 1985). Interestingly, this also appeared to reduce the synthesis of tropoelastin by a repression of elastin mRNA accumulation. These results suggest a possible feedback control mechanism which would couple protein export with synthesis or stability of gene transcripts.

D. Degradation and Turnover

Tropoelastin is very sensitive to proteolysis before cross-linking has occurred. One study suggested that tropoelastin copurified with a serine protease which contributed to this degradation (Mecham and Foster, 1978). There is scant evidence for the intracellular degradation of tropoelastin, although incorporation of amino acid analogs can reduce the production of tropoelastin (Rosenbloom and Cywinski, 1976a), presumably by degradation of defective molecules. Although endogenous protease inhibitors would be expected to reduce proteolysis of secreted tropoelastin, our laboratory has found that human skin fibroblasts from normal (Sephel and Davidson, 1986) and abnormal individuals (Giro *et al.*, 1985) can degrade tropoelastin by a cell-associated process. Similar observations have been made for smooth muscle cells (Nakao *et al.*, 1980) and fibroblasts (Bourdillon *et al.*, 1980). Our data would suggest that normal fibroblasts degrade a very small fraction (~1% per hour) of newly synthesized elastin. It has recently been suggested that a kallikrein-like activity could be responsible for fragmentation of tropoelastin in copper-deficient chicks (Romero *et al.*, 1985).

Degradation of insoluble elastin can have major pathologic consequences and is frequently mediated by inflammatory cells. Polymorphonuclear granulocytes and macrophages harbor elastolytic proteinases which probably account for the majority of elastin destruction. Fibroblast elastases may play a lesser role. Under normal conditions, elastin turnover is minimal. Tracer studies, following the fate of radiolabeled lysine in insoluble elastin, have consistently shown that turnover was incredibly low, with protein half-lives on the order of years (Slack, 1954; Lefevre and Rucker, 1980). Remodeling of elastin must therefore occur at an extremely slow rate. Studies measuring the amount of desmosine in urine (King *et al.,* 1980) confirm that elastin degradation in humans proceeds very slowly.

IV. ASSEMBLY OF ELASTIC FIBERS

A. *Coacervation: A Self-Assembly Process?*

Under physiologic conditions, tropoelastin spontaneously aggregates into an insoluble precipitate. At reduced temperature, cross-link formation by cultured smooth muscle cells was retarded, suggesting that coacervation may be a primary event in the extracellular association of tropoelastin monomers into elastic fibers (Narayanan *et al.,* 1978). It is not known how cells manage to keep tropoelastin in a soluble form prior to secretion, and it is quite likely that accretion of tropoelastin monomers into aggregates occurs very near the cell surface.

B. *Association of Tropoelastin Subunits*

Additional, nonhydrophobic forces may come into play during tropoelastin association. Abraham and Carnes (1978) have described a dimeric form of the molecule, which could represent an assembly intermediate. The presence of two cysteines in an extremely hydrophilic C-terminus (Yoon *et al.,* 1985) could indicate a role for this domain in intermolecular interactions. Recent studies have shown that tropoelastin can assume a fibrillar, banded configuration during coacervation (Bressan *et al.,* 1983), which may indicate the potential for tropoelastin monomers to associate laterally *in vitro.*

C. *Role of Other Matrix Components in Fiber Formation*

The biochemical nature of the morphological entity known as the elastic fiber microfibril is unknown (Cleary and Gibson, 1983). It is clear, however, that there are numerous structural glycoproteins found in association with elastin, and some of these may be involved in determining the actual site of elastic fiber deposition. In certain forms of autosomally inherited cutis laxa, microfibrillar components appear to be dissociated from the amorphous elastin in skin (Holbrook and Byers, 1982). These mutations could be particularly instructive for examining the interaction of elastin with other matrix macromolecules. In elastic cartilage, it would appear that deposition of elastin is facilitated by components of the cartilage matrix (Starcher and Mecham, 1981).

V. Regulation of Production

Because of the exceedingly slow turnover of elastin during adult life, most of the regulation of elastin synthesis occurs during a relatively narrow window of fetal and perinatal maturation. For example, quantitative chemical analyses of insoluble elastin accumulation in the human aorta indicate sharply tapering production by the end of the first year of life, virtually ending by the end of the first decade (Berry *et al.*, 1972). Certain types of pathologies, such as ultraviolet skin damage, pulmonary emphysema, fibrotic liver disease, atherosclerosis, and breast cancer may reactivate abnormal elastin synthesis in humans.

A. Developmentally Regulated Elastin Synthesis

1. Aorta

Insoluble elastin rapidly accumulates in the aorta of the chick (Lee *et al.*, 1977; Keeley, 1979; Keeley and Johnson, 1983; Gardner *et al.*, 1984), pig (Grant, 1967; Davidson *et al.*, 1985a), dog (Harkness *et al.*, 1957; Grant, 1967), and human (Berry *et al.*, 1972; Giro *et al.*, 1974) during the perinatal period. Biosynthetic rates have been determined in the chick (Lee *et al.*, 1977; Keeley and Johnson, 1983; Eichner and Rosenbloom, 1979), the rat (Rucker and Dubick, 1984; Sandberg *et al.*, 1981b), and the pig (Davidson *et al.*, 1985a). Each of these studies confirms the accumulation of insoluble elastin to be closely linked to a rapid induction of elastin synthesis in the medial tissue of the organ. Recent studies from this laboratory have further shown that aortic elastin synthesis varies as a function of distance from the heart, being highest (16% of total protein synthesis) in the thoracic aorta of the neonatal pig. Similar results were obtained in the newborn sheep (J. M. Davidson and G. C. Sephel, 1986). In the developing pig, induction of elastin synthesis progresses down the aorta after birth, reaching its maximal level in the abdominal aorta at 3 weeks (Davidson *et al.*, 1986).

Elastin synthesis has been extensively studied in the chick aorta (Barrineau *et al.*, 1981; Eichner and Rosenbloom, 1979; Burnett *et al.*, 1981; Gardner *et al.*, 1984; Keeley and Johnson, 1983; Lee *et al.*, 1976; Keeley, 1979), where elastin synthesis is dramatically induced between 12 and 14 days of embryonic life. Elastin continues to accumulate rapidly during the first several weeks of postnatal life. Recent studies indicate that the rate of elastin synthesis is largely determined by the availability of functional elastin mRNA (Burnett *et al.*, 1981, 1982; Barrineau *et al.*, 1981). Two forms of elastin appear to be differentially regulated in chick aorta (Barrineau *et al.*, 1981).

Rat aorta also showed a transient, position-dependent burst of elastin synthesis in the perinatal period (Sandberg *et al.*, 1981a; Keeley and Johnson, 1986). The cloning of a cDNA from human fetal aortic mRNA$_e$ indicates a high level of elastin gene expression in this organ as well (Ornstein *et al.*, 1984).

2. LUNG

Elastin plays a critical role in lung function. In the sheep, elastin synthesis is barely detectable at the glandular stage of development (60 fetal days) but rises to about 1.5% of total protein synthesis by the time of birth (Shibahara *et al.*, 1981). Morphologic and immunohistological studies of the tissue confirm this pattern and illustrate the progressive maturation of elastic fibers in the lung interstitium (Fukuda *et al.*, 1984). Elastin accumulation has been evaluated in the rat lung (Myers *et al.*, 1983; Dubick *et al.*, 1981), which appears to be more immature at the time of birth, since the rate of elastin accumulation is highest in the organ 2 weeks after birth.

Elastin synthesis in the chick lung has been shown to commence on about day 14 of development (Eichner and Rosenbloom, 1979; Keeley, 1979; Barrineau *et al.*, 1981; Rucker and Dubick, 1984). Elastin synthesis is virtually unmeasurable in normal adult lung tissue, suggesting that turnover of elastin is insignificant.

3. NUCHAL LIGAMENT

The most highly specialized elastic tissue is the nuchal ligament (ligamentum nuchae) of the ungulates. This is a large cord of elastic tissue which inserts at the back of the skull and on many of the thoracic and lumbar vertebrae. It probably functions to provide passive support to the massive head of grazing animals which frequently sleep standing up. Cleary *et al.* (1967) showed clear chemical evidence for the rapid accumulation of elastin in this structure in the calf during the latter half of fetal life. Elastin comprises nearly 60% by weight of the adult tissue, collagen being the other major protein.

Explant culture of sheep nuchal ligament in the presence of radioactive amino acids demonstrated a logarithmic increase in the rate of elastin synthesis in the latter half of fetal life (Davidson *et al.*, 1982a), which is reflected in increased $mRNA_e$ levels (Davidson *et al.*, 1982a, 1984b). Cells (fibroblasts) derived from nuchal ligament produce substantial quantities of elastin in primary and secondary culture (Sear *et al.*, 1978; Mecham *et al.*, 1981; see below). The studies also showed the progressive differentiation of nuchal ligament from collagen synthesis to elastin synthesis. The nuchal ligament is likely to produce large quantities of the putative microfibrillar component, at least in the early part of its development, but no clear candidate has been identified in biosynthetic or biochemical studies (Cleary and Gibson, 1983).

B. *In Vivo Modulation of Elastic Tissues*

Elastin synthesis per se is difficult to study *in vivo* because of the rapid insolubilization of tropoelastin. However, a number of studies have provided quantitative data on the rates of accumulation of soluble and insoluble elastin in connective tissues.

1. LUNG

Elastin accumulation has been followed in the chick (Barrineau *et al.*, 1981) and rat lung (Dubick and Rucker, 1984) by both chemical and biosynthetic labeling studies. These data indicate a rapid formation of insoluble elastin shortly after birth in both species (Clark *et al.*, 1983). Deprivation of nutritional copper resulted in diminished elastin content of the tissue. Copper deficiency has also been evaluated in the pig (Soskel *et al.*, 1982) and hamster lung (Soskel *et al.*, 1984) with respect to elastin accumulation. Interestingly, despite the increased content of soluble elastin (tropoelastin), total elastin content of the hamster tissues was relatively unaltered.

In the hamster, bleomycin (Clark *et al.*, 1983; Cantor *et al.*, 1983) and elastase (or papain) instillation (Kuhn *et al.*, 1976) have also been used to develop models of lung disease–fibrosis and emphysema, respectively. Both types of lung injury result in increased rates of degradation of elastin, as measured by desmosine, in either lung lavage or urine samples (Clark *et al.*, 1983); however, there appears to be a compensatory mechanism in each case which results in the relatively rapid (1 week) burst of resynthesis of elastin. In the elastase model, turnover of elastin can continue for somewhat longer, likely due to the chronic inflammatory state of these lungs (Kuhn *et al.*, 1976; King *et al.,* 1980). In any case, physiologic indicators would suggest that the newly accumulated elastin is nonfunctional with respect to restoring proper alveolar ventilation.

2. Skin

Few quantitative data are available on the synthesis of elastin by skin. Morphologic studies indicate that elastin accumulation commences at about 20 weeks of gestation in humans (Smith and Holbrook, 1982; Smith *et al.,* 1982) and rises to about 1–2% of skin mass by adulthood. During human aging, the skin gradually becomes less elastic, and histologically there is less elastin found in the superficial dermis (Braverman and Fonferko, 1982; Frances and Robert, 1984) in the so-called elaunin and oxytalan fibers. Part of the loss of elasticity may also be due to fragmentation of the elastic fibers rather than complete destruction.

Several disease states result in the abnormal loss or accumulation of elastin in the skin (Davidson, 1985a; Rÿhanen and Uitto, 1982). Reduced skin elastin content is found in cutis laxa, anetoderma, and a form of atrophoderma. Increased elastin content is suggested in solar elastosis, elastosis perforans serpiginosa, pseudoxanthoma elasticum, the Buschke–Ollendorf syndrome (Rÿhanen and Uitto, 1982; Uitto, 1984; Frances and Robert, 1984), and a newly described condition, elastoderma (Kornberg *et al.,* 1985).

3. Blood Vessels

Elastin appears to accumulate in the atherosclerotic plaque (Ross, 1981). The number of elastic lamellae, and presumably elastin content, is increased in hypertensive blood vessels (Wolinsky and Glagov, 1969), reiterating the possibility that there is a feedback mechanism in the elastic tissue of the aorta and the vascular smooth muscle cell which responds to increased stress. This possibility is reinforced by experimental hypertension studies in the chick (Gardner *et al.,* 1984) and the rat (Keeley and Johnson, 1986).

Elastic fibers are diminished and a lowered desmosine content is reported in Marfan syndrome (Derouette *et al.,* 1981; Abraham *et al.,* 1982; Halme *et al.,* 1982), a heritable connective tissue disease of unknown etiology. Copper deficiency in pigs produces hypertension and aortic hypertrophy (Shields *et al.,* 1962). Large amounts of tropoelastin accumulate in the affected tissue, a major boon to the chemical characterization of the molecule. This laboratory has recently shown that relative elastin synthesis is increased nearly fourfold in the thoracic region of the copper-deficient aorta, probably by the induction of mRNA$_e$ (Hill and Davidson, 1986). It is not known whether hypertension or the failure of elastin to cross-link can directly induce elevated elastin synthesis.

C. In Vitro Expression of Elastin

In the last decade, it has been possible to demonstrate directly the synthesis of elastin by cultured mammalian cells, an important entry into the study of regulation of elastin synthesis.

1. SMOOTH MUSCLE CELLS

Vascular smooth muscle cells from a wide variety of species produce elastin in culture. Initial studies demonstrated the accumulation of elastin or desmosines by primate (Narayanan et al., 1976), pig (Abraham et al., 1974), and rabbit smooth muscle cells (Faris et al., 1976), as well as matrix-free cells from the embryonic chick aorta (Rosenbloom and Cywinski, 1976a; Uitto et al., 1976; Bressan et al., 1977; Myoshi et al., 1976). Subsequently, many of these systems have been used to demonstrate the precursor–product relationship between tropoelastin and elastin (Narayanan et al., 1978; Faris et al., 1976; Narayanan and Page, 1976). Most of these cultured cells will eventually produce an elastin-containing matrix which can be visualized ultrastructurally, but the rat smooth muscle cell (Jones et al., 1979) seems uniquely capable of accumulating large quantities of insoluble elastin in culture, arranged in alternating strata between cell layers reminiscent of the aortic wall (Oakes et al., 1982).

Since smooth muscle cells are capable of accumulating insoluble elastin to varying extents, lysine oxidase activity is present as well as other cofactors which might be required of assembly of elastic fibers.

2. FIBROBLASTS

a. Nuchal Ligament. The nuchal ligament of developing ungulates contains an apparently homogeneous population of fibroblastic cells (Fahrenbach et al., 1966). Initial studies by Sear et al. (1978) and subsequent reports by Mecham and co-workers (1981) established these as elastin-producing cells in culture. Like vascular smooth muscle cells from most species, these fibroblasts are not particularly efficient in accumulating insoluble elastin in the cell matrix, and most of the newly synthesized elastin is found in the culture medium (Mecham, 1981b).

Because nuchal ligament fibroblasts retain their differentiated state for several subcultivations, they have become an important tool in examining the control of elastin synthesis, as discussed further below. A critical observation made by Mecham et al. (1981) pertains to the differentiated state of these cells. Fibroblasts derived from ligaments of mid-gestation calf fetuses ("young" cells) produce low levels of elastin, while cells from near-term calves ("old" cells) produce high levels of soluble elastin. Differentiation, that is the increased production of elastin, can be induced in "young" fibroblasts by cultivation on "old" matrix (Mecham et al., 1984a). These cells also increase their chemotactic activity toward elastin peptides as a function of development (Mecham et al., 1984c).

Other recent studies with nuchal ligament fibroblasts have shown these cells to be chemotactically attracted to a synthetic polyhexapeptide of elastin sequence, VGVAPG (Senior et al., 1984). It is likely that these cells therefore bear cell-surface receptors for elastin. As discussed below, elastin synthesis in nuchal ligament cells is also hormonally responsive.

b. *Skin.* Adult, mammalian skin has a low but significant elastin content ($\leq 2\%$). This laboratory has recently confirmed the long-standing morphologic conclusion that elastin is synthesized by skin fibroblasts (Giro et al., 1985). These studies also demonstrated the presence of elastin mRNA in human skin cells. The further investigation of this property has led us to conclude that elastin production by cultured human skin fibroblasts is a very stable phenotypic property of normal cells, persisting over most of the normal lifespan of the fibroblast population (about 4×10^4 molecules per cell per hour; Sephel and Davidson, 1986). Current evidence would also suggest that *in vitro* aging does cause a diminution of elastin production after 35–40 population doublings. The relationship of this phenomenon to the loss of elastic fibers in aged skin is uncertain. Surprisingly, production levels by human skin fibroblasts in culture (Sephel and Davidson, 1986) approach those of vascular smooth muscle cells from the developing porcine aorta (Giro et al., 1984), which indicates either that human fibroblasts can utilize elastin mRNA more efficiently or that the growth conditions promote the expression of the elastin gene. In addition, cells from human fetal skin show a distinct developmental shift to elastin production between weeks 16 and 20 of gestation (Sephel et al., 1986a), which correlates well with the observed morphologic accumulation of elastin in fetal skin at about 22 weeks.

The human skin fibroblast is a well-established model and source for the biochemical analysis of many metabolic diseases, genetic and acquired, as emphasized by our recent evaluation of potential disease mechanisms in atrophoderma (Giro *et al.*, 1985). These studies have been extended to an evaluation of elastin production by a number of cell strains from patients with autosomal recessive cutis laxa, a disorder characterized by various derangements of and usually loss of dermal elastic fibers. Most of the strains examined show diminished elastin production, at least one defect being associated with abnormal elastin mRNA levels (Sephel *et al.*, 1986b). These studies have also observed the presence of a cell-associated elastolytic activity, perhaps similar to that described by Bourdillon *et al.* (1980). Since human skin fibroblasts produce elastin, they have considerable potential as a system for evaluation of the control of elastin synthesis and the nature of defective elastin synthesis or degradation in human diseases.

Although it seems likely that lung cells produce elastin during development, we have not detected significant quantities of elastin in three strains of human lung fibroblasts (G. Sephel and J. M. Davidson, unpublished results). Other human cell types have not been shown to produce elastin.

3.   Vascular Endothelial Cells

Vascular endothelium lies just inside the internal elastic lamina in normal muscular arteries. Three reports have now demonstrated by either chemical or immunological means the capacity of vascular endothelial cells to synthesize elastin *in vitro* (Carnes and Abraham, 1979; Cantor *et al.*, 1981; Mecham *et al.*, 1983). Little is known of the regulation of elastin synthesis in these cells, except for the observation that conditioned medium from vascular smooth muscle cell cultures stimulated elastin production in pulmonary artery endothelial cells (Mecham *et al.*, 1983).

4.   Chondrocytes

Elastic cartilage contains a population of cells which produce elastin as well as type II collagen and proteoglycans (Quintarelli *et al.*, 1979; Madsen *et al.*, 1983). Two studies have shown that the tropoelastin synthesized by these chondrocytes is immunologically and compositionally indistinguishable from tropoelastin derived from conventional sources (Heeger and Rosenbloom, 1980; Foster *et al.*, 1980b). Elastin appears to be more dispersed in chondrocyte matrix, as little amorphous elastin is seen (Quintarelli *et al.*, 1979). Although elastic fiber microfibrils are not obvious in ultrastructural preparations of elastic cartilage, the presence of excessive amounts of hyaluronate and other glycosaminoglycans may obscure the actual organization of the elastic fibers.

Chondrocytes from elastic cartilage apparently incorporate elastin into the extracellular matrix at a higher efficiency than other cells. It was shown that the bulk of the newly synthesized elastin appears in the cell-associated matrix of cultured ear chondrocytes, independent of the presence of β-aminopropionitrile (Starcher and Mecham, 1981). It is not clear whether the accumulation of proteoglycan can either alter the solubility of tropoelastin or simply "trap" proteins within the matrix. Tropoelastin is a relatively basic protein, which might be expected to interact with a polyanionic environment.

5. MESOTHELIAL CELLS

The pleura of the lungs have a substantial elastin content. Recent studies have shown that cultured mesothelial cells from rat and hamster pleura (Rennard *et al.*, 1984; Mandl *et al.*, 1985) have the capacity to synthesize elastin (desmosines) *in vitro*. These cell strains may be useful for the analysis of pleural elastin metabolism, since at least some experimental models of pulmonary emphysema exhibit accumulation of elastin in this site (Horowitz *et al.*, 1976).

D. *Manipulation of Elastin Synthesis and Accumulation*

Recent advances in experimental methodology and the availability of new reagents have enabled the more detailed examination of the potential regulatory steps in elastin biosynthesis. The key concept in approaching elastin chemistry is the fact that there are a great number of posttranslational modifications, in some cases unique to elastin, which act as potential sites for regulation. Many of the following studies have specifically tried to ask whether there is physiologic regulation at posttranslational steps, or whether chemicals which are known to have a net effect on elastin production or accumulation act at these stages.

1. AMINO ACID ANALOGS

Studies during the early 1960s had suggested that collagen synthesis, being dependent on prolyl hydroxylation and being enriched in

proline, could be regulated by the use of proline analogs (Kivirikko and
Mÿllyla, 1980). Since elastin also contains hydroxyproline, these experiments were extended to ask how elastin production was affected by
proline/hydroxyproline analogs such as azetidine-2-carboxylic acid and
3,4-dehydroproline (Schein *et al.*, 1977). These experiments, together
with results of experiments using α,α'-dipyridyl (Uitto *et al.*, 1976), an
iron chelator, indicated that elastin production was unaffected by
agents altering the presence of hydroxyproline (Rosenbloom and Cywinski, 1976b) but that proline substitution per se would reduce the
amount of elastin synthesized by freshly dissociated embryonic chick
aortic cells (Rosenbloom and Cywinski, 1976a). These studies clearly
established the fact that elastin does not require hydroxylation of proline, or triple-helix formation, to be secreted.

There appears to be some dispute in the literature as to the susceptibility of elastin and tropoelastin to collagenase (bacterial). Most studies have shown that insoluble elastin is totally resistant to this enzyme, but it is conceivable that the susceptible portions of the molecule
have been lost during purification. Nevertheless, hydroxyproline is
present at similar levels in both elastin and tropoelastin. Recently,
Smith *et al.* (1983) have reported a collagen-like sequence in chick
tropoelastin and the susceptibility of this form of the protein to purified
bacterial collagenase. It is not yet known whether this sequence is a
site of enzyme attack or whether the prolyl residues found in this
sequence are hydroxylated.

Valine is an abundant amino acid in elastin, and valine analogs
have a substantial effect on its synthesis (Rosenbloom, 1985).

2. GLUCOCORTICOIDS

Several lines of evidence suggest that glucocorticoids may play a role
in elastin production. Eichner and Rosenbloom (1979) demonstrated
that hydrocortisone acetate, injected into 8-day chick embryos, had a
striking, differential effect on the synthesis of collagen and elastin by
aortic tissue explants and that the normal program of differentiation of
the aorta was markedly altered. Collagen synthesis was strongly suppressed, while elastin synthesis was either unaffected or increased.
These results were confirmed and extended to lung tissue by Foster *et
al.* (1981).

Nuchal ligament fibroblasts from near-term ligament are stimulated by glucocorticoids (Mecham *et al.*, 1984b). Both hydrocortisone
and dexamethasone (10^{-7}–10^{-9} M) were effective, dexamethasone being more potent and stimulating elastin synthesis about twofold in

cultured ligament fibroblasts while depressing total protein synthesis by about 50%. The mechanism of stimulation is uncertain, although nuclear binding was demonstrated. Recent studies on the effects of dexamethasone on collagen metabolism suggest that it may act at a posttranscriptional, pretranslational level (Hamalainen et al., 1985). Thus, a detailed evaluation of elastin mRNA metabolism during steroid induction will be necessary.

3. Ascorbic Acid

Ascorbate is an essential cofactor for polypeptidyl prolyl and lysyl hydroxylation during collagen synthesis, but the role of hydroxyproline in elastin is uncertain. Interesting studies by Dunn and Franzblau (1982) have shown that prolonged exposure of calf arterial smooth muscle cells to ascorbate (50 μg/ml) reduced elastin accumulation substantially. Lower doses (2 μg/ml) seem to produce similar qualitative effects with lower toxicity (Faris et al., 1984). It has been proposed that hydroxyproline could interfere with the stability of the β-spiral structure proposed to exist in the hydrophobic domains of elastin (Bhatnagar et al., 1978). Increased hydroxylation of elastin in hyper-ascorbate-treated cells might have an effect on molecular stability.

Ascorbate has only been shown to alter elastin accumulation, not synthesis. In contrast, primary avian tendon cells (Schwartz et al., 1979) and human skin fibroblasts (Murad et al., 1983) are stimulated to produce more collagen by prolonged ascorbate exposure. Our laboratory, however, has recently tested the effects of ascorbate on elastin production by porcine vascular smooth muscle cells. Short-term exposure (1–3 days) to 50 μg/ml ascorbate reduced elastin production to 50% of controls (J. Alford, P. A. LuValle, and J. M. Davidson, unpublished results), suggesting that hypervitaminosis may have some direct effect on the synthesis of elastin.

4. Cyclic Nucleotides

Elastin-synthesizing cells respond to hormones and other stimuli. Second messengers such as the cyclic nucleotides and calcium could play a role in the regulation of elastin synthesis. Recent studies by Mecham et al. (1985) have shown that elastin synthesis in nuchal ligament cells is specifically stimulated by cyclic GMP and nonspecifically repressed by cyclic AMP. These authors further showed that cyclic AMP could reverse the effects of cyclic GMP, suggesting a potential control mechanism for up- and down-regulation of elastin synthesis.

5. CYTOSKELETAL DRUGS AND IONOPHORES

A number of selective poisons are available to help dissect the elastin secretory mechanism. As with most secretory proteins, colchicine, an antimicrotubular drug, efficiently arrested elastin secretion by chick aortic cells (Uitto *et al.*, 1976). Studies with rat smooth muscle cells have suggested that many agents which alter cell shape, such as cytochalasin B and nonadhesive substrates [poly(hydroxyethyl methacrylate)], can suppress elastin production (Frisch and Werb, 1983).

Consistent with immunohistochemical evidence for the Golgi-dependent secretory pathway, it has recently been shown that monensin, a monovalent cationophore, repressed secretion of elastin by rat smooth muscle cells (Frisch *et al.*, 1985). Interestingly, synthesis of tropoelastin and elastin mRNA levels were both progressively inhibited in secretion-defective cells. These results suggest a possible feedback regulatory mechanism for controlling the rate of tropoelastin gene expression.

6. EXTRACELLULAR MATRIX

Cell–matrix interactions are thought to play many critical roles in embryonic development and disease processes. The phenotype of the bovine nuchal ligament fibroblast is apparently dependent on components of the matrix, since cells derived from mid-gestation nuchal ligament fail to differentiate (produce high levels of elastin) when grown on tissue culture plastic yet increase their elastin production (Mecham *et al.*, 1984a) and chemotactic responsiveness to elastin peptides (Mecham *et al.*, 1984c) when cultivated on killed ligament from near-term fetuses. It is not yet clear which components of the matrix are responsible for this inductive/permissive effect, but purified collagen or elastin substrates were ineffective. This induction elicits a stable change in the ligament cell phenotype, since elastin production is maintained after serial subcultivation on plastic substrates.

E. Extracellular Degradation of Elastin and Elastic Fibers

Because elastin is such a long-lived inert protein, it is clear that destruction of elastic tissue has a major role in determining the physiologic state of most mammals. Many cells, both inflammatory and otherwise, contain elastin-degrading enzymes which have the potential for producing pathologic abnormalities of elastic tissue. Many diseases of the skin, lungs, and blood vessels involve the degradation of elastic tissue.

1. Elastolytic Proteinases

Several review articles have been published recently on the action of elastases and their naturally occurring inhibitors (see Janoff, 1983). A potent elastase is found in the polymorphonuclear granulocyte (neutrophil). This enzyme is very similar in primary structure and biochemical action to the digestive enzyme, pancreatic elastase. Elastin is one of many substrates these serine proteases will cleave, and there is nowhere near the substrate specificity found in collagenase, for example. Neutrophil elastase is thought to be largely regulated by α1-antiprotease levels (Gadek et al., 1981). Macrophages, on the other hand, release a metalloelastase (Banda and Werb, 1981) which appears to be tightly complexed to an endogenous peptide inhibitor (R. M. Senior, personal communication). The presence of the inhibitor may play a role in confining the site of action of elastases to the immediate surroundings of the cell.

Inflammatory cells are unlikely to participate in normal regulation of elastin, but elastin-producing cells such as fibroblasts (Bourdillon et al., 1980; Szendroi et al., 1984; Giro et al., 1985) and smooth muscle cells (Bourdillon et al., 1980) appear to have the potential of degrading both newly synthesized and insoluble elastin. While normal human skin fibroblasts degrade tropoelastin quite slowly (Sephel and Davidson, 1986), it has recently been demonstrated that skin fibroblasts from a patient with a rare skin atrophy produced much higher levels of elastase and were able to degrade tropoelastin in the culture medium, even in the presence of 10% serum (Giro et al., 1985). It is conceivable that elastin turnover takes part in the regulation of elastin accumulation, at least in skin.

2. Age-Related Elastin Destruction/Accumulation

One of the characteristics of human aging is the loss of elasticity and thinning of the skin, i.e., "sags and wrinkles." Histologically, skin of older individuals, especially in sun-exposed areas, shows a fragmentation and thickening of the elastic fibers as well as a loss of elastic fibers from the superficial dermis (Smith et al., 1962). Extremes of ultraviolet radiation exposure, particularly in Caucasians, lead to solar elastosis, in which there is an excessive accumulation of elastic fibers in the skin (Oikarinen *et al.*, 1985). Little is known about the mechanism of elastin destruction although ultraviolet radiation may be able to directly act on elastin (Johnston *et al.*, 1984).

Atherosclerosis involves elastin, since most of the advanced lesions are the result of accumulation of an extracellular matrix produced by vascular smooth muscle cells (Ross, 1981). It is not clear whether these neointimal smooth muscle cells produce abnormal amounts of elastin as a result of their hypertrophy and hyperplasia. Hypertension also induces a marked thickening of the arterial wall and an increase in the number of elastic lamellae (Wolinsky and Glagov, 1969). Recent evidence would suggest that there is a rapid, transient response by the medial smooth muscle cells to increased blood pressure. Elastin synthesis in the aortas of heminephrectomized rat showed a sharp increase within 2 weeks of treatment, whereas collagen content of the tissue continued to rise for several weeks (Keeley and Johnson, 1986). Thus, adult smooth muscle cells may be able to respond specifically to chronic injury (Ross, 1981) or to increased mechanical stress by producing elastin.

3. ELASTIN AND EMPHYSEMA

The most important elastin-associated health problem is pulmonary emphysema (Horowitz *et al.*, 1976; Sandberg *et al.*, 1981b; Clark *et al.*, 1983). There is a morphological loss of elastic tissue, particularly in the interalveolar septa, which inhibits efficient ventilation of the lung air spaces. Patients genetically deficient in α1-antiprotease have provided the best evidence linking destruction of elastin by inflammatory cell proteases to the disease (Gadek *et al.*, 1981). Cigarette smoke may also inactivate antiproteases (Janoff, 1983) or activate inflammatory cells. Emphysema-like diseases can be produced in animals by copper deficiency (Soskel *et al.*, 1983, 1984), enzyme instillation into the lungs (Kuhn *et al.*, 1976), and oxidant (chloramine-T) intoxication (Abrams *et al.*, 1981).

F.   *Abnormal Accumulation of Elastin (Elastoses)*

During pathological conditions, elastin or elastin-like material accumulates in various organs, producing "elastosis." Because the elastin is frequently identified solely on histological grounds, some investigators have used the term "pseudoelastin" to describe elastotic deposits.

The chemical composition of these materials is largely unknown. Diseases which are known to produce excessive amounts of elastin include pseudoxanthoma elasticum, elastosis perforans serpiginosa, actinic (solar) elastosis (Rÿhanen and Uitto, 1983; Uitto, 1984; Davidson, 1985; Oikarinen *et al.*, 1985), and fibrotic breast and liver disease (Davidson, 1985). Abnormal amounts of elastin may also accumulate in the atherosclerotic plaque (Ross, 1981).

What conditions might lead to overproduction of elastin? Hypertension clearly causes increases in the number of elastic lamellae in the major arteries, both in naturally occuring disease and in experimental models using mineralocorticoids with or without salt or heminephrectomy (see Davidson, 1985, for review). Ultraviolet radiation has been reported to cause increased elastin deposition in irradiated mouse skin (Johnston *et al.*, 1984). Chronic inflammatory processes such as sunburn or alcoholic liver damage may act to increase elastin production, or decrease its degradation, in competent cells. Acute experimental injury to lung tissue can elicit a "rebound" in elastin synthesis, but lung function is not restored (Kuhn *et al.*, 1976); this phenomenon may represent another type of elastosis.

VI. Evolution of Elastin

Elasticity is found in many animal tissues, but current evidence suggests that only chordates accumulate detectable amounts of chemically defined elastin. A series of studies by Sage and Gray (reviewed in Sage, 1982, 1983) defined elastin as protein (1) insoluble in 5.2 M guanidinium–HCl/1% β-mercaptoethanol, (2) resistant to bacterial collagenase, (3) desmosine-containing, and (4) positive to Verhoeff's elastic stain and had suggested that elastic tissue was confined to species higher than the jawless fishes; however, a recent reassessment of the histology of lamprey vasculature (Epple *et al.*, 1984) contradicts the presence of an evolutionary boundary at that precise point. The principal difficulty of these studies turns on the question of deciding what constitutes a primordial elastin molecule. Thus, applying the stringent criteria of extreme insolubility, specific cross-links, and particular staining properties may preclude identification of primordial elastins. DNA probes containing presumptive elastin sequences might provide more relaxed criteria.

A. Primitive Elastins

As discussed earlier, elastin in mammals consists of interpersed hydrophobic and cross-link regions which probably function in a three-dimensional array. Several amino acids are consistently absent for reasons which are unclear. Elastin biosynthesis appears to utilize parts of the collagen-synthetic pathway, which itself arose far earlier, during the transition to Metazoan life. Indeed, at least one collagen-like sequence is present in chick tropoelastin (Smith *et al.*, 1981). Sage (1983) has proposed that during the evolution of homeothermic vascular systems, elastin became progressively more hydrophobic, thus more readily undergoing coacervation at physiologic temperatures and perhaps increasing the tendency to form more extensive elastic networks.

Epple and co-workers (1984) have suggested that the unusual cartilage protein isolated from the lamprey (*Petromyzou marinus*) by Wright *et al.* (1983) may correspond to the elastin-like fibers stained in the lamprey blood vessel wall. This protein ("lamprin") is quite different from the known elastins in amino acid composition, but is similarly insoluble. More detailed analyses of such primitive connective tissue proteins may provide new clues into the origin of the elastic protein. Recombinant DNA probes may be an additional way to look at elastin evolution, but the choice of nucleotide sequences would ultimately depend on deciding which parts of the amino acid sequence were most likely to be conserved. It seems unlikely that there would be broad conservation of any noncoding regions of the elastin gene.

B. Invertebrate Elastomers

Elastic proteins appear to have evolved independently in the invertebrates more than once. Bivalve molluscs contain the hinge protein abductin (Kelly and Rice, 1967), and octopus vasculature contains another distinct elastic protein (Shadwick and Gosline, 1981). Insect wings possess an elastic polypeptide, resilin (Weis-Fogh, 1960). The amino acid compositions of these proteins suggest no relationship with elastin, and they presumably arose independently by convergent evolution of protein structure.

C. Interspecific Sequence Homologies

A limited amount of comparative sequence analysis has been made among elastins from different species, based on either amino acid or nucleotide sequences. Compositionally, the elastin of all homeothermic vertebrates is very similar (Sandberg, 1976). A reduced content of hydrophobic residues is found in many of the fishes, and Sage and Gray (Sage, 1982, 1983) have suggested that there is a gradual decline in hydrophobicity in "primordial" elastin. A comparison of the N-terminal sequences of chick (Karr *et al.*, 1981), pig (Gray *et al.*, 1973), and sheep tropoelastins (Davidson *et al.*, 1982b) indicates strong sequence homology. A limited number of chick peptides have now been sequenced (Sandberg *et al.*, 1985), and many of them show near-total homology with the porcine molecule.

DNA sequence analysis of cloned sheep genomic and cDNA indicates a similar extent of homology at the C-terminus of tropoelastin as well (Yoon *et al.*, 1985). Both bovine and human elastin genomic clones have been isolated (Cicila *et al.*, 1984; Ornstein *et al.*, 1985); again, extensive homology seems to be prevalent within the coding regions of these genes. Interestingly, there is an extensive homlogy within the 3′-untranslated region of the elastin mRNA molecule as well, which may indicate either a functional role for this domain or an unusually low rate of genetic rearrangement in this region. Unlike the protein-coding portion of the elastin gene, the 3′ untranslated region contains a large exon.

VII. SUMMARY AND PERSPECTIVES

The biochemistry and biology of elastin have moved forward at a gradual pace, in part due to the very unusual chemistry of the protein. Several excellent biological systems have been exploited within the past several years to address the intriguing questions of how this rubbery substance comes to be expressed during development and how this expression might be regulated in normal and pathological states.

Now that the necessary molecular probes are being developed, we should expect an accelerated understanding of how the protein and gene are organized, which alterations lead to pathological conditions, and how expression of elastin is modulated.

REFERENCES

Aaron, B. B., and Gosline, J. M. (1980). *Nature (London)* **287**, 865–867.
Abraham, P. A., and Carnes, W. H. (1978). *J. Biol. Chem.* **253**, 7973–7975.
Abraham, P. A., Smith, D. W., and Carnes, W. H. (1974). *Biochem. Biophys. Res. Commun.* **58**, 597–604.
Abraham, P. A., Perejda, A. J., Carnes, W. H., and Uitto, J. (1982). *J. Clin. Invest.* **70**, 1245–1252.
Abrams, W. R., Cohen, A. B., Damiano, V. V., Eliraz, A., Kimbel, P., Meranze, D. R., and Weinbaum, G. (1981). *J. Clin. Invest.* **68**, 1132–1139.
Adnet, J. J., Birembaut, P., Sadrin, R., Gaillard, D., Pastisson, C., Robert, L., Dousset, H., and Bogomoletz, W. V. (1981). *In* "New Frontiers in Mammary Pathology" (K. H. Hollman, J. DeBrux, and J. M. Velery, eds). Plenum, New York.
Anwar, R. A. (1977). *Adv. Exp. Med. Biol.* **79**, 329–342.

Anwar, R. A. (1982). *In* "Methods in Enzymology" (L. W. Cunningham and D. W. Frederiksen, eds.), Vol. 82, pp. 606–615. Academic Press, New York.

Banda, M. J., and Werb, Z. (1981). *Biochem. J.* **193**, 589–605.

Barrineau, L. L., Rich, C. B., and Foster, J. A. (1981). *Dev. Biol.* **87**, 46–51.

Benoist, C., and Chambon, P. (1981). *Nature (London)* **290**, 304–310.

Berry, C. L., Looker, T., and Germain, J. (1972). *J. Pathol.* **108**, 265–274.

Bhatnagar, R. S., Rapaka, R. S., and Urry, D. W. (1978). *FEBS Lett.* **95**, 61–64.

Bourdillon, M. C., Brechmeier, D., Blaes, N., Derouette, J. C., Hornebeck, W., and Robert, L. (1980). *Cell Biol. Int. Rep.* **4**, 313–320.

Braverman, I. M., and Fonferko, E. (1982). *J. Inv. Dermatol.* **78**,434–443.

Breathnack, R., & Chambon, P. (1981). *Annu. Rev. Biochem.* **50**, 349–383.

Bressan, G. M., and Prockop, D. J. (1977). *Biochemistry* **16**, 1406–1412.

Bressan, G. M., Castellani, I., Giro, M. G., Volpin, D., Fornieri, C., and Pasquali-Ronchetti, I. (1983). *J. Ultrastruct. Res.* **82**, 335–340.

Brury, R. A. B., and Wallington, E. A. (1976). "Carleton's Histological Technique." Oxford Univ. Press, Oxford.

Burnett, W., and Rosenbloom, J. (1979). *Biochem. Biophys. Res. Commun.* **86**, 478–484.

Burnett, W., Eichner, R., and Rosenbloom, J. (1980). *Biochemistry* **19**, 1106–1111.

Burnett, W., Yoon, K., and Rosenbloom, J. (1981). *Biochem. Biophys. Res. Commun.* **99**, 364–372.

Burnett, W., Finnigan-Bunick, A., Yoon, K., and Rosenbloom, J. (1982a). *J. Biol. Chem.* **257**, 1569–1572.

Burnett, W., Yoon, K., Finnigan-Bunick, A., and Rosenbloom, J. (1982b). *J. Invest. Dermatol.* **79**, 138s–145s.

Byers, P. H., Siegel, R. C., Holbrook, K. A., Narayanan, A. S., Bornstein, P., and Hall, J. G. (1980). *N. Engl. J. Med.* **303**, 61–65.

Cantor, J. O., Keller, S., Parshley, M. S., Darnule, T. V., Darnule, A. T., Cerreta, J. M., Turino, G. M., and Mandl, I. (1980). *Biochem. Biophys. Res. Commun.* **95**, 1381–1386.

Cantor, J. O., Osman, M., Keller, S., Cerreta, J. M., Mandl, I., and Turino, G. M. (1984). *J. Lab. Clin. Med.* **103**, 384–392.

Carnes, W. H., Abraham, P. A., and Buonassisi, V. (1979). *Biochem. Biophys. Res. Commun.* **90**, 1393–1399.

Chipman, S., Faris, B., Barone, L. M., Pratt, C. A., and Franzblau, C. (1985). *J. Biol. Chem.* **260**, 12780–12785.

Cicila, G., Yoon, K., Boyd, C., May., M., and Rosenbloom, J. (1984). *Fed. Proc.* **43**, 1853.

Clark, J. G., Kuhn, C., McDonald, J. A., and Mecham, R. P. (1983). *Int. Rev. Connect. Tissue Res.* **10**, 249–331.

Clark, J. M., and Glagov, S. (1985). *Arteriosclerosis* **5**, 19–34.

Cleary, E. G., and Gibson, M. A. (1983). *Int. Rev. Connect. Tissue Res.* **10**, 97–209.

Cleary, E. G., Sandberg, L. B., and Jackson, D. S. (1967). *J. Cell Biol.* **33**, 469–479.

Cox, D. L., Mecham, R. P., and Sexton, O. J. (1982). *Comp. Biochem. Physiol.* **72**, 619–623.

Damiano, V., Tsang, A., Weinbaum, G., Christner, P., and Rosenbloom, J. (1984). *Collagen Rel. Res.* **4**, 153–164.

Danielsen, L., and Kobayasi, T. (1972). *Acta Derm. Venereol.* **52**, 1–10.

Davidson, J. M. (1986). *In* "Molecular Pathology of Connective Tissue" (J. Uitto and A. Perejda, eds.). Academic Press, New York, in press.

Davidson, J. M., and Crystal, R. G. (1982a). *J. Invest. Dermatol.* **79**, 133S–137S.

Davidson, J. M., and Sephel, G. C. (1986). *In* "Methods in Enzymology" (L. W. Cunningham, ed.). Academic Press, Orlando, in preparation.

Davidson, J. M., Shibahara, S., Smith, K., and Crystal, R. G. (1981). *Connect. Tissue Res.* **8,** 209–212.

Davidson, J. M., Leslie, B., Wolt, T., Crystal, R. G., and Sandberg, L. B. (1982b). *Arch. Biochem. Biophys.* **218,** 31–37.

Davidson, J. M., Smith, K., Shibahara, S., Tolstoshev, P., and Crystal, R. G. (1982c). *J. Biol. Chem.* **257,** 747–754.

Davidson, J. M., Shibahara, S., Boyd, C., Mason, M. L., Tolstoshev, P., and Crystal, R. G. (1984a). *Biochem. J.* **220,** 653–663.

Davidson, J. M., Shibahara, S., Schafer, M. P., Harrison, M., Leach, C., Tolstoshev, P., and Crystal, R. G. (1984b). *Biochem. J.* **220,** 643–652.

Davidson, J. M., Hill, K. E., Mason, M. L., and Giro, M. G. (1985). *J. Biol. Chem.* **260,** 1901–1908.

Davidson, J. M., Hill, K. E., and Alford, J. L. (1986). Submitted for publication.

Derouette, S., Hornebeck, W., Loisance, D., Godeau, G., Cachera, J. P., and Robert, L. (1981). *Pathol. Biol.* **29,** 539–547.

Dubick, M. A., Rucker, R. B., Cross, C. E., and Last, J. A. (1981). *Biochim. Biophys. Acta* **672,** 303–306.

Dunn, D. M., and Franzblau, C. (1982). *Biochemistry* **21,** 4195–4202.

Eichner, R., and Rosenbloom, J. (1979). *Arch. Biochem. Biophys.* **198,** 414–423.

Emanuel, B. S., Cannizzaro, L., Ornstein-Goldstein, N., Indik, Z., Yoon, K., May, M., Olliver, L., Boyd, C., and Rosenbloom, J. (1985). *Am. J. Hum. Genet.* **37,** 873–882.

Epple, A., Hilliard, R. W., and Potter, I. C. (1984). *Comp. Biochem. Physiol.* **79A,** 105–107.

Eyre, D. R., Paz, M. A., and Gallop, P. M. (1984). *Annu. Rev. Biochem.* **53,** 717–748.

Fahrenbach, W., H., Sandberg, L. B., and Cleary, E. G. (1966). *Anat. Rec.* **155,** 563–575.

Faris, B., Salcedo, L. L., Cook, V., Johnson, L., Foster, J. A., and Franzblau, C. (1976). *Biochim. Biophys. Acta* **418,** 93–103.

Faris, B., Ferrera, R., Toselli, P., Nambu, J., Gonnerman, W. A., and Franzblau, C. (1984). *Biochim. Biophys. Acta* **797,** 71–75.

Field, J. M., Rodger, G. W., Hunter, J. C., Serafini-Fracassini, A., and Spina, M. (1978). *Arch. Biochem. Biophys.* **191,** 705–713.

Foster, J. A., Mecham, R. P., Rich, C. B., Cronin, M. F., Levine, A., Imberman, M., and Salcedo, L. L. (1978). *J. Biol. Chem.* **253,** 2797–2803.

Foster, J. A., Rich, C. B., and DeSa, M. D. (1980a). *Biochim. Biophys. Acta* **626,** 383–389.

Foster, J. A., Rich, C. B., Fletcher, S., Karr, S. R., and Przybyla, A. (1980b). *Biochemistry* **19,** 857–864.

Foster, J. A., Rich, C. B., Fletcher, S., Karr, S. R., DeSa, M. D., Oliver, T., and Przybyla A. (1981). *Biochemistry* **20,** 3528–3535.

Foster, J. A., Rich, C. B., and Karr, S. R., (1983). *Int. Rev. Connect. Tissue Res.* **10,** 65–95.

Francis, C., and Robert, L. (1984). *Int. J. Dermatol.* **23,** 166–179.

Franzblau, C. (1971). *In* "Comprehensive Biochemistry" (M. Florkin and E. H. Stotz, eds.), Vol. 26C, pp. 659–712. Elsevier, New York.

Frisch, S. M., and Werb, Z. (1983). *Fed. Proc.* **42,** 1982.

Frisch, S. M., Davidson, J. M., and Werb, Z. (1985). *Mol. Cell. Biol.* **5,** 253–258.

Fukuda, Y., Ferrans, V. J., and Crystal, R. G. (1984). *Am. J. Anat.* **170,** 597–629.

Gadek, J. E., Fells G. A., Zimmerman, R. L., Rennard, S. I., and Crystal, R. G. (1981). *J. Clin. Invest.* **68,** 889–898.

Gardner, R., Heng, H., Penner, M., Sedwick, C., and Rucker, R. (1984). *Res. Commun. Chem. Pathol. Pharmacol.* **43,** 251–264.

Gibson, M. A., and Cleary, E. G. (1983). *Collagen Rel. Res.* **3,** 469–488.

Gilbert, W. (1978). *Nature (London)* **271,** 501.

Giro, M. G., Castellani, I., and Volpin, D. (1974). *Connect. Tissue Res.* **2,** 231–235.

Giro, M. G., Hill, K. E., Sandberg, L. B., and Davidson, J. M. (1984). *Collagen Rel. Res.* **4,** 21–34.

Giro, M. G., Oikarinen, A. I., Oikarinen, H., Sephel, G., Uitto, J., and Davidson, J. M. (1985). *J. Clin. Invest.* **75,** 672–678.

Gomori, G. (1950). *Am. J. Clin. Pathol.* **20,** 665–666.

Grant, R. A. (1967). *J. Atheroscler. Res.* **7,** 463–472.

Gray, W. R., Sandberg, L. B., and Foster, J. A. (1973). *Nature (London)* **246,** 461–466.

Greenlee, T. K., Jr., Ross, R., and Hartman, J. L. *J. Cell Biol.* **30,** 59–71.

Halme, T., Vihersaari, T., Savunen T., Niinikoski, J., Inberg M., and Penttinen, R. (1982). *Biochim. Biophys. Acta* **717,** 105–110.

Hamalainen, L., Oikarinen, J., and Kivirikko, K. J. (1985). *J. Biol. Chem.* **260,** 720–725.

Harkness, M. L. R., Harkness, R. D., and McDonald, D. A. (1957). *Proc. R. Soc. London Ser. B* **146,** 541–551.

Harris, E. D., Blount, J. E., and Leach, R. M., Jr. (1980). *Science* **208,** 55–56.

Heeger, P., and Rosenbloom, J. (1980). *Connect. Tissue Res.* **8,** 21–25.

Heng-Khoo, C. S., Rucker, R. B., and Buckingham, K. W., (1979). *Biochem. J.* **177,** 559–567.

Hill, K. E., and Davidson, J. M. (1986). *Arteriosclerosis,* in press.

Holbrook, K. A., and Byers, P. H. (1982). *J. Invest. Dermatol.* **79,** 7s–16s.

Horowitz, A. L., Elson, N. A., and Crystal, R. G. (1976). *In* "The Biochemical Basis of Pulmonary Function" (R. G. Crystal, ed.), pp. 273–295. Dekker, New York.

Janoff, A. (1983). *Chest* **83,** 54S–58S.

John, R., and Thomas, J. (1972). *Biochem. J.* **127,** 261–269.

Johnston, K. J., Oikarinen, A. I., Lowe, N. J., Clark, J. G., and Uitto, J. (1984). *J. Invest. Dermatol.* **82,** 587–590.

Jones, P. A., Scott-Burden, T., and Gevers, W. (1979). *Proc. Natl. Acad. Sci. U.S.A.* **76,** 353–357.

Kadar, A., Joos, A., and Jellinek, H. (1977). *Arterial Wall* **1,** 45–58.

Kao, W. W.-Y., Bressan, G. M., and Prockop, D. J. (1982). *Connect. Tissue Res.* **10,** 263–274.

Karr, S. R., and Foster, J. A. (1981). *J. Biol. Chem.* **256,** 5946–5949.

Karr, S. R., and Foster, J. A. (1984). *Collagen Rel. Res.* **3,** 459–467.

Keeley, F. W. (1979). *Can. J. Biochem.* **57,** 1273–1280.

Keeley, F. W., and Johnson, D. J. (1983). *Can. J. Biochem. Cell Biol.* **61,** 1079–1084.

Keeley, F. W., and Johnson, D. J. (1986). *Can. J. Biochem.,* in press.

Keith, D. A., Paz, M. A., Gallop, P. M., and Glimcher, M. J. (1977). *J. Histochem. Cytochem.* **25,** 1154–1162.

Kelly, R. E., and Rice, R. V. (1967). *Science* **155,** 208–210.

King, G. S., Mohan, V. S., and Starcher, B. C. (1980a). *Connect. Tissue Res.* **7,** 263–267.

King, G. S., Starcher, B. C., and Kuhn, S. (1980b). *Bull. Eur. Physiopathol. Respir.* **16,** 61–64.

Kivirikko, K. I., and Myllyla, R. (1982). *In* "Methods in Enzymology"(L. W. Cunningham and D. W. Frederiksen, eds.), Vol. 82, pp. 245–304, Academic Press, New York.

Knight, K. R., Ayad, S., Shuttleworth, C. A., and Grant, M. E. (1984). *Biochem J.* **220,** 395–403.

Kornberg, R. L., Hendler, S. S., Oikarinen, A. I., Matsuoka, L. Y., and Uitto, J. (1985). *N. Engl. J. Med.* **312,** 771–774.

Kornblihtt, A. R., Vibe-Pedersen, K., and Baralle, F. E., (1984). *Nucleic Acids Res.* **12,** 5853–5868.

Kuhn, C., Yu, S. Y., Chraplyvy, M., Linder, H. E., and Senior, R. M. (1976). *Lab. Invest.* **34,** 372–380.

Lansing, A. L., Rosenthal, T. B., Alex, M., and Dempsey, B. W. (1952). *Anat. Rec.* **114**, 555–575.

Leach, R. M., Jr., Rucker, R. B., and Van-Dyke, G. P. (1981). *Arch. Biochem. Biophys.* **207**, 353–359.

Lee, I., Yau, M. D., and Rucker, R. B. (1976). *Biochim. Biophys. Acta* **442**, 432–436.

Lefevre, M., and Rucker, R. B. (1980). *Biochim. Biophys. Acta* **630**, 519–529.

Madsen, K., Moskalewski, S., von der Mark, K., and Friberg, U. (1983). *Dev. Biol.* **96**, 63–73.

Mecham, R. P., and Foster, J. A. (1977). *Biochemistry* **16**, 3825–3831.

Mecham, R. P., Foster, J. A., and Franzblau, C. (1976). *Biochim. Biophys. Acta* **446**, 245–254.

Mecham, R. P., Lange, G., Madaras, J. G., and Starcher, B. J. (1981). *J. Cell Biol.* **90**, 322–338.

Mecham, R. P., Madaras, J. G., McDonald, J. A., and Ryan, U. (1983). *J. Cell. Physiol.* **116**, 282–288.

Mecham, R. P., Griffin, G. L., Madaras, J. G., and Senior, R. M. (1984a). *J. Cell Biol.* **98**, 1813–1816.

Mecham, R. P., Madaras, J. G., and Senior, R. M. (1984b). *J. Cell Biol.* **98**, 1804–1812.

Mecham, R. P., Morris, S. L., Levy, B. D., and Wrenn, D. S. (1984c). *J. Biol. Chem.* **259**, 12414–12418.

Mecham, R. P., Levy, B. D., Morris, S. L., Madaras, J. G., and Wrenn, D. S. (1985). *J. Biol. Chem.* **260**, 3255–3258.

Murad, S., Tajima, S., Johnson, G. R., Sivarajah, S., and Pinnell, S. R. (1983). *J. Invest. Dermatol.* **81**, 158–162.

Myers, B., Dubick, M., Last, J. A., and Rucker, R. B. (1983). *Biochim. Biophys. Acta* **761**, 17–22.

Myoshi, M., Kanamori, M., and Rosenbloom, J. (1976). *J. Biochem. (Tokyo)* **79**, 1235–1243.

Nakao, J., Chang, W. G., Murota, S. I., and Orimo, N. (1980). *Atherosclerosis* **36**, 539–544.

Narayanan, A. S., and Page, R. C. (1976). *J. Biol. Chem.* **251**, 1125–1130.

Narayanan, A. S., Sandberg, L. B., Ross, R., and Layman, D. L. (1976). *J. Cell Biol.* **68**, 411–419.

Narayanan, A. S., Page, R. C., Kuzan, F., and Cooper, C. G. (1978). *Biochem. J.* **173**, 857–862.

Nardell, E. A., and Brody, J. S. (1982). *J. Appl. Physiol.* **53**, 140–148.

Oakes, B. W., Batty, A. C., Handley, C. J., and Sandberg, L. B. (1982). *Eur. J. Cell Biol.* **27**, 34–46.

Oikarinen, A., Karvonen, J., Uitto, J., and Hannuksela, M. (1985). *Photodermatol.* **2**, 15–26.

Olliver, L., Mathew, C., LuValle, P. A., Davidson, J. M., and Boyd, C. (1985). In preparation.

Ornstein-Goldstein, N., Indik, Z. K., Yoon, K., Cicila, G., Boyd, C. D., May, M., Morrow, S. D., Rosenbloom, J. C., and Rosenbloom, J. (1984). *J. Cell Biol.* **99**, 406a (Abstr).

Ornstein-Goldstein, M., Indik, Z. K., Yoon, K., Cicila, G., Boyd, C., Morrow, S. D., May, M., Rosenbloom, J. C., and Rosenbloom, J. (1985). *Fed. Proc.* **44**, 662.

Partridge, S. M., Davis, H. F., and Adair, G. S. (1955). *Biochem. J.* **61**, 11–21.

Peltonen, L., Kuivianemi, H., Palotie, A., Kaitila, I., and Kivirikko, K. I. (1983). *Biochemistry* **22**, 6156–6163.

Ponte, P., Ng, S. Y., Engel, J., Gunning, P., and Kedes, L. (1984). *Nucleic Acids Res.* **12**, 1687–1696.

Quintarelli, G., Starcher, B. C., Vocaturo, A., diGranfilippo, L., Gotte, L., and Mecham, R. P. (1979). *Connect. Tissue Res.* **4,** 1–19.

Raghow, R., Lurie, S., Seyer, J. M., and Kang, A. H. (1985). *J. Clin. Invest.* **76,** 1733–1739.

Raju, K., Rampersad, V., Pulleybank, D. E., and Anwar, R. A. (1985). *Fed. Proc.* **44,** 662.

Rennard, S. I., Jaurand, M. C., Bignon, J., Kawanami, O., Ferrans, V. J., Davidson, J., and Crystal, R. G. (1984). *Am. Rev. Respir. Dis.* **130,** 267–274.

Reyes, M. G., Bazile, D. B., Tosch, T., and Rubenstone, A. I. (1982). *Arch. Pathol. Lab. Med.* **106,** 610–614.

Rich, C. B., and Foster, J. A. (1984). *Biochem. J.* **217,** 581–584.

Romero, N., Tinker, D., Hyde, D., and Rucker, R. B. (1986). *Arch. Biochem. Biophys.* **244,** in press.

Rosenbloom, J. (1984). *Lab. Invest.* **51,** 605–623.

Rosenbloom, J., and Cywinski, A. (1976a). *Biochem. Biophys. Res. Commun.* **69,** 613–620.

Rosenbloom, J., and Cywinski, A. (1976b). *FEBS Lett.* **65,** 246–250.

Ross, R. (1981). *Arteriosclerosis,* **1,** 293–311.

Ross, R., and Bornstein, P. (1969). *J. Cell. Biol.* **40,** 366–381.

Rucker, R. B., and Dubick, M. A. (1984). *Environ. Health Perspect.* **55,** 174–191.

Rucker, R. B., and Tinker, D. (1977). *Int. Rev. Exp. Pathol.* **17,** 1–47.

Rucker, R. B., Heng-Khoo, C. S., Dubick, M., Lefevre, M., and Cross, C. E. (1979). *Biochemistry* **18,** 3854–3859.

Rÿhanen, L., and Uitto, J. (1982). In "The Biochemistry and Physiology of the Skin" (L. Goldsmith, ed.), pp. 433–447. Oxford Press, Fairview, New Jersey.

Rÿhanen, L., Graves, P. N., Bressan, G. M., and Prockop, D. J. (1978). *Arch. Biochem. Biophys.* **185,** 344–351.

Sage, H. (1982). *J. Invest. Dermatol.* **79,** 146s–153s.

Sage, H. (1983). *Comp. Biochem. Physiol.* **74,** 373–380.

Sage, E. H., and Gray, W. R. (1977). *Adv. Exp. Med. Biol.* **79,** 291–312.

Sandberg, L. B. (1976). *Int. Rev. Connect. Tissue Res.* **7,** 159–210.

Sandberg, L. B., and Davidson, J. M. (1984). In "Peptide and Protein Reviews" (M. T. W. Hearn, ed.), pp. 169–225. Dekker, New York.

Sandberg, L. B., Hackett, T. N., and Carnes, W. H. (1969a). *Biochim. Biophys. Acta* **181,** 201–207.

Sandberg, L. B., Weissman, N., and Smith, D. W. (1969b). *Biochemistry* **8,** 2940–2945.

Sandberg, L. B., Leach, C. T., Leslie, J. G., Torres, R. A., and Alvarez, V. L. (1980). *Front. Matrix Biol.* **8,** 69–77.

Sandberg, L. B., Leslie, J. G., and Oakes, B. W. (1981a). *Connect. Tissue Res.* **8,** 219–225.

Sandberg, L. B., Soskel, N. T., and Leslie, J. G. (1981b). *N. Engl. J. Med.* **304,** 566–579.

Sandberg, L. B., Leslie, J. G., Leach, C. T., Alvarez, V. L., Torres, A. R., and Smith, D. W. (1985). *Pathol. Biol.* **33,** 266–274.

Saunders, N. A., and Grant, M. E. (1984). *Biochem. J.* **221,** 393–400.

Schein, J., Frankel, L., and Rosenbloom, J. (1977). *Arch. Biochem. Biophys.* **183,** 416–420.

Schwarz, R. I., Farson, D. A., and Bissell, M. J. (1979). *In Vitro* **15,** 941–948.

Schwarzbauer, J. E., Tamkun, J. W., Lemischka, I. R., and Hynes, R. O. (1983). *Cell* **35,** 421–431.

Sear, C. H. J., Kewley, M. A., Jones, C. J. P., Grant, M. E., and Jackson, D. S. (1978). *Biochem. J.* **170,** 715–718.

Senior, R. M., Griffin, G. L., Mechan, R. P., Wrenn, D. S., Prasad, K. U., and Urry, D. W. (1984). *J. Cell Biol.* **99,** 870–874.

Sephel, G. C., and Davidson, J. M. (1986). *J. Invest. Dermatol.*, in press.
Sephel, G. C., Buckley, A., and Davidson, J. M. (1986a). In preparation.
Sephel, G. C., Byers, P. H., Holbrook, K. A., and Davidson, J. M. (1986b). Submitted for publication.
Shadwick, R. E., and Gosline, J. M. (1981). *Science* **213,** 759–761.
Shields, S., Coulson, W. F., Kimball, D. A., Carnes, W. H., Cartwright, G. E., and Wintrobe, M. M. (1962). *Am. J. Pathol.* **41,** 603–617.
Slack, H. G. B. (1954). *Nature (London)* **174,** 512–513.
Smith, D. W., Brown, D. M., and Carnes, W. H. (1972). *J. Biol. Chem.* **247,** 2427–2432.
Smith, D. W., Sandberg, L. B., Leslie, B. H., Wolt, T. B., Minton, S. T., Myers, B., and Rucker, R. B. (1981). *Biochem. Biophys. Res. Commun.* **103,** 880–885.
Smith, J. C., Jr., Davidson, E. A., Sams, W. M., Jr., and Clark, R. D. (1962). *J. Invest. Dermatol.* **39,** 347–350.
Smith, L. T., and Holbrook, K. A. (1982). *Scanning Electron Microsc.* **4,** 1745–1751.
Smith, L. T., Holbrook, K. A., and Byers, P. H. (1982). *J. Invest. Dermatol.* **79,** 93s–104s.
Soskel, N. T., Watanabe, S., Hammod, E., Sandberg, L. B., Renzetti, A. D., Jr., and Crapo, J. D. (1982). *Am. Rev. Respir. Dis.* **126,** 316–325.
Soskel, N. T., Watanabe, S., and Sandberg, L. B. (1984). *Chest* **85,** 70s–73s.
Spina, M., Garbisa, S., Hinnie, J., Hunter, J. C., and Serafini-Fracassini, A. (1983). *Arterioclerosis* **3,** 64–76.
Starcher, B. C. (1977). *Anal. Biochem.* **79,** 11–15.
Starcher, B. C., and Mecham, R. P. (1981). *Connect. Tissue Res.* **8,** 255–258.
Starcher, B. C., Kuhn, C., and Overton, J. E. (1978). *Am. Rev. Respir. Dis.* **117,** 299–305.
Szendroi, M., Meimon, G., Bakala, H., Frances, C., Robert, L., Godeau, G., and Hornebeck, W. (1984). *J. Invest. Dermatol.* **83,** 224–229.
Tamkun, J. W., Schwarzbauer, J. E., and Hynes, R. O. *Proc. Natl. Acad. Sci. U.S.A.* **81,** 5140–5144.
Thung, S. N., and Gerber, M. A. (1982). *Arch. Pathol. Lab. Med.* **106,** 468–469.
Tinker, D., and Rucker, R. B. (1985). *Physiol. Rev.* **65,** 607–657.
Torchia, D. A., and Piez, K. A. (1973). *J. Mol. Biol.* **76,** 419–424.
Uitto, J. (1984). *In* "Dermatology in General Medicine" (T. B. Fitzpatrick, ed.). McGraw-Hill, New York, in press.
Uitto, J., Hoffman, H.-P., and Prockop, D. J. (1976). *Arch. Biochem. Biophys.* **173,** 187–200.
Urry, D. W., Venkatachalam, C. M., Long, M. M., and Prasad, K. U. (1982). *In* "Conformation in Biology" (R. Srinivasan and R. H. Sarma, eds.), pp. 11–27. Adenine Press, New York.
Verhoeff, F. H. (1908). *J. Am. Med. Assoc.* **50,** 876–877.
Volpin, D., Pasquali-Ronchetti, I., Castellani, I., Giro, M. G., Peserico, A., and Mori, G. (1978). *Dermatologica* **156,** 209–223.
Von-der-Mark, H., Aumailley, M., Wick, G., Fleischmajer, R., and Timpl, R. (1984). *Eur. J. Biochem.* **142,** 493–502.
Weis-Fogh, T. (1960). *J. Exp. Biol.* **37,** 880–907.
Wolinsky, H. (1970). *Circ. Res.* **26,** 507–522.
Wolinsky, H., and Glagov, S. *Circ. Res.* **25,** 677–686.
Wright, G. M., and Youson, J. H. (1983). *Am. J. Anat.* **167,** 59–70.
Yoon, K., May, M., Goldstein, N., Indik, Z. K., Olliver, L., Boyd, C., and Rosenbloom, J. (1984). *Biochem. Biophys. Res. Commun.* **118,** 261–269.
Yoon, K., Davidson, J. M., Boyd, C., May, M., LuValle, P., Ornstein-Goldstein, N., Smith, J., Indik Z., Ross, A., Golub, E., and Rosenbloom, J. (1985). *Arch. Biochem. Biophys.* **241,** 684–691.

Elastases: Catalytic and Biological Properties

Joseph G. Bieth

INSERM Unité 237, Faculté de Pharmacie, Université Louis Pasteur, Strasbourg, France

217

I. Introduction

The discovery of elastinolytic proteinases has been triggered by investigations on the pathogenesis of connective tissue diseases. For instance, studies on atherosclerosis led Balo and Banga (1949) to characterize pancreatic elastase. Similarly, the tissue-damaging effect of leukoproteinases prompted Janoff and Scherer (1968) to investigate neutrophil elastase. Besides, the suggestion that this enzyme may promote lung emphysema (Laurell and Eriksson, 1963; Kueppers and Bearn, 1966) brought about an enormous burst of research activity on elastase and on its physiological regulator, α_1-proteinase inhibitor.

This article reviews the molecular and catalytic properties of mammalian and nonmammalian elastases and the possible pathological role of these enzymes. First of all, we define elastases as elastin-solubilizing enzymes. This important definition will be repeated several times in the text. The catalytic properties of porcine pancreatic and human leukocyte elastases will be discussed very thoroughly. It is felt that knowledge of the specificity and mechanism of action of a proteinase is a prerequisite for both delineating its pathological function and designing specific inhibitors of potential therapeutic importance. The section dealing with the catalytic properties also emphasizes that the interpretation of the kinetic parameters describing elastase–substrate interactions is sometimes fraught with unexpected difficulties.

In the section on elastase inhibitors, a large amount of space will be given to α_1-proteinase inhibitor, the physiological antielastase which protects lungs against emphysema. Emphasis will also be made in this section on the way to predict the *in vivo* potency of an inhibitor from *in vitro* measured kinetic constants. Synthetic elastase inhibitors will also be thoroughly discussed.

The sections dealing with other elastases will be mainly devoted to macrophage and *Pseudomonas aeruginosa* elastases. The section on elastase assays will be a critical minireview on available methods and will provide many practical details on how natural or synthetic substrates should be handled.

It was a difficult task for a biochemist to review the pathological role of elastinolytic proteinases. The pathogenic models which are discussed in the present article will therefore necessarily appear to be biochemical oversimplifications of complex biological realities. The therapeutic potential of elastase inhibitors will also be analyzed.

II. Definition and Occurrence

A. *Definition*

A proteinase may be named "elastase" if it possesses the ability to solubilize mature cross-linked elastin. An enzyme that hydrolyzes chemically solubilized elastins or synthetic elastase substrates should not be called an elastase or an "elastase-like" proteinase if it is unable to solubilize fibrous elastin. As will be shown in Section V, elastases do not belong to a homogeneous class of proteinases: they may have variable catalytic sites and widely different primary substrate specificities. In addition, the mechanism by which they solubilize elastin is not well understood. The elastinolytic property of a given proteinase can therefore not be predicted from its ability to cleave a model substrate or even a soluble elastin derivative: it must be verified experimentally. Terms such as "elastase-like" of "elastase-type" enzyme, which are used to name nonelastinolytic proteinases, should no longer be employed (see also Section IX,A). It must also be emphasized here that elastases are not "specific" for elastin since they hydrolyze other proteins as well.

B. *Occurrence*

Table I shows that elastolytic enzymes have been demonstrated in a great variety of mammalian and nonmammalian cells and tissues. As will be shown later, these proteinases have widely different primary substrate specificities. In addition, they do not form a homogeneous

TABLE I

Source and Class of the Various Elastases Reviewed in the Present Chapter

	Proteinase class		
Source of elastase	Serine	Metallo	Thiol
Mammalian cells and tissues			
Pancreas	+		
Polymorphonuclear leukocytes	+		
Macrophage	+	+	+
Monocyte	+	+	
Various normal and tumor cells in culture	+	+	
Nonmammalian cells and tissues			
Bacteria	+	+	
Fungi	?	?	+
Trematodes	+	+	
Snake venoms	+	+	+
Fish pancreas	+	+	

class of enzymes since their catalytic site contains either a serine or a cysteine residue or a metal ion. Papain, a plant thiol-proteinase is also an elastinolytic enzyme (Robert and Robert, 1969).

All the elastases listed in Table I have a neutral or slightly alkaline pH optimum. Pepsin, however, solubilizes elastin with an optimum pH below 2. By contrast, cathepsin D, another carboxyl proteinase, does not solubilize elastin (Collins and Fine, 1981).

III. Pancreatic Elastases: Occurrence and Molecular Properties

Elastase appears to be present in the pancreas of all mammalian or nonmammalian organisms investigated. Like other pancreatic proteinases, it is probably synthesised as an inactive precursor, proelastase, which is activated by limited proteolysis. The presence of proelastase(s) has been demonstrated in swine (Uram and Lamy, 1969; Gertler and Birk, 1970), human (de Caro *et al.*, 1975), dog (Geokas *et al.*, 1980), rat (Largman, 1983), and African lungfish pancreas (de Haën and Gertler, 1974).

A. *Porcine Pancreatic Elastase II*

Activated extracts of hog pancreas contain two different elastases named elastase I and II (Ardelt, 1974). The former, usually referred to as "porcine pancreatic elastase," has been investigated down to the atomic level and is commercially available in pure form. The latter has been studied to some extent (Ardelt, 1974; Gertler *et al.*, 1977), but its covalent and tertiary structures are unknown. It is distinctly different from elastase I in both its molecular properties (e.g., Table II) and substrate specificity (Section V).

B. *Porcine Pancreatic Elastase I*

This is the commercially available elastase on which most structural and kinetic investigations have been performed. We shall give the enzyme its classic name: porcine pancreatic elastase.

1. PURIFICATION

The first preparation of satisfactory purity was obtained by Lewis *et al.* (1956). The best purification method is that described by Shotton (1970), derived from those of Lewis *et al.* (1956) and Smillie and Hartley (1966). It uses Trypsin 1-300 (Nutritional Biochemical Corporation), a commercial acetone powder of porcine pancreas, as the starting material and includes the following steps: (1) extraction, (2) ammonium sulfate precipitation, (3) dialysis and collection of an euglobulin precipitate, (4) batch adsorption of impurities on DEAE–Sephadex, and (5) crystallization. This method takes about 2 weeks, is very easy to carry out since it involves no column chromatography and yields the purest enzyme preparation reported. Depending upon the batch of Trypsin 1-300, the yield varies from 0.7 to 2.5 g of elastase per 500 g of pancreatic powder.

2. THE AMBIGUITY ABOUT "CRYSTALLINE ELASTASE"

The euglobulin precipitate (step 3 of the above procedure) contains substantial amounts of elastase (Lewis *et al.*, 1956; Shotton, 1970). After dissolution of the precipitate and addition of ammonium sulfate, crystallization occurs. However, even after several recrystallizations, an "acidic endopeptidase" (Baumstark, 1970), chymotrypsin C (Thomson and Denniss, 1976), insulinase (Lewis and Thiele, 1957), and car-

TABLE II

AMINO ACID COMPOSITION (RESIDUES PER MOLECULE) OF SOME PANCREATIC
AND LEUKOCYTE ELASTASES

Amino acid	PPE I[a]	PPE II[b]	HPE[c]	RPE[d]	HLE[e]	Cat G[f]	DLE[g]
Asp	24	23	27	26	24	15	21
Thr	19	18	12	17	7	8	8
Ser	22	28	32	27	13	11	11
Glu	19	21	14	21	18	17	18
Pro	7	12	17	9	10	11	12
Gly	25	23	27	28	28	18	26
Ala	17	19	17	16	24	9	23
Val	27	25	23	25	25	16	27
Cys	8	12	8	6	6	4	8
Met	2	2	2	4	2	2	3
Ile	10	13	13	7	11	6	13
Leu	18	21	19	15	20	15	20
Tyr	11	6	12	10	3	4	0
Phe	3	4	3	4	9	5	12
Try	7	10	8		2		3
His	6	4	6	6	4	3	5
Lys	3	5	8	4	1	4	0
Arg	12	6	9	13	22	29	18

[a] Porcine pancreatic elastase I. From Shotton (1970).
[b] Porcine pancreatic elastase II. From Gertler et al. (1977).
[c] Human pancreatic elastase. From Ohlsson and Olsson (1976).
[d] Rat pancreatic elastase. From Largman (1983).
[e] Human leukocyte elastase isoenzyme E$_4$. From Baugh and Travis (1976).
[f] Human leukocyte cathepsin G. From Twumasi and Liener (1977).
[g] Dog leukocyte elastase. From Delshammar and Ohlsson (1976).

boxypeptidase (Koide and Yohizawa, 1981) remain associated with the crystalized elastase.

On the other hand, crystalization of elastase from a low concentration (0.02 M) of sodium sulfate at pH 5 (Shotton, 1970) yields crystals of extremely pure elastase. It is therefore important to understand which crystalline elastase is being provided by commercial suppliers.

3. MOLECULAR PROPERTIES

a. *Stability and Structure.* Porcine pancreatic elastase is remarkably stable at pH 7–8 (Dimicoli *et al.*, 1976) but undergoes rapid inactivation at pH 3 (Lewis *et al.*, 1956) as a possible result of a conformational change (Wasi and Hofmann, 1968). Most of its molecular properties have been reviewed by Shotton (1970), Hartley and Shotton (1971), and Bieth (1978). It is composed of a single polypeptide chain of 240 amino acid residues with four disulfide bridges. Comparison of the covalent structure of porcine pancreatic elastase with that of bovine chymotrypsins and trypsin shows these four proteinases exhibit a high degree of sequence homologies suggesting that they have evolved from a common ancestor. X-Ray crystallography reveals that the elastase molecule is composed of two domains, has a low content of α-helices in its C-terminal part, and is mainly formed of large antiparallel loops.

b. Metal Ion Binding Site. Dimicoli and Bieth (1977) reported that porcine pancreatic elastase has a single calcium-binding site composed of Glu-70 and Glu-80 (chymotrypsin sequence numbering system). The equilibrium association constant for the elastase–calcium complex was found to be $2.2 \times 10^4 \ M^{-1}$ at pH 5 and 35°C. This site is able to bind other metal ions, namely, Gd^{3+} (Dimicoli and Bieth, 1977), Tb^{3+} (Brittain *et al.*, 1976; Duportail *et al.*, 1980; de Jersey and Martin, 1980), Zn^{2+}, and Mg^{2+} (de Jersey and Martin, 1980). Ca^{2+}, Gd^{3+}, and Tb^{3+} have similar affinities for elastase (Duportail *et al.*, 1980) whereas Zn^{2+} and Mg^{2+} bind with association constants 30 and 60 times lower than that of Ca^{2+} (de Jersey and Martin, 1980).

c. Conformation in Solution. The conformation of porcine pancreatic elastase has been extensively investigated using CD, ORD, and infrared spectroscopy (for a review see Bieth, 1978). Elastase is a globular protein with a random coil structure and a very low α-helix content, a result which agrees with the X-ray crystallographic data.

Below pH 4, the protein undergoes conformational changes which are reversible to a certain extent. Between pH 5 and 10.9 or even 12 no gross conformational changes can be detected by CD or ORD. In this respect, elastase does not behave like chymotrypsin, which undergoes a reversible structural transition with a pK_a of 8.3. When the conformation of elastase was studied using circularly polarized luminescence spectroscopy and maximum luminescence intensity of the Tb^{3+}–elastase complex, no conformational change could be detected between pH 5 and 7 or between 5° and 35°C. However, below pH 5 and above pH 7 important conformational changes were diagnosed (Duportail *et al.*, 1980). The structural transition occurring at acidic pH is in agreement with previous data, but the conformational change detected above pH 7 was not seen with other techniques.

C. Human Pancreatic Elastase

1. Occurrence of Only One Major Elastolytic Enzyme in Human Pancreas

According to Clemente *et al.* (1972) human pancreatic juice contains two proenzymes, an anionic and a cationic one, which, upon activation are able to hydrolyze acetyl-(Ala)$_3$ methyl ester, a specific substrate of porcine pancreatic elastase. The cationic proenzyme has been partially purified and is active on insoluble elastin after activation. It is therefore a true proelastase. It is also active on a typical chymotrypsin substrate (de Caro *et al.*, 1975).

Activated extracts of human pancreas contain two enzymes able to hydrolyze acetyl-(Ala)$_3$ methyl ester (Feinstein *et al.*, 1974; Mallory and Travis, 1975; Largman *et al.*, 1976). However, the question as to whether these two proteinases are true elastases is not clear: the two "elastases" isolated by Feinstein *et al.* (1974) have not been tested on elastin, and Mallory and Travis (1975) reported that only one of the two acetyl-(Ala)$_3$ methyl ester hydrolyzing enzymes present in pancreatic extract is active on elastin. On the other hand, Ohlsson and Olsson (1976) reported the occurrence of only one elastase in human pancreatic juice whereas Largman *et al.* (1976) purified two elastases (named 1 and 2) from human pancreas. Elastase 1 is, however, poorly active on elastin (Fujimoto *et al.*, 1980; Largman, 1983). There is therefore apparently only one major elastase in human pancreas.

2. Molecular Properties

Human pancreatic elastase has been isolated in pure form in several laboratories (Ohlsson and Olsson, 1976; Largman *et al.*, 1976; Fujimoto *et al.*, 1980; Rabaud *et al.*, 1980). It is a single-chain molecule of M_r 25,000 (Largman *et al.*, 1976) or 26,000 (Ohlsson and Olsson, 1976). It contains no carbohydrates (Ohlsson and Olsson, 1976) and is a cationic protein (p*I* 9.5, Fujimoto *et al.*, 1980). Its amino acid composition is given in Table II. It does not cross-react immunologically with human leukocyte elastase (Ohlsson and Olsson, 1976).

D. Other Pancreatic Elastases

Elastase activity had been found in the pancreas of cows, cats, chickens (Lewis *et al.*, 1956), dogs (Geokas *et al.*, 1980), rats (Katayama and Ooyama, 1980; Largman, 1983), guinea pigs (Moon and McIvor, 1960),

African lungfishes (de Haën and Gertler, 1974), goosefishes (Lamy and Lansing, 1961), catfishes (Yoshinaka *et al.*, 1984), and moose (Livaart and Stevenson, 1974). Some of these elastases have been isolated and characterized.

Geokas *et al.* (1980) purified two elastases from dog pancreas. The cationic enzyme has a molecular mass of 26.3 kDa and exists as a proenzyme. The second elastase is more anionic. The proteinases differ in substrate specificity (see Section V).

Largman (1983) purified a proelastase from rat pancreas. The activated enzyme has a molecular mass of 27 kDa. Its amino acid composition is given in Table II, and its substrate specificity is similar to that of porcine pancreatic elastase (see Section V). Rat proelastase corresponds to one of the elastase mRNA clones isolated by MacDonald *et al.* (1982).

De Haën and Gertler (1974) isolated two pancreatic proelastases from the African lungfish. The two proteins have molecular masses of about 25 kDa. The activated enzymes have similar substrate specificities (see Section V). Cohen *et al.* (1981a) have isolated a 25-kDa elastase from carp pancreas. Yoshinaka *et al.* (1983, 1984) have purified two elastases from the pancreas of the catfish. Elastase B has a molecular mass of 26 kDa and is a serine proteinase (Yoshinaka *et al.*, 1983). Elastase A has a molecular mass of 24 kDa and is a metalloproteinase requiring Zn^{2+} for activity (Yoshinaka *et al.*, 1984). This is the first report of a pancreatic metalloelastase.

IV. LEUKOCYTE ELASTASES: OCCURRENCE AND MOLECULAR PROPERTIES

Elastase is not present in all white blood cells. Its occurrence in neutrophilic polymorphonuclear leukocytes is now well documented. Recently, elastase activity was also found in monocytes (see Section VIII). The term "leukocyte elastase" used in this review as well as in many other articles, therefore stands for neutrophilic polymorphonuclear leukocyte elastase.

A. Human Leukocyte Elastase

1. LOCALIZATION AND EXTRACELLULAR RELEASE

Leukocyte elastase activity was first reported by Janoff and Scherer (1968). The possible occurrence of a precursor of this enzyme in immature cells has been suggested (Feinstein and Janoff, 1976). Dewald *et al.* (1975) showed that elastase is located in the azurophil granules of polymorphonuclear leukocytes. More recently, Clark *et al.* (1980) designed a sensitive ultrastructural cytochemical substrate of elastase and showed that the enzyme is localized in the nuclear membrane, Golgi complex, endoplasmic reticulum, mitochondria, and granules of human neutrophils. Immunohistochemistry was used to detect elastase in cells of the neutrophilic lineage (Kramps *et al.*, 1984). Only promyelocytes and more differentiated myeloid cells stained positive for elastase (Kramps *et al.*, 1984). The azurophil granules also contain, among others, cathepsin G, cathepsin D, and myeloperoxidase (for a review see Klebanoff and Clark, 1978). The specific granules contain collagenase (Murphy *et al.*, 1977).

Elastase may be released under a great variety of circumstances (for a review see Klebanoff and Clark, 1978). Among these are phagocytosis or reaction of neutrophils with complement components or chemotactic agents. Elastase release *in vitro* has been observed during blood coagulation (Plow, 1982), after reaction of cytochalasin B-treated neutrophils with *N*-formyl-Met-Leu-Phe, a chemotactic peptide (Smith *et al.*, 1980), or with the plasma proteinase kallikrein (Wachfogel *et al.*, 1983). Opsonized zymosan (Campbell *et al.*, 1982) and phorbol myristate acetate (Estensen *et al.*, 1974) may also be used to release elastase. It is worth mentioning that most of these agents also turn on the respiratory burst of the neutrophils (i.e., oxygen consumption and oxidant release).

2. Purification

Elastase isolated from neutrophil granules has been obtained in pure form in several laboratories (for a review see Bieth, 1978). Highly purified enzyme may also be isolated in relatively large quantities from purulent sputum (Martodam *et al.*, 1979). This method involves the following steps: extraction with 1 *M* NaCl, affinity chromatography on Trasylol–Sepharose (Baugh and Travis, 1976) (Trasylol is the trade name for the bovine basic pancreatic trypsin inhibitor), and CM-Sephadex chromatography. The major advantage of this procedure lies in the use of purulent sputum instead of intact neutrophils as a starting material. Sputum is much easier to obtain than intact cells. The procedure of Martodam *et al.* (1979) is successfully used in our and other laboratories.

3. MOLECULAR PROPERTIES

Human leukocyte elastase is a glycoprotein composed of a single polypeptide chain of about 230 amino acid residues (e.g., Baugh and Travis, 1976). Most of the purification procedures yield a mixture of three or four isoenzymes differing in electrophoretic mobility. Ohlsson and Olsson (1974) separated three isoenzymes by repeated preparative electrophoresis on agarose gel and obtained the proteins in a purified form. Baugh and Travis (1976) were able to partially resolve their isoelastases by CM–cellulose chromatography. The most cationic protein called E_4 was obtained in a highly purified form and represents about 60% of the total isoenzymes. Its amino acid composition in reported in Table II (page 222).

The reason for electrophoretic heterogeneity of elastase remains unclear. Ohlsson and Olsson (1974) reported differences in arginine content of their three isoelastases. Baugh and Travis (1976) showed that the mixture of their isoenzymes and isoenzyme E_4 have identical N-terminal sequences and suggested that the isoenzymes may exhibit minor changes in carbohydrate content.

The three isoelastases purified by Ohlsson and Olsson (1974) have similar molecular masses (33, 34, and 36.5 kDa) as determined by SDS–polyacrylamide gel electrophoresis. These values compare favorably with the results of Feinstein and Janoff (1975b) who reported a molecular mass of 34.4 kDa for the mixture of the isoenzymes and with those obtained by Baugh and Travis (1976) for isoelastase E_4: 29.5 (equilibrium centrifugation) or 28.9 kDa (SDS electrophoresis). Molecular masses of 27 (Schmidt and Havemann, 1974; Twumasi and Liener, 1977), 22 (Taylor and Crawford, 1975), and 20 kDa (Starkey and Barrett, 1976) have also been reported.

All isoenzymes are glycoproteins whose electrophoretic mobility does not change after neuraminidase treatment (Baugh and Travis, 1976; Taylor and Crawford, 1975). The isoenzyme E_4 contains 23% sugars (6 kDa), nearly all of which are neutral, with only traces of sialic acid (Baugh and Travis, 1976). Elastase is a very basic protein ($pI > 9$, see Baugh and Travis, 1976; Starkey and Barrett, 1976) due to its high content of arginine residues.

B. Human Leukocyte Cathepsin G

The azurophil granules of neutrophils contain another neutral proteinase named cathepsin G (Starkey and Barrett, 1976) or chymotrypsin-like neutral protease (Schmidt and Havemann, 1974). Although this enzyme is not named "elastase" it exhibits a distinct elastolytic activity (Reilly and Travis, 1980; Boudier et al., 1981b). In addition, it enhances the elastolytic activity of leukocyte elastase (Boudier et al., 1981b). We shall therefore review some of its properties.

According to Ohlsson (1980), granulocytes contain 1–2 μg of cathepsin G per 10^6 cells. This proteinase has been isolated and investigated in several laboratories (Schmidt and Havemann, 1974; Feinstein and Janoff, 1975a; Rindler-Ludwig and Braunstein, 1975; Starkey and Barrett, 1976; Twumasi and Liener, 1977). The most convenient purification procedure is that described by Martodam et al. (1979) which allows both cathepsin G and elastase to be obtained in a highly purified form.

Leukocyte cathepsin G and elastase share many physical–chemical properties: both are basic glycoproteins, occur as isoenzymes, and have comparable molecular masses. Cathepsin G is more basic (Starkey and Barrett, 1976) and contains substantially less carbohydrate than elastase (Twumasi and Liener, 1977). It is composed of a single polypeptide chain whose amino acid composition is given in Table II (page 222).

C. Dog Leukocyte Elastase

Dog leukocyte elastase (Ardelt et al., 1976; Delshammar and Ohlsson, 1976) is composed of a single polypeptide chain with a molecular mass of about 24 kDa. Its amino acid composition is given in Table II. It is a cationic protein with no lysine or tyrosine residues. It is not a glycoprotein and does not exist as isoenzymes like its human counterpart. It exhibits clear-cut elastolytic activity.

D. Other Leukocyte Elastases

Using a synthetic substrate for porcine pancreatic and human leukocyte elastase, Ashe and Zimmerman (1982) were able to detect "elastase-like" activity in the leukocyte granule extracts of hamsters, rats, rabbits, and guinea pigs. Dubin et al. (1976) isolated three proteinases active on a synthetic elastase substrate from horse leukocyte granules, and Virca et al. (1984) partially purified rat leukocyte elastase and showed that it has a substrate specificity similar to that of its human counterpart. As emphasized in Section II, an enzyme cannot be named elastase if it has not been shown to solubilize fibrous elastin. True leukocyte elastolytic activity has been demonstrated in rabbits (Dewald *et al.*, 1975), hamsters (Boudier and Bieth, 1982), and horses (Koj *et al.*, 1976). The elastase content of rabbit and hamster leukocytes is much lower than that of human neutrophils (Dewald *et al.*, 1975; Boudier and Bieth, 1982).

V.   Catalytic Properties of Pancreatic and Leukocyte Elastases

The active center of an enzyme is composed of two parts: the substrate binding site which is responsible for the specificity and the catalytic site which effects the chemical transformation of the bound substrate. For the sake of clarity, we shall discuss these two sites separately.

A.   Catalytic Site and Mechanism of Substrate Hydrolysis

All pancreatic and leukocyte elastases, except catfish pancreatic metalloelastase (Yoshinaka *et al.*, 1984), belong to the family of serine proteinases. This family includes pancreatic trypsin, chymotrypsin, kallikrein, and most of the coagulation and complement proteinases (e.g., plasmin, thrombin, plasminogen activator). Serine proteinases are so named because a particular serine residue is involved in the catalytic breakdown of the substrate. Serine is, however, only one component of the catalytic site of these enzymes. Blow *et al.* (1969) have shown that this site is composed of three hydrogen-bonded amino acid residues, Asp-102, His-57, and Ser-195, which form the so-called charge-relay system or catalytic triad. Electrons are transferred from the buried carboxyl group of Asp-102 to the γ-oxygen of Ser-195 which then becomes a powerful nucleophile able to attack the carbonyl carbon atom of the substrate's peptide bond. Available X-ray crystallographic data demonstrate that the charge-relay system is highly conserved among all serine proteinases.

The hydrolysis of a peptide bond by a serine proteinase involves the minimal steps depicted in Fig. 1. Low-temperature X-ray crystallography was used to confirm the involvement of an acyl–enzyme intermediate during the porcine pancreatic elastase-catalyzed hydrolysis of a model substrate (Alber *et al.*, 1976). The theory of absolute reaction rates predicts that the acylation and the deacylation reactions proceed via a transition state (or activated complex) whose energy is much higher than the ground state. The transition state for acylation is

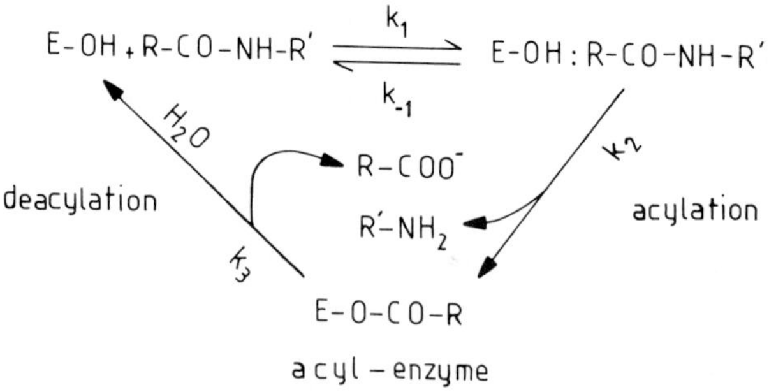

$$E\text{-}OH + R\text{-}CO\text{-}NH\text{-}R' \underset{k_{-1}}{\overset{k_1}{\rightleftharpoons}} E\text{-}OH : R\text{-}CO\text{-}NH\text{-}R'$$

deacylation H_2O k_3 R-COO⁻   R'-NH₂ k_2 acylation

E-O-CO-R

a c y l – enzyme

FIG. 1. Schematic representation of the hydrolysis of a peptide (R—CO—NH—R') by a serine proteinase (E—OH). The initial reversible formation of an adsorption (Michaelis–Menten) complex is followed by a nucleophilic attack of the γ-oxygen of serine on the peptide bond with subsequent formation of an acyl–enzyme intermediate and release of the amine portion of the substrate. The acyl–enzyme then undergoes nucleophilic attack by a polarized water molecule with subsequent regeneration of active enzyme and release of the carboxyl moiety of the substrate. This scheme represents the minimal steps of the enzyme-catalyzed substrate hydrolysis: for both acylation and deacylation reactions a transition state may be postulated.

thought to be a tetrahedral adduct between the γ-oxygen of Ser-195 and the carbonyl group of the substrate (R—CONH—R'):

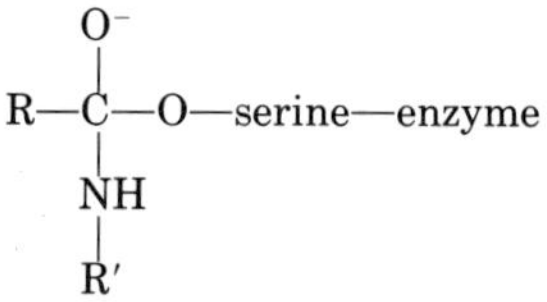

$$R\text{—}\overset{\overset{\textstyle O^-}{|}}{\underset{\underset{\textstyle R'}{\underset{|}{NH}}}{C}}\text{—}O\text{—serine—enzyme}$$

The kinetic constants k_{cat} and K_m describing the enzyme–substrate interaction usually have a complex meaning because (1) the enzymatic reaction proceeds via several intermediates and (2) nonproductive enzyme–substrate binding may occur. If the substrate forms only productive complexes with the enzyme and if the acylation reaction is rate limiting, it may be shown that $K_m = K_s$, the equilibrium dissociation constant of ES, and $k_{cat} = k_2$. If deacylation is rate limiting and/or if nonproductive binding occurs, K_m and k_{cat} do not have simple physical meanings (Bender and Kezdy, 1965; Bieth, 1978). Interestingly, however, $k_{cat}/K_m = k_2/K_s$ whatever the rate-limiting step and the substrate's binding mode.

For most proteinases, the rate of ester hydrolysis is limited by deacylation ($k_{cat} = k_3$) whereas the rate of amide, anilide, or peptide hydrolysis is limited by acylation ($k_{cat} = k_2$). Elastase-catalyzed reactions do not always follow this rule. It has been suggested, for instance, that the porcine pancreatic elastase-catalyzed hydrolysis of esters is limited either by acylation (Gold and Shaltin, 1975) or by deacylation (Thomson and Kapadia, 1979). On the other hand, deacylation appears to be the rate-limiting step of the leukocyte elastase-catalyzed breakdown of good p-nitroanilide or peptide substrates (Stein $et\ al.$, 1984). Great care must therefore be exercised in interpreting the significance of K_m and k_{cat}.

B. Substrate Binding Site and Specificity of Elastases

1. THE SUBSITE NOMENCLATURE OF SCHECHTER AND BERGER

Schechter and Berger (1967) have suggested that the substrate binding site of a proteinase may be divided into a number of subsites each of which accomodates one amino acid residue of the substrate:

$$\text{proteinase:} \quad S_n \ldots S_2 \ S_1 \quad S_1' \ S_2' \ldots S_n'$$
$$\text{substrate:} \quad P_n \ldots P_2 \ P_1 \quad P_1' \ P_2' \ldots P_n'$$

The amino acid residues or the N- or C-terminal blocking groups of the substrate are labeled $P_1 \ldots P_n$ in the N-terminal direction and $P_1' \ldots P_n'$ in the C-terminal direction from the scissile bond. The corresponding subsites of the enzyme are labeled $S_1 \ldots S_n$ and $S_1' \ldots S_n'$. The suggestion of Thompson and Blout (1973a) to abbreviate a binding mode of a peptide which binds, for instance, to S_4, S_3, S_2, and S_1 by the symbol S_{4321} will also be used throughout this review.

2. THE PRIMARY SUBSTRATE SPECIFICITY OF PANCREATIC AND LEUKOCYTE ELASTASES

Strictly speaking, the primary substrate specificity of a proteinase is defined as the specificity of the enzyme for the two amino acid residues adjacent to the scissile peptide bond, i.e., P_1 and P_1'. Experience shows, however, that most proteinases will use only one of these two residues (usually P_1) to express their specificity.

Investigations of the primary substrate specificity of pancreatic and leukocyte elastases with either the oxidized insulin B chain (Sampath-Narayan, 1969; Blow, 1977; Blow and Barrett, 1977; Ardelt $et\ al.$, 1979) or synthetic substrates (e.g. Table III) reveal that these enzymes may be roughly divided into two categories: those which are specific for nonbulky amino acid residues (porcine pancreatic elastase, dog pancreatic elastase, and human and dog neutrophil elastases) and those

TABLE III

INVESTIGATION OF THE PRIMARY SPECIFICITY OF SOME ELASTASES WITH A SERIES OF
Acyl-(Ala)$_2$-Pro-X-p-nitroanilides[a]

	X						
	Ala	Val	Leu	Abu	Met	Phe	Tyr
Porcine pancreatic elastase[b]	29		1	35			10^{-3}
Human pancreatic elastase[b]	0.014	10^{-4}	0.36	0.06			0.27
Dog pancreatic elastase[b]	20		0.38	3.3	46		0.07
Rat pancreatic elastase[b]	2.7	0.06	0.2	3.5	0.01	0.13	2
Human leukocyte elastase[c]	0.4	2.7					
Human leukocyte cathepsin G[c]			0.01		0.015		

[a] The figures are k_{cat}/K_m values expressed as M^{-1} sec^{-1} × 10^{-4}. Values below 1 have been rounded up. Abu = α-aminobutyric acid.

[b] Substrate: succinyl-(Ala)$_2$-Pro-X-p-nitroanilide. From Del Mar et al. (1980) and Largman (1983).

[c] Substrate: acetyl-(Ala)$_2$-Pro-X-p-nitroanilide. From Zimmerman and Ashe (1977).

which preferentially cleave bonds adjacent to bulky aliphatic or aromatic residues (porcine pancreatic elastase II, human pancreatic elastase, and neutrophil cathepsin G). The latter enzymes may be classified in the chymotrypsin family. Rat pancreatic elastase does not exhibit a stringent P_1 specificity: it cleaves P_1 = Ala as fast as P_1 = Tyr (Table III). Horse leukocyte proteinases 2A and 2B preferentially hydrolyze substrates with P_1 = Ala (Koj et al., 1979). The pancreatic elastases isolated from some fishes also exhibit a P_1 = Ala specificity (de Haën and Gertler, 1974; Yoshinaka et al., 1983; Cohen et al., 1981b). The primary specificity of porcine pancreatic elastase is in complete agreement with the X-ray crystallographic structure of the enzyme (Hartley and Shotton, 1971). Table III also shows that the various elastases may have quite different catalytic activities on their best substrate.

3.   SECONDARY SUBSTRATE SPECIFICITY OF PANCREATIC AND
     LEUKOCYTE ELASTASES

We shall define the secondary substrate specificity as the specificity manifested through S–P interactions different from S_1–P_1. The catalytic efficiency of porcine pancreatic elastase considerably increases with the chain length of the substrate (Bieth, 1978; Table IV). Occu-

TABLE IV

EFFECT OF PEPTIDE CHAIN ELONGATION ON THE CATALYTIC ACTIVITY OF PORCINE
PANCREATIC ELASTASE AND HUMAN LEUKOCYTE ELASTASE AND CATHEPSIN G[a]

Size of substrate	Porcine pancreatic elastase[b]		Human leukocyte elastase[c]	Human leukocyte cathepsin G[d]
P_2-P_1-P_1'				1.8 (1)
P_3-P_2-P_1-P_1'	4.2 (1)		740 (1)	22 (12)
P_4-P_3-P_2-P_1-P_1'	12,000	(2,900)	8,700 (12)	430 (240)
P_5-P_4-P_3-P_2-P_1-P_1'	170,000	(40,500)	30,300 (41)	1,370 (770)
P_6-P_5-P_4-P_3-P_2-P_1-P_1'				

[a] The figures are k_{cat}/K_m values in M^{-1} sec^{-1}. Numbers in parentheses are relative values.

[b] Substrate: succinyl-(Ala)$_n$-p-nitroanilide, n = 2 to 4. From Davril et al. (1984).

[c] Substrate: succinyl-(Ala)$_n$-Val-p-nitroanilide, n = 1 to 3. From Wenzel and Tschesche (1981).

[d] Substrate: succinyl-(Ala)$_n$-Phe-p-nitroanilide, n = 1 to 3. From Boudier et al. (1981a).

pancy of subsite S_4 appears to be of critical importance for efficient catalysis. Human leukocyte elastase activity appears to be much less sensitive to substrate size than the former proteinase. With P_1 = Ala substrates, however, the effects are somewhat more pronounced (Lestienne and Bieth, 1980). By contrast, cathepsin G is fairly sensitive to peptide chain elongation. The effect of substrate size on catalysis has not been extensively investigated with other elastases. Porcine pancreatic elastase is much more sensitive to secondary enzyme–substrate interactions than other proteinases.

The substrate binding site of porcine pancreatic elastase extends over 29 Å and is composed of eight subsites, S_5 to S_3' (Bieth, 1978). The specificity of the individual subsites of this enzyme has been rather thoroughly investigated (Bieth, 1978; McRae et al., 1980; Renaud et al., 1983). The substrate binding site of human leukocyte elastase also extends from S_5 to S_3' (McRae et al., 1980; Lestienne and Bieth, 1980). Subsites S_2, S_3, and S_4 are rather large (Yasutake and Powers, 1981). The specificities of S_1' and S_2' of the two elastases are quite similar (Renaud et al., 1983). The active center of other elastases has not been investigated in detail.

4. MULTIPLE PRODUCTIVE BINDING AND NONPRODUCTIVE
BINDING OF SUBSTRATES AND INHIBITORS TO ELASTASES

Multiple productive binding is a binding mode which leads to more than one product as a result of enzyme action. For instance, acetyl-

(Ala)$_4$-NH$_2$ yields a mixture of NH$_3$ of Ala-NH$_2$ in the presence of porcine pancreatic elastase (Thompson and Blout, 1970).

Proline cannot bind at subsite S$_3$ of pancreatic elastase (Thompson and Blout, 1973) or leukocyte cathepsin G (Nakajima et al., 1979). Therefore, synthetic substrates with P$_3$ = proline will mostly bind in a single productive mode.

Nonproductive binding of substrate and inhibitor is a binding mode which does not lead to breakdown of the substrate or to inhibition of the enzyme. If the substrate binds both productively and nonproductively and if these two binding modes are mutually exclusive, the latter is not seen kinetically (Bieth, 1978). For instance, replacement of the succinyl group of succinyl-(Ala)$_3$-p-nitroanilide by a trifluoroacetyl substituent yields a substrate whose reaction with elastase obeys Michaelis–Menten kinetics but whose k_{cat} and K_m values are much lower than those of the succinylated substrate (Lestienne et al., 1982). This behavior is due to the strong affinity of the trifluoroacetyl group for subsite S$_1$ (Hughes et al., 1982) with resultant nonproductive binding of most of the substrate.

If the productive and nonproductive binding modes are not exclusive, and if the ternary enzyme–(substrate)$_2$ complex decomposes at a rate different from that of the binary complex, activation or inhibition by excess substrate may be observed. The former phenomenon exists for pancreatic or leukocyte elastase-catalyzed hydrolyses of some p-nitroanilides (Bieth and Wermuth, 1973; Lestienne and Bieth, 1980).

Nonproductive binding of inhibitors to the active site of porcine pancreatic elastase has been diagnosed by physical methods including X-ray crystallography (Shotton et al., 1971), NMR (Dimicoli et al., 1979), and terbium luminescence spectroscopy (de Jersey and Martin, 1980).

C. Regulation of Elastase Catalysis

In this section we shall consider some effects of secondary enzyme–substrate interactions on elastase catalysis. We shall also deal with other factors that may regulate elastase activity.

1. REGULATION OF ELASTASE CATALYSIS BY SECONDARY ENZYME–SUBSTRATE INTERACTIONS

In Table IV we have shown that the proteolytic coefficient k_{cat}/K_m strongly increases with the chain length of the substrates. The question is now is this increase due to an increase in k_{cat}, to a decrease in K_m, or to a change in both constants? Substrates b of Table IV show that in the case of porcine pancreatic elastase both constants undergo favorable changes upon substrate chain elongation. Human leukocyte elastase behaves in a similar way (Lestienne and Bieth, 1980; Wenzel and Tschesche, 1981), i.e., the longer the substrate, the better the binding ($1/K_m$) and the better the catalysis (k_{cat}). The major difference between the two elastases is the moderate increase in k_{cat} upon occupancy of subsite S_4 of human leukocyte elastase as compared to the enormous enhancement of k_{cat} upon filling of the same subsite of porcine pancreatic elastase (see, for instance, substrates a in Table V). Thompson and Blout (1973d, and refs. therein) have thoroughly investigated the importance of the S_4–P_4 interaction in porcine pancreatic elastase-catalyzed hydrolysis of model substrates. Three of the substrates they used are listed in Table V (substrates b). It can be seen that the P_4 substituents which increase K_m (i.e., which decrease the enzyme–substrate affinity), also increase k_{cat}. Better binding, therefore, does not necessarily lead to better catalysis. Thompson and Blout

TABLE V

TYPICAL EXAMPLES OF REGULATION OF ELASTASE CATALYSIS BY SECONDARY
ENZYME–SUBSTRATE INTERACTION (S–P INTERACTIONS DIFFERENT FROM S_1–P_1)

Substrate						k_{cat} (sec^{-1})	K_m (mM)	k_{cat}/K_m (M^{-1} sec^{-1})
P_5	P_4	P_3	P_2	P_1	P_1'			
Porcine pancreatic elastase								
		Suc - Ala - Ala - NA[a]				0.02	5	4
	Suc	- Ala - Ala - Ala - NA[a]				24	2	12,000
Suc - Ala		- Ala - Ala - Ala - NA[a]				13.6	0.08	170,000
	Ac	- Ala - Pro - Ala - NH$_2$[b]				0.09	4.2	21
	Isobut	- Ala - Pro - Ala - NH$_2$[b]				2.7	8.3	325
	Pival	- Ala - Pro - Ala - NH$_2$[b]				3.7	22	170
Human leukocyte elastase								
MeOSuc - Ala	- Ala	- Pro - Met - NA[c]				0.72	2.4	300
MeOSuc - Ala	- Ile	- Pro - Met - NA[c]				6.8	1.7	4,000
MeOSuc - Ala	- Ala	- Pro - Val - NA[d]				17	0.14	120,000
MeOSuc - Lys(Z) - Ala		- Pro - Val - NA[d]				18	0.026	710,000
MeOSuc - Ala	- Lys(Z) - Pro - Val - NA[d]					12	0.045	260,000

[a] Suc = succinyl; NA = p-nitroanilide. From Davril $et\ al.$ (1984).

[b] Ac = acetyl; Isobut = $(CH_3)_2CHCO$; Pival = $(CH_3)_3CCO$. From Thompson and Blout (1973d).

[c] MeOSuc = succinyl methyl ester; NA = p-nitroanilide. From Nakajima $et\ al.$ (1979).

[d] Lys(Z) = lysine with a carbobenzyloxylated ε NH$_2$; other abbreviations, see footnote c. From Yasutake and Powers (1981).

(1973d) suggested that porcine pancreatic elastase may be an "induced-fit enzyme" (Koshland and Neet, 1968). In such enzymes the substrate may induce conformational changes that favor catalysis. Since part of the substrate binding energy may be utilized to change the enzyme structure, a "good" substrate will have an apparently lower affinity than a "bad" one which does not lose part of its binding energy to induce the enzyme–substrate fit.

Table V also shows two interesting examples of regulation of leukocyte elastase catalysis by secondary enzyme–substrate interactions. In the first example (substrates c), a P_3 substitution leads to a 10-fold increase in k_{cat} without important changes in K_m. By contrast, with substrates d, P_4 or P_3 substitutions lead to substantial increases in enzyme–substrate affinity without important changes in k_{cat}. These two examples illustrate the two mechanisms by which secondary enzyme–substrate interactions may enhance the overall catalytic power of elastase (i.e., k_{cat}/K_m).

An increase in k_{cat} may result either from a good P_1–S_1 fit, with the resultant optimal closeness of the substrate's scissile bond to serine of the catalytic site, or from an S–P induced "activation" of the charge-relay system, with the resultant increase of the nucleophilicity of the oxygen atom of the serine residue. The former mechanism was proposed for porcine pancreatic elastase (Thompson, 1974). The latter was suggested for good substrates of human leukocyte elastase. Stein (1983) used proton inventory data (rate measurements in mixtures of H_2O and D_2O) to determine the number of protons involved in the leukocyte elastase-catalyzed hydrolysis of model substrates. For moderately potent substrates [e.g., succinyl-$(Ala)_2$-Val-p-nitroanilide] only one proton was involved whereas for a good substrate [succinylmethylester-$(Ala)_2$-Pro-Val-p-nitroanilide] the two protons of the charge-relay system were transferred during catalysis. These data suggest that the substrate binding site and the catalytic site are intimately related.

In Section V,B,4 we have shown that catalysis may be activated at high substrate concentrations by the nonproductive binding of a second substrate molecule to elastase. This may be considered as a particular case of regulation of elastase catalysis by enzyme–substrate interactions.

2. Regulation of Elastase Catalysis by Other Factors

Inhibition and activation of elastase activity by interaction of ligands with the enzyme will be reviewed in Section VI. Here we shall discuss the effects of two factors: ionic strength and hydrophobic solvents.

   a. Effect of Ionic Strength.   Ionic strength increases the rate of the porcine pancreatic elastase-catalyzed hydrolysis of benzoyl-Ala-methyl ester: 2 M NaCl increases k_{cat} by a factor of about 3 (Gold and Shaltin, 1975). With the more specific substrate succinyl-(Ala)$_3$-p-nitroanilide, the effect of ionic strength is less pronounced (Boudier *et al.*, 1980). By contrast, the hydrolysis of this substrate by human leukocyte elastase is strongly enhanced by ionic strength: in 5 M NaCl, the reaction rate increases by a factor of 20 (Boudier *et al.*, 1980). The activating effect is mainly on k_{cat}, which increases by a factor of 5 in 2 M NaCl (Lestienne and Bieth, 1980). In addition, ionic strength does not abolish the activation by excess substrate. Moreover, 2 M NaCl increases k'_{cat} of the ternary enzyme–(substrate)$_2$ complex by a factor of 5.7 (Lestienne and Bieth, 1980).

   On other hand, some buffers have an inhibitory effect on the pancreatic elastase-catalyzed hydrolysis of succinyl-(Ala)$_3$-p-nitroanilide. For instance, borate buffer increases K_m and decreases k_{cat}. The borate ion was found to be a competitive inhibitor of pancreatic elastase with a K_i of 50 mM (Davril *et al.*, 1984). As shown in Section III, Ca^{2+} strongly binds to porcine pancreatic elastase. This binding does not, however, influence the catalytic properties of the enzyme (Dimicoli and Bieth, 1977).

   b. Effect of Hydrophobic Solvents.   Most of the synthetic elastase substrates contain hydrophobic amino acid residues. The binding of these substrates to elastase may therefore be hampered by hydrophobic solvents which are often mixed with buffers in order to gain sufficient substrate solubility.

   The porcine pancreatic elastase-catalyzed hydrolysis of succinyl-(Ala)$_3$-p-nitroanilide may be investigated in the absence of organic solvent because of the presence of the hydrophilic succinyl group. In the presence of 1% N-methylpyrrolidone, K_m increases by a factor of 2.2 whereas k_{cat} does not change to a great extent (Bieth *et al.*, 1974). The overall effect of this solvent is therefore inhibition of elastase activity. Acetonitrile and dimethylformamide were also found to inhibit the elastase-catalyzed hydrolysis of model substrates (Bieth and Wermuth, 1973; Geneste and Bender, 1969; Thomson and Kapadia, 1979).

   By contrast, hydrophobic solvents enhance the human leukocyte elastase activity on succinyl-(Ala)$_3$-p-nitroanilide (Lestienne and Bieth, 1980). For instance, 5% N-methylpyrrolidone or dimethylformamide increase the rate by factors of 3.4 and 2.0, respectively. The latter solvent increases k_{cat} and K_m to similar extents i.e., k_{cat}/K_m does not change. As a result, activation of catalysis occurs. On the other hand, with succinyl-$(Ala)_3$-p-nitrophenylester, whose rate-limiting step is deacylation, no activation is observed. This suggests that solvents mainly affect the acylation step of substrate hydrolysis (Lestienne and Bieth, 1980).

D. Action of Elastases on Fibrous Elastin

1. THE CHEMISTRY OF ELASTIN

From a practical point of view, elastin may be defined as the insoluble material which is left after subjecting connective tissues to very harsh treatments such as autoclaving or boiling in NaOH. This residue is insoluble in boiling water and organic solvents. Solubilization occurs only under harsh conditions such as boiling in oxalic acid (Partridge and Davis, 1955), in a mixture of KOH and ethanol (Comte and Robert, 1968), or in 6 N HCl. The two former procedures yield soluble polypeptides called α-elastin or κ-elastin, respectively, whereas the latter method yields the individual amino acids. Solubilization occurs, of course, under mild conditions with catalytic amounts of elastases.

The chemistry and biology of elastin has been the subject of excellent recent reviews (Sandberg *et al.*, 1981; Urry, 1983; Rucker and Dubick, 1984). The amino acid composition of bovine ligamentum nuchae and human lung elastins is given in Table VI. There is a remarkably large proportion of nonpolar amino acids. These amino acids and the cross-linking residues desmosine, isodesmosin, and lysinonorleucine account for the insoluble character of this structural protein. The cross-linking structures all derive from lysine residues. The lysines that form desmosines occur in alanine-rich regions. The sequencing of tropoelastin, the 70-kDa soluble precursor of elastin, is about to be complete and cloning of the elastin cDNA is in active progress (Foster *et al.*, 1983). Tropoelastin contains repeating peptides such as Val-Pro-Gly-Val-Gly or Ala-Pro-Gly-Val-Gly-Val which form β-turns which allow the polypeptide chain to fold back on itself and to form β-spirals, a structure unique to elastin.

The distribution of polar amino acid residues suggests that elastin is an anionic protein. Kagan and Lerch (1976), however, have shown that at least 70% of the dicarboxylic amino acids are amidated. On the other hand, 20–50% of the lysine residues probably occur as $\epsilon(\delta$-adipic acid)-

TABLE VI

AMINO ACID COMPOSITION (NUMBER OF RESIDUES PER 1000
RESIDUES) OF BOVINE LIGAMENTUM NUCHAE AND
HUMAN LUNG ELASTIN[a]

	Elastin source	
	---	---
Amino acid	Bovine ligamentum nuchae	Human lung
Aspartic acid	6	9
Threonine	9	11
Serine	10	10
Glutamic acid	15	25
Proline	120	85
Glycine	324	331
Alanine*	223	258
Cysteine	n.d.	1
Valine*	135	128
Methionine	0	1
Isoleucine	25	21
Leucine*	61	59
Tyrosine*	7	21
Phenylalanine*	30	22
Tryptophan	n.d.	0
Lysine	7	8
Arginine	5	8
Isodesmosine	0.8	0.8
Desmosine	1.2	1.2

[a] The amino acid residues marked by * have been shown to
be P_1 residues of elastase substrates. n.d. = not determined.
From Boudier et al. (1981b).

lysine, the oxidized form of lysinonorleucine (Guay and Lamy, 1981;
Han et al., 1979).

2. COMPARED ACTION OF ELASTASES ON ELASTIN

Table VII shows that elastases of different origin have widely different elastolytic activities. As a rule, pancreatic elastases are significantly more active than leukocyte elastases. For instance, dog and
human neutrophil elastases have identical specific activities (Delshammar and Ohlsson, 1976), and these activities are 14–30 times
lower than those of the corresponding pancreatic enzymes. On the
other hand, the elastolytic activity of a given elastase depends upon

TABLE VII

COMPARED ELASTOLYTIC ACTION OF SOME ELASTASES ON BOVINE
LIGAMENTUM NUCHAE AND HUMAN LUNG ELASTINS

	Relative elastolytic activity	
Elastase	Bovine elastin	Human elastin
Porcine pancreatic elastase[a]	100	78
Human leukocyte elastase[a]	7.2	3.7
Human leukocyte cathepsin G[a]	0.45	0.75
Porcine pancreatic elastase[b]	100	
Human pancreatic elastase[b]	16.6	
Dog pancreatic elastase[b]	199	
Rat pancreatic elastase[b]	67.1	

[a] Substrate: undyed elastin. From Boudier et al. (1981b).
[b] Substrate: Remazol Brilliant Blue elastin. From Largman (1983).

the method used to prepare elastin. For instance, Reilly and Travis (1980) have shown that elastin prepared by guanidine–HCl and collagenase treatment is solubilized four times more quickly by porcine pancreatic elastase, human leukocyte elastase, and cathepsin G than is elastin prepared by hot alkali treatment. Labeling of elastin with dyes or radioactive groups may also alter its susceptibility to elastase digestion. Table VII also shows that the animal origin of elastin influences the rate of elastolysis: it is noteworthy that human leukocyte elastase is only about half as active on human elastin than on bovine elastin. By contrast, cathepsin G is more active on the former than on the latter substrate.

3. MECHANISMS OF ACTION OF ELASTASES ON FIBROUS ELASTIN

a. Correlation between the Rate of Elastolysis and the Catalytic Activity of Elastases. Table VI shows that Ala, Val, Leu, Tyr, and Phe, which constitute the P_1 residues of model substrates of elastases (see Section V,B), account for about 45% of the total amino acid residues of elastin. Gertler et al. (1977) demonstrated that porcine pancreatic elastase cleaves Ala-Ala and Ala-Gly bonds in bovine ligamentum nuchae elastin, a result that confirms, with the natural substrate, the restricted P_1 specificity of this enzyme. Moreover, porcine pancreatic elastase II was found to attack elastin at Leu-Ala, Phe-Ala, and Tyr-

Ala links, again confirming the primary substrate specificity of this elastase and also suggesting a restricted P'_1 specificity.

There is no good correlation, however, between the catalytic activity of elastases on model substrates and their rates of elastolysis. For instance, the best substrates of porcine pancreatic elastase and human leukocyte elastase have similar k_{cat}/K_m values (McRae *et al.*, 1980) suggesting that these two enzymes have similar intrinsic catalytic activities. Yet, they hydrolyze elastin at considerably different rates (Table VII). These differences might be accounted for by differences in the Ala and Val contents of elastin. However, other factors must be important since bovine and human elastins which have similar contents of Val are hydrolyzed with quite different rates by the leukocyte enzyme (Table VII). Canine and porcine pancreatic elastase which are both specific for $P_1 = $ Ala, offer another interesting example: the k_{cat}/K_m value for an oligopeptidic model substrate is higher for the former enzyme than for the latter one and yet canine elastase is twice as active as porcine elastase on fibrous elastin. Lastly, bovine α-chymotrypsin is about 200-fold more active on a long model substrate than human leukocyte cathepsin G, and yet the former enzyme does not solubilize bovine ligamentum nuchae elastin whereas the latter does (Boudier *et al.*, 1981b).

The above discussion shows that the rate at which an elastase solubilizes elastin does not so much depend upon the primary substrate specificity and the intrinsic catalytic activity of the enzyme but may be influenced to a great extent by the nature of elastin itself.

b. Some Features of the Elastase-Catalyzed Solubilization of Elastin. The elastolysis reaction is a special case of heterogeneous catalysis in which the substrate (not the enzyme) is in the particulate phase. From the standpoint of the enzymologist this system appears to be enormously more complex than the reaction of a proteinase with a soluble protein. First, due to its insoluble character, elastin creates high local substrate concentrations which are difficult to rationalize. Second, elastin fibers bear positively and negatively charged groups. Due to their high local concentration, these groups may tightly bind elastase molecules and prevent their elastolytic action (i.e., they may create nonproductive binding). Third, the charged groups may also create an electrostatic microenvironment which may impair productive elastase binding by charge repulsion. Last, the soluble peptides generated by the action of elastase on elastin may themselves serve as elastase substrates and, hence, may inhibit elastolysis. No comprehensive analysis of these multiple phenomena has been performed as yet. Some points, however, have been elucidated.

Gertler *et al.* (1977) have shown that full solubilization of bovine elastin by porcine pancreatic elastase is achieved by hydrolysis of 7.6% of total peptide bonds. Thus, only about one-third of the Ala-X linkages of elastin need to be hydrolyzed in order to get soluble peptides. Kagan *et al.* (1972) have shown that these soluble peptides have molecular masses ranging from 2 to 10 kDa. Moreover, when elastin is pretreated with sodium dodecyl sulfate, 15% fewer peptide bonds need to be cleaved to get full solubilization of elastin, the rate of elastolysis is six times faster, and most of the soluble peptides have a mass of about 30 kDa. These findings clearly suggest that the rate of elastin solubilization is not necessarily related to the catalytic power of a given elastase: a potent enzyme may cleave many more peptide bonds per unit time than a poor one, but the latter may generate much bigger peptides, making it a better "elastase". In addition, the above findings suggest that elastolysis may be enhanced by the concerted action of several proteinases with different substrate specificities. This was found to be the case: cathepsin G, human pancreatic elastase, and bovine α-chymotrypsin are able to significantly enhance the rate of elastin solubilization by human leukocyte elastase (Boudier *et al.*, 1981b, 1984). The stimulation by cathepsin G is particularly important: the rate of solubilization of an equimolar mixture of elastase and cathepsin G is about five times more greater than the sum of the rates observed with the individual enzymes.

Last, we wish to discuss the possible competition between soluble and insoluble elastin for the binding of elastase. Several lines of evidence suggest that this competition is largely in favor of the insoluble material. For instance, porcine pancreatic elastase binds so tightly to fibrous elastin that the complex may be isolated by centrifugation (Hall and Czerkawski, 1961b; Gertler, 1971b). Besides, Gertler *et al.* (1977) have shown that the soluble peptides resulting from elastin digestion do not undergo further proteolytic cleavage. In addition, kinetics of elastin solubilization are usually linear up to at least 50% of substrate hydrolysis (Ardelt *et al.*, 1970; Bieth *et al.*, 1976; Gertler *et al.*, 1977), suggesting that the soluble peptides do not favorably compete with elastin for the binding of elastase.

    c. Possible Nonproductive Binding of Elastases to Elastin. Nonproductive enzyme–substrate binding i.e., binding which does not result in substrate cleavage has already been shown to occur with model substrates of elastase (Section V,B). With elastin, such nonproductive complexes may result from electrostatic interactions between elastase and negatively or positively charged groups of the substrate.

These groups may not only be the side-chains of polar residues but also complexes between Ca^{2+} and neutral amino acid residues (Urry, 1983). In addition, nonproductive hydrophobic elastin–elastase interactions may take place.

Indirect evidence for nonproductive binding is available. Kagan *et al.* (1977) showed that the rate of elastolysis by porcine pancreatic elastase is increased twofold in the presence of an excess of inactive elastase (tosyl elastase) while the amount of active elastase bound to elastin is significantly decreased. These workers suggested that inactive elastase occupied the nonproductive binding sites and forced active elastase to form more productive complexes with elastin.

Lonky and co-workers (Lonky *et al.*, 1978; Lonky and Wohl, 1983) noticed that platelet factor 4 and other lysine-rich ligands are able to strongly enhance the rate of elastolysis of bovine elastin by human leukocyte elastase. There is again competition between these ligands and elastase for the binding to elastin, i.e., there is less elastase bound when these compounds are present. The situation is therefore analogous to that discussed above: the competing molecules force elastase to form more productive complexes with elastin.

   d.   Relative Importance of Electrostatic Interactions in Elastolysis. There is a large body of evidence indicating that electrostatic interactions are of prime importance in elastolysis catalyzed by porcine pancreatic elastase. Many years ago, Hall and Czerkawski (1961a) demonstrated that elastolysis by this enzyme was prevented by esterification of the carboxyl groups of elastin. Gertler has published a series of articles showing the importance of charge complementarity between the negatively charged substrate and the positively charged enzyme. These electrostatic interactions are nonspecific since any protein with a pI > 8.5 readily binds to elastin. The adsorption sharply drops below pH 5 where the carboxyl groups of elastin become protonated and above pH 9.5 where the basic groups of elastase become deprotonated (Gertler, 1971b). The adsorption of elastase to elastin strongly decreases with increasing ionic strength, a result that explains the inhibition of elastolysis by NaCl (Walford and Kickhöfen, 1962). When the ε-amino groups of elastase are maleylated, the enzyme loses its elastolytic activity whereas its action on synthetic substrates is not altered (Gertler, 1971c). On the other hand, the alkaline proteinase of *Aspergillus sojae,* which does not attack elastin but shares the substrate specificity of porcine pancreatic elastase, becomes a powerful elastolytic enzyme after modification of its carboxyl groups (Gertler, 1971a). The importance of electrostatic interactions has been nicely confirmed by Kagan *et al.* (1972), who showed that the increase of the negative charge of elastin by sodium dodecyl sulfate strongly increases both the elastase-binding capacity of elastin and the rate of elastolysis.

On the basis of his findings, Gertler (1971b) suggested that ". . . an enzyme capable of dissolving elastin in the pH range of 7–10 has to fulfil two basic conditions: is has to be basic enough to be adsorbed on elastin, and also its chain specificity has to be directed toward non-polar amino acids. . . ." This hypothesis must now be considered obsolete for the reasons given below.

Jordan *et al.* (1974) have shown that elastin pretreated with a cationic detergent is resistant to native porcine pancreatic elastase but is rapidly solubilized by maleylated, i.e., anionic, elastase. This indicates that, while electrostatic interactions are important, the normal charge complementarity (i.e., anionic elastin + cationic elastase) is not a prerequisite for elastolysis. Therefore, the carboxyl groups of elastin themselves do not contribute to the productive binding of porcine elastase. It may thus be suggested that electrostatic interactions serve merely to attract elastase molecules to the vicinity of elastin fibers and that productive enzyme–substrate binding occurs via nonelectrostatic forces (e.g., hydrophobic interactions). In fact, some elastases are anionic proteins. *Pseudomonas aeruginosa* elastase, for instance, has a p*I* of 5.9, and yet it is a powerful elastolytic enzyme (Morihara *et al.,* 1965). Human pancreatic elastase I is anionic but has a low but distinct elastolytic activity (Largman, 1983). One of the two dog pancreatic elastases is an anionic protein but a powerful elastolytic proteinase (Geokas *et al.,* 1980). The proposal of Gertler (1971b) that elastases have to be basic proteins is therefore not valid for all elastases.

Investigations of the effect of ionic strength on elastolytic activity also suggest that for some elastases electrostatic interactions play a minor role in elastolysis. For instance, the elastolytic activity of *Streptomyces fradiae* elastase is not inhibited by NaCl (Mandl and Cohen, 1960; Morihara and Tsuzuki, 1967). On the other hand, ionic strength strongly stimulates the human leukocyte elastase-catalyzed solubilization of elastin (Boudier *et al.,* 1980) and has little effect on the adsorption of this enzyme on elastin (Lonky and Wohl, 1983). There is further evidence suggesting that electrostatic interactions play a minor role in leukocyte elastase-mediated elastolysis. First, sodium dodecyl sulfate increases the leukocyte elastase activity by only 80% (Lonky and Wohl, 1983) whereas a sixfold stimulation is observed with pancreatic elastase (Kagan *et al.,* 1972). Second, reaction of elastin with polylysine, which interacts electrostatically with the carboxyl groups of this substrate, abolishes the elastolytic activity of porcine pancreatic elastase (Gertler, 1971b) but strongly enhances the activity of human leukocyte elastase (Lonky and Wohl, 1983). Moreover, elastin precoated with lysine-rich ligands binds less leukocyte elastase than does native elastin. This suggests that negatively charged groups of elastin are nonproductive binding sites for leukocyte elastase (Lonky and Wohl, 1983).

e. Conclusions. There is apparently no general mechanism for describing the elastolytic action of all elastases. Productive enzyme–substrate binding certainly occurs via hydrophobic interactions at regions of elastin that fulfil the substrate requirements of a given elastase. These regions might a priori have sequences with polar amino acid residues. However, an antispecificity of pancreatic and leukocyte elastase for P_4 or P_2 = Lys has been described (Yasutake and Powers, 1981). Nonproductive enzyme–substrate binding may be one of the factors that account for the lack of correlation between the catalytic power of an elastase and its ability to solubilize elastin. This binding mode may not only occur via electrostatic interactions, as suggested for human leukocyte elastase, but also via hydrophobic interactions at a locus different from the active site of the enzyme. For enzymes like porcine pancreatic elastase, electrostatic interactions may be the initial driving force that attracts the soluble enzyme to the vicinity of the insoluble substrate. For enzymes like human leukocyte elastase, hydrophobic interactions may be efficient enough to bring enzyme and substrate into close contact.

Last, we wish to point out that the elastin substrate which is usually used to investigate the mechanism of elastolysis cannot be considered as the true natural substrate of elastase because it has been subjected to very harsh treatments during its isolation. As suggested by Kagan and Lerch (1976), most of the carboxylates of "native" elastin may be amidated. Would such a substrate still be solubilized by porcine pancreatic elastase? Reilly and Travis (1980) showed that lung elastin prepared in two different ways was solubilized by elastases with quite different rates. Such observations should be kept in mind when studying the mechanism of elastolysis. Efforts should also be made in the future to prepare "native" elastin. Since cloning of elastin cDNA is currently in progress (Foster *et al.,* 1983) large quantities of tropoelastin, the soluble precursor of elastin, should soon be made available by genetic engineering and converted to truly native elastin by reaction with lysyl oxidase and other posttranslational enzymes.

TABLE VIII

ENDOGENOUS SUBSTRATES OF HUMAN LEUKOCYTE ELASTASE

	Major effects	References	Also cleaved by human leukocyte cathepsin G
Connective tissue macromolecules			
Type I collagen (skin)	Cleavage through the triple helix	Starkey (1977a)	No
Type I collagen (tendon)	Cleavage within the terminal peptides	Starkey (1977a)	No
Type II collagen	Cleavage within the terminal peptides	Starkey et al. (1977)	Yes
Type III collagen	Ile-Thr bond cleaved in the helical region	Gadek et al. (1980a); Mainardi et al. (1980a)	
Type IV collagen (basement membrane)		Mainardi et al. (1980b)	
Fibronectin	Release of biologically active fragments	McDonald and Kelley (1980)	Yes[a]
Cartilage proteoglycans		Malemud and Janoff (1975); Starkey et al. (1977)	Yes
Coagulation factors			
Fibrinogen	Production of a 93-kDa fragment different from that produced by plasmin	Schmidt et al. (1975); Sterrenberg et al. (1983); Plow et al. (1983).	Yes
Factors V, VIII, XII	Inactivated	Schmidt et al. (1975)	Yes, except factor V
Factor XIII	Activation followed by inactivation	Henriksson et al. (1980)	
Plasminogen	Several cleavage products one of which is able to undergo activation by urokinase	Powell and Castellino (1981); Nagamatsu and Soeda (1981)	

Components of the immune system

Immunoglobulins G	IgG1 → Fab + Fc + Fab–Fc	Prince et al. (1979a) Baici et al. (1980a)	Yes
	IgG2 → F(ab)$_2$ + Fab–Fc + Fab + Fc IgG3 → Fab + Fch IgG4 → F(ab)$_2$ + Fab + Fc		
Immunoglobulin M	IgM → F(ab)$_2\mu$-like + Fabμ-like fragments	Prince et al. (1979b); Baici et al. (1980b)	Yes
Complement C3	Cleavage at multiple sites; inactivation	Brozna et al. (1977); Taylor et al. (1977)	Yes
Complement C5	Inactivation	Johnsson et al. (1976); Brozna et al. (1977)	Yes
Plasma proteinase inhibitors			
Antithrombin III	Inactivation	Jochum et al. (1981)	
α_2-Antiplasmin	Inactivation	Brower and Harpel (1982); Gramse et al. (1984)	
Inter-α-trypsin inhibitor	Production of a low molecular mass acid-stable and active fragment	Dietl et al. (1979)	
Cl-Inactivator	Inactivation	Brower and Harpel (1982)	
α_1-Antichymotrypsin[b]	Inactivation	Morii and Travis (1983)	
Miscellaneous proteins			
Latent neutrophil collagenase and gelatinase	Activation	Murphy et al. (1980)	Yes
Plasma apolipoprotein AII[c]	Formation of 7- and 11-kDa fragments by cleavage of Val-X bonds	Byrne et al. (1984)	

[a] From Vartio et al. (1981).
[b] Also inactivated by porcine pancreatic elastase.
[c] Porcine pancreatic elastase also cleaves apolipoproteins (Maeda et al., 1982).

E. Action of Human Leukoproteinases on Endogenous Substrates

Elastases do, of course, hydrolyze not only elastin but also any soluble protein that contains appropriate surface-exposed amino acid sequences. The action of leukocyte elastase on soluble proteins is particularly well documented because of the potential pathological function of this enzyme (see Section X). Table VIII summarizes the most pertinent data that have been reported in this field. It is noteworthy that leukocyte elastase, a serine proteinase, cleaves type III and type IV collagen in their triple-helical regions. This enzyme therefore mimics the action of "true collagenases" which are metalloenzymes. As a rule, leukocyte elastase exerts a harmful action on structural macromolecules and on proteins which play important functions in the organism. This enzyme is, however, an active component of the phagocytic function of polymorphonuclear leukocytes. It has also been shown to cleave bacterial cell walls (Janoff and Blondin, 1973).

Cathepsin G shares some of the proteolytic properties of elastase (Table VIII). In addition, it degrades laminin, another connective tissue protein (Rao et al., 1982). It also possesses the very interesting property of converting angiotensin I to angiotensin II (Reilly et al., 1982) and generating angiotensin II from angiotensinogen, a reaction that normally requires two proteinases: renin and angiotensin-converting enzyme (Wintroub et al., 1984). The physiological relevance of this alternate pathway of angiotensin II generation is not yet clearly understood.

VI. Pancreatic and Leukocyte Elastase Inhibitors

A. Protein Proteinase Inhibitors

1. Human Plasma α_1-Proteinase Inhibitor

Human plasma contains at least seven protein proteinase inhibitors, representing about 10% of the total plasma proteins. Among these, α_1-proteinase inhibitor (formerly called α_1-antitrypsin) has the highest molar concentration and plays a key role in endogenous regulation of elastase activity. Its properties have recently been reviewed by Carrell et al. (1982) and Travis and Salvesen (1983).

a. *Structure and Biosynthesis.* Human plasma α_1-proteinase inhibitor is a 52-kDa glycoprotein (13–15% carbohydrates) with a pI of 4–6. It is formed of a single polypeptide chain of 394 residues with no internal disulfide bonds, a single cysteine residue able to form disulfide interchange reactions with other proteins, and three carbohydrate side-chains N-linked to Asn residues at positions 46, 48, and 247. The amino acid sequence determined by protein chemistry (Carrell *et al.*, 1982) is in good agreement with that deduced from the sequence of the α_1-proteinase inhibitor gene and cDNA (Long *et al.*, 1984, and refs. therein). The precursor molecule contains a 24-amino acid signal peptide. Preliminary X-ray analysis shows that the polypeptide chain of α_1-proteinase inhibitor is highly ordered: it is composed of three β-sheets and eight α-helices (Löbermann *et al.*, 1984). The inhibitor is fairly stable in the neutral pH range, but it rapidly loses its activity at pH values below 4.0.

A striking feature of α_1-proteinase inhibitor is its polymorphism: more than 30 different forms have been diagnosed by acid electrophoresis, and new variants are still being discovered (Sesboüe *et al.*, 1984; Yuasa *et al.*, 1984). This polymorphism is genetically determined (autosomal codominant inheritance) and is referred to as the Pi system. PiMM is the normal phenotype. The S and Z mutants are of particular interest as they are associated with partial plasma inhibitor deficiency and diseases (mainly lung emphysema and neonatal liver cirrhosis). In PiSS and PiZZ individuals the plasma concentration of inhibitor is 60% and 15%, respectively, of the normal (1.3 g/l). PiMS, PiMZ, or PiSZ heterozygotes have intermediate inhibitor levels. It is noteworthy that the S and Z variants are essentially confined to individuals of European descent, 3% of whom are PiMZ. The Z variant accumulates in the hepatocytes. This explains both the occurrence of liver cirrhosis in some PiZZ newborns and the development of early emphysema in some PiZZ adults. The S protein does not accumulate in the liver. The S and Z variants differ from the M protein by one single amino acid residue: in the S protein Val replaces Glu at position 264 and in the Z variant Lys replaces Glu at position 342. The abnormal variants of α_1-proteinase inhibitor are commonly detected by acid electrophoresis of serum proteins. Recently, synthetic oligonucleotide probes (Kidd *et al.*, 1983) and monoclonal antibodies (Wallmark *et al.*, 1984) have been proposed for the sensitive and fast detection of the Z variant.

α_1-Proteinase inhibitor shares 30% of common structure with antithrombin III, another plasma proteinase inhibitor, and ovalbumin, a noninhibitory protein. It has been suggested that these three molecules evolved from a common ancestral proteinase inhibitor some 500 million years ago.

The liver is the major source of plasma α_1-proteinase inhibitors. Biosynthesis of the protein by macrophages (Isaacson *et al.*, 1981), monocytes (Van Furth *et al.*, 1983), lymphocytes (Ikuta *et al.*, 1982), and polymorphonuclear leukocytes (Andersen, 1984) has also been reported.

The α_1-proteinase inhibitor is found not only in plasma but also in lymph and various plasma transudates including the lung alveolar lining fluid, where it plays its most important biological function.

b. Specificity and Mechanism of Action. Plasma α_1-proteinase inhibitor is a nonspecific inhibitor of serine proteinases with which it forms 1:1 complexes resistant to denaturing agents. The molecular mass of the complexes is slightly lower than that of the sum of the individual reactants because a 3.6-kDa peptide is removed from the C-terminal part of the inhibitor during complex formation. The inhibitor therefore behaves in some way like a suicide substrate. Cleavage occurs at a Met(358)-Ser(359) bond called the active center of the inhibitor (P_1–P_1') and located 37 residues from the C-terminus of the molecule. A natural mutant of α_1-proteinase inhibitor in which Met(358) was replaced by Arg has recently been discovered. The genetic variant was a potent thrombin inhibitor, and the child carrying this mutant died from uncontrolled bleeding. Artificial mutants with Val or Arg replacing Met at position 358 have recently been biosynthesized (Rosenberg *et al.*, 1984; Courtney *et al.*, 1985).

Human α_1-proteinase inhibitor has been found to inhibit all elastases tested, whatever their source or their animal origin (e.g., Largman *et al.*, 1976; Delshammar and Ohlsson, 1976; Beatty *et al.*, 1980). In the case of porcine pancreatic elastase, a 1:1 binding stoichiometry may be evidenced by polyacrylamide gel electrophoresis. Yet, inhibition of elastase activity by increasing amounts of inhibitor yielded sometimes 1.8:1 stoichiometries (Baumstark, 1978; James and Cohen, 1978; Satoh *et al.*, 1979). Various mechanisms, have been suggested to explain this discrepancy. Unpublished results from our laboratory show that the enzymatically determined stoichiometry is about 1:1 provided that elastase and inhibitor are reacted for a time sufficient to ensure their complete association before addition of substrate. As shown below, porcine pancreatic elastase and α_1-proteinase inhibitor react relatively slowly. Long preincubation times are therefore required: for instance, with a 50 nM elastase concentration, the preincubation time should be at least 80 min. It is noteworthy that for human leukocyte elastase, which reacts very fast with the inhibitor, a 1:1 binding stoichiometry is found by enzyme inhibition assays (Ohlsson and Olsson, 1974). Binding of proelastase and chymotrypsinogen to α_1-proteinase inhibitor has also been demonstrated (Largman *et al.*, 1979; Brodrick *et al.*, 1980).

Several lines of evidence suggest that the reaction between α_1-proteinase inhibitor and serine proteinases is irreversible. Dissociation of the enzyme–inhibitor complex into native enzyme and inhibitor cannot be achieved. Moreover the complex is not dissociated by denaturating agents, and under second-order conditions, the inhibition reaction follows second-order kinetics for at least five half-lives. It has been suggested that the high binding energy originates from the formation of a high-energy tetrahedral adduct or a covalent linkage between enzyme and inhibitor. The term "irreversible" was used here to emphasize that the complex cannot dissociate into its native components. This does not mean, however, that the inhibition is necessarily permanent. As a matter of fact, transient (or temporary) inhibition has been demonstrated for complexes of α_1-proteinase inhibitor with trypsin, chymotrypsin, and porcine pancreatic elastase (Meyer et al., 1975; Aubry and Bieth, 1977; Oda et al., 1977; Beatty et al., 1982a). The half-lives of these complexes vary between 10 hr (porcine trypsin) and 9 months (human chymotrypsin). The complex formed with porcine pancreatic elastase releases only about 10% enzyme in 1 month (Meyer et al., 1975). The complex formed with human leukocyte elastase is also very stable (Bieth, unpublished results). From the available data concerning the mechanism of action of α_1-proteinase inhibitor, the following reaction scheme may be suggested:

$$\text{E} + \text{I} \underset{k_{-1}}{\overset{k_1}{\rightleftharpoons}} \text{EI} \xrightarrow{k_2} \text{EI*} + \text{fragment} \xrightarrow{k_3} \text{E} + \text{I*}$$

where E = proteinase, I = native inhibitor, I* = proteolytically cleaved inhibitor. The 3.6-kDa fragment is not released into solution but forms tight hydrophobic interactions with EI* (Löbermann et al., 1982). There is only indirect evidence for step 1 (Beatty et al., 1982a). Step 3 (temporary inhibition) is either absent or very low.

α_1-Proteinase inhibitor expresses its specificity through the rate at which it inactivates a given proteinase. Under second-order conditions and low reactant concentrations (i.e., $[\text{E}^0] \simeq [\text{I}^0] < 1\ \mu M$), the inhibition reaction follows second-order kinetics (the reversible EI complex is not kinetically detectable). The reaction scheme is therefore:

$$\text{E} + \text{I} \xrightarrow{k_{\text{assoc}}} \text{EI*}$$

where k_{assoc}, the second-order association rate constant, is related to the above constants by:

$$k_{\text{assoc}} = k_1 \cdot k_2/k_{-1}$$

Measurement of k_{assoc} for 13 serine proteinases of varying specificity and origin has revealed that human leukocyte elastase has the highest rate constant (Beatty *et al.*, 1980). Some values are reported in Table IX. It can be seen that the trypsin-like enzymes react relatively slowly with α_1-proteinase inhibitor. The term "α_1-antitrypsin" is thus misleading. It is noteworthy that human leukocyte and porcine pancreatic elastase which have similar P_1 specificities are inactivated with dramatically different rate constants. It is satisfactory for the kineticist to note that α_1-proteinase inhibitor, which is undoubtly considered as the physiological inhibitor of leukocyte elastase, also exhibits the highest reaction rate with this enzyme.

    c. *Proteolytic Inactivation.*   Some proteinases are resistant to inhibition by α_1-proteinase inhibitor but are able to inactivate this inhibitor by limited proteolysis. Among them are thiol proteinases such as papain and cathepsin B_1 (Johnson and Travis, 1977), metalloproteinases such as *Pseudomonas aeruginosa* elastase (Morihara *et al.*, 1984), mouse peritoneal macrophage elastase (Banda *et al.*, 1980), *Serratia marcescens* metalloproteinases (Virca *et al.*, 1982), *Crotalus adamenteus* venom proteinases (Kress *et al.*, 1979), and *Bacteroides gingivalis* proteinases (Carlsson *et al.*, 1984). The pathological implications of these inactivation reactions will be discussed later.

TABLE IX

INHIBITION OF SOME PROTEINASES BY NATIVE AND
OXIDIZED α_1-PROTEINASE INHIBITOR $(\alpha_1 PI)^a$

Proteinases	Native α_1PI		Oxidized α_1PI	
	k_{assoc}	$d(t)$	k_{assoc}	$d(t)$
Human leukocyte elastase	6.5×10^7	2.9×10^{-3}	3.1×10^4	6.0
Human pancreatic chymotrypsin I	5.4×10^6	3.5×10^{-2}	1.0×10^6	1.9×10^{-1}
Human leukocyte cathepsin G	4.1×10^5	0.47	6.4×10^2	3.0×10^2
Porcine pancreatic elastase	1.0×10^5	—	0	—
Human anionic trypsin	7.3×10^4	2.6	3.2×10^4	5.9
Human cationic trypsin	1.1×10^4	1.7×10^1	3.0×10^3	62.3
Human plasmin	1.9×10^2	1.0×10^3	0	—
Human thrombin	4.8×10^1	4.0×10^3	0	—

   [a] The second-order association rate constants k_{assoc} (Beatty *et al.*, 1980) have been used to calculate the delay times of inhibition $d(t)$ (Bieth, 1980) of the proteinases in plasma assuming a plasma α_1PI concentration of 26 μM. k_{assoc} values are in $M^{-1} sec^{-1}$ and $d(t)$ values in sec.

d. Oxidative Inactivation. The effect of oxidants on α_1-proteinase inhibitor has been reviewed by Matheson *et al.* (1982) and Travis and Salvesen (1983). Methionine residues are readily oxidized into their sulfoxide derivative:

$$
\begin{array}{cc}
\text{—NH—CH—CO—} & \text{—NH—CH—CO—} \\
| & | \\
(\text{CH}_2)_2 & (\text{CH}_2)_2 \\
| & | \\
\text{S} & \text{S}=\text{O} \\
| & | \\
\text{CH}_3 & \text{CH}_3 \\
\text{methionine} & \text{methionine sulfoxide}
\end{array}
$$

It is therefore not surprising that α_1-proteinase inhibitor, whose active center is a Met-Ser bond, undergoes oxidative inactivation to some extent. Oxidation may be brought about by chemicals such as *N*-chlorosuccinimide, chloramine-T or ozone, cigarette smoke condensate, or activated neutrophils or macrophages. The phagocyte-induced oxidation may occur either through a nonenzymatic mechanism (production of O_2^-, H_2O_2, and other reactive species) or through an enzymatic one (production of myeloperoxidase which oxidizes the inhibitor in the presence of $H_2O_2 + Cl^-$).

Studies with chemically oxidized α_1-proteinase inhibitor have revealed that porcine pancreatic elastase, human plasmin, and thrombin are the only proteinases fully resistant to inhibition by the oxidized inhibitor (see Table IX). The former enzyme is able to degrade the modified inhibitor. Other proteinases still react with the modified inhibitor but with reduced rates. The most pronounced decrease in inhibition rate is that observed for human leukocyte elastase: k_{assoc} decreases by a factor of 2,000 upon oxidation of the inhibitor.

The marked effect of methionine oxidation on the reaction of α_1-proteinase inhibitor with elastases has been confirmed by experiments using model substrates with P_1 = either Met or Met(0). The hydrolytic activity of pancreatic elastase, leukocyte elastase, and cathepsin G was markedly reduced following oxidation of the substrates (Nakajima *et al.,* 1979; McRay *et al.,* 1980). An enzyme called methionine sulfoxide peptide reductase is able to reduce the oxidized inhibitor (Abrams *et al.,* 1981b). This enzyme is present in neutrophils (Carp *et al.,* 1983).

2. HUMAN PLASMA α_2-MACROGLOBULIN

The properties of this protein have been recently reviewed by Van Leuven (1982), Travis and Salvesen (1983), and Harpel and Brower

(1983). It is a 725-kDa glycoprotein composed of two noncovalently bound subunits, each of which is formed of two identical chains linked together by disulfide bridges. The amino acid sequence of α_2-macroglobulin has been determined recently. Its concentration in normal plasma is about 3 μM, and it is synthesized by many cell types including fibroblasts and mononuclear phagocytes.

α_2-Macroglobulin forms very tight complexes with nearly all endoproteinases, most of which react with a 2:1 proteinase:macroglobulin stoichiometry. One characteristic feature of this protein–protein interaction is that while the proteinase must be enzymatically active to react with α_2-macroglobulin, it is still active within the final complex. This distinguishes α_2-macroglobulin from other protein proteinase inhibitors where the proteinase active center participates in enzyme–inhibitor binding. The initial step of the proteinase–macroglobulin interaction appears to be a limited proteolytic cleavage at the so-called bait region of α_2-macroglobulin. This region encompasses about 30 amino acid residues located near the middle of the four 180-kDa peptide chains. Each proteinase cleaves the bait region at one or sometimes two specific bonds. For example, porcine elastase hydrolyzes the Val-Gly and Gly-Phe bonds (Sottrup-Jensen et al., 1981) whereas human leukocyte elastase and cathepsin G break a Val-His and a Phe-Tyr linkage, respectively (Virca et al., 1983). The above sites of cleavage are in good accord with the primary substrate specificity of these elastases. Two events follow this initial step: (1) α_2-macroglobulin undergoes an extensive conformational change and (2) four Glu-Cys thioester bonds (one on each peptide chain) are disrupted. The newly available Glu residues may form covalent bonds with Lys residues of proteinases. This reaction occurs to a variable degree and is therefore not responsible for the enormous enzyme–macroglobulin binding energy. The nature of the latter is not known precisely. The two proteinase molecules of the ternary complex are in very close contact (Pochon and Bieth, 1983). The α_2-macroglobulin–proteinase complexes but not native macroglobulin undergo receptor-mediated endocytosis by fibroblasts and macrophages. This explains the rapid clearance of the complexes from plasma.

α_2-Macroglobulin forms a 2:1 complex with porcine pancreatic elastase (Bieth et al., 1970), human pancreatic elastase (Gustavsson et al., 1980), and human and dog leukocyte elastases (Ohlsson and Olsson, 1974; Delshammar and Ohlsson, 1976). For some elastases, the second-order association rate constants k_{assoc} have been measured: $k_{assoc} = 4.4 \times 10^6$ M^{-1} sec^{-1} for pancreatic elastase (Bieth and Meyer, 1984); k_{assoc}

$= 4.1 \times 10^7 \ M^{-1} \ \text{sec}^{-1}$ and $3.7 \times 10^6 \ M^{-1} \ \text{sec}^{-1}$ for human leukocyte elastase and cathepsin G, respectively (Virca and Travis, 1984). The pH dependence of k_{assoc} for the former enzyme suggests that peptide bond cleavage is the rate-limiting step for the elastase–α_2-macro-globulin interaction (Bieth and Meyer, 1984). The conformation of elastase changes upon reaction with the macroglobulin (Duportail *et al.*, 1980).

α_2-Macroglobulin-bound proteinases usually retain their hydrolytic activity on small model substrates but are poorly active or even inactive on proteins. Similarly, binding of small inhibitors readily occurs whereas reaction with large protein proteinase inhibitors is usually impaired or prevented. For instance, macroglobulin-bound porcine pancreatic elastase is almost fully active on *tert*-butoxycarbonyla-lanine-*p*-nitrophenyl ester but completely inactive on elastin and resistant to inhibition by α_1-proteinase inhibitor (Bieth *et al.*, 1970). The bound elastase may, however, by inhibited by protein proteinase inhibitors whose molecular mass is lower than 20 kDa (Bieth *et al.*, 1983). The macroglobulin–human leukocyte elastase complex possesses the intriguing property of being 15-fold more active on succinyl-(Ala)$_3$-*p*-nitroanilide than free elastase (Twumasi *et al.*, 1977). The activating effect is on k_{cat} (Lestienne and Bieth, 1980) and strongly depends on the structure of the substrate (Twumasi *et al.*, 1977). This complex, however, is inactive on elastin (Ohlsson and Olsson, 1974). Its activity on tropoelastin, the soluble precursor of fibrous elastin, is a matter of debate: Galdston *et al.* (1979) reported that the complex retains 6% activity on this protein whereas Kueppers *et al.* (1981) found the complex to be inactive.

3. OTHER HUMAN PLASMA PROTEINASE INHIBITORS

Most of the other plasma inhibitors, namely, antithrombin III, α_2-antiplasmin, Cl-inactivator, and α_1-antichymotrypsin, are inactive on porcine pancreatic and human leukocyte elastases (Travis and Salvesen, 1983). Moreover, the latter enzyme has been shown to inactivate them by proteolytic degradation (see Table VIII). The inter-α-trypsin inhibitor is inactive on porcine pancreatic elastase (Meyer *et al.*, 1975) but inhibits the human leukocyte enzyme (Albrecht *et al.*, 1983). Inter-α-trypsin inhibitor therefore appears to act both as a substrate (Dietl *et al.*, 1979) and as an inhibitor of this elastase. α_1-Antichymotrypsin is a powerful inhibitor of human leukocyte cathepsin G (Beatty *et al.*, 1980).

4. PLASMA PROTEINASE INHIBITORS FROM OTHER SPECIES

Rat plasma contains four proteins able to bind rat pancreatic elastase: α_1-proteinase inhibitor, α_2-macroglobulin, α_2-acute phase protein, and α_1-inhibitor$_3$ (Gauthier *et al.*, 1978). Hamster serum inhibits porcine pancreatic and human leukocyte elastase, but its elastase inhibitory capacity is about four times lower than that of human serum (Boudier and Bieth, 1982). Porcine elastase binds preferentially to hamster α_2-macroglobulin (Stone *et al.*, 1982). Horse plasma α_1-proteinase inhibitor and α_2-macroglobulin bind horse leukoproteinases (Dubin *et al.*, 1984, 1985). Dog plasma α_1-proteinase inhibitor inhibits porcine pancreatic and dog leukocyte elastase (Abrams *et al.*, 1978). Upon treatment with chloramine-T or cigarette smoke extract, this inhibitor loses its elastase inhibitory capacity (Abrams *et al.*, 1980).

5. INHIBITORS FROM VARIOUS ANIMAL AND PLANT TISSUES

Table X lists some protein proteinase inhibitors which are active on pancreatic and/or leukocyte elastase. Unlike plasma proteins, these inhibitors form reversible complexes with their target proteinases. The bronchial mucous inhibitor deserves special comment since it actively participates in the lung defense against neutrophil elastase (see Section X). This inhibitor was isolated from bronchial secretions by Hochstrasser *et al.* (1972) and Ohlsson *et al.* (1977). Both groups of workers used perchloric acid precipitation (the inhibitor is soluble and stable at low pH) followed by affinity chromatography on immobilized trypsin and other conventional chromatographic procedures. Recently, Smith and Johnson (1985) reported a more simple isolation method using only trichloroacetic acid precipitation and chromatography on Sepharose–chymotrypsin. The bronchial inhibitor is a basic protein with a molecular mass of 11–16 kDa (Ohlsson *et al.*, 1977; Kueppers and Bromke, 1983). Its structure is stabilized by seven disulfide bridges (Ohlsson *et al.*, 1977). It inhibits pancreatic trypsin and chymotrypsin, human and dog leukocyte elastase, and cathepsin G (Ohlsson and Tegner, 1976; Tegner *et al.*, 1977; Schiessler *et al.*, 1977). It does not react with porcine pancreatic elastase but inhibits human pancreatic elastase with a K_i of 0.1 μM (Schiessler *et al.*, 1978). Like human plasma α_1-proteinase inhibitor, the bronchial mucous inhibitor is inactivated by cigarette smoke condensate (Carp and Janoff, 1980b; Ohlsson *et al.*, 1980) and *Pseudomonas aeruginosa* elastase (Johnson *et al.*, 1982). It is mainly synthesized in the upper airways (Tegner and Ohlsson, 1977), but its localization in peripheral lung has also been reported (Mooren *et al.*, 1983).

Human seminal plasma inhibitor I closely resembles human bron-

TABLE X

INHIBITION OF PORCINE PANCREATIC ELASTASE (PP ELASTASE) AND HUMAN LEUKOCYTE
ELASTASE (HL ELASTASE) BY PROTEIN PROTEINASE INHIBITORS FROM VARIOUS ANIMAL
AND PLANT TISSUES

Inhibitors (approximate mass)	PP Elastase	HL Elastase
Human bronchial mucous inhibitor (11 kDa)	–	$K_i = 12$ pM^a
Human seminal plasma inhibitor I (11 kDa)	–	$K_i = 2.5$ nM^b
Dog submandibulary gland inhibitor (12 kDa)	$K_i = 0.13 \mu M^c$	$K_i = 5$ nM^d
Bovine pancreatic trypsin inhibitor (6.5 kDa)	$-^e$	$K_i = 1 \mu M^f$
Chicken ovoinhibitor (47 kDa)	$+^e$	$+^g$
Turkey ovomucoid (28 kDa)	$+^e$	$+^g$
Ascaris lumbricoides isoinhibitors (7 kDa)	$K_i = 1$ to 60 pM^h	?
Leech inhibitor (eglin c) (6.8 kDa)	+	$K_i = 0.2$ nM^i
Soybean trypsin inhibitor (Kunitz) (20 kDa)	$-^j$	$+^g$
Soybean inhibitor AA (Bowman–Birk) (8 kDa)	$K_i = 11 \mu M^c$	$K_i \simeq 5$ nM^d
Garden bean trypsin inhibitor II (8 kDa)	$+^k$	?
Lima bean inhibitor (9 kDa)	$-^e$	$+^d$
Chickpea inhibitor (12 kDa)	$-^c$	$K_i \simeq 5$ nM^c
Potato chymotrypsin inhibitor I (39 kDa)	$K_i = 0.29 \mu M^c$	?
Potato chymotrypsin inhibitor II (20 kDa)	$K_i = 0.48 \mu M^c$	?

[a] From Gauthier et al. (1982). [b] From Schiessler et al. (1976). [c] From Bieth et al. (1983). [d] From Schiessler et al. (1977). [e] According to Gertler and Feinstein (1971). [f] From Lestienne and Bieth (1978). [g] According to Starkey (1977b). [h] From Peanasky et al. (1984). [i] From Seemüller et al. (1977). [j] According to Bieth and Frechin (1974). [k] According to Wilson and Laskowski (1975).

chial inhibitor: the two proteins cross-react immunologically and have similar amino acid compositions and proteinase inhibition spectra (see Schiessler et al., 1978, and refs. therein). The two inhibitors might be identical proteins.

The other proteins listed in Table X are all potent pancreatic trypsin and/or chymotrypsin inhibitors. With some exceptions (chicken ovoinhibitor, turkey ovomucoid, Ascaris lumbricoides isoinhibitors, and garden bean trypsin inhibitor II) they are either inactive or poorly efficient on porcine pancreatic elastase. In general, leukocyte elastase appears to be more susceptible to inhibition than pancreatic elastase. On the other hand, the human leukocyte elastase inhibitors also react with dog leukocyte elastase (Ardelt et al., 1976; Schiessler et al., 1977) and eglin c also inhibits horse and rat neutrophil elastase (Dubin et al., 1984; Virca et al., 1984).

Some of the egg white and plant proteins are multiheaded inhibitors i.e., they have separate proteinase binding sites (domains) and are therefore able to bind several enzymes at the same time. Among these, the dog submandibulary gland inhibitor (Geokas *et al.*, 1970; Fritz *et al.*, 1971) and the chicken ovoinhibitor (Gertler and Feinstein, 1971) are noteworthy. The former protein has two independent binding sites: one for trypsin and one for chymotrypsin or leukocyte elastase (Schiessler *et al.*, 1977, 1978). The latter inhibitor has three independent binding sites: one for pancreatic trypsin, one for pancreatic chymotrypsin, and one for pancreatic elastase (Gertler and Feinstein, 1971). It is noteworthy that the elastase binding sites of these two inhibitors have a $P_1 =$ Met residue like α_1-proteinase inhibitor (Shechter *et al.*, 1977; Schiessler *et al.*, 1978). Credit should also be given here to Shechter and co-workers (1977) who were the first to demonstrate an oxidative impairment of the elastase inhibitory capacity of a proteinase inhibitor.

For the sake of completeness, we should note reports describing the inhibition of human leukocyte elastase by proteins present in human polymorphonuclear leukocytes and alveolar macrophages (Janoff and Blondin, 1971; Blondin *et al.*, 1972) and in extracts of *Streptococcus pneumonia* (Vered *et al.*, 1985).

6. PREDICTION OF *IN VIVO* POTENCY OF PROTEINASE INHIBITORS FROM *IN VITRO* MEASURED KINETIC CONSTANTS

The *in vivo* potency (physiological function) of proteinase inhibitors may be predicted to some extent if the kinetic parameters describing the proteinase–inhibitor interaction and the *in vivo* inhibitor concentration $[I^0]$ are known (Bieth, 1980, 1984). The second-order association rate constant k_{assoc} may be used to calcultate $d(t)$, the delay time of inhibition, i.e., the time required for almost complete inhibition of a proteinase *in vivo*: $d(t) \simeq 5/k_{assoc} [I^0]$. Table IX shows that $d(t)$ for α_1-proteinase inhibitor varies from 3 msec (neutrophil elastase) to more than 1 hr (thrombin). This raises the question of how small $d(t)$ should be in order for the inhibitor to efficiently prevent proteolysis of endogenous substrate(s). The fraction of substrate hydrolyzed during the delay time of inhibition depends upon several factors: $d(t)$ itself, the *in vivo* proteinase concentration, k_{cat}, and K_m. It may be shown by trial and error that the highest limit of $d(t)$ is about 1 sec if the proteinase concentration, k_{cat}, and K_m are unknown.

Whereas the $d(t)$ concept allows to predict with some confidence the *in vivo* potency of irreversible inhibitors, it is not sufficient to delineate the physiological function of reversible inhibitors. Due to the reversibility of the binding process, free proteinase will always be present in mixtures of proteinase and inhibitor. In addition, endogenous substrates may dissociate the enzyme–inhibitor complex. It may be shown, however, that if $[I^0]/K_i \geq 1000$, less than 0.1% of free enzyme is present at equilibrium ($[I^0]$ = in vivo inhibitor concentration; K_i = equilibrium dissociation constant of the enzyme–inhibitor complex). If these conditions are fulfilled, the inhibitor exhibits a pseudo-irreversible behavior, the delay time of inhibition concept may be applied, and virtually no substrate-induced dissociation of the enzyme–inhibitor complex occurs. The inhibition of leukocyte elastase by the bronchial mucous inhibitor is described by a K_i of 12 pM and a k_{assoc} of 10^7 M^{-1} sec^{-1} (Gauthier et al., 1982). The in vivo concentration of this inhibitor is not known precisely. However, with such a low K_i, an inhibitor concentration of 10 nM will be sufficient to provide the inhibitor with a pseudo-irreversible character. On the other hand, the limiting value of $d(t)$ defined above [$d(t)$ = 1 sec] will be reached if $[I^0]$ = 0.5 μM. The inhibitor content of alveolar lavage fluid suggests that the latter concentration exists in vivo (Tegner, 1978). The bronchial inhibitor is therefore likely to be a potent physiological inhibitor of leukocyte elastase.

B. Low Molecular Mass Natural and Synthetic Inhibitors

1. ANTIINFLAMMATORY DRUGS AS LEUKOCYTE ELASTASE INHIBITORS

The possible involvement of leukocyte elastase in inflammation (see Section X) led some investigators to assess the leukocyte elastase inhibitory capacity of antiinflammatory drugs. As shown in Table XI, some compounds are potent elastase inhibitors. Gold thiomalate inhibits human leukocyte elastase but not porcine pancreatic elastase (Starkey, 1977). Silver and copper thiomalates are less efficient than the gold derivative (Baici et al., 1984). The efficiency of gold thiomalate and glycosaminoglycan polysulfate is less pronounced when elastase activity is measured with proteoglycan (Stephens et al., 1980) than when a synthetic substrate is used (Baici et al., 1980c, 1981). The reason for this discrepancy is not known. It is also worth mentioning that chondroitin sulfate potentiates the elastolytic activity of leukocyte elastase by reacting with elastin (Lonky et al., 1978). Binding studies show that other glycosaminoglycans, namely heparin, also react with leukocyte elastase (Marossy, 1981).

TABLE XI

INHIBITION OF HUMAN LEUKOCYTE ELASTASE BY SOME ANTIINFLAMMATORY DRUGS

Drug	K_i or I_{50}[a]	Maximum inhibition (%)	Reference
Gold thiomalate	$3.3 \times 10^{-5}\ M$	40	Baici et al. (1981)
Pentosan polysulfate	$1.8 \times 10^{-7}\ M$	60	Baici et al. (1981)
Glycosaminoglycan polysulfate	10^{-7}–$10^{-8}\ M$	75	Baici et al. (1980c)
Chondroitin sulfate	$1.8\ \mu g/ml$[b]	60	Baici and Bradamante (1984)
Phenylbutazone	$2.0 \times 10^{-5}\ M$	85	Stephens et al. (1980)
Indometacin	$1.9 \times 10^{-4}\ M$		Stephens et al. (1980)

[a] Inhibitor concentration for which 50% inhibition is observed.

[b] This result was obtained with a high M_r chondroitin-6-sulfate. The 4-isomer and the low M_r derivative of the 6-isomer are less efficient.

Most of the compounds listed in Table XI form enzymatically active enzyme–inhibitor complexes since full elastase inhibition could not be achieved even with a large excess of drug. On the other hand, the inhibitory power of the sulfated drugs is abolished at an ionic strength higher than 0.4, suggesting that enzyme–inhibitor binding is governed by electrostatic interactions (the K_i values reported in Table XI, however, were measured at a physiological ionic strength). It is noteworthy that polynucleotides also combine with neutrophil elastase to form tight complexes which are held together by electrostatic forces and which have a low residual activity (Lestienne and Bieth, 1983).

Some if not all of the drugs listed in Table XI exhibit sufficient affinity for leukocyte elastase to partially complex this enzyme in vivo when administered at therapeutic doses. Despite their inability to yield full inhibition of enzyme activity, they may therefore be considered as antielastase drugs and this property may, in part, account for their antiinflammatory action.

2. INHIBITORS FROM MICROORGANISMS

The study of proteinase inhibitors produced by microorganisms was initiated by Umezawa. Various Streptomyces species were shown to secrete potent low M_r proteinase inhibitors of varying specificities. Leupeptin and antipain inhibit trypsin-like enzymes; chymostatin, pepstatin, and phosphoramidon are specific for chymotrypsin-like enzymes, carboxyl-proteinases, and metalloproteinases, respectively; elastatinal and elasnin are specific for elastases with a P_1 = Ala or Val primary specificity (Umezawa, 1976).

The structures of elastatinal, chymostatin, elasnin, and phosphoramidon are given in Fig. 2. Elastatinal inhibits porcine, human, dog, and monkey pancreatic elastases with a K_i of $1-3 \times 10^{-7}$ M. By contrast, human, dog, and monkey leukocyte elastases are more resist-

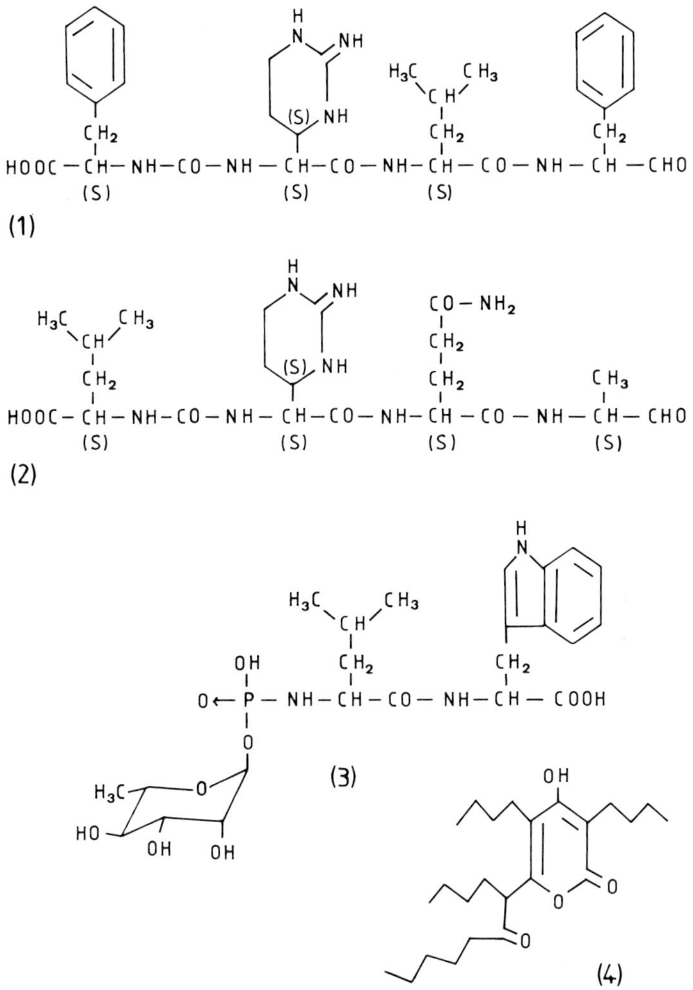

FIG. 2. Elastase inhibitors of microbial origin: 1, chymostatin; 2, elastatinal; 3, phosphoramidon (Umezawa, 1976); 4, elasnin (Omura *et al.*, 1979).

ant to inhibition ($K_i = 0.5$–$1 \times 10^{-4} M$) (Feinstein *et al.*, 1976; Zimmerman and Ashe, 1977; Twumasi and Liener, 1977). Elasnin is rather specific for human leukocyte elastase: the I_{50} value for this enzyme is 1.3 mcg/ml whereas it is 30 mcg/ml for porcine pancreatic elastase (Omura *et al.*, 1978). Chymostatin inhibits human leukocyte cathepsin G with a K_i of $10^{-8} M$ (Feinstein *et al.*, 1976).

The C-terminal amino acid of elastatinal, chymostatin, leupeptin, and antipain has an aldehyde group (CHO) instead of the carboxy group (COOH). This substitution is probably responsible for the high potency of these inhibitors (see paragraph 3 below). It is noteworthy that elasnin, a nonpeptidic compound, inhibits human leukocyte elastase. The mechanism of action of this alkylated α-pyrone is not known as yet but synthetic heterocyclic compounds also inhibit leukocyte elastase (see below).

3.   Synthetic Reversible Inhibitors

The possible involvement of elastase in connective tissue diseases (see Section X) has prompted investigations aimed at designing elastase inhibitors of potential therapeutic use. Table XII lists typical examples of reversible elastase inhibitors. Most of these compounds have peptide-like structures that mimic the normal substrates of these enzymes. However some of them (compounds 9, 10, 11) are heterocycles whose structure is quite unrelated to that of an elastase substrate (see Fig. 3).

Peptide aldehydes such as compound 1 of Table XII or elastatinal are thought to generate transition state analogs of elastase catalysis. Because of the strongly electropositive character of their C-terminal carbonyl carbon, these compounds probably form a hemiacetal with the serine of elastase (Thompson, 1973):

$$\begin{array}{c} O\ H \\ | \\ R{-}C{-}O{-}\text{serine}{-}\text{elastase} \\ | \\ H \end{array}$$

and this complex closely resembles the transition state formed with a substrate (see page 231). It has been shown that the affinity of a substrate for an enzyme is 10^{8}- to 10^{14}-fold higher in the transition state than in the Michaelis–Menten complex (Wolfenden, 1969). A substrate analog which mimics some features of the true substrate in the transition state will therefore be a potent inhibitor of the enzyme. This may account for the high affinity of natural and synthetic aldehydes for elastase and other proteinases.

TABLE XII

TYPICAL EXAMPLES OF REVERSIBLE INHIBITORS OF PORCINE PANCREATIC AND HUMAN LEUKOCYTE ELASTASE[a]

	Inhibitor	K_i (M)		
No.	Structure	Pancreatic elastase	Leukocyte elastase	Reference
1	Ac-Pro-Ala-Pro-Alaninal[b]	8.0×10^{-7}	n.d.	Thompson (1973)
2	MeOSuc-(Ala)$_2$-Pro-NH—CH—B(OH)$_2$[c]	2.5×10^{-10}	5.7×10^{-10}	Kettner and Shenvi (1984)
	$\quad\quad\quad\quad\quad\quad\quad\vert$			
	$\quad\quad\quad\quad\quad\quad CH(CH_3)_2$			
3	C$_6$H$_{11}$CO-Ala-Pro-NHC$_2$H$_5$	1.0×10^{-5}	n.d.	Hassall et al. (1979)
4	Ac-(Ala)$_2$-Pro-Mec-Lac-NHC$_6$H$_5$[d]	4.5×10^{-7}	3.9×10^{-5}	Dorn et al. (1977)
5	CF$_3$CO-Lys-Ala-NHCH$_2$C$_6$H$_5$	2.2×10^{-8}	3.0×10^{-5}	Renaud et al. (1983)
6	CF$_3$CO-Lys-Leu-NHC$_6$H$_4$-p-CH(CH$_3$)$_2$	7.0×10^{-8}	3.0×10^{-7}	Renaud et al. (1983)
7	m-CF$_3$C$_6$H$_4$CO-(Ala)$_2$-C$_6$H$_4$-p-NO$_2$	n.i.	4.0×10^{-6}	Lestienne et al. (1981)
8	Oleic acid	n.i.	9.0×10^{-6}	Ashe and Zimmerman (1977)
9	N-2,4-dinitrophenylbenzisothiazolinone 1,1-dioxide[e]	n.i.	2.1×10^{-6}	Ashe et al. (1981)
10	2-CF$_2$CF$_2$CF$_3$-[4H]-3,1-benzoxazin-4-one[e]	1.6×10^{-6}	9.2×10^{-8}	Teshima et al. (1982)
11	2-CCl$_2$C$_6$H$_5$-4-chloroquinazoline[e]	n.i.	2.7×10^{-7}	Teshima et al. (1982)

[a] Each compound represents the most potent or the most specific of a series of inhibitors tested. n.d. = not determined; n.i. = no inhibition.
[b] Ac = N-acetyl; Alaninal = —NHCH(CH$_3$)CHO.
[c] This inhibitor exhibits the phenomenon of "slow-binding inhibition"; the reported K_i values are steady-state constants.
[d] Ac = N-acetyl; Mec = 2-methylcarbazic acid = azaalanine = —NHN(CH$_3$)CO—; Lac = lactic acid.
[e] The structure of these compounds is shown in Fig. 3.

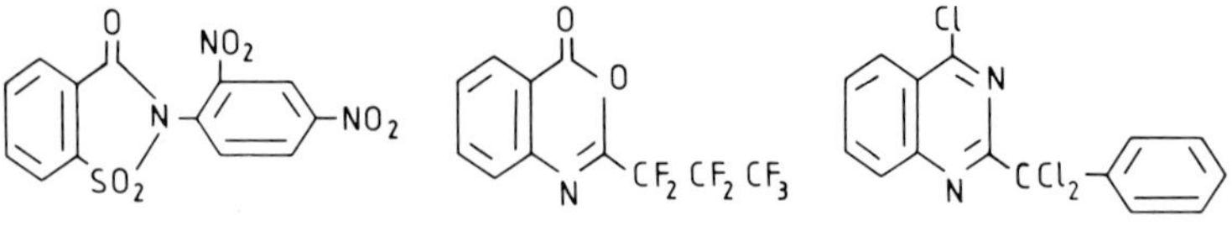

FIG. 3. Synthetic reversible elastase inhibitors. Structures of compounds 9, 10, and 11 of Table XII.

Peptide boronic acid derivatives (e.g., compound 2 of Table XII) are also thought to form tetrahedral adducts with the active site serine residue (Kettner and Shenvi, 1984, and refs. therein). These compounds are the most potent elastase inhibitors ever reported. The series of inhibitors related to compound 10 of Table XII have a potency that correlates well with the degree of polarization of their carbonyl group (see Fig. 3). From this observation it was suggested that part of their affinity may arise from formation of a tetrahedral intermediate with elastase (Teshima *et al.*, 1982).

Thompson (1974) has shown that N-alkylated peptide amides are not hydrolyzed by elastase but do inhibit the enzyme. A series of inhibitors of this class has been designed by Hassall *et al.* (1979). Very high potency could however not be achieved (see compound 3).

The methylcarbazate group of compound 4 is an alanine isostere (see footnote *c* of Table XII) whose carbonyl group may form a relatively stable acyl–elastase if it is previously blocked by *p*-nitrophenol (Powers and Carroll, 1975). Dorn *et al.* (1977) used this property to form acyl–carbazates (e.g., compound 4) that do not undergo enzymatic hydrolysis but retain potent reversible inhibitory activity.

The high potency of trifluoroacetylated peptide anilides (compounds 5 and 6) may in part be due to their tight binding at subsites $S_{11'2'3'}$. The P_3' aromatic ring makes good hydrophobic contacts with S_3', and the P_1' lysine residue makes two strong hydrogen bonds with O-Ser-214 and N-Val-216 of the enzyme (Hughes *et al.*, 1982) and is completely immobilized in the complex (Dimicoli *et al.*, 1984). The CF_3CO group may itself contribute to a significant part of the binding energy. A good hydrophobic S_1–P_1 contact may occur (CF_3 is much more hydrophobic than CH_3). In fact, NMR and X-ray studies have shown that the CF_3CO group is rigidly bound to the enzyme (Dimicoli *et al.*, 1980; Hughes *et al.*, 1982). The strongly electronegative CF_3 group may also increase the electrophilicity of the neighbor carbonyl carbon which might form a tetrahedral adduct with the serine residue of the catalytic site. This view is strengthened by the observation that $CF_3CO\text{-}(Ala)_{2\text{ or }3}$ is hydrolyzed by elastase at their $CF_3CO\text{-}Ala$ bond (Dimicoli *et al.*, 1976).

Unsaturated fatty acids are natural specific inhibitors of leukocyte elastase (e.g., compound 8). It is noteworthy that the corresponding alcohols or nitriles are activators of elastase catalysis. For instance, petroselinyl alcohol increases the rate of substrate hydrolysis by a factor of 12 (Ashe and Zimmerman, 1977).

Compounds 9, 10, and 11 are heterocycles whose structure is depicted in Fig. 3. The two former inhibitors are also active on chymotrypsin while the latter is quite specific for human leukocyte elastase. Substituted α-pyrones which are derivatives of the natural leukocyte elastase inhibitor elasnin (see fig. 2) are being synthesized (Groutas *et al.*, 1984).

4. Synthetic Irreversible Inhibitors

A number of compounds form a stable bond with a catalytically important amino acid residue of elastase and act, therefore, as irreversible inhibitors. They may be classified into two categories (1) active site-directed irreversible inhibitors which already bear the chemical group required for enzyme inactivation and (2) suicide substrates which carry a latent chemical group that is activated in the active site during the catalytic process.

a. Active Site-Directed Irreversible Inhibitors. Irreversible elastase inhibition takes place upon chemical modification of either Ser-195 or His-57 of the catalytic triad. We shall first review the reagents that react with the former residue. Inactivation by the well-known reagent diisopropylphosphorylfluoridate has been reported for all elastases investigated. Alkyl isocyanates also inactive pancreatic elastase (Brown and Wold, 1973) and leukocyte elastase (Ardelt *et al.*, 1976). Phenylmethane sulfonyl fluoride (PMSF) is also frequently used to inactivate proteinases. Powers and co-workers have investigated the specificity and reactivity of a large number of sulfonyl fluorides (Lively and Powers, 1978; Yoshimura *et al.*, 1982). The 2-(CF_3CF_2CONH)-$C_6H_4SO_2F$ derivative was found to be a very fast leukocyte elastase inhibitor ($k_{assoc} = 1700\ M^{-1}\ sec^{-1}$). On the other hand, 2-$(CF_3CF_2CF_2$-$CONH)$- and 2-$(CF_3SNH)C_6H_4SO_2F$ were quite selective for leukocyte elastase.

When a true substrate rapidly acylates Ser-195 and when the acyl–enzyme intermediate deacylates slowly, this substrate may be considered as an irreversible inhibitor. For instance, acetyl-$(Ala)_2$-azaalanine-*p*-nitrophenyl ester acylates elastase within a few seconds but deacylates slowly ($k_{cat} = 3 \times 10^{-3}\ sec^{-1}$) (Powers *et al.*, 1984). The substitution of alanine by azaalanine [—NHN(CH$_3$)CO—] at P$_1$ is responsible for the improved stability of the acyl–enzyme (Powers and Carrol, 1975). This and similar compounds are useful active site titrants of elastase (see Section IX). The inactivation of pancreatic elastase by alkyl p-nitrophenyl pentylphosphonates follows a similar mechanism (Nayak and Bender, 1978). Furoyl saccharin,

is another interesting example of a substrate-like inactivator of elastase. Zimmerman et al. (1980) have shown that this compound irreversibly inhibits elastase within a few seconds. The enzyme cleaves the inhibitor at the —CON< bond of the ring, and the resulting acyl–enzyme deacylates extremely slowly ($k_{cat} = 1.4 \times 10^{-6}$ sec^{-1} for leukocyte elastase).

We shall now deal with peptide chloromethylketones which alkylate one of the nitrogen atoms of His-57. In these compounds the carboxyl group of the C-terminal amino acid residue is replaced by a COCH$_2$Cl substituent which forms a very stable peptide–CH$_2$N(His) bond with the enzyme. These compounds also react with other nucleophiles, but specificity is provided by their reaction at the substrate binding site of proteinases. Their reaction pathway resembles that of a normal substrate up to the acylation step, and a tetrahedral adduct may be postulated as with a normal substrate. Powers and Tuhy (1973) and Thompson and Blout (1973a) were the first to report the inactivation of porcine pancreatic elastase by peptide chloromethyl ketones. Inhibition of other pancreatic elastases as well as of leukocyte elastases was also demonstrated (e.g., Ardelt et al., 1976; Powers et al., 1977). The best inhibitor of human leukocyte elastase was found to be N-succinylmethyl ester-(Ala)$_2$-Pro-Val-CH$_2$Cl (k_{assoc}= 1560 M^{-1} sec^{-1}: Powers et al., 1977). This compound is widely used in animal experiments aimed at testing elastase inhibitors as potential drugs against lung emphysema (see Section XI). Dansylated peptide chloromethyl ketones may be employed to introduce a fluorescent dansyl label into the active site of elastase and other proteinases (Penny and Dyckes, 1980).

b. Suicide Substrates. Several other terms have been used for this class of chemicals: mechanism-based inactivators, suicide inactivators, k_{cat} inhibitors, enzyme-activated irreversible inhibitors and so on. These substrates are latent inhibitors which become activated in the course of their enzyme-catalyzed chemical transformation. They have been widely used for pyridoxal-dependent enzymes (e.g., Jung *et al.*, 1980) but less extensively employed for proteinases (e.g., Béchet *et al.*, 1977; Krafft and Katzenellenbogen, 1981; Hedstrom *et al.*, 1984).

Recently, suicide substrates for pancreatic and leukocyte elastases have also been synthesized. These include alkyl imidazole-N-carbox-amides (Groutas *et al.*, 1980), 3-chloroisocoumarin (Harper *et al.*, 1983), 3-alkoxy-7-amino-4-chloroisocoumarins (Harper and Powers, 1984), and ynenol lactones (Tam *et al.*, 1984). The most efficient inac-tivators of human leukocyte elastase were found to be 3-methoxy-7-amino-4-chloroisocoumarin ($k_{assoc} = 10,000 \ M^{-1} \ sec^{-1}$; no enzyme reac-tivation after standing 100 hr at 25°C) and the ynenol lactone, whose structure and mechanism of action are depicted in Fig. 4 ($k_{assoc} = 28,000 \ M^{-1} \ sec^{-1}$; no enzyme reactivation after gel filtration).

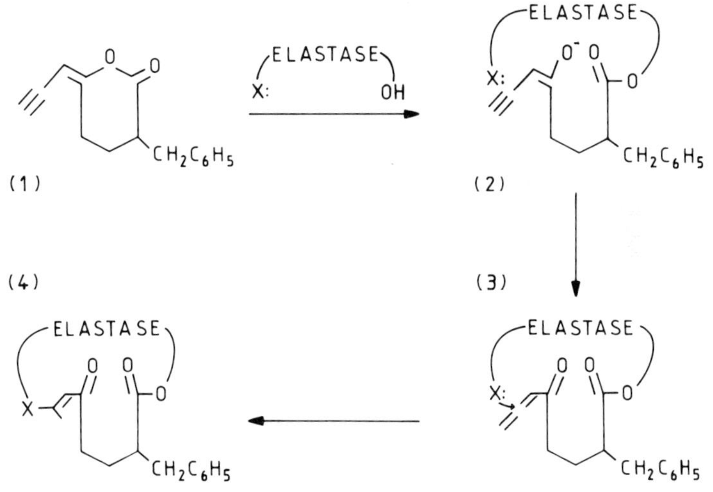

FIG. 4. Proposed pathway for the inactivation of elastase by a suicide substrate. The ynenol lactone 1 forms an acyl–enzyme intermediate 2 by reaction with the serine residue (OH) of the catalytic site. Unmasking of the allenone group (intermediate 3) is followed by a covalent reaction with a nucleophilic residue of the enzyme (X:). (Redrawn from Tam *et al.*, 1984.)

VII. Other Mammalian Elastases

A. Macrophage and Monocyte Elastases

1. Mouse Peritoneal Macrophage Elastase

This enzyme is secreted in substantial amounts into the culture medium of inflammatory macrophages (Werb and Gordon, 1975), from which it may be purified (White et al., 1980b; Banda and Werb, 1981). It is immunologically and catalytically distinct from mouse pancreatic and leukocyte elastase. It occurs as three chromatographically distinct forms, the dominant one having a molecular mass of 22 kDa (Banda and Werb, 1981).

Mouse macrophage elastase is a metalloenzyme requiring Ca^{2+} and another metal for activity (Banda and Werb, 1981). It cleaves the oxidized insulin β-chain at two bonds: Ala-Leu and Tyr-Leu, the latter being hydrolyzed with the highest rate (Kettner et al., 1981). It therefore expresses its primary substrate specificity through the $S_1'-P_1'$ interaction as does Pseudomonas aeruginosa elastase, another metalloproteinase (see section VIII). Mouse macrophage elastase does not cleave succinyltrialanine-p-nitroanilide. It solubilizes elastin by generating fragments that are much bigger than those produced by porcine pancreatic elastase (Banda and Werb, 1981). It also cleaves selected subclasses of IgG immunoglobulins, fibrinogen, proteoglycans, and myelin basic protein (Banda et al., 1983).

Mouse macrophage elastase is inhibited by chelators but not by phosphoramidon, a metalloproteinase inhibitor produced by microorganisms. It is resistant to inhibition by soybean trypsin inhibitor and plasma α_1-proteinase inhibitor (Banda and Werb, 1981). The latter is proteolytically degraded with release of a 4- to 5-kDa peptide (Banda et al., 1980). The inhibitory action of plasma α_2-macroglobulin (Banda and Werb, 1981) is a matter of controversy (White et al., 1981). Banda and Werb (1981) have shown that sodium dodecyl sulfate (SDS) releases elastase from its complex with α_2-macroglobulin so that the latter inhibitor becomes ineffective when elastase activity is measured with SDS-treated elastin (White et al., 1981). Elastase is secreted together with an endogenous inhibitor which masks 80% of its activity. This "latent elastase" may be activated by low ionic strength, SDS (Banda and Werb, 1981), or plasmin in the presence of elastin (Chapman and Stone, 1984b).

Chapman and Stone (1984b) have recently shown that live mouse macrophages also possess a cell-surface-associated cysteine proteinase able to solubilize elastin. Unlike the metalloenzyme, this elastase is not secreted into the macrophage culture medium.

2. Human Alveolar Macrophage Elastase

This is an ill-defined enzyme whose demonstration and characterization have proven to be elusive problems (Rodiguez *et al.*, 1977; de Crémoux *et al.*, 1978; Green *et al.*, 1979; Hinman *et al.*, 1980). Many reasons may account for the difficulties encountered with the study of this elastase: (1) human alveolar macrophages are collected by bronchoalveolar lavage, a procedure which yields 10^7–10^8 macrophages per lavage, and contaminating polymorphonuclear leukocytes are difficult to eliminate exhaustively; (2) human alveolar macrophages have been shown to internalize human leukocyte elastase *in vitro* (Campbell *et al.*, 1979) and *in vivo* (White *et al.*, 1982) and to release active leukocyte elastase (Campbell and Wald, 1983); (3) macrophages are able to synthesize α_1-proteinase inhibitor (Isaacson *et al.*, 1981) and α_2-macroglobulin (White *et al.*, 1980a); and (4) the amount of elastase present in human alveolar macrophages is extremely low.

According to Hinman and co-workers (1980), macrophages are able to synthesize a calcium-dependent elastolytic enzyme that is active on succinyl-(Ala)$_3$-p-nitroanilide. Macrophages from smokers also contain a serine proteinase whose inhibition profile resembles that of human leukocyte elastase.

Recently, Chapman and Stone (1984a) demonstrated that live human alveolar macrophages can degrade elastin if the cells contact the substrate. The enzyme responsible for most of this activity is a cell-surface-associated cysteine proteinase(s). This macrophage-mediated elastolysis reaction still takes place in 10% human serum.

3. Other Macrophage Elastases

Elastase activity has also been found in alveolar macrophages from other species. De Crémoux and co-workers (1978) showed that monkey macrophages secrete a Ca^{2+}-elastase active on succinyl-(Ala)$_3$-p-nitroanilide. Active synthesis of a calcium-dependent elastase was reported for bovine macrophages (Valentine and Fisher, 1984). Elastase activity was also found in rabbit (Janoff *et al.*, 1971), mouse (White *et al.*, 1977), and dog alveolar macrophages (Green *et al.*, 1979).

4. Human Monocyte Elastase

Monocytes are the circulating precursors of macrophages. Immuno-histochemical studies showed that these cells contain leukocyte elastase antigens (Pryzwansky *et al.*, 1978). Enzymatic investigations confirmed that monocytes contain low levels of active leukocyte elastase (Lavie *et al.*, 1980; Hughes *et al.*, 1981). U-937 monocyte-like cells, which resemble immature monocytes, synthesize large quantities of neutrophil elastase (Senior *et al.*, 1982). It is therefore likely that the low levels of elastase found in mature monocytes result from active synthesis rather than from uptake of external enzyme. Circulating and resident cells therefore appear to synthesize two completely different elastases. This was elegantly confirmed by cell culture studies showing that when monocytes differentiate into macrophage-like cells they gradually lose neutrophil elastase and then develop a metalloelastase (Sandhaus *et al.*, 1983).

B. *Miscellaneous Elastases*

Human blood platelets contain an elastase (Robert *et al.*, 1970) which is immunologically different from the neutrophil enzyme (Legrand *et al.*, 1977). The specific activity of this enzyme, however, is less than 0.5% that of neutrophil elastase when fibrous elastin is used as a substrate (Hornebeck *et al.*, 1980).

Bellon and co-workers (1980) have described the isolation of an elastase from human arteries. This enzyme is a serine proteinase whose specific activity on insoluble elastin and on succinyl-$(Ala)_3$-p-nitroanilide is about 10% that of porcine pancreatic elastase. It does not cross-react immunologically with human leukocyte and pancreatic elastases.

The cell extract of cultured human skin fibroblasts is able to solubilize fibrous elastin (Bourdillon *et al.*, 1980). The same is true for cultured rat aorta smooth muscle cells (Hornebeck *et al.*, 1981). The latter elastase was partially purified and characterized. It is a serine proteinase active on succinyl-$(Ala)_3$-p-nitroanilide and on tropoelastin. Its specific activity on insoluble elastin is 0.6% that of porcine pancreatic elastase.

Elastase activity has also been detected in a variety of tumor cell lines in culture (Gilfillan, 1968; Jones and Declerck, 1980; Kao *et al.*, 1982). The human fibrosarcoma cell line HT 1080 possesses a plasma membrane-associated elastolytic enzyme; the cells must be in contact with the extracellular matrix in order to achieve elastolysis (Jones and

Declerck, 1980). The human breast cancer cell line ZR75-31A secretes three elastases into the culture medium, one of which is a metalloenzyme while the two others are serine proteinases (Kao *et al.*, 1982).

VIII. NONMAMMALIAN ELASTASES

A. *Bacterial Elastases*

1. GENERAL SURVEY

Elastolytic activity has been found in a large number of bacteria, including *Flavobacterium elastolyticum* (Mandl and Cohen, 1960), *Pseudomonas pseudomallei, Actinomyces* sp. (Mandl *et al.*, 1962), *Mycobacterium tuberculosis, Clostridium histolyticum, Bacillus anthracoides, B. licheniformis, B. coagulans, B. cereus, B. pumilis,* and *B. mycoides* (Oakley and Bonerjee, 1963; Werb *et al.*, 1982).

Morihara and Tsuzuki (1967) have compared the elastolytic activities of several pure bacterial elastases to that of porcine pancreatic elastase. They found that *Bacillus thermoproteolyticus* proteinase and *Streptomyces fradiae* elastase were four and eight times, respectively, more active than porcine elastase. These two enzymes are thus undoubtedly the most potent elastolytic proteinases ever reported since most mammalian elastases have a specific activity lower than that of the porcine enzyme (see Table VII). Among the other bacterial elastases studied by Morihara and Tsuzuki (1967) are *Bacillus subtilis* alkaline proteinase, *Pseudomonas aeruginosa* elastase, and *Streptomyces griseus* proteinase whose specific activities are about half that of porcine elastase, *B. subtilis* neutral proteinase whose activity is comparable to that of human neutrophil elastase, and *Aspergillus oryzae* and *Pseudomonas chrysogenum* proteinases whose weak elastolytic activity is comparable to that of cathepsin G. The best characterized elastases may be classified into metallo- and serine elastases.

2. METALLOELASTASES

a. Pseudomonas aeruginosa Elastase. About 85% of *P. aeruginosa* strains secrete elastase and two other proteinases (for a review see Wretlind and Pavlovskis, 1983). Most investigations have been done on an elastase isolated from strain IFO 3455, by Morihara and colleagues. This enzyme is now commercially available.

Pseudomonas aeruginosa elastase was first isolated by Morihara *et al.* (1965) using conventional techniques. The enzyme was obtained in a pure crystalline form. It may also be prepared by affinity chromatography on Sepharose–ε-aminocaproyl-D-phenylalanine-methyl ester (Morihara and Tsuzuki, 1975) or HONHCOCH $(CH_2C_6H_5)$CO-Ala-Gly-NH$(CH_2)_3$-agarose (Nishino and Powers, 1980). The molecular mass of this elastase is 35–40 kDa when determined by ultracentrifugation (Morihara et al., 1965) or by SDS–polyacrylamide gel electrophoresis (Kessler et al., 1982). Gel filtration gives a lower measurement. This elastase is one of the rare elastolytic enzymes having an anionic character (pI = 5.9, Morihara et al., 1965).

   Pseudomonas aeruginosa elastase has a typical metallo enzyme inhibition profile with one Zn^{2+} atom per molecule (Morihara and Tsuzuki, 1975). Its elastolytic activity is very low in presence of NaCl concentrations greater than 0.1 M (Morihara et al., 1965). Unlike other elastases, this proteinase expresses its primary substrate specificity through the S_1'–P_1' interaction as shown by specificity studies using either the oxidized insulin B chain (Morihara and Tsuzuki, 1966) or synthetic model substrates (Morihara and Tsuzuki, 1975). The enzyme has a marked specificity for P_1' = Leu, Phe, or Tyr. The S_1' subsite does not show a narrow specificity. This elastase has also an extended substrate binding site as demonstrated with substrates (Morihara and Tsuzuki, 1975) and inhibitors (Nishino and Powers, 1980). It is a powerful catalyst as judged from the high k_{cat} values reported for the hydrolysis of model substrates (see below). Succinyl-(Ala)$_3$-p-nitroanilide is not a substrate for *P. aeruginosa* elastase. This enzyme may be assayed using, for instance, carbobenzoxy-Gly-Leu-Ala, which is cleaved at the Gly-Leu bond (k_{cat} = 945 sec^{-1}, K_m = 1.8 mM). Peptide bond cleavage may be monitored with the ninhydrin assay method (Morihara and Tsuzuki, 1975). Nishino and Powers (1980) have developed a more sensitive assay using 2-aminobenzoyl-Ala-Gly-Leu-Ala-4-nitrobenzylamide containing both a fluorescent and a fluorescence-quenching group which are separated in the course of enzymatic hydrolysis of the substrate with enhancement of fluorescence intensity (k_{cat} = 100 sec^{-1}, K_m = 0.11 mM).

   Pseudomonas aeruginosa elastase also hydrolyzes denatured and native proteins. By so doing it may exert harmful effects on biologically important proteins. It degrades components of the immune system such as IgA and IgG immunoglobulins (Döring et al., 1981) and a variety of complement components (Schultz and Miller, 1974) and it abolishes the bacteriolytic activity of human airway lysozyme by proteolytic cleavage (Jacquot et al., 1985). This elastase also inactivates a number of human protein proteinase inhibitors including α_1-proteinase inhibitor (Morihara et al., 1979), Cl-inhibitor, α_1-antichymotrypsin

(Catanese and Kress, 1984), and bronchial mucous inhibitor (Johnson *et al.*, 1982). Inactivation of α_1-proteinase inhibitor occurs as the result of a single peptide bond cleavage at the Pro(357)-Met(358) link, i.e., the $P_2–P_1$ part of the inhibitor.

Human α_2-macroglobulin appears to be the only protein able to inhibit *P. aeruginosa* elastase (Hochstrasser *et al.*, 1973). The natural metalloenzyme inhibitor phosphoramidon [*N*-α-L-rhamnopyranosyloxy-(hydroxyphosphinyl)-L-leucyl-L-tryptophan, see page 261] inhibits elastase with $K_i = 4 \times 10^{-8}$ *M* (Morihara and Tsuzuki, 1978). Synthetic *N*-α-phosphoryl dipeptides have also been reported (Poncz *et al.*, 1984). All these phosphoric acid derivatives are believed to be transition state analogs of substrate hydrolysis because the enzyme–inhibitor complex may be a tetrahedral phosphorus adduct (Weaver *et al.*, 1977). A series of new inhibitors with hydroxamic acid, *N*-hydroxypeptide, or thiol functional groups have been described by Nishino and Powers (1980). These compounds are ligating agents which bind the Zn^{2+} atom of the active center of elastase. The most potent of these inhibitors, $HSCH_2CH(CH_2C_6H_5)CO$-Ala-Gly-NH_2, has a K_i of 6.4×10^{-8} *M*.

b. Flavobacterium immotum Elastase. The *F. immotum* elastase was purified to homogeneity by Ozaki and Shiio (1975). It is a 13-kDa protein with a p*I* of 8.3–8.9. It hydrolyzes native and denatured proteins in addition to elastin and has a typical metalloproteinase inhibition profile.

Other metalloelastases are found in *Bacillum thermoproteolyticum* and *Clostridium histoliticum*.

3. SERINE ELASTASES

a. Streptomyces griseus Elastases. Gertler and Trop (1971) purified three elastases from a commercial powder of *S. griseus* protease. The three enzymes differed in electrophoretic mobility, molecular mass, and amino acid composition. They hydrolyzed acetyl-(Ala)$_3$ methyl ester with K_m values similar to that of porcine pancreatic elastase and were inhibited by diisopropylfluorophosphate. They showed also a limited reactivity with acetyltyrosine ethyl ester and tosylphenylalanine chloromethyl ketone, two specific reactants of α-chymotrypsin. This chymotrypsin-like specificity was further investigated on elastase III (later called *S. griseus* protease B) with a series a peptide chloromethyl ketones having a Phe residue at P_1 (Gertler, 1974). It was shown that elastase III is much more sensitive to peptide chain elongation than α-chymotrypsin. In particular, a Leu residue at P_2 of the inhibitor considerably increases its reactivity with this enzyme. Elastase II is identical with *S. griseus* protease 3, another member of the chymotrypsin family (Bauer *et al.*, 1976a,b). This enzyme was shown to have a much broader S_1 subsite specificity than bovine α-chymotrypsin since it not only hydrolyzes substrates with Phe or Tyr at P_1 but also cleaves Leu-, Val-, and Ala-containing substrates (Bauer *et al.*, 1976b). In addition, like elastase III, it has a relatively extended substrate binding site (Bauer *et al.*, 1976a).

   b.   Sporangium sp. α-Lytic Protease.   The specific activity of this elastase is half that of porcine pancreatic elastase. These two enzymes have similar substrate and inhibitor specificities. However, the bacterial enzyme probably has a larger S_1 subsite and a smaller substrate binding site (Kaplan *et al.*, 1970; Shaw and Whitaker, 1973). The α-lytic protease of *Steptomyces* sp. is unique among serine proteases in that it has a single histidine residue which participates in the charge-relay system of its catalytic site. Advantage has been made of this feature to investigate the ionization behavior of this residue using ^{13}C-NMR spectroscopy (Hunkapiller *et al.*, 1973; Bachovchin *et al.*, 1981).

   c.   Thermoactinomyces vulgaris Thermitase.   Thermitase has been isolated and studied by Kleine (1982). It is a thermostable serine proteinase with an optimal temperature of 60°C for esterolysis and 85°C for proteolysis. In addition to acting on elastin it hydrolyzes rat tail tendon collagen and other proteins. It hydrolyzes typical chymotrypsin substrates but is also very active on acetyl-(Ala)₃ methyl ester, a behavior that resembles that of α-lytic protease and rat pancreatic elastase.

   d.   Bacillus sp. Ya-B Elastase.   This enzyme has been isolated and investigated by Tsai *et al.* (1983). It is a 25-kDa serine proteinase with a very high pH optimum of activity (11.7). Its specific activity on elastin is higher than that of porcine pancreatic elastase and it also hydrolyzes keratin and collagen.

B.   Other Nonmammalian Elastases

1.   ELASTASES FROM FUNGI

   These have been reviewed by Werb and co-workers (1982). Elastase is produced by fungi species of the genera *Nanizzia, Arthroderma, Trichophyton, Microsporum, Coccidioides, Allesheria,* and *Entomophthora.* It is noteworthy that the human strain of *E. coronata* produces elastase whereas the soil strain does not. *Nanizzia fulva* elastase is a cysteine proteinase.

2. ELASTASE(S) FROM LARVAE OF *SCHISTOSOMA MANSONI*

Several species of schistosomes (blood flukeworms) are highly pathogenic trematodes. Infection of the human host begins by skin penetration of their larval form, the cercaria. Gazinelli *et al.* (1966) have shown that homogenates of whole cercariae possess elastinolytic activity. More recently, McKerrow *et al.* (1982) used a model extracellular connective tissue matrix to demonstrate that cercariae preacetabular gland secretions are able to degrade elastin rapidly. Matrix glycoproteins and collagen were also attacked. These effects were inhibited by α_1-proteinase inhibitor, soybean trypsin inhibitor, and EDTA. One or several elastolytic proteinases are therefore involved in larvae skin penetration. After this initial skin penetration, the larvae transform into a tail-less larval form, the schistosomula. The latter is still able to degrade glycoproteins but has almost completely lost its ability to solubilize elastin (Keene *et al.*, 1983).

3. ELASTASES FROM VENOMS

Bernick and Simpson (1976) have screened the venoms from 25 poisonous snakes for elastolytic activity (12 Crotalidae, 5 Viperidae, and 8 Elapidae). All venoms were more or less active on Congo Red–elastin whereas activity on *tert*-butyloxycarbonyl-Ala-*p*-nitrophenyl ester was present only in venoms from Crotalidae and Viperidae. Interestingly, a correlation was found between elastolytic activity and taxonomy of poisonous snake at the family level. Some of the most active venoms were screened for inhibition of elastase activity by phenylmethane sulfonyl fluoride, EDTA, $HgCl_2$, and cysteine. Surprisingly, inhibition was found with all four componds, suggesting that elastolysis might result from the action of more than one proteinase. Many other snake venoms have proteolytic activity but lack elastolytic activity (Tu, 1977). Some toxic venoms such as that secreted by the cobra (*Naja naja*) or the gila monster (*Heloderma horridum*) have little or no elastase activity (Werb *et al.*, 1982). It is also interesting to note that some venoms from Crotalidae, Viperidae, and Colubridae are able to inactivate α_1-proteinase inhibitor by proteolytic cleavage (Kress and Paroski, 1978). The venom of the Eastern diamondback rattle snake (*Crotalus adamanteus*) contains two proteinases able to inactivate the inhibitor. The elastolytic action of these enzymes, however, is apparently unknown. Venoms of invertebrates (e.g., honey bee, yellow jacket, black widow spider, and Portuguese Man-of-War) contain little or no elastolytic activity (Werb *et al.*, 1982).

4. ELASTASES FROM THE PANCREAS OF FISHES

Elastases have been isolated from the pancreas of the African lung-fish (de Haën and Gertler, 1974), the carp (Cohen *et al.*, 1981a), and the catfish (Yoshinaka *et al.*, 1983, 1984). The molecular and enzymatic properties of these enzymes have been reviewed in Sections III,D and V,B, respectively. Let us simply emphasize here that these elastases are serine proteinases except one of the two catfish elastases, which is a metalloenzyme.

IX. ASSAY OF ELASTASES: A CRITICAL MINIREVIEW

A. *On the Misuse of Soluble Elastins and Succinyltrialanine-p-nitroanilide as Elastase Substrates*

1. ELASTASES ARE ELASTIN-SOLUBILIZING PROTEINASES

A proteinase cannot be named "elastase" if it does not possess the ability to release soluble peptides from insoluble elastin fibers. In the preceding sections we have seen that this property is shared by proteinases with different catalytic sites (serine, metallo-, or cysteine proteinases) and variable primary substrate specificities. We have also emphasized that the mechanism of elastin solubilization is not well understood. As a consequence, one cannot accurately infer the elastolytic capacity of a given proteinase from its molecular properties and its action on soluble proteins or synthetic substrates. Hence, the use of insoluble elastin is mandatory for naming a new proteinase "elastase" or for quantitating "elastase activity" in cell or tissue extracts.

Assays using insoluble elastin are cumbersome, often poorly sensitive, and rarely precise. For these reasons, procedures using soluble elastins or synthetic substrates are largely favored. We shall demonstrate below that such substrates are unvaluable substitutes of fibrous elastin.

2. SPECIFICITY OF SOLUBLE ELASTINS

Two types of chemically solubilized elastins have been reported, α-elastin (Partridge and Davis, 1955) and κ-elastin (Comte and Robert, 1968). The former protein is rapidly cleaved by *Pseudomonas aeruginosa* alkaline proteinase and *P. chrysogenum* proteinase, two enzymes which are unable to solubilize fibrous elastin (Morihara and Tsuzuki, 1967). On the other hand, human serum hydrolyzes κ-elastin but does not attack insoluble elastin (Hornebeck *et al.*, 1983). In addition, platelet elastase is much more active on κ-elastin than on fibrous elastin (Hornebeck *et al.*, 1980). It should also be added that tropoelastin, the soluble precursor of elastin, is rapidly hydrolyzed by trypsin and chymotrypsin (Christner *et al.*, 1978).

3. Specificity of Succinyltrialanime-*p*-nitroanilide

Succinyltrialanine-*p*-nitroanilide is a very sensitive and convenient substrate for porcine pancreatic elastase (Bieth *et al.*, 1974). It is hydrolyzed, however, by nonelastinolytic enzymes present in bile (Ogawa *et al.*, 1979), serum (Sasaki *et al.*, 1981), and synovial fluid (Saklatvala, 1977). It is also rapidly hydrolyzed by human pancreatic protease E, a very poorly elastinolytic enzyme (Mallory and Travis, 1975). It should also be mentioned that another substrate, acetyl-(Ala)$_3$ methyl ester, is rapidly hydrolyzed by the alkaline proteinase of *Aspergillus sojae* which is inactive on fibrous elastin (Gertler and Hayashi, 1971).

On the other hand several elastinolytic proteinases are inactive on succinyl-(Ala)$_3$-*p*-nitroanilide. These include porcine pancreatic elastase II, pancreatic elastase, and mouse macrophage and *P. aeruginosa* elastases.

4. Conclusion

Neither soluble elastins nor synthetic porcine pancreatic elastase substrates may therefore be used as fibrous elastin substitutes to classify an unknown proteinase in the "elastase" family or to quantitate "elastase activity" in cell or tissue extracts. Of course, once a given proteinase has been purified and shown to possess elastinolytic activity, any convenient artificial substrate may be used to study the enzyme.

Nonelastinolytic proteinases active on soluble elastin or on succinyl-(Ala)$_3$-*p*-nitroanilide have sometimes been named "elastase-like" or "elastase-type" enzymes. These denominations are misleading and should be avoided because they suggest that such enzymes have functional properties similar to those of elastases which is obviously not the case.

B. *Methods Using Insoluble Elastins as Substrate*

We shall not review the numerous elastinolytic methods that have been described in the literature. We shall rather recommend a few of them only and give the drawbacks of others. Two kinds of procedures have been developed: those using unlabeled elastins and those employing labeled elastins. We suggest the use of unlabeled rather than dye or radiolabeled elastins whenever possible because the labeled derivatives are chemically modified proteins that may have an altered susceptibility to elastase. In addition, artifacts are much more frequent with labeled than with native elastins.

1. METHODS USING UNLABELED ELASTINS

The most reliable and convenient technique using native elastin is that described by Ardelt and co-workers (1970) in which the solubilized elastin concentration is determined spectrophotometrically at 276 nm, the wavelength of maximal absorption of desmosine, isodesmosine, and tyrosine. The relationship between absorbance and incubation time or enzyme concentration is linear, which is not the case in many other methods. In addition, this method is fairly sensitive since porcine pancreatic elastase concentrations as low as 2 μg/ml (80 nM) may be accurately assayed. This procedure has been successfully used in the reviewer's laboratory with either bovine ligamentum nuchae or human lung elastin. After complete solubilization, the $E_{1cm}^{1\%}$ of the two elastins were found to be 6.0 and 13.3, respectively, at 280 nm (Boudier et al., 1981b). The procedure of Quinn and Blout (1970) in which the soluble digest of native elastin is determined by fluorometry is not significantly more sensitive than the above method. In addition, quenching of fluorescence may interfere with the assay. We therefore recommend the assay of Ardelt et al. (1970) which is now used in several laboratories.

Very convenient semiquantitative methods in which elastin is incorporated into an agar gel have also been proposed (e.g., Senior et al., 1971; Schumacher and Schill, 1972). The elastase sample is poured into wells cut in the elastin–agar, and the diameter of the clear lysis zone which results from the solubilization of elastin particles is measured after a given period of time. These methods are inexpensive, do not require special equipment, and are very sensitive since the plates may be incubated for several days. The elastin–agar plates are now commercially available.

2. METHODS USING DYE-LABELED ELASTINS

When biological samples absorb at 276 nm, the method of Ardelt et al. (1970) cannot be used. Several dye-labeled elastin substrates have been reported. The noncovalently labeled Congo Red– or orcein–elastins are unsuitable for the determination of elastase activity in biological samples containing high concentrations of proteins (e.g., albumin) because such proteins may delabel the substrate (i.e., bring color into solution) and thus mimic enzyme activity (Banga and Ardelt, 1967). We recommend the use of covalently labeled elastin such as Remazol Brilliant Blue–elastin (Rinderknecht *et al.*, 1968; Bieth *et al.*, 1976) or rhodamine–elastin (Huebner, 1976), both of which are commercially available. The soluble peptides may be detected at 595 or 550 nm, respectively. Both methods give linear responses of absorbance to elastase concentration and have detection limits similar to that of the method of Ardelt *et al.* (1970). The sensitivity of the rhodamine–elastin assay may be increased by a factor of 100 if the concentration of soluble peptides is monitored by fluorimetry (Huebner, 1976).

3. Methods Using Radiolabeled Elastins

[125]I-, [14]C-, and ^{3}H-labeled elastins have been proposed for the measurement of elastase activity (Robert and Robert, 1969; Bielefeld *et al.*, 1975; Takahashi *et al.*, 1973). None of these substrates is commercially available. ^{3}H-Labeled elastin is easier to prepare than ^{14}C-labeled elastin. ^{125}I-Labeled elastin must be utilized within a few months and may undergo artificial deiodination by myeloperoxidase (Ragsdale and Arend, 1979). We recommend ^{3}H-labeled elastin, which is the most frequently used radioactive substrate. The labeling reaction is performed with tritiated sodium borohydrate which reduces the aldehydes and the cross-links of elastin (Takahashi *et al.*, 1973). The procedure using this substrate is about three times more sensitive than the fluorescent rhodamine–elastin assay. It is therefore particularly suited for the detection of very low levels of elastase activity.

4. Some Suggestions Concerning the Use of Rhodamine– and ^{3}H-Labeled Elastin

The fluorescence or the radioactivity of the reagent blanks (elastin + buffer) should be as low as possible to avoid artifacts. If necessary, these substrates must be thoroughly washed before use. The total fluorescence or radioactivity of elastin should be determined for each batch of substrate using an excess of porcine pancreatic elastase. This allows the conversion of fluorescence intensity or radioactivity into concentration of solubilized substrate and allows comparison of data obtained with different batches of substrate (this is also true for other elastins).

Due to the high sensitivity of these methods, only a small percentage of substrate need to be solubilized to get reliable fluorescence readings or radioactivity measurements. This high sensitivity might, however, lead to artifacts. For instance, small quantities of soluble proteins might be tightly bound to fibrous elastin and released into solution after a few peptide bonds of elastin have been cleaved. As a consequence, pseudo-elastase activity will be detected during the beginning of the reaction. The radioactivity or the fluorescence intensity associated with these soluble proteins will be negligible after the elastinolytic reaction has taken place to an appreciable extent. We therefore recommend that data representing less than 5% elastin hydrolysis be disregarded. Alternatively, one may determine the kinetics of elastin solubilization and extrapolate the curve to time zero in order to substract any release of nonelastin peptides.

The use of fluorescent or radioactive elastins should be limited to special cases where very low elastase activities are to be detected in cell or tissue extracts. With rhodamine–elastin, fluorescence quenching can occur and should be checked for. Methods using absorbance readings to detect soluble elastin peptides are more accurate and should be used whenever possible. Their sensitivities can be substantially improved by increasing the assay time.

5.   THE MISUSE OF SDS-TREATED ELASTINS

Kagan and co-workers (1972) have shown that SDS-treated elastin is up to sixfold more susceptible to porcine pancreatic elastase than untreated elastin. This observation led many investigators to use SDS-treated elastin for the assay of elastases, whatever their origin. We strongly recommend that elastin without SDS be used. First, it should be recalled that SDS changes the net charge and the conformation of elastin. SDS-treated elastin may therefore be considered as an artificial substrate which can no longer be used to characterize an elastase. It might, for instance, be solubilized by a proteinase that does not attack native elastin. Second, free SDS may be present in assay mixtures containing SDS–elastin. Free SDS inhibits elastase (Kagan *et al.*, 1972) and dissociates elastase–inhibitor complexes (Banda and Werb, 1981). It should also be added that the potentiating effect of SDS is lower with ^{3}H-labeled elastin than with native elastin (Takahashi *et al.*, 1973) and is less pronounced with human leukocyte elastase than with porcine pancreatic elastase (Kagan *et al.*, 1977).

C. Methods Using Synthetic Substrates

1. INTRODUCTORY COMMENTS

Assays using artificial substrates are more convenient, more sensitive, and more reliable than elastinolytic methods. Their use, however, should be restricted to the study of pure enzymes or tissue extracts whose elastinolytic activity has been clearly demonstrated with fibrous elastin. The choice of a synthetic substrate should be governed by factors such as commercial availability, water solubility, stability during the assay, convenience, and sensitivity of detection of reaction products.

Substrates for most of the elastases reviewed in this chapter are now commercially available. These compounds usually contain three to four hydrophobic amino acid residues which render them poorly water soluble. Hence, large amounts of organic solvents must often be included in the reaction mixtures and may interfere with the assays. Water solubility may be increased by using a hydrophilic acid as an N-acylating agent. For instance, N-succinylated substrates are much more water soluble than N-acetylated or N-benzoylated ones and usually require little or no organic solvent in the assay mixture. We therefore recommend substrates with succinyl, gluraryl, or succinylmethyl ester N-blocking groups.

2. THE ADVANTAGES OF p-NITROANILIDES OVER OTHER SUBSTRATES

The stability of the substrate and the convenience and sensitivity of the assay mostly depend on the nature of the substrate's leaving group. Esters are less stable than amides or p-nitroanilides. Esters of p-nitrophenol are so unstable that the assay pH must be around 6.0. Methyl or ethyl esters are moderately stable at pH 7–8, but their hydrolysis requires a pH-stat device to be monitored. We therefore do not recommend such substrates. Compounds with the following leaving groups have been proposed as sensitive and convenient substrates of elastase: p-nitroanilides, 4-methyl-7-coumarylamides (and other fluorogenic substrates) and thiobenzyl esters.

Assays using p-nitroanilides are very convenient because a yellow color develops as the enzymatic reaction proceeds. The action of the enzyme may thus be "seen" and, of course, may be followed spectrophotometrically at 405–410 nm. These substrates are fairly stable to that incubation periods up to 12 hr may used without getting important blank values. In addition, the assays are very sensitive. For instance, with 1 mM succinyl-(Ala)$_3$-p-nitroanilide and 10 nM porcine pancreatic elastase, an absorbance change of 0.04/min is observed (Bieth *et al.*, 1974). The sensitivity may even be increased by a factor of five by converting p-nitroaniline into a diazo dye (Bieth and Wermuth, 1973).

Fluorogenic substrates are also very resistant to autolysis. They are less convenient than the above compounds because special equipment is desired and fluorescence quenching may occur. These substrates are commonly thought to be "supersensitive." This concept must be revised; their k_{cat} values are lower than those of p-nitroanilides because the coumarinylamide bond is more difficult to split than the nitroanilide linkage. Hence, their overall sensitivity is not dramatically higher than that of p-nitroanilides (Castillo *et al.*, 1979, and refs. therein).

Thiobenzyl esters are much less stable than the above substrates; reactions must be performed at neutral pH in nonnucleophilic buffers to ensure reasonable substrate stability during the assay. Spectrophotometric detection of the leaving group (benzyl mercaptan), requires addition of Ellman's reagent or 4,4'-dithiodipyridine to the reaction medium. These reagents combine with benzyl mercaptan to form products which can be detected at 412 or 324 nm but which may also combine with other free thiols present in the assay, thus rendering methods using thiobenzyl esters less reliable than procedures employing p-nitroanilides. The sole advantage of assays using thiobenzyl esters is their sensitivity which is about 10-fold higher than that of the nitroanilide methods (Castillo *et al.*, 1979, and references therein). This advantage does not, however, compensate for the real drawbacks mentioned above. We do not recommend the use of such substrates.

In summary, we suggest the use of p-nitroanilide substrates for their good stability during the assay, their distinct convenience and their fairly good sensitivity. Within the list of commercially available substrates bearing a hydrophilic group, we suggest succinyl-(Ala)$_3$-p-nitroanilide as a porcine pancreatic elastase substrate (Bieth *et al.*, 1974). Succinylmethyl ester-(Ala)$_2$-Pro-Val-p-nitroanilide is the most susceptible substrate for human leukocyte elastase and related proteinases (Nakajima *et al.*, 1979). These enzymes may also be efficiently assayed with the more water soluble and less expensive substrate succinyl-(Ala)$_2$-Val-p-nitroanilide (Wenzel *et al.*, 1980). If high sensitivities are not required, succinyl-(Ala)$_3$-p-nitroanilide may be used: for $[E^0] = 0.4 \mu M$ and $[S^0] = 1$ mM, the absorbance change per minute is about 0.04. For chymotrypsin-like elastases such as procine pancreatic elastase II, human pancreatic elastase, and human leukocyte cathepsin G, substrates of general formula succinyl-(Ala)$_2$-Pro-X-p-nitroanilide (X = Leu, Phe, and Met) are commercially available.

For *Pseudomonas aeruginosa* elastase the fluorogenic substrate 2-aminobenzoyl-Ala-Gly-Leu-Ala-4-nitrobenzylamide is used. This contains both a fluorescent and a fluorescence-quenching group which are separated in the course of enzymatic hydrolysis with resultant enhancement of fluorescence intensity (k_{cat} = 100 sec^{-1}, K_m = 0.11 mM; Nishino and Powers, 1980).

3.   SOME PRACTICAL SUGGESTIONS CONCERNING THE USE OF SYNTHETIC SUBSTRATES

a.   Use Stock Solutions of Substrate.   It is very convenient to store substrates in inert analytical grade solvents (N-methylpyrrolidine, dimethylformamide, or dimethylsulfoxide) at a concentration 100-fold greater than that desired in the final assay. Such solutions will be stable for several months in the refrigerator. A 1:100 dilution in the assay buffer results in a final solvent concentration of 1% which should not impair the enzymatic reaction. A 2% concentration may sometimes be necessary, but 10% solvent (Nakajima *et al.,* 1979; Wenzel *et al.,* 1980) is not required.

b.   Select an Appropriate Substrate Concentration.   In choosing the final substrate concentration [S^0] one should find a compromise between sensitivity requirements (the higher [S^0], the better the sensitivity), water-solubility limitations, cost, and reliability of the assay. An assay is reliable if it gives a linear response of absorbance (e.g., for p-nitroanilides) to enzyme concentration. If the enzyme is stable during the assay, linearity is observed, provided that, under the conditions used, initial reaction rates are measured, i.e., provided that the response of absorbance to time is itself linear. This is easily checked by performing kinetic assays (i.e., recording absorbance versus time curves) or time-dependent end-point assays (e.g., stopping the reaction with acetic acid after various reaction times and reading the absorbancies). It should also be possible to predict the maximal percentage of substrate which may be hydrolyzed under initial rate conditions. We have calculated this percentage for different substrate concentrations. Table XIII shows that the higher the substrate concentration, the higher the percentage of substrate hydrolyzable under initial rate conditions and, of course, the higher the sensitivity of the method. Table XIII also shows the highest absorbancies compatible with the above

TABLE XIII

INFLUENCE OF SUBSTRATE CONCENTRATION ON THE SENSITIVITY AND THE RELIABILITY OF
ELASTASE ASSAYS USING SYNTHETIC p-NITROANILIDE SUBSTRATES

Relative substrate concentration ($[S^0]/K_m$)	Relative reaction rate (v/V_{max})	Extent of substrate hydrolysis compatible with initial rate requirements[a] (%)	Highest absorbance at 410 nm compatible with initial rate requirements[a,b]	
			$K_m = 0.1$ mM	$K_m = 1$ mM
0.1	0.09	4.0	0.003	0.030
1.0	0.50	5.8	0.050	0.500
3.0	0.75	11.3	0.300	3.000

[a]Calculated by trial and error using the Michaelis–Menten equation and assuming that initial rate conditions prevail until the rate decreases by more than 3%.
[b]Calculated using $\varepsilon = 8,800$ M^{-1} cm^{-1} for p-nitroaniline.

requirements when two p-nitroanilide substrates with widely different K_m values are used. It can be seen that for identical $[S^0]/K_m$ values, a "bad substrate" gives a much higher absorbance limit than a "good" one. This demonstrates that K_m should not be the sole factor to take into account when choosing the substrate concentration of the assay. One should rather transform K_m into A_{max}, the highest absorbance compatible with initial rate requirements (i.e., $A_{max} = K_m \times 8,800 \times 0.058$). If A_{max} is too low, the substrate should be used at a concentration higher than K_m. The above analysis also shows that the k_{cat} rather than k_{cat}/K_m is the most important factor for practical purposes. On the other hand, if A_{max} is satisfactory for $[S^0] = K_m$ we do not recommend the use of a substrate concentration higher than K_m because above K_m the reaction velocity increases less and less with $[S^0]$ and water solubility problems may be encountered.

c. *Run Kinetic Assays.* Elastase activity is frequently measured using end-point assays which allow a large number of samples to be tested at the same time. Such methods are less reliable and less informative than kinetic runs where the enzymatic reaction may be directly "seen" on the chart paper of the recorder. End-point assays do not detect deviations from the expected absorbance versus time linearity which may be due to normal or accidental degradation of enzyme or to a slow substrate-induced dissociation of an enzyme–inhibitor complex. We therefore recommend use of at least three different incubation times to perform end-point assays. It is safer to do this than to run a single time point in triplicate.

D. *Active Site Titrants*

The determination of the kinetic constants characterizing an enzyme–substrate interaction necessitates the knowledge of the molar concentration of active enzyme. For instance, the overall catalytic rate constant k_{cat} is obtained by dividing the maximal rate V_{max} by the total concentration of active enzyme $[E^0]$. Even if an enzyme preparation satisfies the usual criteria of protein purity, it may contain some denatured material so that the concentration of active enzyme of a solution will be lower than that determined by weight or by UV absorbance measurement. The determination of the concentration of active enzyme is usually called "active site titration."

Most active site titrants of proteinases are pseudo-substrates whose breakdown follows a scheme identical to that already shown in Section V,A:

$$E + S \underset{k_{-1}}{\overset{k_1}{\rightleftharpoons}} ES \xrightarrow{k_2} EP_2 + P_1 \xrightarrow{k_3} E + P_2$$

A substrate becomes an active site titrant if it fulfills the following requirements: (1) S must be specific for the enzyme, (2) k_2 must be large, (3) k_3 must be small or zero, and (4) P_1 must be observable by absorption or fluorescence spectroscopy.

Powers and his group have developed a series of azapeptide-*p*-nitrophenyl esters which may be used as active site titrants of elastases and other proteinases (Powers and Carrol, 1975; Powers *et al.*, 1984). These peptides have an azaamino acid at the C-terminal position (structure of azaalanine: —NHN(CH$_3$)CO—). The *p*-nitrophenol leaving group (designated P_1 in the above scheme) offers two advantages: first, it forms an unstable activated ester with the C-terminal azaamino acid so that k_2 is extremely fast, and second, it may be detected spectrophotometrically ($\varepsilon = 6{,}250$ at 345 nm; $\varepsilon = 5{,}500$ at 347.5 nm, the isobestic point). The azaamino acid derivatives form stable acyl–enzyme intermediates, designated EP_2 in the above scheme ($k_3 = 10^{-3}$–10^{-4} sec^{-1}). Addition of enzyme to such a pseudo-substrate therefore gives rise to a burst of *p*-nitrophenol whose molar concentration equals that of the active enzyme. For porcine pancreatic and human leukocyte elastase three titrants have been proposed: acetyl-(Ala)$_2$-X-*p*-nitrophenyl ester with X = azaalanine, azanorleucine, or azanorvaline. The latter forms the most stable acyl–enzyme intermediate. When 2 μM leukocyte elastase is reacted with 44 μM acetyl-(Ala)$_2$-azaAla-*p*-nitrophenyl ester at pH 6.0, a burst of about 0.013 absorbance units is observed (Powers *et al.*, 1984).

E. *Immunoassays of Elastases*

Radioimmunoassays or enzyme-linked immunosorbent assays have been described for elastases from porcine pancreas (Ooyama *et al.*, 1977), human pancreas (Geokas *et al.*, 1977), dog pancreas (Carballo *et al.*, 1974), human neutrophils (Ohlsson and Olsson, 1978), dog neutrophils (Kucich *et al.*, 1980), and *Pseudomonas aeruginosa* (Oberness and Döring, 1982). Enzyme-linked immunosorbent assays for the human leukocyte elastase–human α_1-proteinase inhibitor complex have also been reported recently (Neumann *et al.*, 1983; Brower and Harpel, 1983). The elastase–inhibitor complex is sandwiched between two different antibodies, one directed against elastase and the other against the inhibitor. Hence, neither free elastase nor free inhibitor but only their complex are detected.

X. PATHOLOGICAL ROLE OF ELASTASES

A. *Introductory Comments*

1. PATHOLOGICAL VERSUS PHYSIOLOGICAL FUNCTION OF ELASTASES

While reviewing the abundant literature on elastases, the feeling emerges that Nature designed these enzymes for the sole purpose of inducing diseases. Although the physiological function of elastases is poorly documented, we shall attempt to discuss briefly this function to help delineate the pathogenic role of elastinolytic enzymes.

Polymorphonuclear and mononuclear phagocytes have the task of ingesting and digesting foreign substances (bacteria, immune complexes, etc.). Human polymorphonuclear leukocyte elastase has been shown to cleave *E. coli* proteins and to lyse *E. coli* cell walls (Blondin and Janoff, 1976, and refs. therein). The alveolar macrophage elastases may play similar functions. Pancreatic elastases are secreted into the duodenum to digest food.

However, we do not eat much elastin, and bacteria or immune complexes do not contain elastin. So, why did Nature endow these proteinases with elastinolytic properties? Neutrophil-mediated physiological elastinolysis may be required after acute injury of connective tissues, e.g., wounds, as an initial step in the tissue repair mechanism. Chronic elastinolysis of skin, lung, or blood vessel elastin is difficult to consider as a physiological process since the normal turnover of elastin is extremely low. For example, in mice, the turnover of lung elastin is best estimated in years, and in man less than 1% of the total body pool of elastin is turned over in 1 year (for a review see Rucker and Dubick, 1984).

Pathological processes mediated by elastase-carrying cells appear thus to occur as undesirable side-effects of the normal phagocytic and local tissue remodeling function of these cells.

2. NEUTROPHILS AS FAST MOVING BOMBS

It is not always realized that neutrophils are carrying an enormous amount of elastase. Based on 5×10^3 neutrophils per mm^3 and 3 μg elastase per 10^6 cells (see Section IV), there are 75 mg of elastase circulating in the blood stream. This amount does not take into account the marginal cells which may be rapidly released. Local recruitment of neutrophils is very fast due to powerful chemoattractant mechanisms. Thus, very high local concentrations of elastase (and, of course, other leukoproteinases) can be found at sites of inflammation, requiring the organism to provide very efficient mechanisms to control this proteolytic process.

3. THE TARGETS OF NEUTROPHIL ELASTASE

As shown in Table VIII of Section V,E, neutrophil elastase not only cleaves elastin but also other connective tissue proteins such as collagens, proteoglycans, and fibronectin. In addition, it hydrolyzes and inactivates blood coagulation factors, components of the immune system, and plasma proteinase inhibitors. Potential cleavage of all these endogenous substrates must be kept in mind when analyzing the possible pathological role of neutrophil elastase. Consideration should also be given to (1) nonelastinolytic enzymes present in the neutrophil and able to potentiate its action and (2) elastases and proteinases from other cells and tissues, because proteolysis *in vivo* probably results from the cooperative action of several proteinases.

B. Pulmonary Emphysema

1. DEFINITION

According to a committee of the American Thoracic Society, emphysema is defined as "an *anatomic alteration* of the lung characterized by an abnormal enlargement of the airspaces distal to the terminal nonrespiratory bronchiole, accompanied by *destructive changes* of the alveolar walls." The term "destructive changes" is important because it distinguishes emphysema from other lung diseases involving alveolar enlargement. Elastin and collagen fiber disruptions are indeed characteristic features of the emphysematous lung (Sandberg *et al.*, 1981). The term "anatomic alteration" is important too because it emphasizes that lung emphysema is difficult to diagnose in living persons using classical mechanical tests. As a matter of fact, limitation of airflow, which accompanies severe emphysema, also occurs in small airway disease (Bignon and de Crémoux, 1980).

2. The Elastase–Antielastase Theory of the Pathogenesis of Emphysema

A major improvement in the understanding of the pathogenesis of emphysema came from the observation by Laurell and Eriksson (1963) of an association between inherited α_1-proteinase inhibitor deficiency and early emphysema. Later studies indicated that when the deficiency is severe, i.e., when the plasma concentration of α_1-proteinase inhibitor is only 10–15% of the normal level, the frequency of pulmonary emphysema is very high. Such patients usually have the PiZZ phenotype (see Section VI,A,1). Subjects with intermediate plasma inhibitor levels, e.g., with the PiMZ or PiSZ phenotypes, usually exhibit a much lower frequency of severe pulmonary emphysema (Eriksson, 1984).

In 1963, α_1-proteinase inhibitor was named α_1-antitrypsin and its function was unknown. Three years later, Kueppers and Bearn (1966) noticed that leukoprotease is inhibited by α_1-proteinase inhibitor and suggested that this enzyme may promote pulmonary emphysema associated with inherited inhibitor deficiency. This view was favored by animal experiments indicating that elastolytic enzymes (but not other proteinases) were able to produce a pulmonary disorder resembling human emphysema (reviewed by Bignon and de Crémoux, 1980).

Cogenital deficiency of α_1-proteinase inhibitor is, however, a minor cause of emphysema: most patients are smokers. PiZZ individuals who smoke have earlier signs of emphysema and have a lower life expectancy than those who do not smoke (Eriksson, 1984). The first clue for a possible link between smoking and emphysema came from the *in vitro* observation that cigarette smoke condensate impairs the elastase inhibitory capacity of α_1-proteinase inhibitor by an oxidative mechanism (Carp and Janoff, 1978). Later studies revealed that activated neutrophils or macrophages may oxidize the inhibitor *in vitro* and *in vivo* (reviewed by Janoff, 1983) and that dogs treated with chloramine-T, an oxidant, develop emphysematous lesions (Abrams *et al.*, 1981a).

The above findings led to the proposal of the so-called protease–antiprotease imbalance theory of the pathogenesis of emphysema. This theory holds that alveolar structures are normally protected from phagocyte-mediated elastinolysis by α_1-proteinase inhibitor which transudates from plasma into the lung interstitium. Emphysema may occur if the lung elastase burden increases and if the inhibitor is absent (hereditary disease) or oxidized (smokers' emphysema). Even though this hypothesis still requires rigorous proof, it is supported by a large body of circumstantial evidence which will be summarized and discussed below.

3. NEUTROPHIL-MEDIATED PROTEOLYSIS OF LUNG CONNECTIVE TISSUE COMPONENTS

The number of neutrophils collected by bronchoalveolar lavage or detected in biopsy material is higher in smokers than in nonsmokers (Gadek *et al.*, 1980b). This cell recruitment may result from the smoking condition itself but may also be due to macrophage-secreted chemoattractants or to the leukoattractant properties of elastin peptides (Senior *et al.*, 1980; Janoff, 1983). Smokers therefore have more potential elastase in their lungs than nonsmokers.

Release of neutrophil elastase *in situ* is suggested by *in vitro* experiments showing that cigarette smoke, leukoattractants, secretogogues, or phagocytosed particules may stimulate the release of the neutrophil's lysosomal content (reviewed by Gadeck *et al.*, 1980b). In addition to elastases, other proteinases may be secreted, namely cathepsin G, latent collagenase and gelatinase, and plasminogen activator (reviewed by Senior and Campbell, 1983). These proteinases may act in a cooperative fashion to achieve cleavage of elastin fibers. Plasminogen activator may generate plasmin from its ubiquitous substrate, plasminogen. Plasmin readily degrades connective tissue glycoproteins such as fibronectin and laminin and activates latent collagenase (reviewed by Senior and Campbell, 1983). By so doing, it might increase the susceptibility of elastin fibers to elastase-catalyzed degradation. This view is supported by *in vitro* experiments with mouse peritoneal macrophage elastase (Werb *et al.*, 1980) or a cancer cell line elastase (Jones and Declerck, 1980). Cathepsin G and elastase may themselves degrade connective tissue glycoproteins and activate latent collagenase and gelatinase (see Table VIII). Cleavage of collagen by the latter enzymes may be an additional factor that favors the elastinolytic action of elastase. Cathepsin G itself is elastinolytic and strongly enhances the action of elastase *in vitro* (Boudier *et al.*, 1981b); this effect might also occur *in vivo*. Potentiation of elastinolysis by platelet factor 4 might also play a role in elastin degradation (Lonky and Wohl, 1981).

Neutrophil-mediated proteolysis of lung connective tissue components may be controlled in part by α_1-proteinase inhibitor which is present in the lower respiratory tract (see Gadek *et al.*, 1980b). As shown in Section VI,A, this inhibitor is very efficient *in vitro* against neutrophil elastase but reacts slowly with cathepsin G and is very poorly efficient on plasmin. The latter proteinases might be inhibited by their specific plasma inhibitors α_1-antichymotrypsin and α_2-antiplasmin (Travis and Salvesen, 1983) which may transudate from plasma into the lung interstitium. Local synthesis of α_1-antichymotrypsin by alveolar macrophages has also been reported (Burnett *et al.*, 1984). It is doubtful, however, that these two inhibitors may play their function in the lung interstitium since neutrophil elastase is able to inactivate them (see Table VIII). Collagenase and gelatinase activity is probably not controlled by local inhibitors.

4. MACROPHAGE-MEDIATED PROTEOLYSIS OF LUNG CONNECTIVE TISSUE COMPONENTS

Smokers have increased numbers of macrophages within their alveolar structures. Elastin peptides serve also as chemoattractants for these cells (see Gadeck *et al.*, 1980b). As discussed in Section VII,A, human alveolar macrophages contain three elastinolytic proteinases: a metalloenzyme synthesized by these cells, a serine enzyme which is probably neutrophil elastase internalized by the macrophage, and a cell-surface-associated thiol proteinase.

The metalloenzyme is synthesized in very low amounts but is secreted into the culture medium of macrophages and is resistant to the inhibitory action of serum: unrestricted elastolysis may therefore occur. In addition, the levels of this enzyme are higher in smokers than in nonsmokers as measured in macrophage secretions (Hinman *et al.*, 1980) and in bronchoalveolar lavage fluids (Niederman *et al.*, 1984). These observations, taken together with the fact that smokers have great numbers of macrophages in their lungs, suggest the metalloelastase may play a significant role in lung elastinolysis.

By internalizing neutrophil elastase *in situ,* the macrophage may protect this enzyme from inhibition by α_1-proteinase inhibitor and carry it to sites of inflammation where it may be released by various stimuli. One characteristic property of resident macrophages is tight adherence to the extracellular matrix. As shown by *in vitro* experiments (Werb *et al.*, 1980; Jones and Declerck, 1980; Campbell *et al.*, 1982) elastase inhibition by surrounding inhibitors is impaired if the cells that secrete the enzyme are in close contact with the substrate. Therefore, internalized neutrophil elastase may exert its proteolytic action despite the presence of inhibitors. This effect may be particularly important in smokers, whose macrophage content of neutrophil elastase is much higher than that of nonsmokers (Rodriguez *et al.* 1977; Hinman *et al.*, 1980).

The macrophage surface-associated thiol proteinase is a very efficient elastase if the cells contact the substrate since the elastinolytic reaction is not inhibited by serum (Chapman *et al.*, 1984).

In addition to the aforementioned macrophage-mediated elastinolysis, let us mention that these phagocytes can degrade fibronectin (Senior and Campbell, 1983) and may enhance neutrophil-mediated proteolysis by secreting attractants and secretogogues for polymorphonuclear leukocytes (Gadek *et al.*, 1980b).

Lung macrophages are commonly thought to play a minor role in the genesis of pulmonary emphysema because their elastase content is extremely low compared to that of neutrophils. This concept should be revised in view of the above discussion: smokers' activated macrophages have three elastases, two of which are resistant to α_1-proteinase inhibitor. Due to the large number of macrophages present in smokers and to the long life span of these phagocytes, efficient elastinolysis may be brought about by these noninhibitable enzymes. In addition, by acting as a neutrophil elastase reservoir, smokers' macrophages may increase the efficiency of neutrophil-mediated proteolysis since this sequestered elastase may be shielded from the inhibitory action of α_1-proteinase inhibitor.

5. OXIDATIVE INACTIVATION OF α_1-PROTEINASE INHIBITOR AS A POSSIBLE BIOCHEMICAL LINK BETWEEN SMOKING AND EMPHYSEMA

a. Direct Effect of Cigarette Smoke. Cigarette smoke condensate is able to inactivate α_1-proteinase inhibitor *in vitro* and in animals subjected to acute doses of smoke. Elastase is also inactivated by cigarette smoke (Ohlsson *et al.*, 1980) but less than α_1-proteinase inhibitor (for review see Janoff, 1983). Recent studies suggest that cigarette smoke is not very effective in directly inactivating α_1-proteinase inhibitor (Wyss *et al.,* 1984) but decreases the rate constant for the elastase-inhibitor association (Laurent and Bieth, 1985).

 b. *Phagocyte-Mediated Oxidation of α_1-Proteinase Inhibitor.* Activated phagocytes release a number of oxidants which are able to directly inactivate α_1-proteinase inhibitor. The same effect is operated by an enzyme, myeloperoxidase, which inactivates the inhibitor in the presence of H_2O_2 and Cl^- (reviewed by Matheson *et al.,* 1982, and Janoff, 1983). Since smokers have larger numbers of phagocytes than nonsmokers, and since smoking activates these cells, oxidative inactivation of α_1-proteinase inhibitor may occur in these individuals.

 c. *Oxidative Impairment of the Antielastase Function of α_1-Proteinase Inhibitor.* As discussed in Section VI,A,1, oxidation of the methionine residue of the inhibitor active center to methionine sulfoxide leads to a dramatic alteration of the proteinase inhibitory capacity of this protein. Porcine pancreatic elastase and human plasmin become fully resistant to the modified inhibitor. Other enzymes are still able to react with oxidized inhibitor but with considerably reduced rates or increased delay times of inhibition (see Table IX). The most pronounced decrease in inhibition rate is that observed with leukocyte elastase: k_{assoc} decreases by a factor of 2000 upon oxidation of the inhibitor. Theory predicts that with such a reduction in reaction rate, modified α_1-proteinase inhibitor will be poorly effective *in vivo* (see Section VI,A,6). Two sets of experimental evidence favor this view: (1) oxidized α_1-proteinase inhibitor is unable to prevent elastinolysis *in vitro* (Beatty *et al.,* 1984) and (2) dogs treated with the oxidant chloramine-T develop emphysematous lesions (Abrams *et al.,* 1981a).

 d. *Evidence for the Presence of Oxidized α_1-Proteinase Inhibitor in the Lung of Smokers.* *In vivo* oxidized inhibitor has been detected and/or isolated in synovial fluids (Wong and Travis, 1980) and in bronchoalveolar lavage fluids from healthy smokers (Carp *et al.,* 1982) or from patients suffering from adult respiratory distress syndrome (Cochrane *et al.,* 1983). This stands as an unambiguous proof that biological oxidation of the inhibitor takes place. There is, however, some controversy about the occurrence of oxidized α_1-proteinase inhibitor in the lower respiratory tract. The altered inhibitor cannot as yet be directly assessed using monoclonal antibodies, for instance. Therefore indirect methods comparing the elastase inhibitory capacity to the immunochemically determined inhibitor concentration have been used to diagnose a smoke-induced decrease in the functional activity of lung and plasma α_1-proteinase inhibitor. Conflicting results have been obtained with bronchoalveolar lavage fluids (Gadek *et al.*, 1979; Carp *et al.*, 1982; Boudier *et al.*, 1983; Stone *et al.*, 1983) and serum (Beatty *et al.*, 1982b; Cox and Billingsley, 1984). Immunochemical methods using monoclonal antibodies against oxidized inhibitor are being developed. Such methods should be able to solve the above controversies. In addition, immunohistochemical techniques should enable us to have an insight into the state of oxidation of α_1-proteinase inhibitor within the lung interstitium.

   e. Possible Biological Factors Controlling α_1-Proteinase Inhibitor Oxidation. *E. coli* methionine sulfoxide peptide reductase has been found to reduce the oxidized inhibitor and to restore its biological activity (Abrams *et al.*, 1981b). A similar enzyme activity is present in neutrophils (Carp *et al.*, 1983). The neutrophil therefore has the puzzling property of inactivating and reactivating α_1-proteinase inhibitor. The kinetics of these two processes should be investigated in order to better understand this ambiguous function.

   Antioxidants are able to prevent the oxidation of the inhibitor *in vitro*. Such compounds may also regulate the oxidation *in vivo;* ceruloplasmin is a possible candidate for such a function (reviewed by Janoff, 1983).

   While most emphysematous patients are smokers, only about 20% of smokers develop the disease. The presence of variable amounts of methionine sulfoxide peptide reductase or of oxidant scavengers might be one factor that accounts for the variable susceptibility of smokers to this disease.

6. POSSIBLE PROTEOLYTIC INACTIVATION OF α_1-PROTEINASE INHIBITOR

In Section VI,A,1, we have shown that certain thiol or metalloproteinases are able to inactivate α_1-proteinase inhibitor by limited proteolytic cleavage. The metalloelastase from mouse peritoneal macrophages is a typical example of such an inactivating enzyme. It is not known as yet whether the metalloenzyme synthesized by human macrophages is also able to degrade α_1-proteinase inhibitor. On the other hand, thiol proteinase activity is present in neutrophils, in bronchoalveolar lavage fluids (Orlowski *et al.*, 1981), and in macrophages (Burnett *et al.*, 1983; Chapman *et al.*, 1984). Again the effect of these enzymes on α_1-proteinase inhibitor is unknown. It is noteworthy, however, that α_1-proteinase inhibitor collected by bronchoalveolar lavage from healthy nonsmokers is only about 50% active on elastase

(Boudier *et al.*, 1983; Stone *et al.*, 1983). This suggests that proteolytic inactivation of the inhibitor may normally take place *in situ* and could be exacerbated during conditions associated with smoking.

7. THE ROLE OF BRONCHIAL INHIBITOR AND OTHER INHIBITORS

Some properties of bronchial inhibitor have been given in Section VI,A,5. This protein is synthesized mainly in the upper respiratory tract but has also been detected in the peripheral lung (Mooren *et al.*, 1983) and in bronchoalveolar lavage fluids (Stockley *et al.*, 1984; Abrams *et al.*, 1984). From the kinetic constants of its interaction with neutrophil elastase (Gauthier *et al.*, 1982), it may be inferred that it might act as a powerful antielastase *in vivo* (see Section VI,A,6). Although its concentration in the lower respiratory tract is probably lower than that of α_1-proteinase inhibitor (Abrams *et al.*, 1984), it might be occasionally more efficient than the latter inhibitor because of its low molecular mass, which probably aids its diffusion through the highly viscous ground substance of the connective tissue. In addition, as suggested previously (Gauthier *et al.*, 1982) it might inhibit elastin-bound elastase, an action that cannot be achieved by the bulkier α_1-proteinase inhibitor (Reilly and Travis, 1980). This inhibitor might therefore act in concert with the latter molecule. It is noteworthy that its function is also impaired by cigarette smoke and phagocyte-derived oxidants (Carp and Janoff, 1980b).

8. IMPAIRMENT OF THE ELASTIN-REPAIR MECHANISM BY CIGARETTE SMOKE

Although the turnover of elastin is normally very low, elastin biosynthesis is fast in case of injury (e.g., wound healing). Lysyl oxidase is a key enzyme in the biosynthetic process since it catalyzes the oxidation of the ϵ amino groups of lysine residues which is followed by a condensation reaction yielding desmosine and isodesmosine, the major cross-linking amino acids of elastin. Laurent *et al.* (1983) has recently shown that cigarette smoke inhibits the lysyl oxidase-catalyzed oxidation of lysine residues of tropoelastin *in vitro*. The elastin repair mechanism might therefore be impaired in smokers. This view is supported by the observation that chronic exposure of hamsters to smoke alters the incorporation of ^{14}C-lysine into desmosine during the repair of elastase-damaged lung elastin (Osman *et al.*, 1982).

9. SUMMARY AND SPECULATIONS

From the foregoing discussion, smokers' emphysema appears to be a multifactorial disease. The numerous pathogenic factors that have been suggested are difficult to puzzle out. Let us, therefore, attempt to propose a simple scheme that involves the cooperative action of neutrophils and macrophages in the degradation of lung elastin.

Stimulated neutrophils will release their proteinases within the highly viscous ground substance of the connective tissue in which elastin and collagen fibers are embedded. In this medium, elastase will be faced with several targets: α_1-proteinase inhibitor (and perhaps bronchial mucous inhibitor), proteoglycans, glycoproteins, latent collagenase and gelatinase, α_1-antichymotrypsin, α_2-antiplasmin, and macrophage membrane receptors. As shown in Section VI,A,6, the elastase–inhibitor association rate constant k_{assoc} is decreased by competing substrates. In addition, many other factors may decrease k_{assoc}, namely, (1) the oxidation of the inhibitor in the vicinity of the neutrophil, (2) the high viscosity of the ground substance, and (3) the decreased pH at the cell surface during the metabolic burst. On the other hand, a close contact between neutrophils and extracellular matrix may result in high local concentration of elastase which may overcome the local inhibitory capacity.

As a consequence, elastase will be able to achieve some substrate breakdown and to bind to some extent to macrophage receptors during its delay time of inhibition by α_1-proteinase inhibitor. Hence, the plasmin and cathepsin G inhibitors will be partially destroyed and the two enzymes will freely attack connective tissue glycoproteins and activate latent collagenase and gelatinase which, in turn, will solubilize collagen fibers. At this stage, elastase will not have had time enough to reach and to degrade the embedded elastin fibers. In the present model, neutrophil-mediated proteolysis does not, therefore, lead to elastinolysis but is merely used to "clean" the elastin fibers from their surrounding connective tissue macromolecules.

Elastinolysis will then be achieved by the three elastases of the resident macrophages. As already mentioned, these cells will tightly adhere to the matrix and this cell–substrate contact will protect their secreted neutrophil elastase from the inhibitory action of α_1-proteinase inhibitor. The other elastases are per se resistant to inhibition. The low amounts of elastases present in macrophages will be compensated for by the long life span of these resident cells. Hence, efficient elastinolysis of "nude" elastin fibers will occur.

Our model hypothesizes that the large number of phagocytes present in smokers' lungs and their continuous recruitment and activation by smoke, chemoattractants, and secretogogues may be sufficient to rationalize the development of emphysema in smokers. Although we do not disregard oxidative processes, we feel that the oxidative inactivation of α_1-proteinase inhibitor is not the principal link between smoking and emphysema. We are not unaware that this view contradicts commonly accepted proposals. To be of major importance, the oxidative process should be efficient enough to oxidize the totality of the inhibitor present in lung, i.e., to create an "acquired α_1-proteinase inhibitor deficiency" comparable in magnitude to the inherited deficiency. This is apparently not the case since (1) α_1-proteinase inhibitor collected by bronchoalveolar lavage from smokers contains a substantial proportion of active inhibitor and (2) smokers do not develop early emphysema. Even a 50% oxidative inactivation of lung α_1-proteinase inhibitor would not necessarily lead to emphysema per se since PiMZ or PiSZ subjects have only about 50% inhibitor and yet do not frequently develop emphysema. For these reasons, we believe that the oxidative inactivation of α_1-proteinase inhibitor, while favoring to some extent neutrophil-mediated proteolysis, is not of major importance in the genesis of smokers' emphysema.

C. Infections and Inflammatory Diseases

1. Pseudomonas aeruginosa Infections

Pseudomonas aeruginosa is an opportunistic pathogen which may cause fatal infections in vulnerable hosts such as individuals with severe burns, cancer patients under immunosuppressive therapy, children with cystic fibrosis, or postoperative patients under respirators (reviewed by Wretlind and Pavloskis, 1983). About 85% of *P. aeruginosa* strains secrete elastase and alkaline proteinase. This bacterium also secretes exotoxin A. In addition, neutrophils are recruited to sites of infection, and their phagocytic action releases elastase and other enzymes which will amplify the pathogenic action of the bacteria by inactivating biologically important proteins (see Table VIII). As discussed in Section VIII,A,2, *P. aeruginosa* elastase may inactivate a variety of proteins including IgG and IgA immunoglobulins, complement components, lysozyme, α_1-proteinase inhibitor, Cl-esterase inhibitor, α_1-antichymotrypsin, and human bronchial mucous inhibitor. By so doing, it will lower the natural antibacterial defense mechanisms of the host and weaken the host's natural antileukoproteinase screen. Plasma α_2-macroglobulin, the only human protein able to inhibit the bacterial elastase, does not readily transudate into tissues because of its high molecular mass. Hence, *P. aeruginosa* infections may be accompanied by uncontrolled proteolysis operated by both bacterial and neutrophil proteinases. The pathogenic role of *P. aeruginosa* elastase has been confirmed by experiments showing that strains deficient in active elastase are less virulent than elastase-producing strains (Blackwood *et al.*, 1983).

Pulmonary infections caused by *P. aeruginosa* are not uncommon. *Pseudomonas* pneumonia is accompanied by intraalveolar hemorrhage and necrosis (Fetzer *et al.*, 1967). These effects may be induced in animals by instillation of the bacterial proteinases (Gray and Kreger, 1979). Children with cystic fibrosis commonly develop *P. aeruginosa* infections with resulting airway damage. Their bronchial secretions are so purulent that they may be used as starting material for the isolation of leukoproteinases (Martodam *et al.*, 1979). Within this medium, the neutrophil and the bacterial elastases act in concert to inactivate the C3 component of complement (Suter *et al.*, 1984) and immunoglobulins (Fick *et al.*, 1984), thus preventing phagocytosis of the bacteria. *In vivo* release of bacterial elastase in cystic fibrosis is also evidenced by the production of antielastase antibodies in infected patients (Cho *et al.*, 1978).

Pseudomonas aeruginosa infections of burn wounds are frequent. Immunization of animals with bacterial elastase affords partial protection against experimental bacterial infection, confirming the pathogenic role of elastase (Kawaharajo and Homma, 1977).

Pseudomonas aeruginosa infections of human cornea are rare but may lead to loss of vision due to corneal scarring and perforation. Similar lesions may be produced in other animals (e.g., Kessler *et al.*, 1977). In addition, phosphoramidon, a *P. aeruginosa* elastase inhibitor (see Section VIII,A,2) is able to prevent elastase-induced corneal ulceration in animals (Kawaharajo *et al.*, 1982).

The pathogenic role of *P. aeruginosa* in some enteritis is suggested by animal experiments (Okada *et al.*, 1976). By contrast, this bacterium appears to play a minor role in septicemia (Wretlind and Pavloskis, 1983).

2. Other Infections

The inflammatory reaction which accompanies infections may lead to leukocyte recruitment, phagocytosis, and release of neutrophil oxidants and proteinases, whose deleterious action on plasma proteins are summarized in Table VIII of Section V,E. For instance, *in vitro* experiments show that phagocytosis of yeast cells or immune complexes by granulocytes results in a significant release of elastase, collagenase, and myeloperoxidase (Ohlsson and Olsson, 1977). On the other hand, injection of *E. coli* endotoxin in dogs results in the appearence of plasma immunoreactive leukocyte elastase bound to α_1-proteinase inhibitor (Aasen and Ohlsson, 1978) and partial destruction of plasma antithrombin III, prothrombin, factor XIII, plasminogen, α_2-antiplasmin, and complement component C3 (Jochum *et al.*, 1984a). Severe septicemia is accompanied by an increase in plasma levels of elastase–α_1-proteinase inhibitor complex correlated with a decrease of antithrombin III, factor XIII (Jochum *et al.*, 1984a), and other coagulation factors (Egbring *et al.*, 1977). These findings indicate that during the delay time of inhibition of elastase by α_1-proteinase inhibitor (defined in Section VI,A,6), partial breakdown of endogenous elastase substrates takes place. This effect will be discussed later. Immunoreactive neutrophil elastase has also been detected in pleural empyema (Suter *et al.*, 1981). The α_1-proteinase inhibitor collected by bronchoalveolar lavage in patients with acute bacterial pneumonia has a very low functional activity and some patients have free neutrophil elastase activity (Abrams *et al.*, 1984).

Leukoproteinases liberated in the course of the inflammatory reaction that accompanies infections may therefore be considered as aggravating factors of infections. Plasma α_1-proteinase inhibitor, while complexing neutrophil elastase *in vivo,* does apparently not react fast enough to fully prevent elastase-catalyzed breakdown of endogenous substrates despite its extremely low delay time of inhibition (3 msec). Inspection of the equation

$$[P\infty]/[S^0] = k_{cat}[E^0] \, d(t)/5K_m$$

developed in Section VI,A,6, reveals that several factors may account for the observed extent of substrate breakdown ($[P\infty]/[S^0]$) during the delay time of inhibition [$d(t)$], namely, (1) [E^0], the elastase concentration, may be high in the vicinity of the neutrophil, (2) the elastase–plasma substrate interaction may have large k_{cat}/K_m ratios, and (3) the inhibitor may be oxidized in the vicinity of the neutrophil so that $d(t)$ will be 6 sec instead of 3 msec.

3. Rheumatoid Arthritis and Other Inflammatory Processes

According to Jochum *et al.* (1984b) plasma elastase–α_1-proteinase inhibitor complex is a reliable marker of inflammatory processes, such as multiple trauma or septicemia, and may be considered a better indicator than the classical C-reactive protein. This demonstrates that neutrophil elastase is released during inflammation and confirms that α_1-proteinase inhibitor is a physiological antielastase.

Rheumatoid arthritis also gives rise to elevated levels of elastase–α_1-proteinase inhibitor complex (Schnebli et al., 1984). This invalidating disease is characterized by an extensive proteolytic degradation of the articular cartilage. During the acute phases of this disease, there is a massive infiltration of neutrophils in the joint space. It has been suggested that as many as 10^8 cells may be permanently present in a knee. Due to their high turnover, these cells may liberate ~4 mg of leukoproteinases per day (Barrett and Starkey, 1977). The joint is apparently protected against these enzymes by α_1-proteinase inhibitor whose plasma concentration rises during inflammation (this inhibitor is an "acute phase reactant") and which readily transudates into the joint space as a result of increased vascular permeability accompanying the local inflammatory reaction. In vitro experiments document the degradation of cartilage proteoglycans and collagen by neutrophil elastase, cathepsin G, and collagenase (Malemud and Janoff, 1975; Janoff et al., 1976; Barrett and Starkey, 1977; Starkey, 1977a; Starkey et al., 1977; Baici et al., 1982). Neutrophil elastase reduces the tensile strength and stiffness of articular cartilage as a result of its action on proteoglycans and collagen (Bader et al., 1981). Immunohisto-chemistry has been used to localize elastase in articular cartilage from patients with rheumatoid arthritis (Velvart et al., 1981).

It may be hypothesized that articular cartilage degradation occurs because elastase (and other proteinases) overcome the local elastase inhibitory capacity. This apparently is not true because rheumatoid arthritis synovial fluids have no free elastase activity (Velvart et al., 1981) and possess active α_1-proteinase inhibitor (Virca et al. 1984). In addition, the inhibitor does apparently play its physiological function since synovial fluids contain large amounts of elastase–inhibitor complex in addition to low amounts of free inhibitor (Virca et al., 1984). The latter observation, together with the finding that synovial fluids contain oxidized α_1-proteinase inhibitor (Wong and Travis, 1980), suggest that the concentration of active inhibitor might be too low to fully inhibit elastase before it reaches the cartilage structures (as shown in Section VI,A,6, the delay time of inhibition is inversely proportional to the inhibitor concentration). An alternative possibility is that elastase is protected from inhibition because α_1-proteinase inhibitor cannot penetrate into the articular cartilage (Janoff et al., 1976).

Adult respiratory distress syndrome (ARDS) is another disease where neutrophil elastase may play a pathological function. This syndrome may result from leukocyte sequestration in the pulmonary microcirculation. Lee and co-workers (1981) found high elastase activity in the bronchoalveolar lavage fluids of about 50% of their ARDS patients. The functional activity of α_1-proteinase inhibitor was considerably decreased. According to Cochrane et al. (1983), the α_1-proteinase inhibitor from the lower respiratory tract of ARDS patients exists in three inactive forms, namely, oxidized, elastase-bound and proteolytically inactivated. ARDS may therefore be considered as an example of a pathological state where the high elastase load has been able to overcome the local elastase inhibitory capacity and to lead to acute lung damage.

The peritoneal exudate of acute peritonitis also contains significant amounts of elastase bound to α_1-proteinase inhibitor (Ohlsson and Olsson, 1977).

D. Atherosclerosis

The pathogenesis of this multifactorial disease is largely unknown. The involvement of elastase(s) in atherosclerotic lesions is suggested by the observed fragmentation of elastin fibers within the media of arterial walls. For instance, Hornebeck and co-workers (1978) showed that the content of aorta cross-linked elastin decreased with the degree of atherosclerosis.

Several lines of evidence suggest that elastolytic enzymes are indeed present in the arterial wall. For instance, human arteries contain an elastase that is immunologically different from the human pancreatic and neutrophil enzymes (Bellon et al., 1980). Pig aortic elastase cross-reacts with pig pancreatic elastase but has a lower specific activity than the latter enzyme (Hornebeck et al., 1975). Solid-phase-bound antibodies against porcine pancreatic elastase may be used to isolate an elastase from pig aorta (Rabaud et al., 1981). Rat aorta contain immunoreactive rat pancreatic elastase (Katayama and Ooyama, 1980).

Some of the above results raise the question of how pancreatic elastase migrates into blood vessels. Katayama and Fujita (1972) have shown that the intestinal absorption of intact pancreatic elastase is extremely low. Besides, plasma contains fast acting elastase inhibitors. It is therefore unlikely that pancreatic elastase uses the intestinal $\rightarrow$ blood pathway to reach the arteries. A more direct route may be suggested. It is well established that a small fraction of the pancreatic exocrine secretions leak into the blood circulation (e.g., amylase, lipase, and immunoreactive proteinases may be detected in plasma). Geokas and co-workers (1980) have demonstrated free and α_1-protein-ase inhibitor-bound pancreatic proelastase in dog plasma. Part of the plasmatic zymogen may therefore reach the large blood vessels and undergo activation *in situ*.

Additional elastase activity may be generated locally by smooth muscle cells (Hornebeck *et al.*, 1981) or imported by platelets which are known to invade the intima and the media of aortae (Sandberg *et al.*, 1981) and which exhibit low but detectable elastinolytic activity (Hornebeck *et al.*, 1980).

In summary, only circumstantial evidence is available for the role of elastase in atherosclerosis. The elastase pathogenic model is, however, favored by the finding that elastin is fragmented in the atherosclerotic arterial wall and that elastase(s) is present *in situ*. In addition, lipids and calcium ions which are present in atherosclerotic lesions may enhance elastinolysis as suggested by Kagan *et al.* (1972, 1977), and platelet factor 4 might have the same effect (Lonky and Wohl, 1981).

E. Cancer

Malignant cells synthesize and release significant amounts of proteinases (Van den Hooff, 1983). Tumor invasion, a prerequisite for metastasis, is facilitated by proteolytic breakdown of the extracellular matrix, and a prominent role in this process has been ascribed to collagenases (reviewed by Liotta *et al.*, 1983). As discussed in Section VII,B, elastolytic activity has been found in some tumor cells in culture. The human fibrosarcoma cell line investigated by Jones and DeClerck (1980) is of particular interest since it synthesizes an elastase that is not secreted but bound at the surface of the cell. Elastolysis does not take place if the cells do not contact the extracellular matrix. This appears to be an interesting mechanism of regulation of proteolysis: (1) when the cells do not contact the matrix, their elastase is harmless and (2) once the cells contact the matrix, catalysis becomes very efficient due to the high local elastase concentration at the cell–matrix interface. Further investigations are required to delineate the role of elastase and other connective-tissue hydrolyzing proteinases in tumor invasion.

F. Miscellaneous Diseases

Cutis laxa is a rare and unique disease characterized by a fragmentation of elastin fibers and a decrease in elastin content of a variety of connective tissues with resultant cutis laxa, emphysema, and aortic aneurysms (Harris *et al.*, 1978). Although cutis laxa is also named "generalized elastolysis" there is no evidence for the participation of elastases in the pathogenesis of this disease.

As already discussed in Section VIII,B, elastolytic enzymes may participate in the pathogenesis of fungi and some snake venoms. It is noteworthy that in some families of snakes a correlation was found between elastolytic activity and taxonomy of poisonous snakes. Snake venom elastases may facilitate the penetration of the toxins into blood circulation; hence, they may hasten the toxic effects. Elastolysis, however, is not a prerequisite for venom toxicity as evidenced by the absence of elastase activity in the venom of the cobra. The elastase which facilitates the skin penetration of the larvae of *Schistosoma mansoni* is a splendid example of a "disposable" enzyme.

XI.   ELASTASE INHIBITORS AS POTENTIAL DRUGS

The possible pathogenic role of elastases (see Section X) led several research groups to design elastase inhibitors as potential therapeutic agents. Most efforts are presently spent on leukocyte elastase inhibitors because there is convincing evidence that diseases such as pulmonary emphysema or rheumatoid arthritis are promoted or at least exacerbated by neutrophil elastase.

Pulmonary emphysema may be induced in animals by intratracheal instillation of elastase (reviewed by Bignon and de Crémoux, 1980). The pulmonary disorders may be prevented by prior administration of elastase inhibitors such as peptide chloromethyl ketones (Janoff and Dearing, 1980; Ip *et al.*, 1981). These experiments merely confirm that animal emphysema results from the proteolytic action of elastase used to induce the disease. They do not prove that elastase inhibitors may cure emphysema or decrease the progression of the emphysematous process. The latter pharmacological investigations require long-term treatments with elastase inhibitors and cannot, therefore, be done with chloromethyl ketones which are not devoid of toxicity. Compounds such as elasnin (Omura *et al.*, 1978) or suicide substrates (Harper *et al.*, 1983; Harper and Powers, 1984; Tam *et al.*, 1984) are likely to be less toxic and should prove to be useful for such long-term experiments.

Protein inhibitors may also be potential drugs for the treatment of emphysema. For instance, eglin c, a potent leukoproteinase inhibitor isolated from the leech (see Section VI,A,5) and now produced by genetic engineering, is devoid of toxicity and is able to prevent elastase-induced emphysema in hamsters (Schnebli *et al.*, 1985). Recently, Gadeck *et al.* (1981) administed human α_1-proteinase inhibitor to PiZZ emphysematous patients. Bronchoalveolar lavage showed that the parenterally administred inhibitor had transudated into the alveolar lining fluid. The effect of such a replacement therapy on the progression of the disease will require long-term clinical trials on large numbers of patients. These trials will be rendered easier by the availability of α_1-proteinase inhibitor produced by genetic engineering (Courtney *et al.*, 1984; Cabezon *et al.*, 1984). Moreover, Met-358 → Val-358 mutants of α_1-proteinase inhibitor have recently been biosynthesized (Rosenberg *et al.*, 1984; Courtney *et al.*, 1985). These molecules are as active on neutrophil elastase as the natural inhibitor, but, unlike the latter, they do not undergo oxidative inactivation. Since oxidative processes play a role in emphysema, the Val-358 inhibitor may prove to be of greater therapeutic value than the native molecule in replacement therapy for PiZZ individuals or even in the treatment of genetically sufficient emphysematous patients. Results from recent *in vitro* experiments tend to favor this view: George *et al.* (1984) have shown that the degradation of basement membrane collagen by stimulated neutrophils was efficiently inhibited by a 10-fold lower dose of Val-358 α_1-proteinase inhibitor than of the natural inhibitor, the differences in efficiency of the two molecules being related to the resistance of the mutant inhibitor to neutrophil-mediated oxidation.

Rheumatoid arthritis is another disease whose progression might be significantly retarted by neutrophil elastase inhibitors. In this respect, the fairly potent elastase inhibitory capacity of some antiinflammatory drugs (Table XI, Section VI,B,1) should be considered as encouraging. Direct instillation of elastase inhibitors in the joint should prove useful for the treatment of acute phases of the disease. The aforementioned nonoxidizable Val-358 mutant of α_1-proteinase inhibitor should be an efficient drug since part of the natural inhibitor occurs as an oxidized derivative in synovial fluids from rheumatoid arthritis patients (Wong and Travis, 1980). On the other hand, it may be advisable to use low molecular mass inhibitors (e.g., elasnin or suicide substrates) together with protein inhibitors because the latter apparently have difficulties penetrating into the articular cartilage (Janoff *et al.*, 1976).

Antielastases might also prove useful in the treatment of acute inflammatory reactions in general, as suggested by animal experiments. For instance, peptide aldehydes (see Section VI,B,2) have been shown to inhibit carrageenin-induced edema (Umezawa, 1976). Soybean trypsin inhibitor AA (Table X, Section VI,B,5) is able to partially prevent *E. coli* endotoxin-induced shock in the dog (Jochum *et al.*, 1984a). As shown in Section X, *Pseudomonas aeruginosa* elastase appears to play a well-defined pathogenic role in *Pseudomonas* infections. Animal experiments again suggest that antielastases may have beneficial effects. For instance, phosphoramidon, a metalloenzyme inhibitor (see Section VIII,A,2), is able to prevent elastase-induced corneal ulceration (Kawaharajo *et al.*, 1982). On the other hand, treatment of burned, *P. aeruginosa*-infested mice with α_2-macroglobulin enhances the survival of the animals (Holder, 1983). Also, immunization of animals with *P. aeruginosa* elastase affords partial protection against experimental bacterial infection (Kawaharajo and Homma, 1977). Phosphoramidon or synthetic *P. aeruginosa* elastase inhibitors (Nishino and Powers, 1980) may therefore be considered as potential therapeutic agents in *P. aeruginosa* infections. Administration of such drugs should be favorably complemented by neutrophil elastase inhibitors since infections are always accompanied by leukocyte recruitment and leukoproteinase release at sites of infection.

As suggested by Glaser (1983), α_1-proteinase inhibitor may prove of value in the treatment of adult respiratory distress syndrome (ARDS), where free neutrophil elastase has been detected in bronchoalveolar lavage fluids (Lee *et al.*, 1981). Moreover, the nonoxidizable Val-358 inhibitor mutant should be preferentially used since part of the α_1-proteinase inhibitor of the lower respiratory tract of ARDS patients occurs as an oxidized derivative (Cochrane *et al.*, 1983).

Much effort is presently spent on the design of synthetic neutrophil elastase inhibitors (see Section VI,B). As emphasized by Schnebli *et al.* (1985), several criteria need to be met by a proteinase inhibitor in order to have therapeutic potential, namely: specificity, potency, low toxicity, lack of antigenicity, and bioavailability. We believe that suicide substrates such as those recently developed (see Section VI,B,4) are very promising because (1) they are latent inhibitors which need to be activated by the target enzyme (see Fig. 4) and should, therefore, have a narrow specificity, and (2) they have a nonpeptidic structure which should render them resistant to most peptidases and, therefore, endow them with bioavailability.

Let us now apply the theory outlined in Section VI,A,6 to the question of the potency of drugs. If a compound is or behaves like an irreversible inhibitor (e.g., suicide substrates) we may use the delay time of inhibition concept, $d(t)$, to define its potency. For instance, the suicide substrate shown in Fig. 4 has a k_{assoc} of 2.8×10^4 M^{-1} sec^{-1} for neutrophil elastase. We have demonstrated that $d(t)$ should not exceed 1 sec for efficient inhibition to take place. The $d(t) = 5/k_{assoc}$ $[I^0]$ relationship shows then that $[I^0]$, the *in vivo* drug concentration, should be at least $2 \times 10^{-4} \ M$. Pharmacologists would probably consider this to be too high a concentration. The best suicide substrate ever reported, therefore, is far from being potent enough for therapeutic use (the reader who is surprised by this statement should realize that the k_{assoc} of this compound is almost identical to that of oxidized α_1-proteinase inhibitor shown in Table IX). To analyze the potency of reversible inhibitors, let us use eglin c as an example (Schnebli et al., 1985). This compound has a K_i of $8 \times 10^{-11} \ M$ for neutrophil elastase. We have shown that a reversible inhibitor may behave like an irreversible one in vivo provided that $[I^0]/K_i \geq 1000$. This indicates that eglin c has a pseudo-irreversible behavior provided that $[I^0]$, its in vivo concentration, is higher or equal to $10^{-7} \ M$. Such drug concentrations may be easily obtained. Since the $d(t)$ concept also applies to pseudo-irreversible inhibitors, we may use the value of k_{assoc} for the eglin c–neutrophil elastase system ($1.4 \times 10^7 \ M^{-1} \ sec^{-1}$) to calculate the minimal $[I^0]$ required for having a $d(t)$ not larger than 1 sec. This calculation yields $[I^0] = 3 \times 10^{-7} \ M$. This demonstrates that eglin c is a highly potent neutrophil elastase inhibitor since it is predictably efficient at a very low concentration.

The foregoing discussion demonstrates that the $d(t)$ and the pseudo-irreversible inhibition concepts we have developed in Section VI,A,6 to delineate the physiological function of natural proteinase inhibitors may also serve as useful guidelines for the design of proteinase inhibitors of potential therapeutic use.

XII. CONCLUDING REMARKS

Comparison of the data discussed above with those compiled in a previous review (Bieth, 1978) indicates that during the past decade little progress has been achieved in the elucidation of the structure of porcine pancreatic elastase and human leukocyte elastase while enormous strides have been made in areas such as the design of synthetic elastase inhibitors, the structure and function of α_1-proteinase inhibitor, and the pathogenesis of lung emphysema. The best synthetic reversible elastase inhibitor quoted in the previous review had a K_i of 0.8 μM whereas the most potent compound listed in Table XII has a K_i of 0.25 nM! Only 6 years have elapsed between the discovery of the oxidative inactivation of α_1-proteinase inhibitor and the production of a genetically engineered nonoxidizable mutant of this protein! The enormous progress that has been made in the field of lung emphysema argues well for the future unraveling of the mysteries of this disease.

The amino acid sequence of human neutrophil elastase is about to be established (J. Travis, personal communication). This, together with X-ray analyses of the molecule and computer graphics, should rapidly improve our knowledge of the active center of elastase and will aid the future design of elastase inhibitors. The area of suicide elastase substrates, a very promising class of inhibitors, is just developing, and it can be anticipated that more potent and more specific compounds will soon emerge. Active research is being conducted on the crystal structure of α_1-proteinase inhibitor. In the next few years we should have better insight into the nature of the forces which are responsible for the enormous affinity of this inhibitor for elastase. This, in turn, may provide new ideas for the design of synthetic inhibitors.

Since elastases are defined according to their elastin-solubilizing capacity, the state of the substrate is of critical importance to the recognition of the enzyme, and efforts should be made to prepare a kind of "native" elastin which would more closely resemble matrix elastin than the fibrous material we are presently using. This should soon be possible since tropoelastin is about to be fully sequenced and may thus be prepared in large quantities by genetic engineering and converted into cross-linked elastin. In the meantime, we strongly advise the use of extracellular matrices prepared by cell culture, especially if cell-surface-associated elastinolytic activity is investigated.

ACKNOWLEDGMENTS

I wish to thank Sylvie Dirrig for her very efficient assistance in the preparation of this article, Dr. Michael Courtney (Transgène, Strasbourg), Dr. Robert P. Mecham (Washington University, St Louis, Missouri), and Dr. James C. Powers (Georgia Institute of Technology, Atlanta) for reading and improving the manuscript and Danièle Spielberger for diligently typing it.

REFERENCES

Aasen, A. O., and Ohlsson, K. (1978). *Hoppe-Seyler's Z. Physiol. Chem.* **359**, 683–690.
Abrams, W. R., Kimbel, P., and Weinbaum, G. (1978). *Biochemistry* **17**, 3556–3561.
Abrams, W., Eliraz, A., Kimbel, P., and Weinbaum, G. (1980). *Exp. Lung Res.* **1**, 211–223.
Abrams, W., Cohen, A. B., Damiano, V., Eliraz, A., Kimbel, P., Meranze, D. R., and Weinbaum, G. (1981a). *J. Clin. Invest.* **68**, 1132–1139.
Abrams, W. R., Weinbaum, G., Weissbach, L., Weissbach, H., and Brot, N. (1981b). *Proc. Natl. Acad. Sci. U.S.A.* **78**, 7483–7486.
Abrams, W. R., Fein, A. M., Kucich, U., Kueppers, F., Yamada, H., Kuzmowycz, T., Morgan, L., Lippmann, M., Goldberg, S. K., and Weinbaum, G. (1984). *Am. Rev. Respir, Dis.* **129**, 735–741.
Alber, T., Petsko, G. A., and Tsernoglou, D. (1976). *Nature (London)* **263**, 297–300.
Albrecht, G. J., Hochstrasser, K., and Salier, J.-P. (1983). *Hoppe-Seyler's Z. Physiol. Chem.* **364**, 1703–1708.

Andersen, M. M. (1984). *Scand. J. Clin. Lab. Invest.* **44**, 257–265.

Ardelt, W. (1974). *Biochim. Biophys. Acta* **341**, 318–326.

Ardelt, W. (1975). *Biochim. Biophys. Acta* **393**, 267–273.

Ardelt, W., Kzienzy, S., and Nidzwiecka, N. (1970). *Anal. Biochem.* **34**, 180–187.

Ardelt, W., Tomczak, Z., Ksiezny, S., and Dudek-Wojciechowska, G. (1976). *Biochim. Biophys. Acta* **445**, 683–693.

Ardelt, W., Tomczak, Z., and Dudek-Wojciechowska, G. (1979). *Acta Biochim. Pol.* **26**, 267–273.

Ashe, B. M., and Zimmerman, H. (1977). *Biochem. Biophys. Res. Commun.* **75**, 194–199.

Ashe, B. M., and Zimmerman, M. (1982). *Biochem. Int.* **5**, 487–494.

Ashe, B. M., Clark, R. L., Jones, H., and Zimmerman, M. (1981). *J. Biol. Chem.* **256**, 11603–11606.

Aubry, M., and Bieth, J. (1977). *Clin. Chim. Acta* **78**, 371–380.

Bachovchin, W. W., Kaiser, R., Richards, J. H., and Roberts, J. D. (1981). *Proc. Natl. Acad. Sci. U.S.A.* **78**, 7323–7326.

Bader, D. L., Kempson, G. E., Barrett, A. J., and Webb, W. (1981). *Biochim. Biophys. Acta* **677**, 103–108.

Baici, A., and Bradamante, P. (1984). *Chem. Biol. Interact.* **51**, 1–11.

Baici, A., Knöpfel, M., Fehr, K., Skvaril, F., and Böni, A. (1980a).*Scand. J. Immunol.* **12**, 41–51.

Baici, A., Knöpfel, M., Fehr, K., and Böni, A. (1980b). *Immunol. Lett.* **2**, 47–51.

Baici, A., Salgam, P., Fehr, K., and Böni, A. (1980c). *Biochem. Pharmacol.* **29**, 1723–1727.

Baici, A., Salgam, P., Fehr, K., and Böni, A. (1981). *Biochem. Pharmacol.* **30**, 703–708.

Baici, A., Salgam, P., Cohen, G., Fehr, K., and Böni, A. (1982). *Rheumatol. Int.* **2**, 11–16.

Baici, A., Camus, A., and Marsich, N. (1984). *Biochem. Pharmacol.* **33**, 1859–1865.

Balo, J., and Banga, I. (1949). *Nature (London)* **164**, 491–494.

Banda, M. J., and Werb, Z. (1981). *Biochem. J.* **193**, 589–605.

Banda, M. J., Clark, E. J., and Werb, Z. (1980). *J. Exp. Med.* **152**, 1563–1570.

Banda, M. J., Clark, E. J., and Werb, Z. (1983). *J. Exp. Med.* **157**, 1184–1196.

Banga, I., and Ardelt, W. (1967). *Biochim. Biophys. Acta* **146**, 284–286.

Barrett, A. J., and Starkey, P. M. (1977). *In* "Rheumatoid Arthritis" (J. L. Gordon and B. L. Hazleman, eds.), pp. 211–221. North-Holland Publ., Amsterdam.

Bauer, C. A., Thompson, R. C., and Blout, E. R. (1976a). *Biochemistry* **15**, 1291–1295.

Bauer, C. A., Thompson, R. C., and Blout, E. R. (1976b). *Biochemistry* **15**, 1296–1299.

Baugh, R. J., and Travis, J. (1976). *Biochemistry* **15**, 836–841.

Baumstark, J. S. (1970). *Biochim. Biophys. Acta* **220**, 534–551.

Baumstark, J. S. (1978). *J. Immunol. Methods* **23**, 79–89.

Beatty, K., Bieth, J., and Travis, J. (1980). *J. Biol. Chem.* **255**, 3931–3934.

Beatty, K., Travis, J., and Bieth, J. (1982a). *Biochim. Biophys. Acta* **704**, 221–226.

Beatty, K., Robertie, P., Senior, R. M., and Travis, J. (1982b). *J. Lab. Clin. Med.* **100**, 186–192.

Beatty, K., Matheson, N., and Travis, J. (1984). *Hoppe-Seyler's Z. Physiol. Chem.* **365**, 731–736.

Béchet, J.-J., Dupaix, A., and Blagoeva, I. (1977). *Biochimie* **59**, 231–239.

Bellon, G., Ooyama, T., Hornebeck, W., and Robert, L. (1980). *Artery* **7**, 290–302.

Bender, M. L., and Kezdy, F. J. (1965). *Annu. Rev. Biochem.* **34**, 49–76.

Bernick, J. J., and Simpson, J. W. (1976). *Comp. Biochem. Physiol.* **54B**, 51–54.

Bielefeld, D. R., Senior, R. M., and Yu, S. S. (1975). *Biochem. Biophys. Res. Commun.* **67**, 1553–1559.

Bieth, J. G. (1978). *In* "Frontiers of Matrix Biology" (J. G. Bieth, G. M. Collin-Lapinet, and L. Robert, eds.), Vol. VI, pp. 1–82. Karger, Basel.

Bieth, J. G. (1980). *Bull. Eur. Physiopathol. Respir.* **16**, (Suppl.), 183–195.

Bieth, J. G. (1984). *Biochem. Med.* **32**, 387–397.

Bieth, J., and Frechin, J. C. (1974). *Biochim. Biophys. Acta* **364**, 97–102.

Bieth, J. G., and Meyer, J. F. (1984). *J. Biol. Chem.* **259**, 8904–8906.

Bieth, J. G., and Wermuth, C. G. (1973). *Biochem. Biophys. Res. Commun.* **53**, 383–390.

Bieth, J., Pichoir, M., and Métais, P. (1970). *FEBS Lett.* **8**, 319–321.

Bieth, J. G., Spiess, B., and Wermuth, C. G. (1974). *Biochem. Med.* **11**, 350–357.

Bieth, J., Pichoir, M., and Metais, P. (1976). *Anal. Biochem.* **70**, 430–433.

Bieth, J. G., Kandel, M.-J., Zreika, M., and Pochon, F. (1983). *Ann. N.Y. Acad. Sci.* **421**, 209–217.

Bignon, J., and de Crémoux, H. (1980). *Bull. Eur. Physiopathol. Respir.* **16** (Suppl.), 13–25.

Blackwood, L. L., Stone, R. M., Iglewski, B. H., and Pennington, J. E. (1983). *Infect. Immun.* **39**, 198–201.

Blondin, J., and Janoff, A. (1976). *J. Clin. Invest.* **58**, 971–979.

Blondin, J., Rosenberg, R., and Janoff, A. (1972). *Am. Rev. Respir. Dis.* **106**, 477–479.

Blow, A. M. J. (1977). *Biochem. J.* **161**, 13–16.

Blow, A. M. J., and Barrett, A. J. (1977). *Biochem. J.* **161**, 17–19.

Blow, D. M., Birktoft, J. J., and Hartley, B. S. (1969). *Nature (London)* **221**, 337–340.

Boudier, C., and Bieth, J. G. (1982). *Biochem. Med.* **28**, 41–50.

Boudier, C., Andersson, K. K., Balny, C., and Bieth J. G. (1980). *Biochem. Med.* **23**, 219–222.

Boudier, C., Jung, M. L., Stambolieva, N., and Bieth, J. G. (1981a). *Arch. Biochem. Biophys.* **210**, 790–793.

Boudier, C., Holle, C., and Bieth, J. G. (1981b). *J. Biol. Chem.* **256**, 10256–10258.

Boudier, C., Pelletier, A., Pauli, G., and Bieth, J. G. (1983). *Clin. Chim. Acta* **132**, 309–315.

Boudier, C., Laurent, P., and Bieth, J. G. (1984). *Adv. Exp. Med.* **167**, 313–317.

Bourdillon, M. C., Brechemier, D., Blaes, N., Derouette, J. C., Hornebeck, W., and Robert, L. (1980). *Cell Biol. Int. Rep.* **4**, 313–320.

Brittain, H. G., Richardson, F. S., and Martin, R. B. (1976). *J. Am. Chem. Soc.* **98**, 8255–8260.

Brodrick, J. W., Glaser, C. B., Largman, C., Geokas, M. C., Graceffo, M., Fassett, M., and Maeda, H. (1980). *Biochemistry* **19**, 4865–4870.

Brower, M. S., and Harpel, P. C. (1982). *J. Biol. Chem.* **257**, 9849–9854.

Brower, M. S., and Harpel, P. C. (1983). *Blood* **61**, 842–849.

Brown, W. E., and Wold, E. (1973). *Biochemistry* **12**, 828–834.

Brozna, J. P., Senior, R. M., Kreutzer, D. L., and Ward, D. A. (1977). *J. Clin. Invest.* **60**, 1280–1288.

Burnett, D., Crocker, J., and Stockley, R. A. (1983). *Am. Rev. Respir. Dis.* **128**, 915–919.

Burnett, D., McGillivray, D. H., and Stockley, R. A. (1984). *Am. Rev. Respir. Dis.* **129**, 473–476.

Byrne, R. E., Polacek, D., Gordon, J. I., and Scanu, A. M. (1984). *J. Biol. Chem.* **259**, 14537–14544.

Cabezón, T., De Wilde, M., Herion, P., Loriau, R., and Bollen, A. (1984). *Proc. Natl. Acad. Sci. U.S.A.* **81**, 6594–6598.

Campbell, E. J., and Wald, M. S. (1983). *J. Lab. Clin. Med.* **101**, 527–536.

Campbell, E. J., White, R. R., Senior, R. M., Rodriguez, R. J., and Kuhn, C. (1979). *J. Clin. Invest.* **64,** 824–833.

Campbell, E. J., Senior, R. M., McDonald, J. A., and Cox, D. L. (1982). *J. Clin. Invest.* **70,** 845–852.

Carballo, J., Kasahara, K., Appert, H. E., and Howard, J. M. (1974). *Proc. Soc. Exp. Biol. Med.* **146,** 997–1002.

Carlsson, J., Herrmann, B. F., Höfling, J. F., and Sundqvist, G. K. (1984). *Infect. Immun.* **43,** 644–648.

Caro, A., de, Figarella, C., and Guy, O. (1975). *Biochim. Bipophys. Acta* **379,** 431–443.

Carp, H., and Janoff, A. (1978). *Am. Rev. Respir. Dis.* **118,** 617–621.

Carp, H., and Janoff, A. (1980a). *J. Clin. Invest.* **66,** 987–995.

Carp, H., and Janoff, A. (1980b). *Exp. Lung Res.* **1,** 225–237.

Carp, H., Miller, F., Hoidal, J. R., and Janoff, A. (1982). *Proc. Natl. Acad. Sci. U.S.A.* **79,** 2041–2045.

Carp, H., Janoff, A., Abrams, W., Weinbaum, G., Drew, R. I., Weissbach, H., and Brot, N. (1983). *Am. Rev. Respir. Dis.* **127,** 301–305.

Carrell, R. W., Jeppsson, J. O., Laurell, C. B., Brennan, S. O., Owen, M. C., Vaughan, L., and Boswell, D. R. (1982). *Nature (London)* **298,** 329–334.

Castillo, M. J., Nakajima, K., Zimmerman, M., and Powers, J. C. (1979). *Anal. Biochem.* **99,** 53–64.

Catanese, J., and Kress, L. F. (1984). *Biochim. Biophys. Acta* **789,** 37–43.

Chapman, H. A., and Stone, O. L. (1984a). *J. Clin. Invest.* **74,** 1693–1700.

Chapman, H. A., and Stone, O. L. (1984b). *Biochem. J.* **222,** 721–728.

Chapman, H. A., Stone, O. L., Vavrin, Z. (1984). *J. Clin. Invest.* **73,** 806–815.

Cho, Y. J., Oh, Y. H., Abe, C., Homma, J. Y., Usui, M., and Matsuhashi, T. (1978). *Jpn. J. Exp. Med.* **48,** 491–496.

Christner, P., Weinbaum, G., Sloan, B., and Rosenbloom, J. (1978). *Anal. Biochem.* **88,** 682–688.

Clark, J. M., Vaughan, D. W., Aiken, B. M., and Kagan, H. M. (1980). *J. Cell Biol.* **84,** 102–119.

Clemente, F., de Caro, A., and Figarella, C. (1972). *Eur. J. Biochem.* **31,** 186–193.

Cochrane, C. G., Spragg, R., and Revak, S. D. (1983). *J. Clin. Invest.* **71,** 754–761.

Cohen, T., Gertler, A., and Birk, Y. (1981a). *Comp. Biochem. Physiol.* **69B,** 639–646.

Cohen, T., Gertler, A., and Birk, Y. (1981b). *Comp. Biochem. Physiol.* **69B,** 647–653.

Collins, J. F., and Fine, R. (1981). *Biochim. Biophys. Acta* **657,** 295–303.

Comte, P., and Robert, L. (1968). *Bull. Soc. Chim. Biol.* **50,** 1349–1351.

Courtney, M., Buchwalder, A., Tessier, L.-H., Jaye, M., Benavente, A., Balland, A., Kohli, V., Lathe, R., Tolstoshev, P., and Lecocq, J. P. (1984). *Proc. Natl. Acad. Sci. U.S.A.* **81,** 669–673.

Courtney, M., Jallat, S., Tessier, L.-H., Benavente, A., Crystal, R. G., and Lecocq, J.-P. (1985). *Nature (London)* **313,** 149–151.

Cox, D. W., and Billingsley, G. D. (1984). *Am. Rev. Respir. Dis.* **130,** 594–599.

Crémoux, H., de, Hornebeck, W., Jaurand, M. C., Bignon, J., and Robert, L. (1978). *J. Pathol.* **125,** 171–177.

Davril, M., Jung, M. L., Duportail, G., Lohez, M., Han, K. K., and Bieth, J. G. (1984). *J. Biol. Chem.* **259,** 3851–3857.

Del Mar, E. G., Largman, C., Brodrick, J. W., Fassett, M., and Geokas, M. C. (1980). *Biochemistry* **19,** 468–472.

Delshammar, M., and Ohlsson, K. (1976). *Eur. J. Biochem.* **69,** 125–131.

Dewald, B., Rindler-Ludwig, R., Bretz, U., and Baggiolini, M. (1975). *J. Exp. Med.* **141,** 709–723.

Dietl, T., Dobrinski, W., and Hochstrasser, K. (1979). *Hoppe-Seyler's Z. Physiol. Chem.* **360,** 1313–1318.

Dimicoli, J. L., and Bieth, J. G. (1977). *Biochemistry* **16,** 5532–5537.

Dimicoli, J. L., Bieth, J., and Lhoste, J. M. (1976). *Biochemistry* **15,** 2230–2236.

Dimicoli, J. L., Renaud, A., Lestienne, P., and Bieth, J. G. (1979). *J. Biol. Chem.* **254,** 5208–5218.

Dimicoli, J. L., Renaud, A., and Bieth, J. (1980). *Eur. J. Biochem.* **107,** 423–432.

Dimicoli, J. L., Lam-Tanh, H., Toma, F., and Fermandjian, S. (1984). *Biochemistry* **23,** 3173–3180.

Döring, G., Obernesser, H.-J., and Botzenhart, K. (1981). *Ztrbl. Bakteriol. Mikrobiol. Hyg. (A)* **249,** 89–98.

Dorn, C. P., Zimmerman, M., Yang, S. S., Yurewicz, E. C., Ashe, B. M., Frankshun, R., and Jones, H. (1977). *J. Med. Chem.* **20,** 1464–1468.

Dubin, A., Koj, A., and Chudzik, J. (1976). *Biochem. J.* **153,** 389–396.

Dubin, A., Potempa, J., and Koj, A. (1984). *Symp. Biol. Hung.* **25,** 233–248.

Dubin, A., Potempa, J., and Silberring, J. (1985). *Int. J. Biochem.,* in press.

Duportail, G., Lefèvre, J. F., Lestienne, P., Dimicoli, J. L., and Bieth, J. G. (1980). *Biochemistry* **19,** 1377–1382.

Egbring, R., Schmidt, W., Fuchs, G., and Havemann, K. (1977). *Blood* **49,** 219–231.

Eriksson, S. (1984). *Schweiz. Med. Wschr.* **114,** 893–894.

Estensen, R. D., White, J. G., and Holmes, B. (1974). *Nature (London)* **248,** 347–348.

Feinstein, G., and Janoff, A. (1975a). *Biochim. Biophys. Acta* **403,** 477–492.

Feinstein, G., and Janoff, A. (1975b). *Biochim. Biophys. Acta* **403,** 493–505.

Feinstein, G., and Janoff, A. (1976). *Proc. Soc. Exp. Biol. Med.* **152,** 36–41.

Feinstein, G., Hofstein, R., Hoifmann, J., and Sokolovsky, M. (1974). *Eur. J. Biochem.* **43,** 569–581.

Feinstein, G., Malemud, C. J., and Janoff, A. (1976). *Biochim. Biophys. Acta* **429,** 925–932.

Fetzer, A. E., Werner, A. S., and Hagstrom, J. W. C. (1967). *Am. Rev. Respir, Dis.* **96,** 1121–1125.

Fick, R. B., Jr, Naegel, G. P., Squier, S. U., Wood, R. E., Gee, B. L., and Reynolds, H. Y. (1984). *J. Clin. Invest.* **74,** 236–248.

Foster, J. A., Rich, C. B., and Karr, S. R. (1983). *In* "International Review of Connective Tissue Research" (D. A. Hall and D. S. Jackson, eds.), Vol. 10, pp. 65–95. Academic Press, New York.

Fritz, H., Jaumann, E., Meister, R., Pasquay, P., Hochstrasser, K., and Fink, E. (1971). *In* "Proceedings of the International Research Conference on Proteinase Inhibitors" (H. Fritz and H. Tschesche, eds.), pp. 257–270. De Guyter, Berlin.

Fujimoto, K.-I., Ogawa, M., Saito, N., Kosaki, G., Minamiura, N., and Yamamoto, T. (1980). *Biochim. Biophys. Acta* **612,** 262–267.

Gadek, J. E., Fells, G. A., and Crystal, R. G. (1979). *Science* **206,** 1315–1316.

Gadek, J. E., Fells, G. A., Wright, D. G., and Crystal, R. G. (1980a). *Biochem. Biophys. Res. Commun.* **95,** 1815–1822.

Gadek, J. E., Hunninghake, G. W., Fells, G. A., Zimmerman, R. L., Keogh, B. A., and Crystal, R. G. (1980b). *Bull. Eur. Physiopathol. Respir.* **16** (Suppl.), 27–40.

Gadek, J. E., Klein, H. G., Holland, P. V., and Crystal, R. G. (1981). *J. Clin. Invest.* **68,** 1158–1165.

Galdston, M., Levytska, V., Liener, I. E., and Twumasi, D. Y. (1979). *Am. Rev. Respir. Dis.* **119,** 435–441.

Gauthier, F., Genell, S., Mouray, H., and Ohlsson, K. (1978). *Biochim. Biophys. Acta* **526,** 218–226.

Gauthier, F., Frysmark, U., Ohlsson, K., and Bieth, J. G. (1982). *Biochim. Biophys. Acta* **700,** 178–183.

Gazinelli, G., Ramalho-Pinto, F. J., and Pellegrino, J. (1966). *Comp. Biochem. Physiol.* **18,** 689–700.

Geneste, P., and Bender, M. L. (1969). *Proc. Natl. Acad. Sci. U.S.A.* **64,** 683–685.

Geokas, M. C., Silverman, P., and Rinderknecht, H. (1970). *Experientia* **25,** 942–943.

Geokas, M. C., Brodrick, J. W., Johnson, J. H., and Largman, C. (1977). *J. Biol. Chem.* **252,** 61–67.

Geokas, M. C., Largman, C., Brodrick, J. W., and Fassett, M. (1980). *Am. J. Physiol.* **238,** G 238- G 246.

George, P. M., Vissers, M. C. M., Travis, J., Winterbourn, C. C., and Carrel, R. W. (1984). *Lancet* **2,** 1426–1428.

Gertler, A. (1971a). *FEBS Lett.* **19,** 255–258.

Gertler, A. (1971b). *Eur. J. Biochem.* **20,** 541–546.

Gertler, A. (1971c). *Eur. J. Biochem.* **23,** 36–40.

Gertler, A. (1974). *Fed. Eur. Biochem. Soc. Lett.* **43,** 81–85.

Gertler, A., and Birk, Y. (1970). *Eur. J. Biochem.* **12,** 170–176.

Gertler, A., and Feinstein, G. (1971). *Eur. J. Biochem.* **20,** 547–552.

Gertler, A., and Hayashi, K. (1971). *Biochim. Biophys. Acta* **235,** 378–380.

Gertler, A., and Trop, M. (1971). *Eur. J. Biochem.* **19,** 90–96.

Gertler, A., Weiss, Y., and Burstein, Y. (1977). *Biochemistry* **16,** 2709–2716.

Gilfillan, R. F. (1968). *Cancer Res.* **28,** 137–143.

Glaser, C. (1983). *Am. Rev. Respir. Dis.* **127,** S47–S53.

Gold, R., and Shaltin, Y. (1975). *Biochim. Biophys. Acta* **410,** 421–426.

Gramse, M., Egbring, R., and Havemann, K. (1984). *Hoppe-Seyler's Z. Physiol. Chem.* **365,** 19–26.

Gray, L., and Kreger, A. (1979). *Infect. Immun.* **23,** 150–159.

Green, M. R., Lin, J. S., Berman, L. B., Osman, M. M., Cerreta, J. M., Mandl, I., and Turino, G. M. (1979). *J. Lab. Clin. Med.* **94,** 549–562.

Groutas, W. C., Badger, R. C., Ocain, T. D., Felker, D., Frankson, J., and Theodorakis, M. (1980). *Biochem. Biophys. Res. Commun.* **95,** 1890–1894.

Groutas, W. C., Abrams, W. R., Carroll, R. T., Moi, M. K., Miller, K. E., and Margolis, M. T. (1984). *Experientia* **40,** 361–362.

Guay, M., and Lamy, F. (1981). *Connect. Tissue Res.* **9,** 127–130.

Gustavsson, E. L., Ohlsson, K., and Olsson, A. S. (1980). *Hoppe-Seyler's Z. Physiol. Chem.* **361,** 169–176.

Haen, A., de, and Gertler, A. (1974). *Biochemistry* **13,** 2673–2677.

Hall, D. A., and Czerkawski, J. W. (1961a). *Biochem. J.* **80,** 128–134.

Hall, D. A., and Czerkawski, J. W. (1961b). *Biochem. J.* **80,** 134–136.

Han, K. K., Davril, M., Lohez, M., Moczar, M., and Moczar, E. (1979). *Arterial Wall* **5,** 69–74.

Harpel, P. C., and Brower, M. S. (1983). *Ann. N.Y. Acad. Sci.* **421,** 1–9.

Harper, J. W., and Powers, J. C. (1984). *J. Am. Chem. Soc.* **106,** 7618–7619.

Harper, J. W., Hemmi, K., and Powers, J. C. (1983). *J. Am. Chem. Soc.* **105,** 6518–6520.

Harris, R. B., Heaphy, M. R., and Perry, H. O. (1978). *Am. J. Med.* **65,** 815–822.

Hartley, B. S., and Shotton, D. M. (1971). *In* "The Enzymes" (P. D. Boyer, ed.), 3rd Ed, Vol. III., pp 323–375. Academic Press, New-York.

Hassall, C. H., Johnson, W. H., and Roberts, N. A. (1979). *Bioorg. Chem.* **8**, 299–309.

Hedstrom, L., Moorman, A. R., Dobbs, J., and Abeles, R. H. (1984). *Biochemistry* **23**, 1753–1759.

Henriksson, P., Nilsson, I. M., Ohlsson, K., and Stenberg, P. (1980). *Thromb. Res.* **18**, 343–351.

Hinman, L. M., Stevens, C. A., Matthay, R. A., and Gee, J. G. L. (1980). *Am. Rev. Respir. Dis.* **121**, 263–271.

Hochstrasser, K., Reichert, R., Schwarz, S., and Werle, E. (1972). *Hoppe-Seyler's Z. Physiol. Chem.* **353**, 221–226.

Hochstrasser, K., Theopold, H. M., and Brandt, O. (1973). *Hoppe-Seyler's Z. Physiol. Chem.* **54**, 1013–1016.

Holder, I. A. (1983). *Rev. Infect. Dis.* **5** (Suppl. 5), S914–S921.

Hornebeck, W., Derouette, J. C., and Robert, L. (1975). *FEBS Lett.* **58**, 66–70.

Hornebeck, W., Adnet, J. J., and Robert, L. (1978). *Exp. Gerontol.* **13**, 293–298.

Hornebeck, W., Starkey, P. M., Gordon, J. L., Legrand, Y., Pignaud, G., Robert, L., Caen, J. P., Ehrlich, H. P., and Barrett, A. J. (1980). *Thromb. Haemostasis* **42**, 1681–1683.

Hornebeck, W., Brechemier, D., Bourdillon, M. C., and Robert, L. (1981). *Connect. Tissue Res.* **8**, 245–249.

Hornebeck, W., Potazman, J. P., de Crémoux, H., Bellon, G., and Robert, L. (1983). *Clin. Physiol. Biochem.* **1**, 285–292.

Huebner, P. F. (1976). *Anal. Biochem.* **74**, 419–429.

Hughes, K. T., Coles, G. A., Harry, T. R., and Davies, M. (1981). *Biochim. Biophys. Acta* **662**, 111–118.

Hughes, D. L., Sieker, L. C., Bieth, J. G., and Dimicoli, J. L. (1982). *J. Mol. Biol.* **162**, 645–658.

Hunkapiller, M. W., Smallcombe, S. F., Whitaker, D. R., and Richards, J. H. (1973). *Biochemistry* **12**, 4732–4743.

Ikuta, T., Okubo, H., Kudo, J., Ishibashi, H., and Inoue, T. (1982). *Biochem. Biophys. Res. Commun.* **104**, 1509–1516.

Ip, M. P. C., Kleinerman, J., Ranga, V., Sorensen, J., and Powers, J. C. (1981). *Am. Rev. Respir. Dis.* **124**, 714–717.

Isaacson, P., Jones, D. B., Millward-Sadler, G. H., Judd, M. A., and Payne, S. (1981). *J. Clin. Pathol.* **34**, 982–990.

Jacquot, J., Tournier, J.-M., and Puchelle, E. (1985). *Infec. Immun.* **47**, 555–560.

James, H., and Cohen, A. (1978). *J. Clin. Invest.* **62**, 1344–1353.

Janoff, A. (1983). *J. Appl. Physiol: Respir. Environ. Exercise Physiol.* **55**, 285–293.

Janoff, A., and Basch, R. S. (1971). *Proc. Soc. Exp. Biol. Med.* **136**, 1054–1058.

Janoff, A., and Blondin, J. (1971). *Proc. Soc. Exp. Biol. and Med.* **136**, 1050–1053.

Janoff, A., and Blondin, J. (1973). *Lab. Invest.* **29**, 454–458.

Janoff, A., and Dearing, R. (1980). *Am. Rev. Respir. Dis.* **121**, 1025–1029.

Janoff, A., and Scherer, J. (1968). *J. Exp. Med.* **128**, 1137–1140.

Janoff, A., Rosenberg, R., and Galdston, M. (1971). *Proc. Soc. Exp. Biol. Med.* **136**, 1054–1058.

Janoff, A., Feinstein, G., Malemud, C. J., and Elias, J. M. (1976). *J. Clin. Invest.* **57**, 615–624.

Jencks, W. P. (1969). "Catalysis in Chemistry and Enzymology." McGraw-Hill, New York.

Jersey, J., de, and Martin, R. B. (1980). *Biochemistry* **19**, 1127–1132.

Jochum, M., Lander, S., Heimburger, N., and Fritz, H. (1981). *Hoppe-Seyler's Z. Physiol. Chem.* **362**, 103–112.

Jochum, M., Duswald, K. H., Neumann, S., Witte, J., and Fritz, H. (1984a). *Adv. Exp. Med. Biol.* **167**, 391–404.

Jochum, M., Duswald, K.-H., Dittmer, H., and Neumann, S. (1984b). *In* "Marker Proteins in Inflammation" (P. Arnaud, J. Bienvenu, and P. Laurent, eds.), Vol. 2, pp. 51–55. De Gruyter, Berlin.

Johnson, D., and Travis, J. (1977). *Biochem. J.* **163**, 639–641.

Johnson, D. A., Carter-Hamn, B., and Dralle, W. M. (1982). *Am. Rev. Respir. Dis.* **126**, 1070–1073.

Johnsson, U., Ohlsson, K., and Olsson, I. (1976). *Scand. J. Immunol.* **5**, 421–426.

Jones, P. A., and Declerck, Y. A. (1980). *Cancer Res.* **40**, 3222–3227.

Jordan, R. E., Hewitt, N., Lewis, W., Kagan, H., and Franzblau, C. (1974). *Biochemistry* **13**, 3497–3503.

Jung, M. J., Koch-Weser, J., and Sjoerdsma, A. (1980). *In* "Enzyme Inhibitors as Drugs" (M. Sandler, ed.), pp. 95–114. Macmillan, London.

Kagan, H. M., and Lerch, R. M. (1976). *Biochim. Biophys. Acta* **434**, 223–232.

Kagan, H. M., Grombie, G. C., Jordan, R. E., Lewis, W., and Franzblau, C. (1972). *Biochemistry* **11**, 3412–3418.

Kagan, H. M., Jordan, R. E., Lerch, R. M., Mukherjee, D. P., Stone, P., and Franzblau, C. (1977). *Adv. Exp. Med. Biol.* **79**, 189–207.

Kao, R. T., Wong, M., and Stern, R. (1982). *Biochem. Biophys. Res. Commun.* **105**, 383–389.

Kaplan, H., Symonds, V. B., Dugas, H., and Whitaker, D. R. (1970). *Can. J. Biochem.* **48**, 649–658.

Katayama, K., and Fujita, T. (1972). *Biochim. Biophys. Acta* **288**, 181–189.

Katayama, K., and Ooyama, T. (1980). *Chem. Pharm. Bull.* **28**, 3422–3426.

Kawaharajo, K., and Homma, J. Y. (1977). *Jpn. J. Exp. Med.* **47**, 495–500.

Kawaharajo, K., Homma, J. Y., Aoyagi, T., and Umezawa, H. (1982). *Jpn. J. Exp. Med.* **52**, 271–272.

Keene, W. E., Jeong, K. H., McKerrow, J. H., and Werb, Z. (1983). *Lab. Invest.* **49**, 201–207.

Kessler, E., Kennah, H. E., and Brown, S. I. (1977). *Invest. Ophthalmol. Vis. Sci.* **16**, 488–497.

Kessler, E., Israel, M., Landshman, N., Chechick, A., and Blumberg, S. (1982). *Infect. Immun.* **38**, 716–723.

Kettner, C., Shaw, E., White, R., Janoff, A. (1981). *Biochem. J.* **195**, 369–372.

Kettner, C. A., and Shenvi, A. B. (1984). *J. Biol. Chem.* **259**, 15106–15114.

Kidd, V. J., Wallace, R. B., Itakura, K., and Woo, S. L. C. (1983). *Nature* **304**, 230–234.

Klebanoff, S. J., and Clark, R. A. (1978). "The Neutrophil: Function and Clinical Disorders." North-Holland Publ., Amsterdam.

Kleine, R. (1982). *Acta Biol. Med. Ger.* **41**, 89–102.

Koide, A., and Yoshizawa, M. (1981). *Biochem. Biophys. Res. Commun.* **100**, 1091–1098.

Koj, A., Chudzik, J., and Dubin, A. (1976). *Biochem. J.* **153**, 397–402.

Koshland, D. E., and Neet, K. E. (1968). *Annu. Rev. Biochem.* **37**, 359–410.

Krafft, G. A., and Katzenellenbogen, J. A. (1981). *J. Am. Chem. Soc.* **103**, 5459–5466.

Kramps, J. A., van der Valk, P., van der Sandt, M. M., Lindeman, J., and Meijer C. J. L. M. (1984). *J. Histochem. Cytochem.* **32**, 389–394.

Kress, L. F., and Paroski, E. A. (1978). *Biochem. Biophys. Res. Commun.* **83**, 649–656.

Kress, L. F., Kurecki, T., Chan, S. K., and Laskowski, M., Sr. (1979). *J. Biol. Chem.* **254,** 5317–5320.

Kucich, U., Abrams, W. R., and James, H. L. (1980). *Anal. Biochem.* **109,** 403–409.

Kueppers, F., and Bearn, A. G. (1966). *Proc. Soc. Exp. Biol. Med.* **121,** 1207–1209.

Kueppers, F., and Bromke, B. J. (1983). *J. Lab. Clin. Med.* **101,** 747–757.

Kueppers, F., Abrams, W. R., Weinbaum, G., and Rosenbloom, J. (1981). *Arch. Biochem. Biophys.* **211,** 143–150.

Lamy, F., and Lansing, A. I. (1961). *Proc. Soc. Exp. Biol. Med.* **106,** 160–162.

Largman, C. (1983). *Biochemistry* **22,** 3763–3770.

Largman, C., Brodrick, J. W., and Geokas, M. C. (1976). *Biochemistry* **15,** 2491–2500.

Largman, C., Brodrick, J. W., Geokas, M. C., Sischo, W. M., and Johnson, J. H. (1979). *J. Biol. Chem.* **254,** 8516–8524.

Laurell, C. B., and Eriksson, S. (1963). *Scand. J. Clin. Lab. Invest.* **15,** 132–140.

Laurent, P., and Bieth, J. G. (1985). *Biochem. Biophys. Res. Commun.* **126,** 275–281.

Laurent, P., Janoff, A., and Kagan, H. M. (1983). *Am. Rev. Respir. Dis.* **127,** 189–192.

Lavi, G., Zucker-Franklin, D., and Franklin, E. C. (1980). *J. Immunol.* **125,** 175–180.

Lee, C. T., Fein, A. M., Lippmann, M., Holtzman, H., Kimbel, P., and Weinbaum, G. (1981). *N. Engl. J. Med.* **304,** 192–196.

Legrand, Y., Caen, J. P., Robert, L., and Wautier, J. L. (1977). *Thromb. Haemostasis* **37,** 580–582.

Lestienne, P., and Bieth, J. (1978). *Arch. Biochem. Biophys.* **190,** 358–360.

Lestienne, P., and Bieth, J. G. (1980). *J. Biol. Chem.* **255,** 9289–9294.

Lestienne, P., and Bieth, J. G. (1983). *Biochimie* **65,** 49–52.

Lestienne, P., Dimicoli, J. L., and Bieth, J. (1978). *J. Biol. Chem.* **253,** 3459–3460.

Lestienne, P., Dimicoli, J. L., Wermuth, C. G., and Bieth, J. G. (1981). *Biochim. Biophys. Acta* **658,** 413–416.

Lewis, U. J., and Thiele, E. H. (1957). *J. Am. Chem. Soc.* **79,** 755–756.

Lewis, U. J., Williams, D. E., and Brink, N. G. (1956). *J. Biol. Chem.* **222,** 705–720.

Lievaart, P. A., and Stevenson, K. J. (1974). *Can. J. Biochem.* **52,** 637–641.

Liotta, L. A., Rao, C. N., and Barsky, S. H. (1983). *Lab. Invest.* **49,** 636–649.

Lively, M. O., and Powers, J. C. (1978). *Biochim. Biophys. Acta* **525,** 171–179.

Löbermann, H., Lottspeich, F., Bode, W., and Huber, R. (1982). *Hoppe-Seyler's Z. Physiol. Chem.* **363,** 1377–1388.

Loebermann, H., Tokuoka, R., Deisenhofer, J., and Huber, R. (1984). *J. Mol. Biol.* **177,** 531–556.

Long, G. L., Chandra, T., Woo, S. L. C., Davie, E. W., and Kurachi, K. (1984). *Biochemistry* **23,** 4828–4837.

Lonky, S. A., and Wohl, H. (1981). *J. Clin. Invest.* **67,** 817–826.

Lonky, S. A., and Wohl, H. (1983). *Biochemistry* **22,** 3714–3720.

Lonky, S. A., Marsh, J., and Wohl, H. (1978). *Biochem. Biophys. Res. Commun.* **85,** 1113–1118.

McDonald, J. A., and Kelley, D. G. (1980). *J. Biol. Chem.* **255,** 8848–8858.

McDonald, R. J., Swift, G. H., Quinto, C., Swain, W., Pictet, R. L., Nikovits, W., and Rutter, W. J. (1982). *Biochemistry* **21,** 1453–1463.

McKerrow, J. H., Keene, W., Jeong, K., and Werb, Z. (1982). *Lab. Invest.* **49,** 195–200.

McRae, B., Nakajima, K., Travis, J., and Powers, J. C. (1980). *Biochemistry* **19,** 3973–3978.

Maeda, H., Nakamura, N., and Uzawa, H. (1982). *J. Biochem.* **92,** 1213–1218.

Mainardi, C. L., Hasty, D. L., Sayer, J. M., and Kang, A. H. (1980a). *J. Biol. Chem.* **255,** 12006–12010.

Mainardi, C. L., Dixit, S. N., and Kang, A. H. (1980b). *J. Biol. Chem.* **255,** 5435–5441.

Malemud, C. J., and Janoff, A. (1975). *Arthritis Rheum.* **18,** 361–368.

Mallory, P. A., and Travis, J. (1975). *Biochemistry* **14,** 722–730.

Mandl, I., and Cohen, B. B. (1960). *Arch. Biochem. Biophys.* **91,** 47–53.

Mandl, I., Keller, S., and Cohen, B. (1962). *Proc. Soc. Exp. Biol. Med.* **109,** 923–925.

Marossy, K. (1981). *Biochim. Biophys. Acta* **659,** 351–361.

Martodam, R. R., Baugh, R. J., Twumasi, D. Y., and Liener, I. E. (1979). *Prep. Biochem.* **9,** 15–31.

Matheson, N. R., Janoff, A., and Travis, J. (1982). *Mol. Cell. Biochem.* **45,** 65–71.

Meyer, J. F., Bieth, J., and Métais, P. (1975). *Clin. Chim. Acta,* **62,** 43–53.

Moon, H. D., and McIvor, B. C. (1960). *J. Immunol.* **85,** 78–80.

Mooren, H. W. D., Kramps, J. A., Franken, C., Meijer, C. J. L. M., and Dijkman, J. A. (1983). *Thorax,* **38,** 180–183.

Morihara, K., and Tsuzuki, H. (1966). *Arch. Biochem. Biophys.* **114,** 158–165.

Morihara, K., and Tsuzuki, H. (1967). *Arch. Biochem. Biophys.* **120,** 68–78.

Morihara, K., and Tsuzuki, H. (1975). *Agric. Biol. Chem.* **39,** 1123–1128.

Morihara, K., and Tsuzuki, H. (1978). *Jpn. J. Exp. Med.* **48,** 81–84.

Morihara, K., Tsuzuki, H., Oka, T., Inouie, H., and Ebata, M. (1965). *J. Biol. Chem.* **240,** 3295–3304.

Morihara, K., Tsuzuki, H., and Oda. K. (1979). *Infect. Immun.* **24,** 188–193.

Morihara, K., Tsuzuki, H., Harada, M., and Iwata, T. (1984). *J. Biochem.* **95,** 795–804.

Morii, M., and Travis, J. (1983). *J. Biol. Chem.* **258,** 12749–12752.

Murphy, G., Reynolds, J., Bretz, U., and Baggiolini, M. (1977). *Biochem. J.* **162,** 195–197.

Murphy, G., Bretz, U., Baggiolini, M., and Reynolds, J. J. (1980). *Biochem. J.* **192,** 517–523.

Nagamatsu, A., and Soeda, S. (1981). *Chem. Pharm. Bull.* **29,** 1121–1129.

Nakajima, K., Powers, J. C., Ashe, B. M., and Zimmerman, M. (1979). *J. Biol. Chem.* **254,** 4027–4032.

Nayak, P. L., and Bender, M. L. (1978). *Biochem. Biophys. Res. Commun.* **83,** 1178–1182.

Neumann, S., Hennrich, N., Gunzer, G., and Lang, H. (1983). *In* "Progress in Clinical Enzymology II" (D. M. Goldberg and M. Werner, eds.), pp. 293–298. Masson, New York.

Niederman, M. S., Fritts, L. L., Merrill, W. W., Fick, R. B., Matthay, R. A., Reynolds, H. Y., and Gee, J. B. L. (1984). *Am. Rev. Respir. Dis.* **129,** 943–947.

Nishino, N., and Powers, J. C. (1980). *J. Biol. Chem.* **255,** 3482–3486.

Oakley, C. L., and Bonerjee, N. G. (1963). *J. Pathol. Bacteriol.* **85,** 489–506.

Obernesser, H.-J., and Döring, G. (1982). *Zbl. Bakt. Hyg. I. Abt. Orig.* **252,** 248–256.

Oda, K., Laskowski, M., Sr., Kress, L. F., and Kowalski, D. (1977). *Biochem. Biophys. Res. Commun.* **76,** 1062–1070.

Ogawa, M., Kosaki, G., Tanaka, S., Iwaki, K., and Nomoto, M. (1979). *Clin. Chim. Acta* **93,** 235–238.

Ohlsson, K. (1980). *Bull. Eur. Physiopathol. Resp.* **16,** (Suppl.), 209–222.

Ohlsson, K., and Olsson, I. (1974). *Eur. J. Biochem.* **42,** 519–527.

Ohlsson, K., and Olsson, A. S. (1976). *Hoppe Seyler's Z. Physiol. Chem.* **357,** 1153–1161.

Ohlsson, K., and Olsson, I. (1977). *Scand. J. Haematol.* **19,** 145–152.

Ohlsson, K., and Olsson, A. S. (1978). *Hoppe-Seyler's Z. Physiol. Chem.* **359,** 1531–1539.

Ohlsson, K., and Tegner, H. (1976). *Scand. J. Clin. Lab. Invest.* **36,** 437–445.

Ohlsson, K., Tegner, T., and Åkesson, U. (1977). *Hoppe-Seyler's Z. Physiol. Chem.* **358,** 583–589.

Ohlsson, K., Fryksmark, U., and Tegner, H. (1980). *Eur. J. Clin. Invest.* **10**, 373–379.

Okada, K., Kawaharajo, K., Homma, J. Y., Aoyama, Y., and Kubota, Y. (1976). *Jpn. J. Exp. Med.* **46**, 245–249.

Omura, S., Ohno, H., Saheki, T., Yoshida, M., and Nakagawa, A. (1978). *Biochem. Biophys. Res. Commun.* **83**, 704–709.

Omura, S., Nakagawa, A. and Ohno, H. (1979). *J. Am. Chem. Soc.* **101**, 4386–4388.

Ooyama, T., Kawamura, K., and Katayama, K. (1977). *FEBS Lett.* **77**, 61–64.

Orlowski, M., Orlowski, J., Lesser, M., and Kilburn, K. H. (1981). *J. Lab. Clin. Med.* **97**, 467–476.

Osman, M., Cantor, J., Roffman, S., Turino, G. M., and Mandl, I. (1982). *Am. Rev. Respir. Dis.* **125**, 213–217.

Ozaki, H., and Shiio, I. (1975). *J. Biochem.* **77**, 171–180.

Partridge, S. M., and Davis, H. F. (1955). *Biochem. J.* **61**, 21–33.

Peanasky, R. J., Bentz, Y., Paulson, B., Graham, D. L., and Babin, D. R. (1984). *Arch. Biochem. Biophys.* **232**, 127–134.

Penny, G. S., and Dyckes, D. F. (1980). *Biochemistry* **19**, 2888–2894.

Plow, E. F. (1982). *J. Clin. Invest.* **69**, 564–572.

Plow, E. F., Gramse, M., and Havemann, K. (1983). *J. Lab. Clin. Med.* **102**, 858–869.

Pochon, F., and Bieth, J. G. (1983). *Ann. N.Y. Acad. Sci.* **421**, 81–89.

Poncz, L., Gerken, T. A., Dearborn, D. G., Grobelny, D., and Galardy, R. E. (1984). *Biochemistry* **23**, 2766–2772.

Powell, J. R., and Castellino, F. J. (1981). *Biochem. Biophys. Res. Commun.* **102**, 46–52.

Powers, J. C., and Carroll, D. L. (1975). *Biochem. Biophys. Res. Commun.* **67**, 939–944.

Powers, J. C., and Tuhy, P. M. (1973). *Biochemistry* **12**, 4767–4774.

Powers, J. C., Gupton, B. F., Harley, A. D., Nishino, N., and Whitley, R. J. (1977). *Biochim. Biophys. Acta* **485**, 156–166.

Powers, J. C., Boone, R., Carroll, D. L., Gupton, B. F., Kam, C.-M., Nishino, N., Sakamoto, M., and Tuhy, P. M. (1984). *J. Biol. Chem.* **259**, 4288–4294.

Prince, H. E., Folds, J. D., and Spitznagel, J. K. (1979a). *Clin. Exp. Immunol.* **37**, 162–168.

Prince, H. E., Folds, J. D., and Spitznagel, J. K. (1979b). *Mol. Immunol.* **16**, 301–306.

Pryzwansky, K. B., Martin, L. E., and Spitznagel, J. K. (1978). *J. Reticuloendothel. Soc.* **24**, 295–310.

Quinn, R. S., and Blout, E. R. (1970). *Biochem. Biophys. Res. Commun.* **40**, 328–330.

Rabaud, M., Tribouley-Duret, J., Lefebvre, F., Desgranges, C., and Bricaud, H. (1980). *C.R. Acad. Sci. Paris,* **291**, 825–828.

Rabaud, M., Desgranges, C., Lefebvre, F., and Bricaud, H. (1981). *Connect. Tissue Res.* **9**, 11–17.

Ragsdale, C. G., and Arend, W. P. (1979). *J. Exp. Med.* **149**, 954–968.

Rao, C. N., Margulies, I. M. K., Goldfarb, R. H., Madri, J. A., Woodley, D. T., and Liotta, L. A. (1982). *Arch. Biochem. Biophys.* **219**, 65–70.

Reilly, C. F., and Travis, J. (1980). *Biochim. Biophys. Acta* **621**, 147–157.

Reilly, C. F., Tewksbury, D. A., Schechter, N. M., and Travis, J. (1982). *J. Biol. Chem.* **257**, 8619–8622.

Renaud, A., Lestienne, P., Hugues, D. L., Bieth, J. G., and Dimicoli, J. L. (1983). *J. Biol. Chem.* **258**, 8312–8316.

Rinderknecht, H., Geokas, M. C., Silverman, P., Lillard, Y., and Haverback, B. J. (1968). *Clin. Chim. Acta.* **19**, 327–339.

Rindler-Ludwig, R., and Braunsteiner, H. (1975). *Biochim. Biophys. Acta* **379**, 606–617.

Robert, B., and Robert, L. (1969). *Eur. J. Biochem.* **11**, 62–67.

Robert, B., Szigeti, M., Robert, L., Legrand, Y., Pignaud, G., and Caen, J. (1970). *Nature,* **227,** 1248–1249.

Rodriguez, R. J., White, R. R., Senior, R. M., and Levine, E. A. (1977). *Science,* **198,** 313–314.

Rosenberg, S., Barr, P. J., Najarian, R. C., and Hallewell, R. A. (1984). *Nature (London)* **312,** 77–80.

Rucker, R. B., and Dubick, M. A. (1984). *Environ. Health Perspect.* **55,** 179–191.

Saklatvala, J. (1977). *J. Clin. Invest.* **59,** 794–801.

Sampath-Narayan, A., and Anvar, R. A. (1969). *Biochem. J.* **114,** 11–17.

Sandberg, L. B., Soskel, N. T., and Leslie, J. G. (1981). *N. Eng. J. Med.* **304,** 566–579.

Sandhaus, R. A., McCarthy, K. M., Musson, R. A., and Henson, P. M. (1983). *Chest,* **83,** 60S–62S.

Sasaki, M., Yoshikane, K., Nobata, E., Katagiri, K., and Takeuchi, T. (1981). *J. Biochem.* **89,** 609–614.

Satoh, S., Kurecki, T., and Laskowski, M. Sr. (1979). *Biochem. Biophys. Res. Commun.* **86,** 130–137.

Schechter, I., and Berger, A. (1967). *Biochem. Biophys. Res. Commun.* **27,** 157–162.

Schiessler, H., Arnhold, M., Ohlsson, K., and Fritz, H. (1976). *Hoppe-Seyler's Z. Physiol. Chem.* **357,** 1251–1260.

Schiessler, H., Ohlsson, K., Olsson, I., Arnhold, M., Birk, Y., and Fritz, H. (1977). *Hoppe-Seyler's Z. Physiol. Chem.* **358,** 53–58.

Schiessler, H., Hochstrasser, K., and Ohlsson, K. (1978). *In* "Neutral Proteases of Human Polymorphonuclear Leukocytes" (K. Havemann and A. Janoff, eds.), pp. 195–207. Urban & Schwartzenberg, Munich.

Schmidt, W., and Havemann, K. (1974). *Hoppe Seyler's Z. Physiol. Chem.* **335,** 1077–1082.

Schmidt, W., Egbring, R., and Havemann, K. (1975). *Thromb. Res.* **6,** 315–321.

Schnebli, H. P., Christen, P., Jochum, M., Mallya, R. K., and Pepys, M. B. (1984). *Adv. Exp. Med. Biol.* **167,** 355–362.

Schnebli, H. P., Liersch, M., Virca, G. D., Bodmer, J. L., Snider, G. L., Lucey, E. C., and Stone, P. G. (1985). *Eur. J. Respir. Dis.* **66,** 66–70.

Schultz, D. R., and Miller, K. D. (1974). *Infect. Immun.* **10,** 128–135.

Schumacher, G. F. B., and Schill, W. B. (1972). *Anal. Biochem.* **48,** 9–26.

Seemüller, U., Meier, M., Ohlsson, K., Müller, H.-P., and Fritz, H. (1977). *Hoppe-Seyler's Z. Physiol. Chem.* **358,** 1105–1117.

Senior, R. M., and Campbell, E. J. (1983). *Clin. Lab. Med.* **3,** 645–666.

Senior, R. M., Huebner, P. F., and Pierce, J. A. (1971). *J. Lab. Clin. Med.* **77,** 510–516.

Senior, R. M., Griffen, G. L., and Mecham, R. P. (1980). *J. Clin. Invest.* **66,** 859–962.

Senior, R. M., Campbell, E. J., Landis, J. A., Cox, F. R., Kuhn, C., and Koren, H. S. (1982). *J. Clin. Invest.* **69,** 384–393.

Sesboüé, R., Vercaigne, D., Charlionet, R., Lefebvre, F., and Martin, J.-P. (1984). *Hum. Hered.* **34,** 105–113.

Shaw, M. C., and Whitaker, D. R. (1973). *Can. J. Biochem.* **51,** 112–114.

Shechter, Y., Burstein, Y., and Gertler, A. (1977). *Biochemistry* **16,** 992–997.

Shotton, D. M. (1970). *In* "Methods in Enzymology" (G. E. Perlmann and L. Lorand, eds.), Vol. 19, pp. 113–140. Academic Press, New York.

Shotton, D. M., White, N. J., and Watson, H. C. (1971). *Cold Spring Harbor Symp. Quant. Biol.* **36,** 91–105.

Smillie, L. B., and Hartley, B. S. (1966). *Biochem. J.* **101,** 232–241.

Smith, C. E., and Johnson, D. A. (1985). *Biochem. J.* **225,** 463–472.

Smith, R. J., Wierenga, W., and Iden, S. S. (1980). *Inflammation,* **4,** 73–88.

Sottrup-Jensen, L. Lønblad, P. B., Stepanik, T. M., Petersen, T. E., Magnusson, S., and Jörnvall, H. (1981). *FEBS Lett.* **127,** 167–173.

Starkey, P. M. (1977a). *Acta Biol. Med. Ger.* **36,** 1549–1554.

Starkey, P. M. (1977b). *In* "Proteinases in Mammalian Cells and Tissues" (A. Barrett, ed.), pp. 57–89. North-Holland Publ., Amsterdam.

Starkey, P. M., and Barrett, A. J. (1976). *Biochem. J.* **155,** 255–264.

Starkey, P. M., Barrett, A. J., and Burleigh, M. C. (1977). *Biochim. Biophys. Acta* **483,** 386–397.

Stein, R. L. (1983). *J. Am. Chem. Soc.* **105,** 5111–5116.

Stein, R. L., Viscarello, B. R., and Vildonger, R. A. (1984). *J. Am. Chem. Soc.* **106,** 796–798.

Stephens, R. W., Walton, E. A., Ghosh, P., Taylor, T. K. F., Gramse, M., and Havemann, K. (1980). *Drugs Res.* **30,** 2108–2112.

Sterrenberg, L., Nieuwenhuizen, W., and Hermans, J. (1983). *Biochim. Biophys. Acta* **755,** 300–306.

Stockley, R. A., Morrison, H. M., Smith, S., and Tetley, T. (1984). *Hoppe-Seyler's Z. Physiol. Chem.* **365,** 587–595.

Stone, P. J., Calore, J. D., Snider, G. L., and Franzblau, C. (1982). *J. Clin. Invest.* **69,** 920–931.

Stone, P. J., Calore, J. D., McGowan, S. E., Bernardo, J., Snider, G. L., and Franzblau, C. (1983). *Science* **221,** 1187–1189.

Suter, S., Nydegger, U. E., Roux, L., and Waldvogel, F. A. (1981). *J. Infect. Dis.* **144,** 499–508.

Suter, S., Schaad, B., Roux, L., Nydegger, E., and Waldvogel, F. A. (1984). *J. Infect. Dis.* **149,** 523–531.

Takahashi, S., Seifter, S., and Yang, F. C. (1973). *Biochim. Biophys. Acta* **327,** 138–146.

Tam, T. F., Spencer, R. W., Thomas, E. M., Copp, L. J., and Krantz, A. (1984). *J. Am. Chem. Soc.* **106,** 6849–6851.

Taylor, J. C., and Crawford, I. P. (1975). *Arch. Biochem. Biophys.* **169,** 91–101.

Taylor, J. C., Crawford, I. P., and Hugli, T. E. (1977). *Biochemistry* **16,** 3390–3396.

Tegner, H. (1978). *Acta Otolaryngol..* **85,** 282–289.

Tegner, H., and Ohlsson, K. (1977). *Hoppe-Seyler's Z. Physiol. Chem.* **358,** 427–429.

Tegner, H., Ohlsson, K., and Olsson, I. (1977). *Hoppe-Seyler's Z. Physiol. Chem.* **358,** 431–433.

Teshima, T., Griffin, J. C., and Powers, J. C. (1982). *J. Biol. Chem.* **257,** 5085–5091.

Thompson, R. C. (1973). *Biochemistry* **12,** 47–51.

Thompson, R. C. (1974). *Biochemistry* **13,** 5495–5501.

Thompson, R. C., and Blout, E. R. (1970). *Proc. Natl. Acad. Sci. U.S.A.* **67,** 1734–1740.

Thompson, R. C., and Blout, E. R. (1973a). *Biochemistry* **12,** 44–47.

Thompson, R. C., and Blout, E. R. (1973b). *Biochemistry* **12,** 51–57.

Thompson, R. C., and Blout, E. R. (1973c). *Biochemistry* **12,** 57–66.

Thompson, R. C., and Blout, E. R. (1973d). *Biochemistry* **12,** 66–71.

Thomson, A., and Denniss, I. S. (1976). *Biochim. Biophys. Acta* **429,** 581–590.

Thomson, A., and Kapadia, S. B. (1979). *Eur. J. Biochem.* **102,** 111–116.

Travis, J., and Salvesen, G. S. (1983). *Annu. Rev. Biochem.* **52,** 655–709.

Tsai, Y.-C., Yamasaki, M., Yamamoto-Suzuki, Y., and Tamura, G. (1983). *Biochem. Int.* **7,** 577–583.

Tu, A. T. (1977). "Proteolytic Enzymes of Venoms: Chemistry and Molecular Biology." Wiley, New-York.

Twumasi, D. Y., and Liener, I. E. (1977). *J. Biol. Chem.* **252,** 1917–1926.
Twumasi, D. Y., Liener, I. E., Galdston, M., and Levytska, V. (1977). *Nature* **267,** 61–63.
Umezawa, H. (1976). *In* "Methods in Enzymology" (L. Lorand, ed.), Vol. 45, pp. 678–695. Academic Press, New York.
Uram, M., and Lamy, F. (1969). *Biochim. Biophys. Acta* **194,** 102–111.
Urry, D. W. (1983). *Ultrastruct. Pathol.* **4,** 227–251.
Valentine, R., and Fisher, G. L. (1984). *J. Leukocyte Biol.* **35,** 449–457.
Van den Hooff, A. (1983). *Int. Rev. Connect. Tissue Res.* **10,** 395–432.
Van Furth, R., Kramps, J. A., and Diesselhof-Den Dulk M. M. C. (1983). *Clin. Exp. Immunol.* **51,** 551–557.
Van Leuven, F. (1982). *Trends Biochem. Sci.* **7,** 185–187.
Vartio, T., Seppa, H., and Vaheri, A. (1981). *J. Biol. Chem.* **256,** 471–477.
Velvart, M., Fehr, K., Baici, A., Sommermeyer, G., Knöpfel, M., Cancer, M., Salgam, P., and Böni, A. (1981). *Rheumatol. Int.* **1,** 121–130.
Vered, M., Schutzbank, T., and Janoff, A. (1984). *Am. Rev. Respir. Dis.* **130,** 1118–1124.
Virca, G. D., and Travis, J. (1984). *J. Biol. Chem.* **259,** 8870–8874.
Virca, G. D., Lyerly, D., Kreger, A., and Travis, J. (1982). *Biochim. Biophys. Acta* **704,** 267–271.
Virca, G. D., Salvesen, G. S., and Travis, J. (1983). *Hoppe-Seyler's Z. Physiol. Chem.* **364,** 1297–1302.
Virca, G. D., Mallya, R. K., Pepys, M. B., and Schnebli, H. P. (1984). *Adv. Exp. Med. Biol.* **167,** 345–353.
Wachtfogel, Y. T., Kucich, U., James, H. L., Scott, C. F., Schapira, M., Zimmerman, M., Cohen, A. B., and Colman, R. W. (1983). *J. Clin. Invest.* **72,** 1672–1677.
Walford, R. L., and Kickhöfen, B. (1962). *Arch. Biochem. Biophys.* **98,** 191–196.
Wallmark, A., Alm, R., and Eriksson, S. (1984). *Proc. Natl. Acad. Sci. U.S.A.* **81,** 5690–5693.
Wasi, S., and Hofmann, T. (1968). *Biochem. J.* **106,** 926–930.
Weaver, L. H., Kester, W. R., and Matthews, B. W. (1977). *J. Mol. Biol.* **114,** 119–132.
Wenzel, H. R., and Tschesche, H. (1981). *Hoppe-Seyler's Z. Physiol. Chem.* **362,** 829–831.
Wenzel, H. R., Engelbrecht, S., Reich, H., Mondry, W., and Tschesche, H. (1980). *Hoppe-Seyler's Z. Physiol. Chem.* **361,** 1413–1416.
Werb, Z., and Gordon, S. (1975). *J. Exp. Med.* **142,** 361–377.
Werb, Z., Banda, M. J., and Jones, P. A. (1980). *J. Exp. Med.* **152,** 1340–1357.
Werb, Z., Banda, M. J., McKerrow, J. H., and Sandhaus, R. A. (1982). *J. Invest. Dermatol.* **79,** 154s–159s.
White, R., Lin, H.-S., and Kuhn, C. (1977). *J. Exp. Med.* **146,** 802–808.
White, R., Janoff, A., and Godfrey, H. P. (1980a). *Lung,* **158,** 9–14.
White, R., Norby, D., Janoff, A., and Dearing, R. (1980b). *Biochim. Biophys. Acta* **612,** 233–244.
White, R., Lee, D., Habicht, G., and Janoff, A. (1981). *Am. Rev. Respir. Dis.* **123,** 447–449.
White, R., Janoff, A., Gordon, R., and Campbell, E. (1982). *Am. Rev. Respir. Dis.* **125,** 779–781.
Wilson, K. A., and Laskowski, M. Sr. (1975). *J. Biol. Chem.* **250,** 4261–4267.
Wintroub, B. U., Klickstein, L. B., Dzau, V. J., and Watt, K. W. K. (1984). *Biochemistry* **23,** 227–232.
Wolfenden, R. (1969). *Nature,* **223,** 704–705.
Wong, P. S., and Travis, J. (1980). *Biochem. Biophys. Res. Commun.* **96,** 1449–1454.
Wretlind, B., and Pavlovskis, O. R. (1983). *Rev. Infect. Dis.* **5,** (Suppl. 5) S998–S1004.

Wyss, A., Virca, G. D., and Schnebli, H. P. (1984). *Hoppe-Seyler's Z. Physiol. Chem.* **365,** 511–516.

Yasutake, A., and Powers, J. C. (1981). *Biochemistry* **20,** 3675–3679.

Yoshimura, T., Barker, L. N., and Powers, J. C. (1982). *J. Biol. Chem.* **257,** 5077–5084.

Yoshinaka, R., Tanaka, H., Sato, M., and Ikeda, S. (1983). *Bull. Jpn. Soc. Sci. Fish.* **49,** 637–642.

Yoshinaka, R., Sato, M., Tanaka, H., and Ikeda, S. (1984). *Biochim. Biophys. Acta* **798,** 240–246.

Yuasa, I., Suenaga, K., Gotoh, Y., Ito, K., Yokoyama, N., and Okada, K. (1984). *Hum. Genet.* **67,** 209–212.

Zimmerman, M., and Ashe, B. M. (1977). *Biochim. Biophys. Acta* **480,** 241–245.

Zimmerman, M., Morman, H., Mulvey, D., Jones, H., Frankshun, R., and Ashe, B. M. (1980). *J. Biol. Chem.* **255,** 9848–9851.

Characterization and
Regulation of Lysyl Oxidase

Herbert M. Kagan

Department of Biochemistry, Boston University School of Medicine, Boston, Massachusetts

REGULATION OF MATRIX ACCUMULATION

I. Introduction

Collagen and elastin play unique roles in the structure and function of connective tissues by virtue of their ability to serve as insoluble stress-bearing structures with high tensile strength or elasticity and as matrices for tissue growth and development. The unusual mechanical properties of these proteins are largely dependent on their contents of inter- and intrachain lysine-derived covalent cross-linkages. These cross-linkages derive from peptidyl α-aminoadipic-δ-semialdehyde (AAS), the formation of which occurs by the oxidative deamination of lysine in these proteins by lysyl oxidase (Fig. 1). Spontaneous condensations between these side-chain aldehyde functions with other vicinal aldehydes and unreacted ε-amino groups can yield the variety of intra- and intermolecular cross-linkages which exist in these connective tissue proteins, thus accounting for the metabolic conversion of soluble precursors of collagen or elastin into continuously cross-linked, insoluble fibers. The cross-linkages can provide mechanical limits to the tensile and elastic stresses placed upon fibers of these connective tissue proteins.

The existence of an enzyme with lysyl oxidase activity had long been implied by the observations that the administration of specific agents, notably including β-aminopropionitrile (BAPN), various carbonyl-modifying reagents, or the depletion of copper from the diet can induce lathyrism, a condition characterized by a variety of connective tissue abnormalities, including aortic rupture, skeletal deformities, and skin fragility. Biochemical analyses of lathyritic tissues subsequently revealed that collagen was unusually soluble while defects were also noted in elastic fibers, concomitant with decreased lysine-derived cross-linkages and increased lysine content in these proteins. Pinnell and Martin (1968) were the first to demonstrate the enzyme-catalyzed formation of the aldehyde and cross-linkages in connective tissue substrates *in vitro* using a preparation of chick cartilage as the enzyme source. This enzyme activity was strongly inhibited by BAPN and by copper chelators *in vitro* and thus appeared to be a copper-

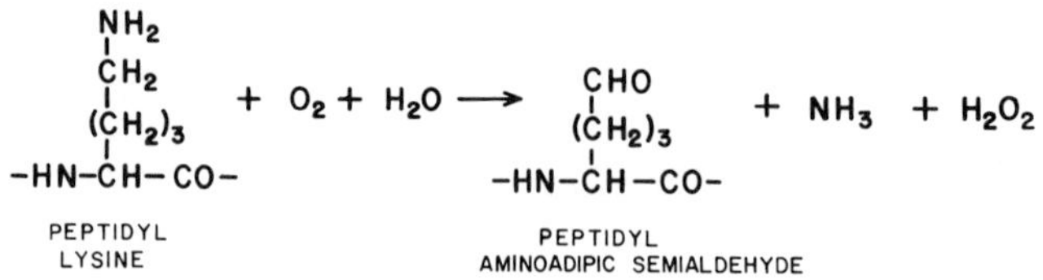

$$
\begin{array}{c}
NH_2 \\
| \\
CH_2 \\
| \\
(CH_2)_3 \\
| \\
-HN-CH-CO-
\end{array}
+ O_2 + H_2O \longrightarrow
\begin{array}{c}
CHO \\
| \\
(CH_2)_3 \\
| \\
-HN-CH-CO-
\end{array}
+ NH_3 + H_2O_2
$$

PEPTIDYL LYSINE   PEPTIDYL AMINOADIPIC SEMIALDEHYDE

Fig. 1. Reaction catalyzed by lysyl oxidase.

dependent amine oxidase consistent with the properties expected of the enzyme assumed to synthesize the cross-linkages in elastin and collagen *in vivo*. The present article intends to review progress made in our understanding of this unusual catalyst following upon the most recent review of its properties and function in 1979 (Siegel, 1979).

II. POSTTRANSLATIONAL MODIFICATIONS OF CONNECTIVE TISSUE PROTEINS

A. Collagen

The biosynthesis of collagen consists of an integrated and complex series of intracellular and extracellular biochemical events. Reviews of this subject have appeared to which the reader is referred for details beyond those summarized here (Bornstein and Traub, 1979; Prockop *et al.*, 1979; Minor, 1980). Collagen is initially synthesized as preprocollagen chains on membrane-bound polysomes on the rough endoplasmic reticulum. These monomeric chains contain an N-terminal signal peptide segment approximately 100 residues long which is apparently involved in the initiation of synthesis and the extension of nascent polypeptide chains into the rough endoplasmic reticulum (RER). This prepropeptide segment is removed by a membrane-bound "signal peptidase" activity in the RER. The product pro-α-chain has a molecular weight (MW) of approximately 154,000 and consists of N-terminal and C-terminal noncollagenous propeptide regions of 20,000 and 34,000 MW, respectively, which in turn flank a central collagenous region, (Gly-X-Y)$_{334}$, of approximately 100,000 MW.

Collagen is subject to at least eight known posttranslational modifications, including that catalyzed by lysyl oxidase. The first of these involves the hydroxylation of proline by prolyl-4- and prolyl-3-hydroxylases and of lysine residues by lysyl hydroxylase. Each of these enzymes require free oxygen, Fe^{2+}, α-ketoglutarate, and ascorbic acid. These hydroxylations begin on nascent preprocollagen chains and are completed in the lumen of the RER on free pro-α-chains before the helix is formed. Following hydroxylation, specific hydroxylysine residues of pro-α-chains are glycosylated to galactosylhydroxylysine which may be further processed to glucosylgalactosylhydroxylysine residues by Mn^{2+}-dependent glucosyl- and galactosyltransferases utilizing UDP-sugars as substrates. Hydroxylation of proline residues stabilizes the collagen triple helix so that its denaturation occurs at higher than body temperature. The sugar substituents on hydroxylysine residues are thought to affect the orderly packing of collagen into fibrils and may be involved in interactions of collagen with other macromolecules and cell membranes. Three monomeric hydroxylated and glycosylated pro-α-chains then interact in the RER forming interchain disulfide bonds between the C-terminal propeptide regions, following which the three covalently linked chains spontaneously wind around each other to form the collagen triple helix structure. The procollagen triple helix is then transported to the Golgi complex and packaged for secretion in condensed Golgi vacuoles. These vacuoles are transported to the cell surface, apparently by a microtubule-dependent process, and are secreted by exocytosis. The N- and C-terminal propeptide regions of procollagen molecules are cleaved at or near the cell surface, yielding triple helical tropocollagen monomers which retain short telopeptide non-triple helical segments at each end of their component α-chains. These cleavages are catalyzed by different proteolytic enzymes each selective for the N- or C-terminal propeptide regions. The tropocollagen monomers then undergo intermolecular associations to form oligomeric nucleation aggregates which subsequently undergo lateral and longitudinal aggregation to form the quarter-staggered fibrillar structure of extracellular collagen. Cross-linking of collagen appears to occur predominantly in the extracellular space. Interaction of lysyl oxidase with collagen is presumably precisely integrated with specific stages in fibril formation in view of steric restrictions imposed on the accessibility of tropocollagen units to lysyl oxidase as the fiber dimensions increase. It appears that oxidation of lysine in the interstitial collagens is restricted to one lysine in the N-terminal and one in the C-terminal telopeptide regions, respectively, while those in the triple helix do not normally become oxidized.

B. *Elastin*

Details of intracellular events in the biosynthesis of elastin are not as completely understood as are those of collagen, at this writing. The reader is referred to recent reviews on the structure and biosynthesis of elastin and its precursor (Sandberg *et al.*, 1981; Franzblau and Faris, 1982; Foster *et al.*, 1983). The existence of tropoelastin, the soluble precursor to insoluble elastin, has been documented by several investigators. Consistent with its precursor role, a monomeric tropoelastin species of approximately 72,000 MW can be isolated from tissue or cell culture sources in which lysyl oxidase activity is inhibited by lathyrogenic agents or by copper depletion, while pulse–chase experiments reveal its eventual incorporation into extracellular elastin fibers. In contrast to the extensive hydroxylation of proline in collagen, only 7–

8% of the approximately 100 proline residues per 800 residues in tropoelastin and mature elastin are hydroxylated, while there appears to be no hydroxylysine nor glycosylated hydroxylysine in soluble or insoluble elastin. In further dissimilarity to collagen, elastin does not contain extensive repeat structures of the Gly-X-Y triplet, although evidence for a short collagen-like sequence in elastin has been reported (Smith *et al.*, 1981). There is some controversy concerning the presence of ordered conformation and the conformational bases of the elastic properties of elastin. Thermodynamic analyses of its elastic behavior (Gosline, 1976) and NMR studies of the insoluble protein (Fleming *et al.*, 1980) point toward a high degree of mobility and structural randomness in its polypeptide chains. On the other hand, ultrastructural studies (Gotte *et al.*, 1974; Cleary and Cliff, 1978), circular dichroism (Urry *et al.*, 1969), and electron spin resonance techniques (Urry and Long, 1977; Urry, 1982) on elastin or of coacervated aggregates of soluble elastin peptides, tropoelastin, or elastin-like synthetic peptides are consistent with some degree of secondary and higher ordered structures in this protein. Elastin appears to contain the potential for at least two differing structural domains, one of which stems from its presence of repeating hydrophobic valine-containing peptide sequences such as pentapeptide sequence (VPGVG), which repeats 11 times in one portion of elastin, and the hexapeptide unit (PGVGVA), which repeats 6 times in one tryptic peptide isolated from tropoelastin (Urry, 1982). Synthetic polypeptide models of these sequences behave similarly to soluble forms of elastin in that they can undergo coacervation with an inverse temperature dependency. Further, these repeat polypeptides exhibit the β-turn structural feature which when repeated on the helical axis forms the β-spiral structure. Structures consistent with the β-spiral have been observed in elastic fibers generated from partial hydrolysates of elastin (Cleary and Cliff, 1978). Elastin has been envisioned to consist of regions of such "loose" helical structures which alternate with alanine-rich, lysine-containing regions postulated to contain short runs of the tighter, α-helical structure (Sandberg *et al.*, 1981). These alanine-rich sequences are the sites of lysine oxidation and cross-linkage formation. Tropoelastin isolated from copper-deficient pig aorta contains approximately 47 lysine residues whereas mature insoluble elastin contains approximately 5 lysine residues per 800 residues (Sandberg *et al.*, 1981; Sandberg and Wolt, 1982), the difference being accounted for by the oxidation of approximately 30 of the lysines in tropoelastin and by condensations of unmodified lysines in cross-linking reactions, in contrast to the oxidation of only two lysine residues per α1-chain of type I collagen, for example.

Since lysine oxidation eliminates many sites of positive charge and thus changes the net polarity of elastin to a considerable extent, it is likely that the extensive oxidation of tropoelastin by lysyl oxidase may markedly influence the degree of ordered structure in this protein.

C. Chemistry and Biosynthesis of the Cross-Linkages

The biosynthesis of the cross-linkages is initiated by the enzymatic oxidation of lysine to α-aminoadipic-δ-semialdehyde in tropoelastin and tropocollagen units while oxidation of lysine evidently continues in the accreting elastin and collagen fibrils that accumulate in the extracellular space. Many different cross-linkage compounds which may be intrachain or join 2, 3, or 4 polypeptide chains have been identified or strongly implicated in elastin and collagen. The summary schemes for their chemistry and formation (Fig. 2A, B, and C) can account for the biosynthesis of those cross-linkages indicated. Recent reviews on the chemistry and biosynthesis of the cross-linkages have appeared (Eyre *et al.*, 1984; Robins, 1983; Paz *et al.*, 1982; Rucker and Murray, 1978).

1. Elastin Cross-Linkages

The aldol condensation product and dehydrolysinonorleucine compounds appear to be intramolecular products, the former arising from the condensation of aldehydes generated from two lysine residues separated by three intervening alanine residues and the latter arising from Schiff base formation between an unmodified lysine and an oxidized lysine residue between which two alanine residues intervene, as deduced from sequencing of cross-linked elastin peptides (Fig. 2A; Foster *et al.*, 1974). The desmosine-type cross-linkages are proposed to arise from various possible condensation reactions (Davis, 1978; Rucker and Murray, 1978), one of which is shown (Fig. 2B), between the aldol and Schiff base cross-linkage, the product of which, following dehydration of the condensed product, is a peptidyl dihydrodesmosine structure linking two chains. Dihydrodesmosine may be a quantitatively important form of the desmosine-type cross-linkages in elastin (Paz *et al.*, 1982), while studies with model compounds indicate that the required oxidation of the dihydro compound prerequisite to desmosine formation can occur simply with molecular oxygen as the oxidant (Davis, 1978). It also appears that both sodium borohydride-reducible (dehydrolysinonorleucine) and prereduced (lysinonorleucine) forms of the Schiff base cross-linkage are found in elastin (Lent and Franzblau,

1967). It has been suggested that dehydrolysinonorleucine might serve as an electron acceptor for the oxidation of dihydrodesmosine to desmosine (Piez, 1968), although this has apparently not been experimentally tested.

2. COLLAGEN CROSS-LINKAGES

Both the aldol condensation product and the dehydrolysinonorleucine cross-linkages are common to elastin and collagen. In types I,

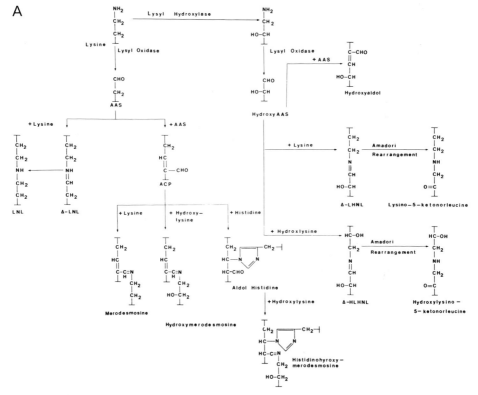

FIG. 2. (A) Summary of cross-linkage biosynthesis. Abbreviations: AAS, α-aminoadipic-δ-semialdehyde; ACP, aldol condensation product; LNL, lysinonorleucine; Δ-LNL, dehydrolysinonorleucine; Δ-LHNL, dehydrolysinohydroxynorleucine; Δ-HLHNL, dehydrohydroxylysinohydroxynorleucine. *Note:* Cross-linkages involving only lysine precursors are found in elastin and collagen; cross-linkages involving hydroxylysine precursors are restricted to collagen. (B) Proposed pathway for desmosine biosynthesis. (Adapted from the review of Rucker and Murray, 1978.) (C) Proposed pathway of hydroxypyridinium cross-linkage of collagen (Eyre *et al.*, 1984).

B

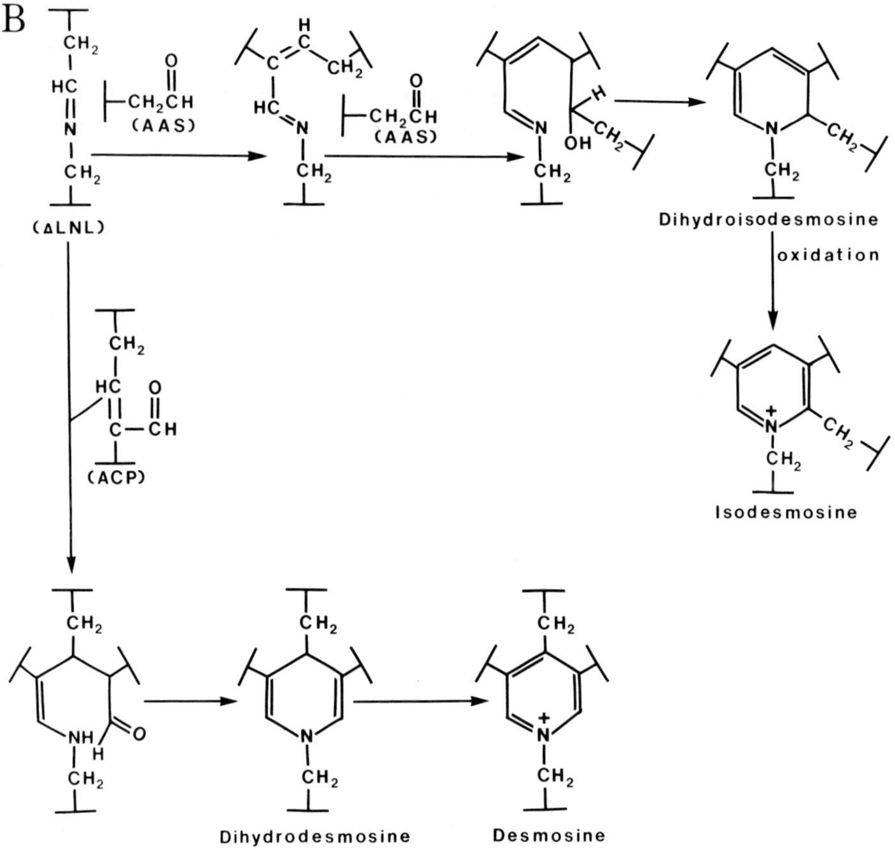

(ΔLNL)

(AAS)

(AAS)

Dihydroisodesmosine

oxidation

Isodesmosine

(ACP)

Dihydrodesmosine

Desmosine

C

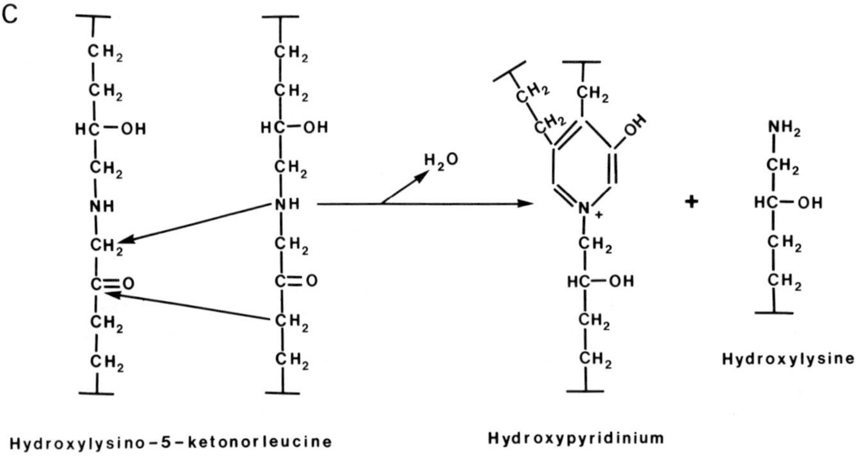

H_2O

Hydroxylysino-5-ketonorleucine

Hydroxypyridinium

NH_2

Hydroxylysine

II, and III collagens, the former predominantly serves as an intramolecular cross-linkage between N-terminal telopeptide regions of alpha chains within tropocollagen units while Schiff base as well as more complex, multivalent cross-linkages, each of which may involve lysine or hydroxylysine and the aldehydes derived therefrom, predominantly participate in intermolecular condensations (Fig. 2A; Eyre *et al.*, 1984; Rucker and Murray, 1978). In contrast to elastin, naturally reduced forms of Schiff base or of other more complex cross-linkages have yet to be identified in collagen, as recently reviewed (Eyre *et al.*, 1984). As noted, cross-linking in collagen and elastin differ by virtue of the presence of hydroxylysine in collagen and its participation in the formation of certain collagen cross-linkages. The hydroxylated amino acid may be oxidized to the corresponding semialdehyde or it may directly participate in Schiff base formation through its ε-amino group with a hydroxylysine- or lysine-derived aldehyde residue. Thus, hydroxylysinonorleucine and dihydrosylysinonorleucine each are intermolecular cross-linkages in collagen (Bailey and Fowler, 1969; Kang, 1972; Mechanic *et al.*, 1971). Such hydroxylated cross-linkages also exist as glycosylated derivatives, as noted by the finding that 80% of the DHLNL of bovine amnion type III collagen exists as the glucosylgalactosyl derivative (Cannon and Davison, 1978), while glycosylated cross-linkages have also been found in type I and type II collagens as well (Robins and Bailey, 1974). Cross-linkages derived from hydroxylysine may undergo Amidori rearrangement to keto forms, as illustrated in Fig. 2A, providing additional stability to the collagen molecule. Thus, 5-ketolysinonorleucine is more stable to hydrolysis than is dehydrolysinonorleucine (Robins and Bailey, 1974). Collagen also contains a polyfunctional fluorescent cross-linkage identified as the 3-hydroxypyridinium moiety (Fujimoto *et al.*, 1978) proposed to derive from two hydroxylysyl aldehydes and a hydroxylysine residue (Fig. 2C; Eyre and Oguchi, 1980). Siegel *et al.* (1982) have supported the conclusion that this is a natural component of collagen by demonstrating that it is synthesized *in vitro* following the oxidation of isolated chick calvaria collagen by purified lysyl oxidase. In similar fashion, Siegel and Lian (1975) demonstrated the lysyl oxidase-dependent synthesis of the tetrafunctional cross-linkage, dehydrohistidinohydroxymerodesmosine, in collagen *in vitro,* the existence of which as a natural component of collagen had been questioned (Robins and Bailey, 1973). In addition to these processes of cross-linkage synthesis, Rigby *et al.* (1977) and Bailey *et al.* (1977) have found evidence for the further, oxygen-mediated nonenzymatic oxidation of Schiff base linkages in collagen to isopeptide linkages, resulting in the isolation of aminoadipic acid from collagen hydrolysates. Such peptide linkages between lysine-derived side chains would be expected to stabilize and further insolubilize collagen, consistent with connective tissue changes occurring in ageing. The effect of increased cross-linkage content on collagen stability was emphasized by the demonstration that the generation of as little as 0.1 cross-linkage per mole of collagen consequent to lysyl oxidase action markedly increases the resistance of collagen fibrils to digestion by human synovial collagenase (Vater *et al.,* 1979).

D. *Cross-Linkages in Other Macromolecules*

Citations have now appeared in the literature which indicate that elastin and collagen are likely not the only macromolecules to contain lysine-derived peptidyl aldehydes and cross-linkages. Thus, Diedrich and Schnaitman (1978) and Mirelman and Siegel (1979) independently reported the existence of peptidyl α-aminoadipic-δ-semialdehyde in the major outer membrane proteins of *Escherichia coli.* Diedrich and Schnaitman (1978) speculated that the aldehyde may subsequently form a Schiff base cross-linkage with diaminopimelic acid of the peptidoglycan layer which lies between the outer layer and the cytoplasmic membrane of *E. coli.* Indeed, Mirelman and Siegel (1978) identified AAS and two additional products in hydrolysates of cell envelopes, the latter two consistent with Schiff base products derived in part from AAS. These authors further demonstrated the time-dependent release of tritium from cell envelopes labeled with [6-³H]lysine, consistent with the enzyme-catalyzed oxidation of peptidyl lysine.

The observation that egg shell membranes from copper-deficient hens show structural defects and faulty shell deposition (Baumgartner *et al.,* 1978) raised the possibility that egg shell membrane protein may also contain cross-linkages similar to those in connective tissue proteins. Indeed, desmosine, isodesmosine, AAS, and the aldol condensation product, as well as hydroxylated proline and lysine residues (Starcher and King, 1980; Leach *et al.,* 1978; Crombie *et al.,* 1981), have been identified in preparations of egg shell membrane protein. The contents of AAS and the aldol each far exceed the relatively small contents of desmosine, leading to the suggestion that the desmosine cross-linkage may not be critical to the function of this protein or may develop slowly with time (Crombie *et al.,* 1981; Starcher and King, 1980). It is of particular interest that there appears to be no lysyl oxidase activity in the membrane but that this enzyme activity and copper content are discretely located in the isthmus of the oviduct (Harris *et al.,* 1980a), raising the interesting possibility that the oviduct enzyme may catalyze lysine oxidation on the egg membrane as it passes through the isthmus. Since shell deposition occurs subsequent to the passage of the egg past the site of lysyl oxidase activity at the isthmus, it may be that the oxidation of lysine is a prerequisite to shell deposition.

III. ASSAY AND PURIFICATION OF LYSYL OXIDASE

A. Methods of Assay

Methods of assay have been developed which permit definition of the activity of lysyl oxidase against collagen or elastin substrates *in vitro* (Pinnell and Martin, 1968; Siegel *et al.*, 1970b; Siegel, 1974) as well as against nonpeptidyl amines (Trackman and Kagan, 1979; Trackman *et al.*, 1981) and other protein substrates (Kagan *et al.*, 1984). The former method is discontinuous and most commonly utilizes forms of collagen or elastin biosynthetically labeled in organ culture with [6-^{3}H]- or [4,5-^{3}H]lysine in the presence of the lysyl oxidase inhibitor BAPN. Addition of lysyl oxidase to the [6-^{3}H]- or [4,5-^{3}H]lysine-containing forms of elastin or collagen leads to the catalytic release of a tritium ion which can exchange with water. The ^{3}HHO formed can be isolated from the assay mixture by distillation, and its radioactivity can be quantified by liquid scintillation spectrometry. Modifications which facilitate this assay method have been described (Misiorowski *et al.*, 1976; Melet *et al.*, 1977). Tritiated collagen substrates are commonly prepared from 16-day chick embryo calvaria pulsed in culture with tritiated lysine and are optimally active as substrates as reconstituted collagen fibrils (Siegel, 1974). Elastin substrates are prepared from similarly cultured and pulsed 16-day chick embryo aortae (Pinnell and Martin, 1968). The saline insoluble aortic pellet is 88% elastin and 12% collagen, but the collagen can be removed by treatment with purified bacterial collagenase (Narayanan *et al.*, 1974b; Stassen, 1976). Background rates of tritium release may be substantial due to endogenous lysyl oxidase tightly bound to the isolated elastin pellet, but this can be controlled by prior inactivation of the pellet with 1 N HCl (Kagan *et al.*, 1974). Siegel and Fu (1976) similarly noted that endogenous enzyme in calvarial collagen substrates may be inactivated by inclusion of 5 mM BAPN during preincubation of the collagen at 37°C while forming reconstituted fibrils. Purified tropoelastin is also oxidized by lysyl oxidase *in vitro* and incorporated into a preexistent elastin matrix (Narayanan *et al.*, 1978). Desmosine formation was favored at temperatures which enhance coacervation of the tropoelastin substrate. A tritiated, soluble substrate for lysyl oxidase, presumably composed of soluble forms of elastin and collagen, is released into the medium during incubation of chick embryo aortae with [^{3}H]lysine in culture (Harris et al., 1974). Although the specific substrate proteins of these preparations have not been characterized, this soluble material, normally a by-product in the preparation of the insoluble aortic elastin substrate, is a useful substrate for the assay of lysyl oxidase activity.

Although of limited use for establishing initial or relative rates of activity, elastin or collagen substrates labeled with [^{14}C]lysine are of value in assessing the specific aldehyde or crosslinkage products generated by the enzyme in vitro (Pinnell and Martin, 1968). Enzymatically generated [^{14}C]α-aminoadipic-δ-semialdehyde is oxidized with performic acid to the acid-stable [^{14}C]α-aminoadipic acid product which can be identified upon amino acid analysis of the hydrolyzed substrate analyzing both for ninhydrin-reactive peaks and by monitoring radioactivity in fractions collected from the column effluent. Similarly, aldehyde or cross-linkage products of enzyme activity in vitro may be assessed by split-stream amino acid analysis of base- or acid-hydrolyzed aliquots of sodium borohydride-reduced [^{3}H]lysine- or [^{14}C]lysine-labeled substrates (Lent and Franzblau, 1967). Reduction with the borohydride reagent converts aldehydes to base-stable alcohol derivatives and Schiff base adducts to acid- or base-stable secondary amines. It is always advisable to confirm that tritium release from [^{3}H]lysine-labeled substrates reflects aldehyde and/or cross-linkage formation by such analytical procedures.

The finding that lysyl oxidase can also utilize soluble nonpeptidyl alkyl mono- or diamines (Trackman and Kagan, 1979) permitted the development of a continuous fluorometric peroxidase-coupled assay for H_2O_2 release which stoichiometrically accompanies aldehyde formation (Trackman et al., 1981; Fig. 3). Initial rates of product release are linear with time and, if purified enzyme is used, with the amount of enzyme assayed. Further, the assay is quite sensitive (0.1–5 nmol min^{-1}). However, the reaction kinetics deviate from linearity as the assay continues, reflecting the fact that lysyl oxidase undergoes self-catalyzed inactivation coincident with the processing of amines (Kagan et al., 1983a). Partial protection against autoinactivation is afforded by the inclusion of certain antioxidants in the assay, consistent with evidence for the release of hydroxy radical during amine oxidation (Kagan et al., 1983a). Optimal rates in this assay system are obtained in 1.2 M urea, likely due to the prevention of the formation of enzyme aggregates which are presumed not to be catalytically efficient (Kagan et al., 1983a; Jordan et al., 1977). Activity toward 1,5-diamino-

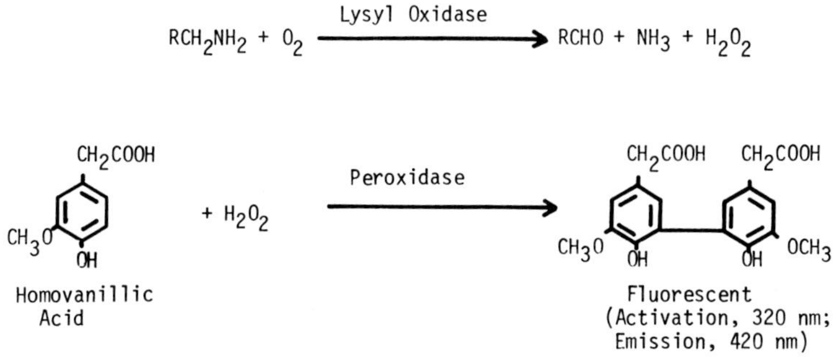

$$\text{RCH}_2\text{NH}_2 + \text{O}_2 \xrightarrow{\text{Lysyl Oxidase}} \text{RCHO} + \text{NH}_3 + \text{H}_2\text{O}_2$$

FIG. 3. Peroxidase-coupled assay for lysyl oxidase activity.

pentane is inhibited by BAPN with a K_i of 6 μM (Tang et al., 1983) thus approximating the sensitivity of oxidation of elastin or collagen substrates to inhibition by this agent. This assay has proven to be valuable for explorations of the specificity and mechanism of the purified enzyme.

B. Methods of Purification

Most purification schemes thus far employed for the isolation of lysyl oxidase have followed similar patterns. Each takes advantage of the stability of lysyl oxidase in 6 M urea solutions and the fact that inclusion of 6 M urea in elution buffers improves chromatographic recoveries and resolution of the enzyme (Narayanan et al., 1974b). The use of urea proved to be of even greater advantage when it was found that lysyl oxidase is largely insoluble in saline buffers but is readily solubilized by buffers supplemented with 4 to 6 M urea (Harris et al., 1974; Kagan et al., 1974; Stassen, 1976; Shieh and Yasunobu, 1976; Siegel and Fu, 1976; Jordan et al., 1977). Discrete quantities of saline-soluble lysyl oxidase activity can be extracted from connective tissues, including chick embryo bone (Siegel et al., 1970b), mature chicken aorta (Harris et al., 1974), and chick embryo aorta (Kagan et al., 1974). The saline-soluble fraction represents only a small fraction (~6%) of the total activity in chicken aorta (Harris et al., 1974). The saline-extractable enzyme was partially purified from chick embryo bone in the complete absence of urea (Siegel et al., 1970b). As eventually proved to be true of the urea-solubilized enzyme, this preparation required enzyme-bound copper and molecular oxygen for activity and exhibited a pH optimum of approximately 7.7. The salt-soluble enzyme of chick embryo aorta also demonstrates these catalytic properties and is inhibited by carbonyl reagents (Kagan *et al.*, 1974), in further similarity to the urea-soluble enzyme. The molecular weight of the partially purified cartilage enzyme approximated 170,000 under native conditions by gel exclusion chromatography. This value is considerably larger than that found for the urea-solubilized enzyme in sodium dodecyl sulfate (SDS) and may reflect enzyme aggregates (Jordan *et al.*, 1977) or complexes of enzyme with soluble macromolecular substrates. Although the urea- and saline-soluble forms exhibit catalytic similarities, the fact that continued extraction with saline does not solubilize that enzyme fraction eventually solubilized by urea is suggestive of a discrete difference between the two forms, the nature of which remains unknown.

The urea-soluble enzyme has been purified from chick embryo cartilage (Siegel and Fu, 1976; Stassen, 1976; Rowe *et al.*, 1977), chicken aorta (Harris *et al.*, 1974), bovine aorta (Vidal *et al.*, 1975; Kagan *et al.*, 1979), bovine ligament (Jordan *et al.*, 1977), bovine lung (Shieh and Yasunobu, 1976; Cronlund, 1983), bovine cartilage (Sullivan and Kagan, 1982), turkey aorta (Narayanan *et al.*, 1982), and human placenta (Kuivaniemi *et al.*, 1984). Most of these studies have taken advantage of the solubility properties of the enzyme by first extracting the bulk of saline-soluble components before solubilizing lysyl oxidase with urea. Data of several purification studies are summarized in Table I. As noted, most purification methods follow similar patterns, employing various sequences of application of urea extracts, after dilution to lower the urea concentration, to collagen–Sepharose and DEAE–cellulose chromatography (Siegel and Fu, 1976). The tendency of bovine ligament and aortic lysyl oxidase to self-aggregate in the absence of urea but to disocciate to 32,000-Da species in 6 M urea (Jordan *et al.*, 1977) led to the use of molecular exclusion chromatography in 6 M urea as an effective final purification of enzyme partially purified by passage through collagen–Sepharose CL 4B and then DEAE–cellulose (Kagan *et al.*, 1979; Cronlund, 1983; Kuivaniemi *et al.*, 1984). Lysyl oxidase is not eluted from DEAE or collagen–Sepharose by neutral salt buffers but is eluted from the collagen affinity support by 6 M urea and from DEAE by salt in 6 M urea buffers. While enzyme binding to DEAE doubtlessly involves ionic interactions with the cationic matrix, the requirement for urea implies that other nonionic, possibly hydrophobic bonds are also involved. Alternatively, conformational changes induced by high urea concentrations may alter the state of aggregation and the charge density of the matrix-bound enzyme to facilitate elution from collagen–Sepharose directly and from DEAE in the presence of salt.

TABLE I

Purification of Lysyl Oxidase from Various Tissues[a]

Reference[b]	Source	Purification sequence	Heterogeneity (variants)	Molecular weight(s) $\times 10^{-3}$	Inhibitors
1	Chick embryo cartilage	PBS; AS ppn; pH ppn; BioGel		170 (Native)	
2	Chick aorta	U; DE; Affin-OCMP	2	61; 59 (SDS)	Carbonyl reagents
3	Bovine lung	U; AS ppn; DE; Affin	2	80; 160 (Native) 53; 28 (SDS)	BAPN (>1 mM); Cu chelators
4	Turkey aorta	U; Affin		100; 77; 52; others (SDS)	BAPN
5	Chick cartilage	U; Affin; DE; DE	4	28 (SDS)	
6	Bovine aorta	U; Affin; DE; Sephacryl	4	32 (SDS)	Carbonyl reagents; Cu chelators; BAPN
7	Bovine ligament	U; Affin; DE; Sephacryl	4	32 (SDS)	
8	Bovine lung	U; Affin; DE; Sephacryl	4	29–34 (SDS)	BAPN
9	Human placenta	U; Affin; DE; Sephacryl	4	30	
10	Calf aorta smooth muscle cells	Elastin–Hydrogel; HPLC		~30	

[a] Abbreviations are as follows: Affin, chromatography or collagen–Sepharose affinity columns; Affin-OCMP, chromatography with chick embryo aorta organ culture media proteins coupled to Sepharose; AS ppn, ammonium sulfate precipitation; BAPN, β-aminopropionitrile; BioGel, chromatography with BioGel; DE, DEAE–cellulose chromatography; Elastin–Hydrogel, chromatography with elastin coupled to Hydrogel; HPLC, high performance liquid chromatography; PBS, phosphate-buffered saline extraction; SDS, sodium dodecyl sulfate gel electrophoresis; Sephacryl, chromatography with Sephacryl. U, 4 or 6 M urea extraction.

[b] Numbered references are as follows: 1, Siegel et al. (1970); 2, Harris et al. (1974); 3, Shieh and Yasunobu (1976); 4, Narayanan et al. (1982); 5, Stassen (1976); 6, Kagan et al. (1979); 7, Jordan et al. (1977); 8, Cronlund (1983); 9, Kuivaniemi et al. (1984); 10, Ferrara et al. (1982).

In addition to these preparations of lysyl oxidase, Serrafini-Fracassini *et al.* (1981) isolated a 34.4-kDa glycoprotein from bovine ligamentum nuchae by extraction in guanidine in 2-mercaptoethanol while further purification involved alcohol precipitation. Although these approaches are distinctly different from the more common procedures summarized in Table I, this preparation displayed lysyl oxidase activity toward the chick embryo aortic elastin substrate as well as toward free lysine. However, this enzyme was unusually resistant to BAPN ($I_{50} > 270$ μM versus an I_{50} of 5–10 μM for the aortic enzyme). The urea-soluble bovine aortic lysyl oxidase does not appear to be a glycoprotein (Sullivan and Kagan, 1982), in further dissimilarity to this preparation. Nevertheless, similarities between the isolated guanidine soluble enzyme with structural glycoproteins apparently closely associated with nascent elastic fibers (Robert *et al.*, 1971; Pasquali-Ronchetti, 1981, 1984; Gibson and Cleary, 1982) raises possibilities concerning the role of the catalytically active glycoprotein isolated by Serrafini-Fracassini *et al.* (1981) in connective tissue fiber synthesis.

IV. PHYSICAL PROPERTIES

A. *Molecular Weight*

There is a long-standing ambiguity in the assessment of the molecular weight of lysyl oxidase, as inspection of Table I clearly demonstrates. Thus, the enzyme purified from chick embryo cartilage has been reported to have a molecular weight in SDS of 28,000 (Stassen, 1976) and 62,000 (Siegel and Fu, 1976). It may not be coincidental that those preparative schemes which first apply enzyme to collagen–Sepharose and then to DEAE–cellulose, followed either by rechromatography on DEAE or by gel exclusion chromatography in urea yield apparently homogeneous products with molecular weights between 28,000 and 34,000 (preparations 5 through 10, Table I). Conversely, purification schemes first employing chromatography through DEAE (preparations 1 through 4) yield single (preparation 1) or double (preparation 2) bands approximating 60,000 MW or result in multiple bands, the most prominent of which equal or exceed 52,000. Preparation 8 of bovine lung (Table I) yielded enzyme unusually resistant to BAPN ($I_{50} > 1$ mM) and thus may have contained other amine oxidases, while preparation 4 of turkey aorta employed purification conditions usually insufficient to completely purify aortic lysyl oxidase of other species and they may have contained other proteins in the final product. Narayanan *et al.* (1982) employed a mixture of synthetic protease inhibitors in Preparation 4 and suggested that the higher molecular weight products obtained were due to inhibition of proteolysis during the purification which may otherwise lead to the 30,000-MW band. Nevertheless, purifying the bovine aortic enzyme in the PMSF–EDTA–iodoacetamide mixture used by Narayanan et al. (1982) employing the purification sequence indicated in preparation 6 still yields the 32,000-MW product in approximately 95% purity (H. Kagan, unpublished observations). Nevertheless, it has been noted that the 32,000-MW band slowly degrades in vitro yielding a 24,000-MW band and other products (Sullivan and Kagan, 1982) while the human placenta enzyme (MW 30,000) copurifies with a band of approximately 24,000 MW which also appears to derive from the 30,000-MW product (Kuivaniemi et al., 1984). Thus, it remains possible that the varied molecular weights for the enzyme isolated from the same tissue by different chromatographic sequences (e.g., preparation 1 versus preparation 5) may be due to proteolysis since one sequence may concentrate a protease together with the enzyme while another may separate such a protease from the enzyme early in the preparative procedure. While the tendency of the enzyme to aggregate in the absence of urea (Jordan et al., 1977) may also account for higher molecular weights obtained, such aggregates would of necessity be linked by nondisulfide covalent bonds since the higher molecular weight bands were observed in SDS gels in disulfide reductants. It does appear, however, that the purification sequence utilized for the bovine aortic enzyme results in products of ~30,000 MW from different tissues.

Uncertainty also remains about the molecular weight of the functional unit of lysyl oxidase in vivo. Further, it should be noted that the use of denaturing levels of urea in the isolation of the enzyme coupled with the separation methods employed may well result in the resolution and ultimate loss of a regulatory subunit yet to be identified. Since lysyl oxidase is secreted as a soluble protein in cell culture (Layman et al., 1972; Ferrera et al., 1982), although urea-extractable enzyme also exists in such cultures apparently in tight association with the extracellular matrix (Ferrera et al., 1982), cell culture systems seem to offer opportunities for characterizing physical properties under urea-free conditions and to compare saline-soluble and urea-soluble enzyme forms.

B. Enzyme Variants

As noted in Table I, lysyl oxidase of various tissues resolves into multiple functional enzyme species upon gradient elution from DEAE in 6 M urea. At least four peaks resolve from urea extracts of chick cartilage (Stassen *et al.*, 1976), bovine aorta (Kagan *et al.*, 1979), or human placenta (Kuivaniemi *et al.*, 1984) if a sufficiently shallow salt gradient is employed. The four peaks individually purified from bovine aorta are closely related species as evidenced by the nearly identical peptide maps obtained from trypsin or *Staphylococcus aureus* V8 protease digests of each, by their common N-terminal Asx residue, by their common subunit molecular weight of 32,000 ± 800, and by their essentially identical substrate specificities toward collagen, elastin, and alkylamines (Sullivan and Kagan, 1982). The amino acid compositions of the first three and most prominent bovine aortic peaks, the mean compositions of the first two and last two peaks, respectively, of the DEAE chromatogram of the human placental enzymes, and one of the purified chick cartilage peaks are compared in Table II. The compositions of these enzymes are similar although not identical to each other. Although amide contents have not been established, the enzymes appear to be predominantly anionic in character, consistent with their affinities for DEAE–cellulose. The origin of the enzyme variants remains obscure although it seems reasonable, given the potential for proteolysis of lysyl oxidase, as noted, that the multiple peaks might arise by proteolytic modifications of a common precursor, although multiple genomic origin also remains a possibility. The very similar if not identical substrate specificities of each form argues against a unique biological role for each species. Studies on the sequence and biosynthesis of lysyl oxidase should provide further insights into this matter.

C. Cofactors of Lysyl Oxidase

1. COPPER

Nutritional copper deficiency results in connective tissue defects quite similar to those seen in BAPN-induced experimental lathyrism, notably including fragmentation and dissolution of aortic elastic laminae eventually resulting in aortic aneurysm (Shields *et al.*, 1962; O'Dell *et al.*, 1961). The biochemical correlates also parallel those seen in BAPN-treated animals and include decreased aldehyde and increased soluble collagen in tendon (Chou *et al.*, 1969) and increased lysine and decreased desmosines in aortic (Miller *et al.*, 1965) and lung elastin (Buckingham *et al.*, 1981). Early reports had implicated copper-dependent monoamine or diamine oxidases as the molecular sites which are affected by copper deficiency since activity of these enzymes decreased in parallel with the development of connective tissue abnor-

TABLE II

AMINO ACID COMPOSITIONS OF LYSYL OXIDASE OF DIFFERENT TISSUES

	Residues per 1000 residues					
	Bovine aorta[a]			Human placenta[b]		Chick cartilage[c]
Residue	Peak I	Peak II	Peak III	Pool I	Pool II	
Asx	121	125	122	125	123	136
Thr	57	57	55	59	55	53
Ser	104	86	104	98	101	82
Glx	113	136	136	133	130	106
Pro	60	51	50	57	58	58
Gly	120	87	108	114	111	97
Ala	71	81	83	77	75	66
Val	39	42	35	51	48	39
Cys	27	24	18	ND[d]	ND	30
Met	15	16	15	ND	ND	15
Ile	30	27	31	33	33	40
Leu	64	86	78	73	77	67
Tyr	25	31	21	24	22	65
Phe	27	30	26	31	34	27
Lys	31	36	36	46	47	31
His	39	25	27	27	29	29
Arg	56	61	56	52	57	59

[a] Data of Kagan et al. (1979).

[b] Data of Kuivaniemi et al. (1984), presented as the means of compositions of DEAE peaks I and II (pool I) and of DEAE peaks III and IV (pool II).

[c] Data of Stassen (1976). Represents composition of fourth enzymatically active peak eluted from DEAE–cellulose.

[d] ND, not determined.

malities (Kim and Hill, 1966; Page and Benditt, 1967; Rucker et al., 1970; Rucker and Goetlich-Reimann, 1972), while an aortic monoamine oxidase preparation had been shown to oxidize both benzylamine and peptidyllysine (Rucker et al., 1970). A more highly purified preparation of an aortic benzylamine oxidase did not oxidize lysine in a tritiated elastin substrate, however, suggesting that the earlier report reflected contamination by lysyl oxidase (Shieh et al., 1975). However, other preparations of monoamine oxidases of bovine serum (Oda et al., 1981) and dental pulp (Nakano et al., 1974) were weakly active against endopeptidyl lysine in various synthetic oligopeptides although the enzyme of dental pulp was inactive against collagen and elastin and was less sensitive to inhibition by BAPN than urea-soluble lysyl oxidase (Nakano et al., 1974). In this regard, a copper-requiring diamine oxidase of human placenta was found to utilize tropocollagen as a substrate (Crabbe, 1979). Although this enzyme was inhibited by BAPN, the inhibition was only expressed after several minutes of incubation at 37°C and appeared to require levels of BAPN in excess of the usual sensitivity of urea-soluble lysyl oxidase. A water-extractable histaminase activity of pig aorta has been shown to oxidize lysine in synthetic polypeptides and in an elastin substrate. This enzyme activity is similarly inhibited by copper chelators and carbonyl reagents (Buffoni and Raimondi, 1981; Buffoni et al., 1981). Thus, although each of these amine oxidases are copper dependent, their importance in the oxidation of lysine in collagen and elastin is not immediately evident although the possibility that these varied amine oxidases may oxidize peptidyllysine in vivo is intriguing.

The report of Pinnell and Martin (1968) of an amine oxidase in chick cartilage which oxidized lysine in an elastin substrate appears to be the first demonstration in vitro of enzyme activity apparently specific for the oxidation of lysine in connective tissue proteins and which exhibited the expected sensitivity to BAPN. Subsequent studies on this enzyme established its requirement for copper for catalytic function (Siegel et al., 1970b), as illustrated by the inhibition of this enzyme as well as preparations of lysyl oxidase of other chick connective tissues by various copper chelators, including α,α'-dipyridyl (Siegel et al., 1970b; Kagan et al., 1974), 8-hydroxyquinoline (Kagan et al., 1974), and diethyldithiocarbamate (Harris et al., 1974; Shieh and Yasunobu, 1976). More direct evidence for a catalytic role of enzyme-bound copper was shown by the inactivation of enzyme upon removal of copper by dialysis against chelators (Siegel et al., 1970b) or by acid precipitation (Harris et al., 1974) and by the restoration of enzyme activity by addition of cupric ion to the apo-lysyl oxidase preparation. Both cobaltous and ferrous ion (Siegel et al., 1970b) were partially effective in restoring activity. Direct measurements of enzyme-bound copper revealed that the highly purified chicken aortic enzyme contains 0.75 g atom of copper per 60,000-MW subunit (Harris et al., 1974) while the bovine aortic enzyme contained 0.7 g atom per 32,000-MW subunit (Tang et al., 1983). Since the stoichiometries differ from unity, it is possible that these values reflect partial loss of cofactor in vivo or during purification. The peptidyl amine oxidase isolated from bovine lung (Shieh and Yasunobu, 1976) contained approximately 1 g atom of copper per 70,000-MW subunit, which ESR analysis indicated to be predominantly in the cupric state. As noted, this enzyme preparation was unusually resistant to BAPN, thus cautioning against extrapolation of its properties to more typically sensitive forms of lysyl oxidase.

The bovine aortic enzyme yielded EPR parameters consistent with the conclusion that the copper in the resting enzyme is in the copper(II) state in a tetragonally elongated octahedral environment with at least two nitrogen ligand atoms (Greenaway et al., 1984).

2. CARBONYL COFACTOR

The presence of a second cofactor with carbonyl reactivity in lysyl oxidase has long been suspected. Thus, the administration of compounds with reactivity toward carbonyl functions, including ureides, hydrazines, and hydrazides, caused severe defects in connective tissues and increased the solubility of collagen in chick embryos (Levene, 1961). Among these agents, administration of iproniazid decreased and/or altered the ratio of cross-linkages in chick aortic elastin and tendon collagen (Chou et al., 1970; Wimmerova et al., 1980). Inhibition of lysyl oxidase activity in vitro by micro- to millimolar concentrations of isoniazid, iproniazid, phenylhydrazine, hydroxylamine, cyanide, or bisulfite further supported the presence of a functional carbonyl in this enzyme (Harris et al., 1974; Kagan et al., 1974; Arem and Misiorowski, 1976). The antituberculous efficacy of isoniazid (INH) appears related to its lathyrogenic capacity by its ability to inhibit collagen deposition around tubercles (Levene, 1961; Arem and Misiorowski, 1976). Hydralazine, a substituted hydrazine analogous to INH, has antihypertensive properties and proved to be a potent (I_{50} 30 μM), irreversible inhibitor of chick aortic lysyl oxidase in vitro (Numata et al., 1981). Since this compound also inhibits prolyl hydroxylase (Bhatnagar et al., 1972), the lathyrogenic activity of hydralazine may reflect its interference both with hydroxylation of collagen and with cross-linkage formation. Reduced forms of disulfhydryl compounds, e.g., dithiothreitol (DTT), inhibit lysyl oxidase irreversibly in vitro (Misiorowski and Werner, 1978; Harris et al., 1974). It was suggested that the inhibition was due to complexing of DTT with an enzyme carbonyl, since disulfhydryl compounds can form stable bifunctional derivatives of aldehydes, while the enzyme was not inhibited by corresponding concentrations of 2-mercaptoethanol or by iodoacetamide, arguing against disulfides or free sulfhydryls as the DTT-susceptible target (Misiorowski and Werner, 1978).

The lathyrogenic effects of ureides, hydrazides, and hydrazines were significantly reversed by treatment with pyridoxal (PL) (Levene, 1961) or pyridoxal phosphate (PLP) in vivo or in organ culture (Rucker and O'Dell, 1970) thus implicating PL or PLP as a carbonyl cofactor of lysyl oxidase. Consistent with this hypothesis, pyridoxine-deficient diets decreased the levels of newly synthesized cross-linkages in aortic elastin in chicks (Starcher, 1969) and in skin and bone collagens of chick or rat (Fujii *et al.*, 1979), while vitamin B_6 deficiency (Murray *et al.*, 1978) or administration of isoniazid (Carrington *et al.*, 1984) also decreased the activities of salt- or urea-soluble cartilage lysyl oxidase. Administration of pyridoxine restored enzyme levels in the dietary model of vitamin B_6 deficiency (Murray *et al.*, 1978) in isoniazid-treated but not in BAPN-treated embryos (Carrington *et al.*, 1984). It is notable that the urea-soluble aortic enzyme activity was not significantly changed by vitamin B_6 deficiency (Murray *et al.*, 1978) while administration of 4-deoxypyridine, a vitamin B_6 antagonist, reduced urea-extractable chick cartilage enzyme activity only by 26% (Bird and Levene, 1983). Notably, lysyl oxidase levels respond to dietary changes in other vitamins as well. Thus, chick bone enzyme activity increased twofold in response to reduction of vitamin D levels (Gonnerman *et al.*, 1976) while deprivation of thiamin lowered both skin lysyl oxidase activity and wound breaking strength, the latter consistent with decreased cross-linkage content (Alvarez *et al.*, 1982).

While these studies suggest the participation of PL or PLP as a carbonyl cofactor in lysyl oxidase, they do not eliminate indirect effects which may underlie the changes seen in cross-linkage biosynthesis and enzyme activity. Thus, as noted by Levene (1961), free PL or PLP might transiently protect the enzyme against such carbonyl reagents by forming Schiff base complexes with these reagents in solution. It also seems relevant to note that lysyl oxidase activity of rat bone and skin (Sanada *et al.*, 1978) and mouse cervix (Ozasa *et al.*, 1981) increase in response to 17β-estradiol while enzyme activity of new born rat skin was decreased by administration of the glucocorticoid triamcinolone acetate (Benson and LuValle, 1981). Thus, PLP interacts with glucocorticoid (Cake *et al.*, 1978) and estrogen (Muldoon and Cidlowski, 1980) membrane receptors while those glucocorticoid receptors that are capable of being activated are increased as is the rate of steroid translocation to the nucleus in vitamin B_6-deficient rats (DiSorbo *et al.*, 1980). It seems possible, therefore, that alteration in vitamin B_6 levels may indirectly alter levels of lysyl oxidase by perturbation of steroid hormone metabolism. Notably, it has been observed that the content of α-aminoadipic-δ-semialdehyde, the immediate product of lysyl oxidase, is not significantly altered, although the aldol condensation product increases while desmosine content decreases in lung elastin of vitamin B_6-deficient rats (Rucker *et al.*, 1985). These vitamin B_6-deficient animals also exhibited elevated plasma levels of sulfur amino acids, including homocysteine and the disulfide of homocysteine (Myers *et al.*, 1985). Notably, connective tissue defects are also apparent in homocystinuria, including skeletal abnormalities and lens dislocation, suggestive of defects in collagen cross-linking (Rosenberg and Scriver, 1980). One of the three predominant homocystinuric phenotypes appears to involve a deficiency of the vitamin B_6-dependent enzyme, cystathionine-β-synthase (Fig. 4). Since this enzyme utilizes homocysteine as a substrate, increases in homocysteine in vitamin B_6 deficiency or in homocystinuria can be accounted for by the decreased activity of this vitamin B_6-dependent enzyme (Mudd, 1980). Myers *et al.* (1985) noted that the alteration in cross-linkage distribution in elastin of vitamin B_6-deficient rats paralleled those seen in homocystinuria (Jackson, 1973) and those resulting from administration of D-penicillamine (Siegel, 1977). D-Penicillamine can alter and/or decrease cross-linkage formation by virtue of its ability to reversibly derivatize aldehyde functions in elastin and collagen as thiazolidine adducts (Nimni, 1968; Siegel, 1977) and seems to selectively prevent polyfunctional cross-link formation from Schiff base precursors in collagen (Siegel, 1977). Since homocysteine and penicillamine are each aminothiols capable of participating in thiazolidine formation (Fig. 5), it seems possible that cross-linkage defects in vitamin B_6 deficiency could result from the accumulated affect of homocysteine consequent to inhibition of cystathionine-β-synthase (Myers *et al.*, 1985). Since thiazolidine formation is reversible, supplementation of deficient animals with vitamin B_6 could reverse these equilibria upon reactivation of cystathionine-β-synthase thus depleting excess homocysteine levels.

Thus, it is clearly essential to directly characterize a catalytically functional carbonyl at the active site of lysyl oxidase to overcome such possible indirect affects. Such support stems in part from the finding of Murray and Levene (1977) that radioactivity derived from [^{3}H]pyridoxine injected into chick embryos eluted from DEAE coincident with the eluted peak of the chick embryo cartilage lysyl oxidase activity. Treatment of the labeled enzyme preparation with isoniazid eliminated most of the protein-associated label and an equivalent degree of

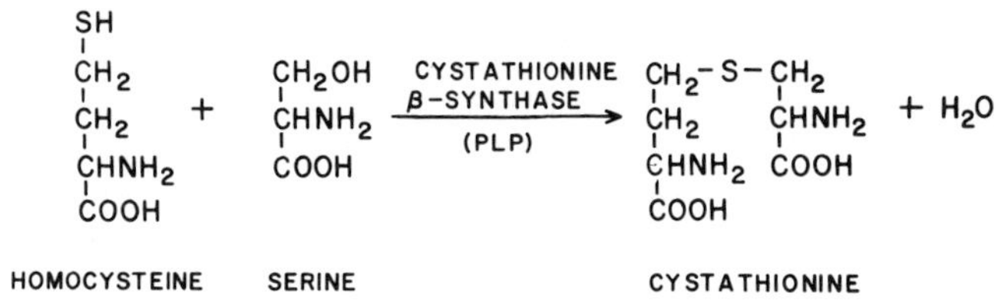

FIG. 4. Reaction catalyzed by cystathionine-β-synthase.

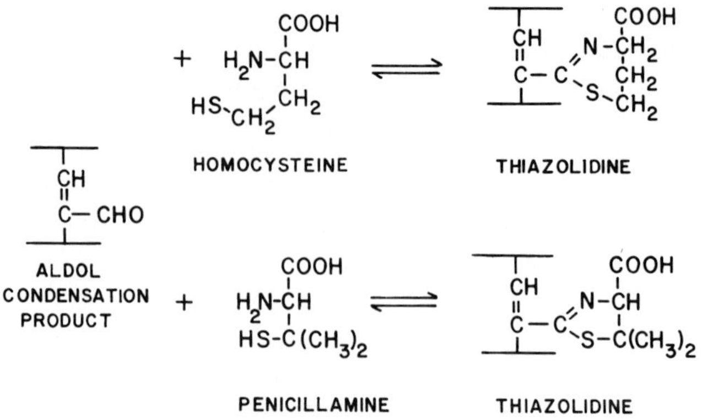

FIG. 5. Thiazolidine formation from homocysteine or D-penicillamine.

enzyme activity. While this result is consistent with the nutritional studies cited, these chemical effects might still reflect the formation of a Schiff base between [^{3}H]pyridoxal and a nonactive site ϵ-amino function of the enzyme which in turn should be displaceable by transimination upon subsequent treatment with isoniazid. Loss of enzyme activity could result from the independent modification of an active site carbonyl by the hydrazide reagent.

The strongest support to date for a cofactor role of PL or PLP in lysyl oxidase is found in the report of Bird and Levene (1982) demonstrating that the loss of activity accompanying illumination or dialysis of the chick embryo aortic enzyme against urea-free buffers is reversed by dialysis against PLP. The fluorescence spectrum of the semicarbazide derivative solubilized from the enzyme after modification with semicarbazide closely resembled that of authentic PLP semicarbazone although the cyanide derivative of the enzyme exhibited a fluorescence emission maximum at 390 nm while that of the cyanide adduct of PLP was at 415 nm. The authors calculated that the chick enzyme contains 2.26 mol of PLP per 31,000-MW subunit. While this study does support a cofactor role for PLP, the unexpected stoichiometry of the cofactor remains to be understood and integrated into a catalytic mechanism, as does the discrepancy of the cyanide spectra.

The characterization of a residue with carbonyl reactivity has also been explored with the urea-extractable enzyme purified from bovine aorta (Williamson et al., 1985) in part by applying a highly sensitive immunoassay procedure specific for protein-bound PLP described by Viceps-Madore et al. (1983). Proteins to be analyzed by this procedure are reduced with sodium borohydride to convert Schiff base linkages by which PLP is commonly bound to apoproteins to secondary amines thus generating stable phosphopyridoxyl protein derivatives. Such samples are then reacted with a monoclonal antibody specific for the phosphopyridoxyl hapten. As shown in Fig. 6, immunoblot analysis of 2.5 nmol of borohydride-reduced bovine aortic lysyl oxidase is completely negative toward this antibody, while positive reactions result with enzyme reduced in the presence of authentic PLP as a control and with 1.1 or 11 pmol of reduced glycogen phosphorylase, a PLP-dependent enzyme. The absorption spectrum of the bovine enzyme differs considerably from that of aspartate aminotransferase, a PLP-dependent enzyme (Fig. 7). Further, [^{14}C]phenylhydrazine forms a covalent bond with lysyl oxidase which is not displaced by dialysis or by dilute acid or base at room temperature (Williamson et al., 1985), a result inconsistent with an aldimine linkage between PLP or another carbonyl with an enzyme amino function in the absence of substrate,

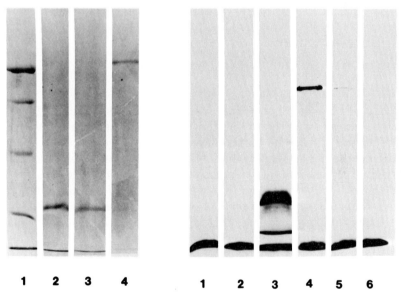

1   2   3   4   1   2   3   4   5   6

FIG. 6. Immunoblot analysis for pyridoxal 5′-phosphate in lysyl oxidase. Left: Coomassie Blue-stained SDS–PAGE gel. Lane 1, molecular weight markers; lane 2, 10 μg reduced lysyl oxidase; lane 3, 10 μg lysyl oxidase reduced in the presence of 5 mM PLP; lane 4, 10 μg reduced phosphorylase *b*. Right: Western immunoblot analysis of SDS–PAGE gel using monoclonal antibody E6(2)2. Lanes 1 through 4 correspond to the same lanes as above; lanes 5 and 6 contain 1.0 and 0.1 μg of reduced phosphorylase *b*, respectively.

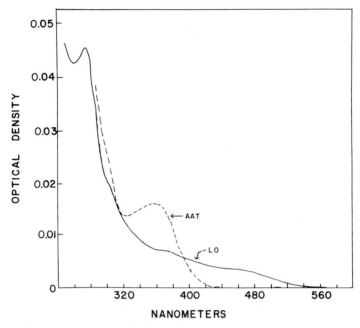

FIG. 7. Absorption spectra of lysyl oxidase (LO, 8×10^{-7} M) and aspartate amino transferase (AAT, 1.3×10^{-6} M). Spectra were recorded at pH 7.7.

although PLP is commonly linked to PLP-dependent proteins through such a linkage. In further dissimilarity to the results obtained with the chick aorta enzyme, the partial loss of activity accompanying dialysis of the bovine aortic enzyme against urea-free phosphate buffer is not prevented or restored by dialysis against or addition to assays of PLP and/or $CuCl_2$. These results thus point toward the presence of a carbonyl compound different from PLP in the bovine enzyme. Research on this aspect of lysyl oxidase thus appears to be following the path taken over several years in the investigation of the carbonyl cofactor of bovine serum monoamine oxidase which was initially thought to be PLP-dependent (Yamada and Yasunobu, 1962). More recent analyses disputed this conclusion (Suva and Abeles, 1978), however. Indeed, Lobenstein-Verbeek *et al.* (1984) have recently isolated a carbonyl chromophore as the dinitrophenylhydrazone from this enzyme whose spectral and chromatographic properties were identical to those of the dinitrophenylhydrazone of pyrroloquinoline quinone (PQQ) (Fig. 8). PQQ shows both carbonyl group functionality and redox behavior and thus could serve an electron accepting role in amine oxidase catalysis

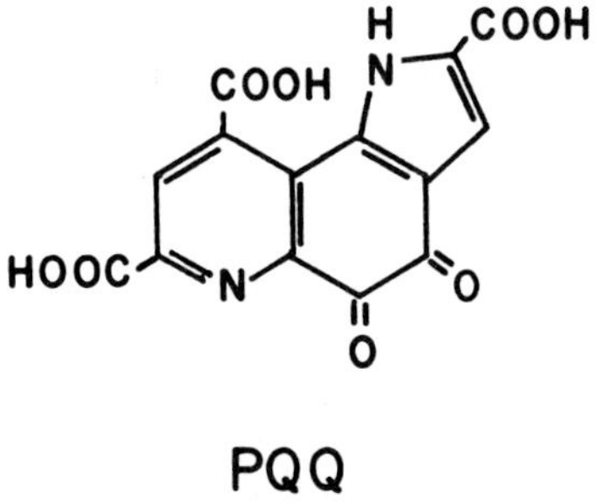

PQQ

FIG. 8. Structure of pyrroloquinoline quinone. (From Duine and Frank, 1981.)

(Duine and Frank, 1981). Further investigation should resolve the possibility that this or a related chromophore is functional in the bovine aortic enzyme while it will also be essential to assess the possibility that lysyl oxidase of different sources may have different functional carbonyls in view of the conclusions of Bird and Levene (1982) concerning the presence of PLP in the chick cartilage enzyme.

V. Catalytic Properties

A. Assay Optima

1. pH

Enzyme prepared from chick or bovine tissues has a bell-shaped pH-rate profile with an optimum approximating pH 8 with elastin or collagen substrates (Pinnell and Martin, 1968; Siegel, 1974; Kagan et al., 1974) or with simple mono- or diamine substrates (Trackman and Kagan, 1979; Trackman et al., 1981).

2. Substrate Concentration

a. *Proteins and Amines.* Saturating kinetics have been obtained with soluble or insoluble elastin (Harris et al., 1974) and with fibrillar collagen substrates (Siegel, 1974). Apparent K_m values of collagen substrates have been reported as 0.85 (Siegel, 1976), 2.4 (Stassen, 1976), and 1.05 μM (Narayanan et al., 1982) while the K_m for tropoelastin assayed with the turkey aortic enzyme is 11.1 μM (Narayanan et al., 1982). Corresponding values for insoluble elastin substrates are more difficult to assess since the enzyme may oxidize both newly incorporated [³H]lysine as well as preexistant unlabeled lysine residues in the insoluble substrate and with an indeterminate and likely differing degree of accessibility of each thus complicating assessment of the effective substrate concentration. Apparent K_m values for mono- or diamine substrates vary from 0.7 to 6.2 mM, depending upon the specific compound in use. 1,5-Diaminopentane is among the more effective of these substrates, with a K_m of 1.1 mM (Tang *et al.*, 1984). These K_m values are 100 to 1000 times greater than those for the various forms of collagen or elastin substrates, consistent with the expectation that peptidyllysine is an optimal substrate for lysyl oxidase. Indeed, the bovine aortic enzyme effectively oxidizes lysine in synthetic oligopeptides with K_m values of approximately 70 to 300 μM depending upon the sequence vicinal to lysine in each peptide (Kagan *et al.*, 1984).

b. Oxygen. Removal of oxygen by purging assay mixtures with nitrogen gas reduces or eliminates enzyme activity against collagen (Siegel *et al.*, 1970b) or elastin (Kagan *et al.*, 1974; Narayanan *et al.*, 1974) substrates, supporting the role of oxygen as a substrate and presumably as an electron acceptor in the lysyl oxidase-catalyzed reaction. Indeed, use of varied oxygen–nitrogen gas mixtures as the gaseous environment for assays of the bovine aortic enzyme activity against the tritiated insoluble elastin substrate yields a hyperbolic curve (Fig. 9) indicative of saturation kinetics and a specific substrate role for oxygen in this enzymatic reaction (Sullivan and Kagan, 1985). Several such experiments have yielded a $K_{m_{app}}$ for oxygen of 17.5 $\pm$

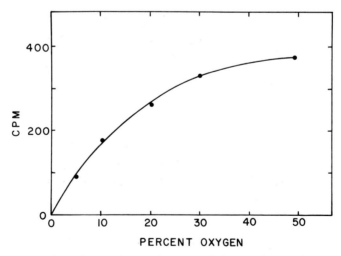

FIG. 9. Oxygen-dependent oxidation of a tritiated elastin substrate by lysyl oxidase. Ordinate: counts per minute of enzyme-dependent ^{3}HHO formed in assay.

3.5%. Since this value approximates or exceeds the concentration of oxygen in the lung and other connective tissues, the rate of the enzyme reaction should be responsive to variations within the physiological range of oxygen concentrations.

3. TEMPERATURE OPTIMUM AND THERMAL STABILITY

The temperature profile for the oxidation of insoluble aortic elastin by lysyl oxidase exhibits an optimum of 52°C, with activity persisting up to 65°C (Kagan et al., 1974). The relatively high optimal temperature likely does not reflect stabilization of the enzyme by its tight association with elastin nor a temperature-dependent change in the structure of elastin since the temperature optimum for the bovine aortic enzyme against the 1,5-diaminopentane substrate is 55°C, quite similar to the optimum with elastin (Trackman et al., 1981). The bovine aortic enzyme exhibits a remarkable degree of thermal stability since irreversible denaturation occurs at approximately 92°C (Trackman et al., 1981). Thus, the 52°C assay optimum would appear to represent the onset of a reversible conformational change in the enzyme which decreases activity. In contrast to the bovine aortic enzyme, the purified chick cartilage enzyme loses 50% of its activity in 15 min at 37°C (Siegel, 1979). This may reflect structural differences between the enzymes of these two sources while the possibility of destabilization of the cartilage enzyme by a contaminating protease cannot be excluded.

4. OTHER FACTORS

As noted, the native molecular weight of the optimally functional oligomeric or monomeric state of lysyl oxidase is unknown. Indeed, prospects of determining this information are hampered by the tendency of even moderately concentrated solutions of the enzyme (30–50 μg ml^{-1}) in urea to polymerize upon dialysis into urea-free buffer (Jordan et al., 1977). The nearly threefold stimulation of rates of oxidation of alkylamines by the presence of 1 to 2 M urea in assay mixtures suggests that higher polymers are inactive toward these simple substrates (Trackman et al., 1981), although such urea concentrations inhibit oxidation of the insoluble elastin substrate presumably by interference with binding interactions between this protein substrate and the enzyme (Kagan et al., 1979). Clearly, definition of specific assay optima can vary considerably with the nature of the substrate. Indeed, 2 M concentrations of KCl, KBr, NaCl, and $(NH_4)_2SO_4$ accelerated rates of oxidation of secreted soluble chick aortic proteins by as much as 10-fold over rates at low ionic strength while stimulation was considerably less with an insoluble elastin substrate (Harris *et al.*, 1974). The stimulation of activity correlated with an increase in the fraction of enzyme capable of binding to and oxidizing the substrate possibly reflecting alterations in the state of aggregation of the substrate or of lysyl oxidase (Harris *et al.*, 1974).

B.   Mechanism of Action

As noted, the reaction catalyzed by lysyl oxidase appears to proceed as follows:

$$RCH_2NH_2 + O_2 + H_2O \rightarrow RCHO + NH_3 + H_2O_2$$

Precedents derived from studies on other amine oxidases predict that the electrons released upon the oxidative deamination of carbon 6 of peptidyllysine are transferred to oxygen reducing this acceptor to the peroxide state, ultimately to be released from the enzyme as hydrogen peroxide, while the oxygen of the aldehyde product would stem from water (Walsh, 1979). Although this mechanistic course has not been experimentally verified with lysyl oxidase, electron transfer almost certainly involves a role for an intermediate electron acceptor at the active site which can be fulfilled by a carbonyl cofactor. In spite of the residual uncertainty about its identity, it seems probable that such a prosthetic group at least shares chemical features with PLP and thus a mechanism is illustrated invoking PLP modeled after mechanisms suggested for other copper-dependent, carbonyl-reactive amine oxidases (Hamilton, 1971; Walsh, 1979) (Fig. 10). Formation of the substrate–carbonyl imine (**II**) provides a conjugated system of double bonds for electron flow from carbon 6 of lysine to the electrophilic pyridinium nitrogen to yield intermediate **III**. The reduced cofactor may be reoxidized by passage of an electron pair to oxygen mediated by copper yielding intermediate **IV**. While the scheme illustrates the hydrolysis of intermediate **IV** to yield the free peptidyl aldehyde product, it is also possible that the aldehyde may be hydrolyzed from intermediate **III** prior to reoxidation of the cofactor. In either event, intermediate (**IV**) produced after passage of electrons to reduce oxygen to peroxide may then tautomerize to the pyridoximine intermediate (**VI**) from which ammonia can be released by hydrolysis completing the catalytic cycle. The nature of the interaction of copper with the carbonyl cofactor while mediating electron passage is hypothetical, as, indeed, is the entire proposed mechanism. However, some precedent is found for the

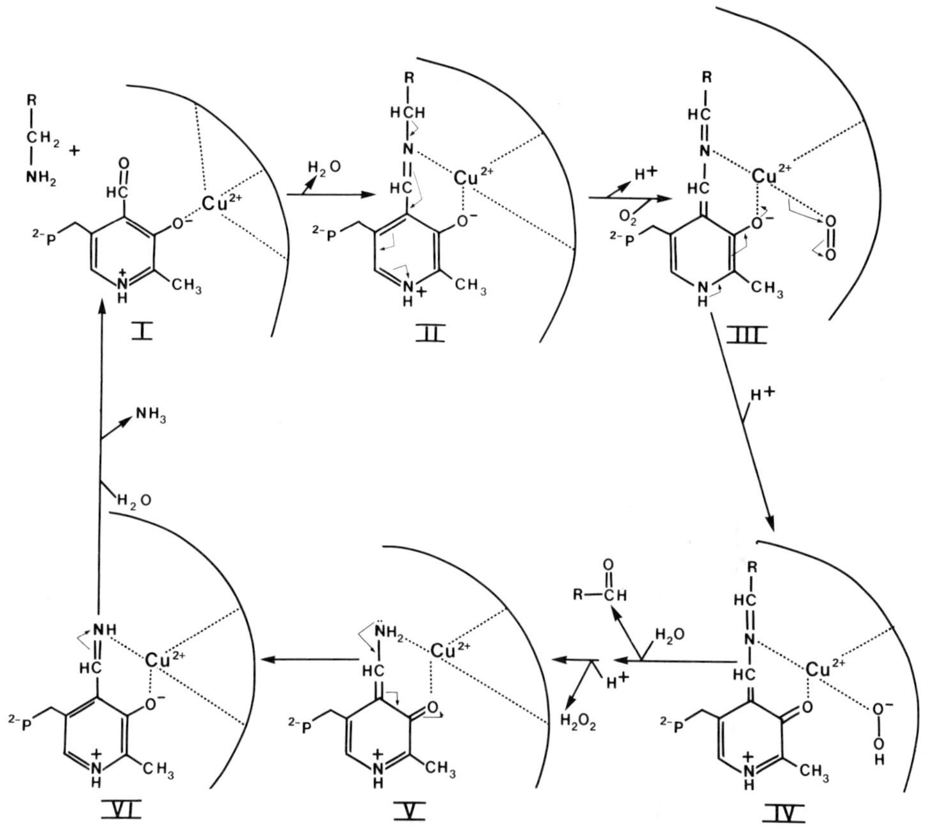

FIG. 10. Hypothetical mechanism of amine oxidation.

participation of copper in such a mechanism in model studies of the copper-dependent oxidation of Schiff base complexes of β-phenyl-α-aminomalonic acid with 5-deoxypyridoxal (Blum *et al.*, 1976). In any such instance, electron transfer from the reduced cofactor may occur by simultaneous passage of two electrons or by consecutive one-electron steps, the latter implicating superoxide ion as an intermediate stage in the reduction of oxygen. Although superoxide dismutase does not alter the rate of catalysis by lysyl oxidase, traces of hydroxy radical have been detected during the processing of alkylamine substrates, indicative of the potential of one-electron transfer at the active site (Kagan *et al.*, 1983a). It is possible that superoxide dismutase may be sterically prevented from processing O_2^- at the active site of lysyl oxidase. Clearly, definition of the precise mechanism of action of lysyl oxidase remains an important but as yet incompleted aspect of research. It is equally clear that this goal in turn awaits the unequivocal identification of the organic cofactor of lysyl oxidase.

C. Inhibition by β-Aminopropionitrile and Related Compounds

1. BAPN-INDUCED LATHYRISM

Early evidence for the existence of lysyl oxidase arose from descriptions of the deleterious effects on connective tissues resulting from the administration *in vivo* of lathyrogenic agents which were subsequently shown to inhibit lysyl oxidase activity *in vitro*. Thus, β-aminopropionitrile is a potent naturally occurring lathyrogen found in the sweat pea *Lathyratus odoratus*. Growing animals fed this legume, or treated with BAPN itself, develop spinal curvature, costochondral junction enlargement, and aortic rupture among other sequelae (Geiger *et al.*, 1933; Levene, 1961). There is now abundant evidence that these effects stem from the inhibition of lysyl oxidase with consequent inhibition of cross-linkage formation in elastin and collagen. The reversibly associated fibrillar aggregates of these proteins may ultimately be resolubilized and/or proteolytically degraded thus generating the macroscopic pathology typical of lathyrism (Levene and Gross, 1959; Page and Bendit, 1966; Tanzer, 1965; Barrow *et al.*, 1974; Bornstein *et al.*, 1966; Kang *et al.*, 1969; Miller *et al.*, 1965, 1967; Partridge *et al.*, 1964, 1966; Kadar *et al.*, 1976). Although BAPN is the active inhibitor of lysyl oxidase, this compound occurs in *Lathyratus odoratus* as β-(γ-glutamyl)aminopropionitrile (Schilling and Strong, 1954). Since the β-amino group of BAPN must be available for effective inhibition of lysyl oxidase *in vitro* or to induce lathyrism *in vivo* (Tang *et al.*, 1983; Levene and Gross, 1959), the γ-amide bond of β-(γ-glutamyl)aminopropionitrile is presumably cleaved by an amidase or protease to release the effective agent *in vivo*.

2. INHIBITION MECHANISMS

Studies by Siegel *et al.* (1970b) and Narayanan *et al.* (1972) established that BAPN is a potent and irreversible inhibitor of lysyl oxidase with I_{50} values approximating 3–5 μM. Narayanan *et al.* (1972) found evidence for the covalent incorporation of BAPN into lysyl oxidase by noting that ^{14}C-labeled BAPN coelutes with enzyme activity by gel exclusion chromatography of a partially purified enzyme preparation. The extent of labeling of a homogeneous preparation of bovine aortic lysyl oxidase by [1,2-14C]BAPN and [3-14C]BAPN were essentially identical (Tang *et al.*, 1983), consistent with the covalent incorporation of the entire carbon chain of BAPN and indicating that the nitrile moiety is apparently not cleaved from BAPN during the development of irreversible inhibition. Tang *et al.* (1983) also established that inhibition by BAPN is competitive with different substrates and that the development of irreversible inhibition accompanying covalent incorporation is temperature and time dependent and follows site-saturation kinetics, while covalent incorporation is largely prevented by prior inactivation of the enzyme by 2,4-dinitrophenylhydrazine. These results are consistent with a mechanism of inactivation in which BAPN binds at the active site and is then enzymatically processed to a chemically reactive species which covalently derivatizes the enzyme, typical of enzyme inhibitors categorized as suicide inactivators (Rando, 1975). Tang *et al.* (1983) proposed that the processing of BAPN involves Schiff base formation between the β-amino function and a functional enzyme carbonyl, presumably following the course of substrate processing (Fig. 11). α- and β-Proton abstraction from the bound inhibitor can then yield the electrophilic ketenimine species (intermediate d, Fig. 11) which can subsequently be covalently attacked by an enzyme nucleophile to derivatize and inactivate the enzyme. This scheme predicts that the nitrile moiety plays an essential electrophilic role in the tautomeric changes occurring in the enzyme-bound inhibitor. Consistent with this concept, it was found that other

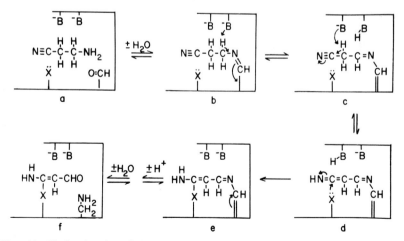

FIG. 11. Mechanism-based inactivation of lysyl oxidase by β-aminopropionitrile (BAPN). (From Tang *et al.*, 1983.)

TABLE III
MECHANISM-BASED IRREVERSIBLE
INHIBITORS OF LYSYL OXIDASE

Inhibitor	K_i $M \times 10^6$	$k_2{}^a$ min^{-1}
BrCH$_2$CH$_2$NH$_2$	7	1.07
ClCH$_2$CH$_2$NH$_2$	10	0.40
N≡CCH$_2$NH$_2$	6	0.16

[a] k_2 = apparent first order rate-limiting inactivation rate constant (Tang *et al.*, 1984).

electrophilic substituents, including bromine, chlorine, or the nitro moiety can substitute for the nitrile function in the BAPN structure to yield new suicide inhibitors of lysyl oxidase (Tang *et al.*, 1984). As shown in Table III, β-chloro- and β-bromoethylamine prove to inactivate lysyl oxidase more rapidly than BAPN but with affinities as indicated by K_i values similar to that of BAPN (Tang *et al.*, 1984). Further manipulation of the chemistry of such compounds may yield antifibrotic agents even more effective than BAPN.

D. Substrate Specificity

There is abundant evidence that lysyl oxidase purified from various sources oxidizes both elastin and collagen substrates (Siegel, 1974, 1979; Stassen, 1976; Narayanan *et al.*, 1974; Sullivan and Kagan, 1982; Kuivaniemi *et al.*, 1984). Moreover, each of the multiple, catalytically functional forms of lysyl oxidase of chick cartilage (Stassen, 1976), bovine aorta (Kagan and Sullivan, 1982), and human placenta (Kuivaniemi *et al.*, 1984) oxidize both proteins at approximately the same relative rates, negating the hypothesis that the ability of the enzyme to oxidize two such structurally different proteins may be accounted for by the enzyme heterogeneity. The physical–chemical basis of the apparent specificity of this enzyme for these two connective tissue proteins remains a subject of interest and of investigative efforts.

1. OXIDATION OF LYSINE IN COLLAGEN

Aldehyde products formed in type I collagen by lysyl oxidase *in vitro* have been located at the amino-terminal non-triple helical telopeptides of the α1- and α2-chains (Siegel and Martin, 1970), consistent with the locus of the aldol condensation product intramolecular cross-link formed *in vivo* (Bornstein *et al.*, 1966). Incubation of type I collagen with highly purified chick cartilage enzyme was shown also to result in the formation of the bifunctional cross-linkages N^6:6'-dehydro-5,5'-dihydroxylysinonorleucine and N^6:6'-dehydro-5-hydroxylysinonorleucine (Siegel, 1976). These cross-linkages are the expected derivatives of the aldehyde derived from telopeptide lysine 17^C and triple helical lysine 87, one or both of which may be hydroxylated (Rauterberg *et al.*, 1972; Kuboki *et al.*, 1981), thus indicating that lysine 17^C in the C-terminal telopeptide of the α1-chain was also a site of oxidation by the enzyme. Levels of borohydride-reducible Schiff base cross-linkages formed from enzyme-generated aldehydes in the presence or absence of BAPN in fibrillar bone collagen *in vitro* reached a maximum level and then decreased while levels of polyfunctional cross-linkages continued to rise (Siegel, 1976). Thus, formation of complex cross-linkages from aldehydes can occur independently of enzyme action with the specific cross-linkage ultimately produced reflecting the steric relationships imposed on the cross-linkage progenitors by the structure of collagen.

The initial expression of enzyme activity toward lysine in collagen is also strongly dependent on the structural features of this substrate. Thus, highly purified chick cartilage lysyl oxidase was only minimally active against denatured type I collagen, isolated α1-and α2-chains, or against triple helical pepsin-treated collagen lacking the N- and C-terminal telopeptides, while rates of oxidation were maximal with reconstituted fibrils of native collagen molecules (Siegel, 1974). Although activity is not directed against lysine in the triple helical region, the oxidation of the fibrillar collagen substrate was inhibited by triple helical pepsin-treated collagen suggesting that the enzyme might interact with the triple helix even though lysine oxidation seems restricted to the telopeptide lysine (Siegel, 1974; Siegel and Fu, 1976). Collagen prepared from calvaria in which proline hydroxylation had been inhibited was also a poor substrate, likely because of inefficient fibril formation *in vitro* (Siegel and Fu, 1976). These results suggest the requirement of an intermolecularly organized arrangement of collagen monomers for the appropriate binding and orientation of lysyl oxidase to susceptible lysine residues. This structural requirement is apparently met by the quarter-staggered relationship between monomers in native collagen fibrils. Siegel (1979) has suggested that the enzyme may bind to the two nearly homologous sequences near the N- and C-terminal ends of the triple helices of collagen molecules which are most proximal to the lysine residues in the N- and C-terminal telopeptides of adjacent quarter-staggered molecules. Indeed, these two triple helical sequences are highly conserved in types I, II, and III collagens (Fietzek *et al.*, 1977; Butler *et al.*, 1976), as shown in Fig. 12.

It appears that posttranslational enzymatic modifications of collagen occurring prior to lysine oxidation may also influence the susceptibility of lysine in collagen to lysyl oxidase. Although purified chick cartilage lysyl oxidase may oxidize both lysine and hydroxylysine in collagen *in vitro* (Siegel, 1974), glycosylation of hydroxylysine in collagen to residues of glucosylgalactosylhydroxylysine may inhibit lysine oxidation. Thus, Yamauchi *et al.* (1982) have noted that ^{3}H-labeled glycosylated dihydroxynorleucine, the NaB^{3}H$_4$-reduced derivative of a glycosylated hydroxylysine aldehyde, has apparently not been found in NaB^{3}H$_4$-reduced preparations of various collagen types, while nonglycosylated dihydroxylysinonorleucine is abundant in reduced collagens.

a. *Genetic Types of Collagen as Substrates for Lysyl Oxidase.* Urea-extractable lysyl oxidase purified from chick embryo cartilage (Siegel, 1974; Stassen, 1976), chicken or bovine aorta (Harris *et al.*, 1974; Sullivan and Kagan, 1982), and human placenta (Kuvaneimi *et al.*, 1984) each oxidatively deaminate type I collagen *in vitro* producing aldehydes from which the aldol, Schiff base, and hydroxypyridinium-type cross-linkages can form spontaneously (Siegel and Martin, 1970; Siegel, 1976; Siegel and Lian, 1975). Studies with renatured artificial mixtures of α1(I)- and α2(I)-chains *in vitro* (Siegel, 1979) and assessment of the time dependency of aldehyde formation in collagen *in vitro* (Fukae and Mechanic, 1980) suggest that the α2(I)-chain is more readily oxidized by lysyl oxidase than the α1(I)-chain. Evidence that type II collagen is oxidized *in vivo* is clear from its content of intermolecular 3-

```
                    (85)                            (92)
    a1(I)   -Gly-Met-Hyl-Gly-His-Arg-Gly-Phe-ᵃ

    a1(II)  -Gly-Val-Hyl-Gly-His-Arg-Gly-Phe-ᵇ

    a1(III) -Gly-Met-Hyl-Gly-His-Arg-Gly-Phe-ᵃ


                   (925)                           (932)
    a1(I)   -Gly-Ile-Hyl-Gly-His-Arg-Gly-Phe- ᵃ

    a1(III) -Gly-Ile-Hyl-Gly-His-Arg-Gly-Phe-ᵃ
```

FIG. 12. Sequences near N- and C-terminal regions of collagen triple helices. References: a, Fietzek *et al.* (1976); b, Butler *et al.* (1976).

hydroxypyridinium residues (Wu and Eyre, 1984b) while cross-linkages derived from lysyl and hydroxylysyl residues have also been identified in type III collagen (Bailey and Sims, 1976; Glanville and Fietzek, 1976; Cannon and Davison, 1978), although there does not appear to have been a direct demonstration that types II or III collagens are oxidized by lysyl oxidase *in vitro*. Evidence has been obtained for an intermolecular cross-linkage between type I and type III collagens of human leiomyoma (Henkel and Glanville, 1982). Siegel (1979) noted that type I and III procollagens labeled with [6-^{3}H]lysine in human fibroblast cultures are substrates for chick cartilage lysyl oxidase *in vitro,* although they are not nearly as rapidly oxidized as fibrils reconstituted from soluble type I collagen monomers. However, type I procollagen isolated from chick tendon is not a substrate for purified human placental lysyl oxidase (Kuivaniemi *et al.,* 1984). Since the extension peptides of procollagen interfere with the formation of quarter-staggered fibrils (Helseth and Veis, 1981; Miyahara *et al.,* 1984), it seems unlikely that procollagen is a preferred substrate for lysyl oxidase *in vivo* in view of the evident preference of the enzyme for fibrillar forms of collagen substrates.

It appears that type IV collagen also is stabilized by lysine-derived cross-linkages, as initially described for preparations of Descemet's membrane, renal glomerulus, and anterior lens capsule collagens (Tanzer and Kefalides, 1973). Dihydroxylysinonorleucine and hydroxyaldolhistidine have been identified in type IV collagen (Wu and Cohen, 1982) while the ketoimine hydroxylysino-5-oxonorleucine appears to be the principal $NaBH_4$-reducible cross-linkage in basement membrane collagen (Heathcote *et al.,* 1980; Le Pape *et al.,* 1981; Wu and Cohen, 1982). Bailey *et al.* (1984) localized this ketoimine predominantly in the N- and C-terminal regions of type IV molecules and concluded that this compound is converted to a nonreducible, presumably polyvalent cross-linkage with time. Further analyses of type IV collagen should reveal whether type IV contains the conserved Hyl-Gly-His-Arg sequence found in the triple helices of types I, II, and III collagens, the hydroxylysine residue of which participates in intermolecular cross-linkage formation in these interstitial collagens, and which may be a recognition sequence for the binding of lysyl oxidase, as previously discussed. It also remains to be established that lysyl oxidase isolated from interstitial connective tissues oxidizes type IV collagen or whether there is an enzyme with specificity toward basement membrane collagen. Similar considerations apply to cartilage type IX collagen in which hydroxypyridinium residues have recently been found (Wu and Eyre, 1984b).

2. OXIDATION OF LYSINE IN ELASTIN

Consistent with its role as the precursor to cross-linked, insoluble elastin, tropoelastin accumulates and insoluble elastin synthesis is reduced when tissue lysyl oxidase activity is inhibited by copper deprivation or by the administration of BAPN. Purified tropoelastin is oxidized and covalently incorporated through newly formed desmosine cross-linkages into an aortic elastin matrix upon incubation with purified lysyl oxidase *in vitro* (Narayanan *et al.*, 1974a; Narayanan and Page, 1976). Although the formation of desmosines requires an oxidative step to convert the dihydrodesmosine intermediate to the desmosine product, molecular oxygen is apparently not required for the final assembly of these pyridinium-type cross-linkages *in vitro* once the aldehyde precursors are generated in tropoelastin by lysyl oxidase (Narayanan *et al.*, 1974).

It is of interest that hydroxyproline content can have opposing effects on the control of the synthesis and cross-linking of elastin, on the one hand, and collagen, on the other. Approximately 5 to 10% of the imino acid content of tropoelastin is hydroxylated while 40 to 50% of the imino acid residues of types I, II, or III collagens exist as hydroxyproline. Interference with intracellular proline hydroxylation destabilizes the structure of procollagen (Rosenbloom and Cywinski, 1976), thus reducing intracellular transport and secretion and ultimately the amount of collagen cross-linked in the extracellular compartment. In contrast, while the substrate potential of underhydroxylated tropoelastin for lysyl oxidase is not significantly different from that of tropoelastin containing the normal complement of hydroxyproline (Narayanan *et al.*, 1978), increasing the hydroxyproline content of newly synthesized elastin by supplementing cultured aortic smooth muscle cells with ascorbate markedly reduces the cross-linkage content and amount of elastin which accumulates in the extracellular matrix (Dunn and Franzblau, 1982). Notably, the optimal temperature for coacervation of the elastin-like polymer (Val-Pro-Gly-Val-Gly)$_n$, increases markedly with increasing hydroxylation of its proline residues, presumably as a result of interference by the polar hydroxyproline side chains with hydrophobic interactions which normally favor interpeptide alignment during the coacervation process (Urry *et al.*, 1979). Since coacervation seems to favor oxidation and cross-linking of tropoelastin (Narayanan *et al.*, 1974) and of elastin-like synthetic peptides (Kagan *et al.*, 1980), it seems likely that the interference of elastin deposition in ascorbate-stimulated cultures may similarly reflect decreased coacervation and, consequently, reduced oxidation and cross-linking of excessively hydroxylated tropoelastin. The hypothesis that coacervation is essential to oxidation must be tempered by the finding of a cross-linked dimer of tropoelastin from copper-deficient pig aorta, suggesting that monomeric as well as coacervated multimers of tropoelastin may be oxidized *in vivo* (Abraham and Carnes, 1978).

3. Effects of Charge and Sequence on the Specificity of Lysyl Oxidase

As noted, the primary and higher-ordered structures of collagen and elastin differ considerably, although both are substrates for lysyl oxidase. Since lysine-derived cross-linkages are not broadly distributed among other proteins, the basis of this restricted enzyme specificity is not immediately evident. However, both net substrate charge and sequence vicinal to lysine appear to influence the specificity of this enzyme.

a. Electrostatic Charge. The activity of purified aortic lysyl oxidase toward an insoluble elastin substrate is stimulated as much as fivefold by elastin-bound cationic amphiphiles such as dodecyltrimethylammonium chloride but is completely inhibited by elastin-bound anionic amphiphiles, including saturated and unsaturated free fatty acids and sodium dodecylsulfate. The cationic elastin ligands increase the catalytic rate by markedly lowering the K_m of the substrate, while neither the anionic nor cationic agents alter the rate of oxidation of *n*-butylamine by lysyl oxidase, consistent with an elastin substrate-directed effect (Kagan *et al.,* 1981b). Thus, the enzyme activity is qualitatively responsive to the net charge of the insoluble elastin substrate. It is of interest that this ionic relationship is precisely the inverse of that between pancreatic elastase and elastin, since those cationic ligands which stimulate oxidation of elastin by lysyl oxidase completely inhibit the degradation of elastin by pancreatic elastase while anionic ligands which inhibit the expression of lysyl oxidase toward elastin strongly stimulate elastolysis (Kagan *et al.,* 1972). Since elastase is a cationic protein while lysyl oxidase is anionic at physiological pH, it appears that the metabolism of insoluble elastin by soluble polar enzymes may be limited by the degree of electrostatic attraction or repulsion existing between the attacking enzyme and this extremely hydrophobic, largely apolar insoluble substrate. It should be noted that the oxidation of peptidyl lysine to the aldehyde eliminates this source of cationic charge. Since approximately 60% of the lysines of tropoelastin become oxidized, the polarity of elastin is changed considerably by the cross-linking process. Continued cross-linking of maturing elastin fibers might then be influenced by interactions with other more polar molecules in the matrix. In view of the charge relationships noted between lysyl oxidase and elastin, it is of interest that microfibrillar components of the developing elastic matrix appear to be composed of anionic glycoproteins (Ross and Bornstein, 1969; Cleary *et al.*, 1981; Robert *et al.*, 1971; Pasquali-Ronchetti *et al.*, 1981, 1984). Various roles have been speculated upon for this microfibrillar material in elastogenesis, including that of providing a framework for the growing elastic fiber, and a relationship to lysyl oxidase has been considered (Cleary *et al.*, 1981), although the precise nature, role, and heterogeneity of microfibrillar proteins has yet to be clarified. Interactions between this anionic glycoprotein material and cationic lysines of tropoelastin units may serve to anchor the elastin precursor during fibrogenesis and possibly prevent the oxidation of key lysines whose ϵ-amino functions are destined to be incorporated as the pyridinium nitrogens of the desmosine cross-linkages. In view of the electrostatic relationships noted in elastin oxidation, it is of interest that anionic components of tobacco smoke inhibit lysyl oxidase activity toward elastin *in vitro* by a substrate-directed mechanism (Laurent *et al.*, 1983). Further, elastin resynthesis is inhibited by tobacco smoke *in vivo* in hamsters in which an emphysematous response had been induced by a single intratracheal administration of elastase (Osman *et al.*, 1982). Desmosine resynthesis was reduced by 40% in the smoke-exposed hamsters, suggesting that lysyl oxidase and/or cross-linkage formation was inhibited, possibly in part reflecting the effects noted *in vitro* by Laurent *et al.* (1983).

The general importance of electrostatic charge in enzyme–substrate interactions was emphasized by the finding that lysyl oxidase can oxidize a variety of basic but not acidic proteins *in vitro* (Kagan *et al.*, 1983, 1984). Indeed, the enzyme generates α-aminoadipic-δ-semialdehyde as well as lysine-derived cross-linkages in lysine-rich histone H1 (Kagan *et al.*, 1983) and oxidizes lysine in a variety of basic proteins whose isoelectric points occur at or higher than pH 8 while none of various acidic proteins tested were substrates for the enzyme (Fig. 13) (Kagan *et al.*, 1984). It was of particular interest to note that bovine serum albumin is not a substrate, but it is readily oxidized if its carboxylate functions are first chemically converted to neutral amide functions (Fig. 13). The generation of substrate potential accompanies the resultant change in pI from 4.7 for native albumin to 11.4 for amidated albumin. Clearly, electrostatic potential between the en-

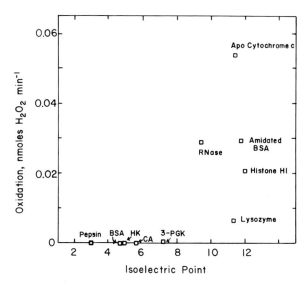

FIG. 13. Correlation of substrate potential of various proteins with isoelectric points of the substrate. Abbreviations: BSA, bovine serum albumin; CA, carbonic anhydrase; HK, hexokinase; 3-PGK, 3-phosphoglycerokinase; RNase, ribonuclease. (From Kagan *et al.*, 1984.)

zyme and its substrates is of considerable importance to the specificity of lysyl oxidase.

b. Amino Acid Sequence. Consistent with the fact that lysyl oxidase utilizes proteins as substrates, the amino acid sequence vicinal to lysine influences the susceptibility of peptidyllysine in synthetic oligo- and polypeptides to oxidation by lysyl oxidase *in vitro* (Kagan *et al.*, 1984). Rates of oxidation of various random or ordered sequence peptides were maximal if lysine was in an alanine-rich sequence and tended to decrease as the molecular size or anionic character of neighboring side chains increased in the order Ala > Val > Leu > Phe > Tyr > Glu. Vicinal glutamate residues were particularly inhibitory to lysine oxidation. Analysis of the K_m and V_{max} values for lysine oxidation in various ordered polypeptides (Table IV) assembled by solid phase synthesis (Kagan *et al.*, 1984) reveal that a second cationic lysine or arginine residue increases the V_{max} value relative to that of peptide I, consistent with the prior evidence cited that net cationic charge of the substrate facilitates oxidation. Arginine one or three residues C-terminal to lysine also increases K_m, however, pointing toward enzyme–substrate interactions at least three residues distant from the lysine to

TABLE IV

Oxidation of Ordered Oligopeptides by Lysyl Oxidase[a]

Peptide	K_m $(M \times 10^{-5})$	V_{max} [nmol H_2O_2 $(10 \ min)^{-1}]$	V_{max}/K_m
I Ala$_2$-Lys-Ala$_2$	8.2	0.43	0.053
II Ala$_2$-Lys-Ala$_2$-Lys-Ala$_2$	6.8	0.66	0.097
III Ala$_2$-Lys-Ala$_2$-Arg-Ala$_2$	29.6	0.97	0.032
IV Ala$_2$-Lys-Arg-Ala$_2$	20.	0.93	0.047
V Ala$_2$-Lys-Gly-Ala$_2$	75.9	0.47	0.006
VI Ala$_2$-Glu-Lys-Ala$_2$	14.4	0.21	0.014
VII Ala$_2$-Lys-Tyr-Ala$_2$	41.	0.79	0.019

[a] From Kagan et al. (1984).

be oxidized, consistent with an extended substrate recognition site. Notably, glutamate C-terminal to lysine (peptide V) markedly inhibits oxidation, increasing K_m nearly 10-fold over that of peptide I, while glutamate N-terminal to lysine reduces V_{max}/K_m to a lesser degree, producing a much smaller increase in K_m while reducing V_{max} by one-half that of peptide I. Thus, anionic sites vicinal to lysine inhibit the expression of enzyme activity but with some degree of steric specificity. These results also suggest that the substrate binds to an extended active site in a preferred directional sense, for example, in the N → C rather than the C → N direction, and supports the concept that there may be multiple E–S contacts at and at a distance from the susceptible lysine residue.

Inspection of specific sequences in which lysine is oxidized in elastin and collagen (Fig. 14) provides interesting comparisons with the results obtained with synthetic polypeptides. Oxidizable lysine residues are predominantly found in alanine-rich sequences in elastin. The general absence of bulky or anionic side chains in these sequences could account for the extensive oxidation of lysine in this protein, consistent with the results cited above. Sequence studies on cross-linked elastin peptides (Foster et al., 1974) predict that the lysine residue in elastin peptide (1) (Fig. 14) bonded to the amino group of tyrosine [or phenylalanine (Baig et al., 1980)] is resistant to oxidation since its ε-amino function condenses as such with the aldehyde generated by oxidation of the other lysine residue in this sequence forming an intrachain Schiff base cross-linkage. Subsequent condensation of this cross-linkage with a neighboring aldol condensation product cross-

Elastin Peptides[a, b]

(1)   X-X-Ala-Ala-Ala-Ala-Ala-**LYS**-Ala-Ala-Ala-Lys-Tyr-X-

(2)   X-X-Ala-Ala-Ala-**LYS**-Ala-Ala-Ala-Ala-**LYS**-Ala-X-X-

Collagen Peptides

N-Terminal Telopeptides

a(I)   pGlu-Leu-Ser-Tyr-Gly-Tyr-Asp-Glu-**LYS**-Ser-Thr-Gly-[c]

a(I)   pGlu-Phe-Asp-Ala-**LYS**-Gly-Gly-[d]

a(III) pGlu-Tyr-Gly-Ala-Tyr-Asp-Val-**LYS**-Ser-Gly-Val-[e]

C-Terminal Telopeptides

*a*1(I) Ser-Gly-Gly-Phe-Asp-Phe-Ser-Phe-Leu-Pro-Gln-Pro-Pro-Gln-Glu-**LYS**-Ala-His-Asp-Gly-Gly-Arg-Tyr-Tyr-Arg-Ala-[c, f]

*a*2(I)Gly-Gly-Tyr-Glu-Val-Gly-Phe-Asp-Ala-Glu-   –   –   –   –   –   –Tyr-Tyr-Arg-Ala-[f]

*a*1(II) Gly-Thr-Gly-Ile-Asp-Met-Ser-Ala-Phe-Ala-Gly-Leu-Gly-Gln-Thr-Glu-**Lys**-Gly-Pro-Asp-Pro-Ile-Arg-Tyr-Met-Arg-Ala-[g]

*a*1(III) Gly-Pro-Cys-Cys-Gly-Gly-   –Val-Ala-Ser-Leu-Gly-Ala-Gly-Glu-**LYS**-Gly-Pro-Val-Gly-Tyr-Gly-Tyr-Glu-Tyr-Arg-[h]

FIG. 14. Lysine-containing sequences susceptible to lysyl oxidase in elastin and collagen. LYS, oxidized by lysyl oxidase. References: a, Sandberg *et al.* (1981); b, Foster *et al.* (1974); c, Fietzek and Kuhn (1976); d, Fietzek *et al.* (1974); e, Glanville and Fietzek (1976); f, Fuller and Boedtker (1981); g, Sandell *et al.* (1984); h, Yamada *et al.* (1983).

linkage can account for the appearance of this lysine residue as the source of the pyridinium nitrogen in the desmosine ring (Foster *et al.*, 1974). The hypothesis that C-terminal tyrosine may prevent oxidation by lysyl oxidase (Foster *et al.*, 1974) is supported by the significant increase in K_m induced by this residue in peptide VII of Table IV, although the consequent inhibitory effect is modulated by the accompanying increase in V_{max}, indicating that the effects in the accreting elastin fiber would of necessity be more complex to account for complete prevention of the oxidation of lysine in this sequence. In contrast to the selective oxidation of one lysine in elastin peptide (1), both lysines in the sequence of peptide (2) can be oxidized and their aldehyde products can spontaneously condense to yield the aldol condensation product (Foster *et al.*, 1974).

As noted, the oxidation of lysine in collagen is restricted to the single lysine residues in each of the non-triple helical telopeptides. It is of interest that lysine in the N-terminal telopeptide of $\alpha 1$(I) follows an -Asp-Glu- sequence while those in the $\alpha 2$(I)- and $\alpha 1$(III)-chains follow -Asp-Ala- or -Asp-Val-, respectively (Fig. 14). Similarly, the oxidizable lysine occurs in -Glu-Lys-Ala- or -Glu-Lys-Gly- sequences in the C-terminal telopeptides of $\alpha 1$(I), $\alpha 1$(II), or $\alpha 1$(III) (Fig. 14). Thus, lysine is proximal to anionic sites in each of these telopeptide sequences, although it is of interest that lysine is always bonded through its α-amino and not its α-carboxy function to glutamate when that residue is next to the lysine residue. This arrangement appears most consistent with the results obtained with the synthetic peptides in Table IV since the -Lys-Glu- sequence is much less susceptible to oxidation than is the -Glu-Lys- sequence. It is of interest in this regard that lysine in the C-terminal telopeptide is oxidized before lysine 9^N in $\alpha 1$(I) in guinea pigs *in vivo* (Fukae and Mechanic, 1982). This temporal sequence of oxidation is consistent with the fact that there are two anionic residues adjacent to lysine 9^N while there is one anionic residue adjacent to lysine 17^C in $\alpha 1$(I), assuming that the affinity and/or the rate of oxidation would be less in regions of higher anionic charge density. It is also noteworthy that the C-terminal telopeptide of $\alpha 2$(I) lacks a lysine residue (Table IV), indicated by sequencing of the gene for $\alpha 2$(I) (Fuller and Boedtker, 1981). Further, lysine in each of the telopeptides sequences described is bonded through its carboxyl group to residues with small R groups, i.e., serine, glycine, and alanine, consistent with the results obtained with the synthetic random and ordered polypeptides (Kagan *et al.*, 1984) and with the inhibitory effect of C-terminal tyrosine (Foster *et al.*, 1974) or phenylalanine (Baig *et al.*, 1980) on lysine oxidation in elastin. Thus, it is the C-terminal side of substrate lysine which appears to be most sensitive to interference by bulky or anionic side chains with optimal enzyme-substrate contacts. It is also of interest that lysine in the N-terminal telopeptides occurs in -Asp-X-Lys-Y- sequences, while -X-Glu-Lys-Y- sequences are characteristic of the C-terminal region (Fig. 14). Conceivably, these anionic residues may be involved in the appropriate alignment of the peptidyl substrate with the enzyme, as suggested. However, definition of a specificity-determining role for vicinal anionic residues in collagen must consider the fact that lysine in elastin occurs most frequently in alanine-rich sequences deficient in anionic residues, although Mecham and Foster (1979) have reported the isolation of the peptide fragment -Ala-Glu-AAS-(Glu)- from aortic elastin of copper deficient pigs.

While there doubtlessly are other effects of sequence on the enzyme specificity yet to be established, it appears that sequence alone will not account for the evident selectivity of lysyl oxidase for elastin and collagen at the apparent exclusion of other proteins *in vivo*. As noted, the preference of lysyl oxidase for structural organization at the quaternary level, as in quarter-staggered collagen fibrils and in coacervates of tropoelastin, suggests that the enzyme specificity may also be influenced by binding sites unique to specific quaternary structures present in fibrillar arrays of these molecules. In light of the sequence and charge effects noted, the two conserved triple helical sequences which align opposite to the N- and/or C-terminal telopeptide lysines in D-staggered fibrils of types I, II, or III collagens (Fig. 12) may well be involved in the interaction of lysyl oxidase with collagen but possibly not as direct binding sites for enzyme as had been previously suggested (Siegel, 1979). Notably, these sequences (Fig. 12) each contain hydroxylysine, histidine, and arginine and thus are sites of at least two and potentially three cationic charges. While such cationic charge density should provide attractive forces for lysyl oxidase binding, it also seems possible that these residues may interact with the neighboring tropocollagen unit to neutralize the unfavorable anionic charge density proximal to the N- and C-terminal telopeptide lysine residues. This would be expected to enhance lysyl oxidase reactivity without invoking interpeptide enzyme binding phenomena. Recent analyses of the elastin gene also point toward the presence of sequences in elastin with grouped cationic residues (J. Rosenbloom, personal communication). Further investigation of such factors as vicinal charge should ultimately provide a more complete understanding of the unique specificity of lysyl oxidase.

4. TEMPORAL AND STERIC RELATIONSHIPS IN FIBRILLOGENESIS

It is generally assumed that lysyl oxidase functions primarily in the extracellular compartment, and, indeed, lysyl oxidase is secreted into the medium of cell cultures (Layman *et al.*, 1972; Gonnerman *et al.*, 1981). It is of interest to consider the topologic relationships which might exist between the enzyme and its collagen substrate as collagen fibers are formed in the extracellular milieu. Postulated interactions between the enzyme and collagen must account for the steric restrictions which can prevent access of telopeptide lysines within accreting fibrils to lysyl oxidase. Thus, Siegel and Fu (1976) noted that enzymatic rates of oxidation of preformed fibrillar collagen substrates *in vitro* reached a plateau considerably before all of the telopeptide lysines in the fibrils were oxidized even though the enzyme which had been initially added to the fibrils was bound as a sedimentable complex to the fibrillar substrate. Initial rates were resumed, however, upon the addition of fresh substrate aliquots, suggesting that the enzyme binds to molecules at the surface of the fiber and may then act on newly accreting collagen molecules. The likelihood that the enzyme cannot penetrate into the preformed fibrillar structure was supported by direct binding studies noting that the ratio of bound enzyme to type I collagen fibril mass decreases markedly as the collagen concentration increases (Cronlund *et al.*, 1985). The inability of the enzyme to penetrate the inner domain of native collagen fibers predicts that cross-linking must occur at an early stage of collagen fibrillogenesis. Direct binding studies have also demonstrated that the enzyme binds to the triple helical portion of collagen molecules, as suggested by earlier kinetic studies (Siegel, 1976), since the apparent binding constants for the formation of sedimentable complexes between enzyme and native fibrils or fibrils from which the telopeptides had been removed by proteolytic modification were quite similar (Cronlund *et al.*, 1985).

Recent years have witnessed considerable progress in the analysis of collagen fibrillogenesis. Native collagen fibrils *in vivo* and those formed by thermal induction from collagen monomers *in vitro* reveal a periodicity (D) of 67 nm, or 1/4.4 times the length of the molecule. It appears that the conversion of collagen molecules to the quarter- or D-staggered fibrillar array is an entropy-driven self-assembly process, the information for which resides in the structure of collagen. Turbidometric analyses of fibrillogenesis *in vitro* have described a lag phase followed by a sigmoidal increase in turbidity. There is evidence for the formation of linear 4D-staggered dimeric or trimeric (Silver *et al.*,

1979; Silver, 1981) or longer (Gelman *et al.,* 1979) aggregates of collagen molecules during the lag phase. These linear oligomers or "nuclei" may subsequently undergo lateral aggregation during the growth or secondary phase characteristic of turbidity–time curves, finally yielding D-staggered collagen fibrils. It seems likely that lysyl oxidase may first utilize a species of collagen which is predominant before a significant degree of lateral aggregation has occurred, in light of features of the collagen–enzyme complexes previously described. Such candidates include the linear 4-D staggered dimeric or trimeric nuclei, or, possibly, the earliest products of lateral aggregation between such nuclei. Since the enzyme appears specific for lysine in the telopeptide extensions, it is important to note that the telopeptide extensions appear to play critical roles in collagen fibrillogenesis (Gelman *et al.,* 1979; Helseth and Veis, 1981; Capaldi and Chapman, 1982). Thus, pepsin- or pronase-digested collagen, lacking most or all of the two telopeptide regions, initiates fibrillogenesis very slowly (Gelman *et al.,* 1979; Helseth and Veis, 1981) and forms fibrils with abnormal morphology (Gelman *et al.,* 1979). Helseth and Veis (1981) noted that the isolated amino telopeptide specifically accelerated the nucleation of collagen molecules from which the telopeptides had been proteolytically removed, indicating that the amino telopeptide is likely involved in the nucleation phenomenon. Similar evidence points to a role for the C-terminal telopeptide in the formation of 4-D staggered nuclei (Capaldi and Chapman, 1982) as well as in the lateral growth phase in fibrillogenesis (Helseth and Veis, 1981; Capaldi and Chapman, 1982). It seems that the temporal relationship of lysine oxidation may well be critical to fibrillogenesis since the aldehyde derivative of the amino telopeptide was not effective in promoting nucleation suggesting a role for the epsilon amino group of lysine 9^N in the nucleation process (Helseth and Veis, 1981). Further, comparisons of the kinetics of fibrillogenesis of native and sodium borohydride-reduced collagen indicated that collagen aldehydes play a role in stabilizing nucleating species of unknown structure which are present at the end of the lag phase (Brennan and Davison, 1980). As noted, oxidation of the C-terminal telopeptide lysine seems to precede that at the N-telopeptide region *in vivo* (Fukae and Mechanic, 1980). Thus, it is possible that lysyl oxidase may initially oxidize lysine in the C-terminal telopeptide of early lateral aggregates. Intermolecular condensation of the resultant aldehyde with lysine (or hydroxylysine) 87 in the adjacent D-staggered tropocollagen unit should stabilize these nuclei as they undergo lateral aggregation. Further intra- and intermolecular cross-linking would then of necessity be limited to initial aggregates of these nuclei, possibly mediated by lysyl oxidase bound to the surface of the early aggregates. This suggests that the rate of maturation of early lateral aggregates to fibers composed of several collagen molecules would be limited in rate by the rate of dissociation of lysyl oxidase from fibrillar surfaces.

VI. PATHOLOGY

In view of the essential and potentially controlling role exerted by lysyl oxidase in the biosynthesis and deposition of fibrous proteins of connective tissue, it is not surprising that there has been considerable interest in the quantitation of the expression of this enzyme in connective tissue diseases. Deficiencies in lysyl oxidase are found in certain inherited diseases of connective tissue whose symptoms mimic those of experimental lathyrism. In contrast, the fibrotic response of affected tissues to various agents generally includes significant elevations in levels of lysyl oxidase activity. Indeed, this circumstance offers promise that appropriate chemotherapeutic agents targeted toward lysyl oxidase may be of benefit in controlling fibrotic diseases.

A.   Lysyl Oxidase Deficiency in Inherited Metabolic Disease

1.   THE ANEURYSM-PRONE MOTTLED MOUSE

At least five mutations can occur at the mottled locus on the X-chromosome of the mouse to yield the tortoise (Mo^{to}), dappled (Mo^{dp}), brindled (Mo^{br}), viable brindled (Mo^{vbr}), and Blotchy (Mo^{blo}) variants (Rowe *et al.*, 1974). The viable male $Mo^{blo/Y}$ hemizygote exhibits depigmented hair, bone deformities, extensible skin, aortic aneurysms (Andrews *et al.*, 1975), and defects in lung elastin and develops panacinar emphysematous-like lung lesions (Fisk and Kuhn, 1976). Rowe *et al.* (1974) reported marked decreases in the contents of desmosine and aldol condensation product cross-linkages in the aortic elastin of the Mo^{vbr} strain, suggestive of a lysyl oxidase deficiency. Urea-soluble lysyl oxidase activity was reduced against a collagen substrate, relative to C3H littermate controls, to 20% in Mo^{vbr} males, to 33% in Mo^{blo}, and to 71% in the male Mo^{br} (Rowe *et al.*, 1974). Of this series, only the male Mo^{br} did not exhibit connective tissue abnormalities, suggesting that 29% reduction in the enzyme activity was insufficient to induce biochemical changes in elastin and collagen. Starcher *et al.* (1977) noted markedly decreased levels of lysyl oxidase in the lung tissue and cultured fibroblasts derived from blotchy mice, consistent with the tendency of this variant to develop lung lesions resembling panacinar emphysema. There also appears to be an inherited defect in alveolar macrophage function in the blotchy mouse which could contribute to the emphysematous reaction (Ranga and Kleinerman, 1981).

It appears, however, that the primary biochemical defect in this disease involves mechanisms of intestinal absorption and transport of dietary copper (Hunt, 1974, 1976) and accumulation and retention of copper in the cells of affected tissues (Camakaris *et al.*, 1979; Mann *et al.*, 1979a). Thus, intestinal copper absorption is severely reduced in $Mo^{br/Y}$ (Evans and Reis, 1978; Mann *et al.*, 1979a) while copper which is absorbed is abnormally distributed among the tissues, with excess accumulations in kidney, gut mucosa, and intestine and depleted levels of copper in liver, brain, plasma, and most other organs (Hunt, 1974; Camakaris *et al.*, 1979). The disturbances in copper metabolism, the reduction in levels of lysyl oxidase and the pathology seen in connective tissues are quite analogous to effects noted in Menkes' syndrome in humans. The mottled mouse mutant thus assumes importance as a model of this human disease. Cultured fibroblasts of Menkes' patients and of $Mo^{br/Y}$ mice accumulate excess amounts of copper (Goka *et al.*, 1976; Starcher *et al.*, 1978; Royce *et al.*, 1980), and it has been suggested on this basis that the fundamental defect in both cases involves the complexing of intracellular copper by a copper-binding protein in a fashion which renders the metal ion unavailable for copper-requiring enzymes including lysyl oxidase (Danks, 1977). Indeed, Starcher *et al.* (1978) found that the major portion of ^{64}Cu incorporated into cultured normal, $Mo^{blo/Y}$, and Menkes' fibroblasts was associated with a 12,000-MW protein in each case. However, the control of copper availability may be specific for different copper proteins within the spectrum of these diseases of copper metabolism since ceruloplasmin, dopamine-β-hydroxylase and lysyl oxidase are all severely reduced in the $Mo^{br/Y}$ mutant while only lysyl oxidase is deficient in the $Mo^{blo/Y}$ variant (Starcher *et al.*, 1978). Notably, a single subcutaneous injection of 50 μg of copper retained as Cu(I) in an alkyl polyether–sebacic acid solution increased the survival rate of $Mo^{br/Y}$ mice and elevated levels of lysyl oxidase in these mutants from 50–60% of control levels to 84–150% of the level of normal mice (Royce *et al.*, 1982; Mann *et al.*, 1979b). Such treatment, however, was less effective with $M^{blo/Y}$ mice (Mann *et al.*, 1981).

2. MENKES' SYNDROME

Menkes' syndrome is a lethal X-linked recessive human disorder. Patients exhibit severe cerebral degeneration, pili torti, hypothermia, scurvy-like bone changes, subdural hematoma, and generalized arterial disease manifested as grossly abnormal arterial elastic laminae. Such features are consistent with those occurring in copper deficiency while the defects in connective tissue proteins point toward decreased function of lysyl oxidase (Danks, 1983). Lysyl oxidase activity in the medium of cultured Menkes' fibroblasts was markedly reduced, displaying 3 to 42% of the activity of controls against collagen or elastin substrates, while the copper content of the cell layers was significantly elevated relative to control cultures (Royce et al., 1980).

As a true of the mottled mouse variants, the primary defect in Menkes' disease appears to be one of abnormal availability and metabolic disposition of copper, rendering it inaccessible to copper enzymes, including lysyl oxidase, and presumably other enzymes, including tyrosinase, dopamine-β-hydroxylase, cytochrome oxidase, and superoxide dismutase, thus accounting for connective tissue abnormalities, depigmentation, and neurologic disturbances seen in the murine and human diseases (Danks, 1983). The increased copper content in cultured Menkes' fibroblasts appears to accumulate in metallothionein or a metallothionein-like protein (Bonewitz and Howell, 1981; Labadie et al., 1981; Peltonen et al., 1983). Notably, copper is a more potent inducer of metallothionein mRNA in Menkes' fibroblasts than in normal fibroblasts (Schmidt et al., 1984), suggesting a mechanism whereby copper is rendered inaccessible by increased levels of a copper-induced, normal, or mutant metallothionein species. However, metallothionein gene sequences are not found on the X chromosome, indicating that perturbations in metallothionein levels in X-linked Menkes' disease must occur by a trans-acting alteration in transcriptional regulation or indirectly by a Menkes'-induced alteration in copper homeostasis (Schmidt et al., 1984). Assuming that the reduction in levels of lysyl oxidase activity is secondary to lack of copper availability, it remains important to distinguish between the possibilities that the lack of appropriately accessible copper decreases the biosynthesis of lysyl oxidase protein, consistent with the proposal of Rayton and Harris (1979), and/or that newly synthesized enzyme protein is rendered more susceptible to proteolysis by the absence of bound copper at its active site and thus may be rapidly degraded. Assessment of changes in lysyl oxidase protein by immunological titration has yet to be reported in

Menkes' cells or tissues, but this approach should yield further insight into the molecular mechanisms of control of lysyl oxidase in this and related disease states. It remains possible that the genes coding for lysyl oxidase and an intracellular copper transport protein may be closely located on the X chromosome with both being affected by a single mutation (Starcher *et al.*, 1978; Rowe *et al.*, 1977; Kuivaniemi *et al.*, 1982).

3. EHLERS–DANLOS SUBTYPE IX

Ehlers–Danlos subtype IX is a heritable, presumably X-linked connective tissue disorder whose clinical symptoms closely resemble those of Menkes' but which differ from Menkes' in that the hair is coarse but not kinky and there are no distinct neurological abnormalities (Kuivaniemi *et al.*, 1982; Peltonen *et al.*, 1983). Copper concentrations and ^{64}Cu uptake were markedly elevated in cultured skin fibroblasts, but copper content was decreased in skin and hair while serum ceruloplasmin levels were also low. In further analogy to Menkes' disease, copper accumulated in a metallothionein-like protein within the fibroblasts. Lysyl oxidase levels were markedly reduced in the media of the fibroblast cultures as was insolubilization of collagen into the culture matrix (Kuivaniemi *et al.*, 1982; Peltonen *et al.*, 1983). Thus, there seems to be a pattern of diseases relating disturbances in copper metabolism and lysyl oxidase deficiencies.

4. X-LINKED CUTIS LAXA

Cutis laxa is a heterogeneous group of systemic connective tissue disorders all characterized by lax skin. The dominantly inherited of the two forms described involves only the dermis while the recessively inherited form additionally may display emphysema, pulmonary infection, diverticula of the gastrointestinal and genitourinary tracts, hernias, and can result in early death (Danks, 1983). Cultured dermal fibroblasts of a symptomatic 6-year-old male lacked lysyl oxidase activity against elastin or collagen substrates, whereas those derived from the mother had levels intermediate between those of the child and normal fibroblasts (Byers *et al.*, 1976). The lack of apparent cardiovascular or cartilage abnormalities in the child implied that cross-linking proceeded normally in these tissues (Byers *et al.*, 1976). In other instances, lysyl oxidase activity was severely reduced in extracts of skin

biopsies and in the medium of cultured fibroblasts while dermal collagen extractability was increased in affected males (Byers *et al.*, 1980).
Enzyme protein was virtually undetectable in skin biopsies by im-
munodiffusion assay thus indicating that loss in enzyme activity is due
to decreased synthesis or increased degradation of lysyl oxidase (Byers
et al., 1980). Both serum copper and serum ceruloplasmin were markedly reduced in a cutis laxa patient (Byers *et al.*, 1980). Similar reductions in lysyl oxidase activity and abnormalities in copper metabolism
have been described in another connective tissue disease which appears related to X-linked cutis laxa (Kaitila *et al.*, 1982). Hence, reduction in lysyl oxidase activity and lysyl oxidase protein may be secondary to a primary defect in copper metabolism in these instances, again
similar to Menkes' disease.

5.   OTHER GENETIC DISEASES

Marfans' syndrome is a heritable connective tissue disease exhibiting skeletal, ocular, and cardiovascular abnormalities with the cause
of death usually due to aortic aneurysm in the fourth decade of life
(McKusick, 1972). Collagen is unusually soluble in skin biopsies
(Scheck *et al.*, 1979) and cultured skin fibroblasts (Priest *et al.*, 1973)
suggestive of defective cross-linking and implicating defects in lysyl
oxidase in this disease. However, lysyl oxidase activity was equivalent
to controls in cultured fibroblasts of Marfans' patients in two studies
(Layman *et al.*, 1972; Royce and Danks, 1982), indicating that this
enzyme is likely not the metabolic site of this disease. Scheck *et al.*
(1979) observed anomalous patterns of migration of the $\alpha2$ chains of
type I collagen isolated from the aorta of a patient with Marfan's syndrome, suggesting that a defect in the biosynthesis of this chain leading to inefficient cross-linking between α-chains may be at the basis of
this disease.

Although an early report indicated a deficiency of lysyl oxidase activity in the media of cultured dermal fibroblasts of Ehlers–Danlos
syndrome subtype V (diFerrante *et al.*, 1975), the activity and antigen-
ically titrable levels of lysyl oxidase as well as reducible cross-linkage
profiles of skin biopsies were equivalent to those of biopsied normal
skin (Siegal *et al.*, 1979). Lyophilization of media samples prior to
assay in the earlier study may have contributed to the low activities
found in the fibroblast cultures, as suggested (Siegel *et al.*, 1979). It
thus appears unlikely that this disease entity is based upon a primary
defect in the lysyl oxidase gene.

B. *Fibrotic Diseases*

1. CARDIOVASCULAR DISEASE

a. Atherosclerosis. Early lesions in atherosclerotic arterial walls are characterized by excessive accumulation of intracellular and extra-cellular lipid deposits. Total collagen and elastin subsequently increase in the affected intima-media. The raised lesion may eventually become covered by a collagenous fibrous cap (Ross and Glomset, 1976). Increases in rates of collagen synthesis have been demonstrated with cultured aortic segments taken from rabbits fed atherogenic diets (Erhart and Holderbaum, 1980). Apparently concomitant with these changes in connective tissue proteins, lysyl oxidase activity increases 2.5 times over control values in the rabbit aortic arch within the first 90 days of feeding an atherogenic, fibrogenic diet containing 8% peanut oil and 2% cholesterol. In contrast, there was little change in enzyme activity in the abdominal aorta, consistent with the primary locus of lesions in the aortic arch of this animal model (Kagan *et al.*, 1981a) and suggesting that the increased enzyme activity reflects metabolically activated smooth muscle cells which proliferate at the sites of atherosclerotic lesions. Chvapil *et al.* (1976) observed that lysyl oxidase as well as prolyl hydroxylase, collagenase, and collagen content remained unchanged in the aortae of chickens fed a 2% cholesterol diet for 6 weeks, however. These contrasting results may reflect the absence of the fibrogenic peanut oil component in the diet of the latter study, as well as species differences.

b. Hypertension. Vascular wall fibrosis contributes importantly to increased flow resistance in hypertension (Wolinsky, 1972). Indeed, rates of collagen biosynthesis and deposition increase in hypertensive rats in a manner which is reversible by antihypertensive agents (Ooshima *et al.*, 1974). It is thus of interest that administration of BAPN (50–100 mg/kg) prevented the rise in blood pressure induced by deoxycorticosterone–salt in rats while BAPN administered after the onset of hypertension lowered the blood pressure (Iwatsuki *et al.*, 1977). Consistent with this ameliorative effect of BAPN, Sheridan *et al.* (1979) determined that the aortic lysyl oxidase activity of 12-week-old spontaneously hypertensive rats was slightly increased (1.3 to 1.4-fold) over the control values and more elevated (2.3-fold) in the DOCA–salt induced disease in 20-week-old rats, the variations in increase in enzyme correlating with the higher degree of hypertension in the induced model. Treatment with BAPN also returned the levels of both collagen and total protein synthesis to normotensive values. It thus seems that lysyl oxidase, although not the primary site of the molecular defect in hypertension, may play a regulatory role in the severity of the disease by controlling the degree of collagen fibrosis. In turn, the degree of hypertension as influenced by the extent of vascular fibrosis may modulate protein synthetic activity, including that of collagen biosynthesis, suggesting a potentially beneficial effect of antifibrotic agents in the control of hypertension.

Administration of propranalol, an antihypertensive agent, increased reactive aldehydes and altered the distribution of cross-linkages in aortic elastin and collagen of hypertension- and aneurysm-prone turkeys (Boucek *et al.*, 1983). Although evidence for the mechanism of these effects is not available, it was suggested that this may be due to interactions between this agent and the enzyme and/or its elastin and collagen substrates.

c. Myocardial Infarction. The activities of myocardial lysyl oxidase and prolyl hydroxylase increase significantly over a 2- to 6-day period following the induction of myocardial infarction in rabbits by coronary ligation (Lerman *et al.*, 1983). The deposition and cross-linking of collagen fibers at the ischemic site during healing apparently accounts for the increased mechanical strength of the damaged portion of the cardiac wall in comparison to the unaffected portions of the wall (Lerman *et al.*, 1983).

2. Models of Fibrotic Lung Disease

a. Bleomycin-Induced Pulmonary Fibrosis. Total urea-soluble lysyl oxidase activity increased approximately sixfold over controls in response to the intratracheal instillation of rats with bleomycin sulfate (Counts *et al.*, 1981), an agent known to induce severe lung fibrosis. The maximal increase in enzyme activity preceded those of lung collagen and elastin by as much as 4 weeks. Activities fell to near normal levels by 4 weeks (Counts *et al.*, 1981) while elevated collagen synthesis rates approximate control levels at 10 weeks (Clark *et al.*, 1982). A heat-stable factor was identified in the conditioned medium of lung explants of control and bleomycin-exposed lungs which suppressed collagen biosynthesis and lung fibroblast proliferation. Since there was more suppressive factor activity in bleomycin-exposed than in control lung explants (Clark *et al.*, 1982), this factor may represent a means of limiting collagen accumulation and possibly influence the return of lysyl oxidase to control levels following lung injury.

b. Cadmium Inhalation. Consistent with the localized fibrotic bronchitic changes seen in human lungs following exposure to airborne cadmium, rat lung lysyl oxidase activity increased 14-fold while prolyl hydroxylase was elevated 3.5-fold over controls by 4 days after a single exposure of rats to cadmium vapors (Chichester *et al.*, 1981). Activities returned to control levels by 21 days while lung collagen content was measurably elevated by 4 days and continued to increase for at least 10 days after exposure (Chichester *et al.*, 1981). Cadmium appears to selectively increase collagen as opposed to noncollagen protein synthesis in the lung of this rat model (Sampson *et al.*, 1984). The increase in connective tissue enzymes and collagen synthesis likely stems from the activation of interstitial fibroblasts proliferating in apparent response to a variety of inflammatory signals emanating from infiltrating monocytes and neutrophils evident in cadmium-exposed lungs (Sampson *et al.*, 1984; Asvadi and Hayes, 1978). The fibrotic response to repeated daily exposures of cadmium aerosol is less than that of a single, acute exposure (Sampson *et al.*, 1984) possibly as a result of the protection afforded to the lung against cadmium by the nearly linear induction in lung metallothionein levels seen during repeated daily exposures to cadmium vapors (Sampson *et al.*, 1984). The course of cadmium-induced pathology in hamster lungs is dramatically altered if lysyl oxidase is inhibited by dietary BAPN prior to and after the intratracheal administration of $CdCl_2$ (Niewohner and Hoidal, 1982). Control animals develop a diffuse lung fibrosis while BAPN-treated animals develop bullous emphysema, clearly demonstrating that the activity of lysyl oxidase is critical to the specific response to cadmium. There is evidently a balance between elastolysis caused by elastases of infiltrating monocytes and neutrophils (Padmanabhan *et al.*, 1982) and connective tissue synthesis during the repair response which may be altered by inhibition of lysyl oxidase. In contrast to the stimulation of lysyl oxidase in cadmium-exposed lungs, the enzyme in rat bone is reduced by 40 to 89% by maintenance on a diet supplemented with 50 ppm $CdCl_2$. This may reflect the ability of cadmium to directly inhibit the rat bone enzyme activity *in situ* as demonstrated in assays *in vitro* (Iguchi and Sano, 1982). The solubility of bone collagen was increased by this dietary manipulation, consistent with the inhibition of lysyl oxidase (Iguchi and Sano, 1982). It is possible that the bone enzyme is inhibited by replacement of the active site copper atom by ambient tissue cadmium. Metallothionein-mediated protection against such an effect may be less efficient in bone than in lung while the much more prolonged exposure of the animals to cadmium in this dietary model likely leads to greater accumulation of this toxic agent than is true of the aerosol model.

3. LIVER FIBROSIS

Hepatic fibrosis contributes to progressive hepatic disfunction and occurs in response to a variety of agents, notably including chronic, excess consumption of alcohol. Collagen synthesis and deposition is significantly increased in biopsied percutaneous human liver specimens taken from alcoholic patients (Chen and Leevy, 1975). The normally low levels of hepatic lysyl oxidase activity increased as much as 30-fold in response to the induction of liver fibrosis in rats by repeated injections of CCl_4, while prolyl and lysyl hydroxylase increased 3.5- and 1.7-fold, respectively (Siegel et al., 1978; McPhie, 1981). The marked increase in liver lysyl oxidase activity was paralleled by an increase in the plasma of approximately 16-fold. Immunofluorescence studies indicated that lysyl oxidase was associated with extracellular collagen fibers in the diseased liver (Siegel et al., 1978). The marked response and the ease of detection of lysyl oxidase in biopsy and plasma samples suggest that this enzyme might serve as a marker for the development of fibrosis. In this regard, increased lysyl oxidase activity has also been detected in lung lavage fluid of rats exposed to cadmium vapors (Chichester et al., 1981). Carter et al. (1982) noted that the development of hepatic fibrosis, increased hepatic and serum lysyl oxidase activity and increased hepatic collagenase activity were characteristic of chronic but not of a single acute administration of CCl_4 to rats. The apparent resistance to collagenolysis of the excess hepatic collagen deposited while collagenolytic activity was increased could be due to extensive cross-linking (Carter et al., 1982; Feinman et al., 1979).

4. DIABETES

Connective tissue defects are among the sequelae of the diabetic condition, evidenced by the thickening of capillary basement membrane, indicative of increased deposition of type IV collagen, and by increased arterial sclerosis, suggestive of changes in interstitial collagen biosynthesis and deposition (Prockop et al., 1979). The activities of kidney prolyl hydroxylase, lysyl hydroxylase and collagen glycosyltransferases (Khalifa and Cohen, 1975; Grant et al., 1976; Ristelli et al., 1976) as well as the activity of lung lysyl oxidase (Madia et al., 1979) are each increased in drug-induced diabetes in rats, consistent with increases in collagen synthesis and deposition.

There is some discrepancy concerning the extent of cross-linking of collagens in different diabetic tissues, however. Chang et al. (1980)

reported increased cross-linking as evidence by decreased collagen solubility and increased ratio of β- to α-chains in newly synthesized type I collagen in subcutaneous polyester implants in streptozotocin-diabetic rats. In contrast, LePape et al. (1981) noted reduced levels of NaB^3H_4-reducible intermolecular cross-linkages in the glomerular basement membranes of streptozotocin-diabetic rats, while there was an accumulation of the reducible linkage between C-1 of ambient glucose and the ϵ-amino functions of lysyl and hydroxylysyl residues known to form spontaneously in collagens and other proteins in diabetes (Higgins and Bunn, 1981). Such N-glycosylation would be expected to interfere with cross-linkage formation, and, in fact, the content of interstitial collagens is lessened in wounds and skin of diabetic subjects (Goodson and Hunt, 1977). Decreased cross-linking in turn may account for accelerated catabolism noted in skin collagen in diabetic animals (Schneir et al., 1982). Additional insight into the potentially adverse effect of high ambient glucose levels on collagen stability was provided by the finding that glucose inhibits collagen fibril formation in vitro thus preventing the formation of the optimal substrate configuration for lysyl oxidase and thereby inhibiting the oxidation of collagen by the enzyme (Lien et al., 1984). This effect was believed to reflect specific noncovalent interactions of glucose at sites of collagen monomers which normally are involved in intermolecular collagen–collagen interactions necessary for formation of the quarter-staggered fibrillar structure. Thus, it appears that collagen biosynthesis may be influenced at several levels which involve cross-linkage formation in diabetes. Increased lysyl oxidase activity may or may not result in increased cross-linkage formation and thus more stable collagen deposition, depending upon the concentration of and access to ambient glucose of specific sites of interstitial and/or basement membrane collagens in diabetes.

C. Chemotherapeutic Control of Fibrosis

There have been long-standing efforts to reduce scarring in wound repair and fibrosis by the inhibition of lysyl oxidase by administration of BAPN, as previous reviews have noted (Chvapil, 1975; Siegel, 1979; Fuller, 1981). Doses of BAPN which have been employed vary from 10–40 mg/kg/day (Arem et al., 1979) in the rat to 1 g/day in man (Peacock and Madden, 1978) with resultant antifibrotic effects exerted in liver (Haney et al., 1972), lung (Kuhn and Starcher, 1980; Percarpio and Fischer, 1976; Chichester et al., 1981), tumors (Cohen et al., 1979), dermal wounds (Arem et al., 1979), urethrial strictures (Peacock and

Madden, 1978), keloid (Fleisher *et al.*, 1976), flexor tendons (Peacock and Madden, 1969), and in healing peripheral nerve tissue (Rankin *et al.*, 1983). BAPN is most effective in reducing enzyme activity and cross-linking *in vivo* when topically applied as the free base as opposed to the fumarate salt (Fleisher *et al.*, 1981). Topical application of BAPN effectively enhanced the desired corneal-flattening effect of radial keratotomy presumably by preventing fibrotic scarring and resultant corneal contracture (Kogan and Katzen, 1983). BAPN also limited the degree of posttraumatic vitreous proliferation after double proliferating injury (Moorhead, 1981).

Lysyl oxidase activity of postburn (Hayakawa *et al.*, 1976) and postsurgery scar tissue (Knapp *et al.*, 1977) remains elevated for extended periods of time during the healing period. Enzyme activity in hypertrophic and keloid tissues was elevated, although the collagen of these tissues appeared to be less cross-linked than in normal or mature scar tissues, possibly due to proteolytic remodeling of inappropriately ordered collagen fibers (Knapp *et al.*, 1977).

The potential reduction of the fibrotic response to the inhibition of lysyl oxidase activity by agents as BAPN must be balanced against reductions in wound tensile strength or other undesirable effects which may result from such treatment (Arem *et al.*, 1975). For example, atherosclerotic-resistant rats developed severe atheroma by supplementation of a hyperlipidemic diet with BAPN (Bouissou *et al.*, 1978). Myocardial hypertrophy develops in BAPN-treated, aorta-constricted rats (Bing *et al.*, 1978). Injection of mice with BAPN during the first 4 weeks of life produces large lungs, a deficient number of alveoli, and a loss in lung elastic recoil. Much of the damage to the lungs appeared to be irreversibe (Kida and Thurlbeck, 1980). In contrast, a slight but statistically significant increase was found in the longevity of mice fed BAPN in drinking water at a 1 mg/ml concentration (LaBella and Vivian, 1978). Clearly, dose management, mode of administration, and stage of growth are critical to the effect of BAPN.

VII. Physiological Control of Lysyl Oxidase

In addition to the changes in lysyl oxidase activity seen in various pathological conditions, the enzyme is responsive to a variety of endogenous and exogenous physiological perturbations, including those involved in growth, development, changes in nutrition, and other transient alterations in homeostasis not conventionally associated with disease.

A. Hormonal Influences

1. Hypophysectomy

Following upon evidence that hypophysectomy led to decreased levels of cross-linked collagen (Everitt and Delbridge, 1972; Deyl et al., 1967), Howarth and Everitt (1974) noted that saline-soluble aortic benzylamine oxidase activity was decreased in hypophysectomized rats as was the aldehyde content of soluble collagen. Treatment of the hypophysectomized rats with growth hormone or cortisone restored this amine oxidase activity to normal levels. Although lysyl oxidase can oxidize benzylamine (H. M. Kagan, unpublished observations), the use of this substrate and the assay of the saline-soluble fraction compromises the conclusion that lysyl oxidase activity was altered by hypophysectomy. Shoshan and Finkelstein (1976) subsequently demonstrated that urea-extractable skin lysyl oxidase activity against an elastin substrate as well as the cross-linking of implanted lathrytic collagen in vivo were each markedly reduced in hypophysectomized rats indicating an influence of pituitary hormone(s) on lysyl oxidase. Following upon the observation that glucocorticoids decrease both collagen synthesis and the activities of prolyl hydroxylase and collagen glucosyltransferase (Newman and Cutroneo, 1978), it was noted that intraperitoneal injection of triamcinolone diacetate (6 mg/kg), a synthetic glucocorticoid, reduced urea-soluble rat skin lysyl oxidase activity by 91% and prolyl hydroxylase by 51% (Benson and LuValle, 1981). Since corticosteroids suppress release of adrenocorticotropic hormone from the adenohypophysis, the mechanism of reduction in lysyl oxidase activity by the synthetic glucocorticoid may converge on that of hypophysectomy since both decrease the availability of ACTH. Lysyl oxidase activity in the medium of cultured human smooth muscle cells tended to increase but only minimally upon incubation of the cells with cortisol in culture (Jarvelainen et al., 1982), indicative of little if any direct influence of this hormone on the production and/or secretion of enzyme in these cells.

2. Modulation by Estrogen

Steroid hormones and estrogen in particular are known to influence connective tissue proteins. Estrogen increases protocollagen prolyl hydroxylase activity and collagen accumulation in the rat uterus (Salvador and Tsai, 1973; Kao et al., 1969). Consistent with the several instances noting coordinated effects of connective tissue perturbations on the activity of lysyl oxidase, the activities of the enzyme extracted from ovariectomized rat skin and bone (Sanada *et al.*, 1978) or ovariectomized mouse cervix (Ozasa *et al.*, 1981) increased severalfold in response to injections of 17β-estradiol. Testosterone increased the activity of the enzyme of skin but not that of bone of ovariectomized rats (Sanada *et al.*, 1978). Estrogen also increased the insolubility of dermal collagen, consistent with increased cross-linking (Sanada *et al.*, 1978). Cervical lysyl oxidase activity increased markedly in intact mice during estrus and was lowest during diestrus evidently in response to changes in estrogen levels characteristic of the estrus cycle (Ozasa *et al.*, 1981). In contrast with estrogen-induced elevations of collagen synthetic capacity in the uterus, estrogens have a collagen-lowering effect in the aorta possibly due in part to increased turnover (Woessner, 1969). Collagen synthesis is decreased, however, by 17β-estradiol in cultures of aortic smooth muscle cells (Beldekas *et al.*, 1981), emphasizing the potential of organ-specific effects of estrogens on connective tissue protein synthesis. It will be of interest to assess whether the response of the enzyme to estradiol is similarly cell or tissue specific. The marked response of the cervical enzyme activity to control by steroid hormones presumably reflects hormone-induced alterations in the biosynthesis of lysyl oxidase protein, but, as in other instances cited, this has yet to be directly demonstrated. The mechanism of action of steroid hormones apparently entails the accumulation of steroid–receptor complexes in the nucleus. These complexes may then bind to specific DNA sites adjacent to regulated genes subsequently stimulating gene transcription (Jensen *et al.*, 1968; Gorski *et al.*, 1968) or, possibly, transcription may be activated indirectly by a protein mediator of the interaction of hormone–receptor complex with DNA (Vannice *et al.*, 1984). These models predict that lysyl oxidase synthesis may also be transcriptionally modulated by hormones.

B. Nutritional Effects and Turnover

The inhibitory effects of the deprivation of dietary copper and PLP on tissue lysyl oxidase activity have been noted. In addition to deficiencies of these specific nutrients, complete starvation alters enzyme levels. Thus, lysyl oxidase activity of rat lung decreases to approximately 25% of the level in fed animals, with a $t_{1/2}$ for the decrease in activity of 14–16 hr (Madia *et al.*, 1979). This value agrees reasonably well with the $t_{1/2}$ of 16–18 hr for the loss of lysyl oxidase *in vivo* in response to the administration of BAPN (Harris *et al.*, 1977). Starvation is known to increase proteolysis activity in lung (Thet *et al.*, 1977), and thus the similar values for $t_{1/2}$ suggest that lysyl oxidase may be modulated by proteolytic turnover, although this has yet to be directly demonstrated. The decrease in enzyme in response to dietary or cofactor deprivation also might reflect increased proteolytic susceptibility of the apoenzyme accumulating in the absence of required cofactor(s). Overall, these results raise the possibility that relatively short-term nutritional deprivation may have measurable effects on the development of connective tissues. Indeed, although the depressed level of lung lysyl oxidase activity returns to above normal levels within 3 hours of refeeding (Madia et al., 1979), starved rats exhibit decreased lung elasticity which does not return to normal upon refeeding (Sahebjami and Vassalo, 1979).

C. Regulatory Effects of Copper

Copper deficiency has long been recognized as a primary, diet-related cause of connective tissue pathology coupled with growth retardation. Extensive reviews on this subject have appeared (Carnes, 1971; Tinker and Rucker, 1985) to which the reader is referred. As previously noted, the evidence is clear that connective tissue pathology seen in copper deficiency predominantly reflects a deficiency in functional lysyl oxidase consequent to the deprivation of the metal ion cofactor. Copper deficiency in growing animals commonly results in skeletal and vascular tissue abnormalities, including osteoporosis, joint deformation, and bone fragility while internal hemorrhage and aortic aneurysms may develop with continued deprivation, the latter consistent with impaired maturation of elastin and collagen in the arterial wall (Rucker et al., 1975). An apparent correlation has been noted in humans between low levels of hepatic copper and the development of aortic aneurysms possibly reflective of a heritable copper deficiency (Tilson, 1982). A heritable diet-related defect in copper metabolism may similarly be involved in the tendency of a scoliosis-susceptible line of chickens to develop spinal curvature when fed a diet low in copper (6–10 μg g^{-1}), since this diet did not cause this defect in nonsusceptible chicks (Opsahl et al., 1984). However, lysyl oxidase activity and copper levels were within normal limits in bone tissue of susceptible animals fed the low copper diet, although reducible cross-linkage content of bone collagen was reduced in the affected animals (Opsahl et al., 1984). This syndrome is thus suggestive of a defect in collagen cross-linking mechanisms, although the involvement of alterations in lysyl oxidase is not readily apparent.

In some cases, the effects of copper deprivation may not be entirely irreversible. Copper supplementation can partially reverse the cardio-vascular pathology and mechanical defects in bone of copper-deprived chicks (Rucker *et al.*, 1975; Opsahl *et al.*, 1982). However, the emphysematous increases in alveolar size induced in rats by copper deprivation *in utero* and for 6 to 10 weeks after birth was not reversed by replenishment of the diet with copper, indicative that copper exerts a critical role in lung development (O'Dell *et al.*, 1978). In this case, the irreversibility likely reflects the incomplete cross-linking of elastin at a time crucial to the partitioning of the primitive alveolar sacs (O'Dell *et al.*, 1978). Soskel *et al.* (1982, 1984) have described a model of emphysema induced in growing pigs by a copper-deficient, zinc-supplemented diet, reasoning that zinc, which can inhibit lysyl oxidase activity in granulomatous implants *in vivo* (Chvapil and Misiorowski, 1980), would synergistically enhance the effects of copper deprivation on connective tissue development. Although there was focal damage in alveolar elastic fibers, the total content of lung elastin was not altered leaving some uncertainty about the central role of lysyl oxidase deficiency in this model (Soskel *et al.*, 1982). Indeed, neither urea-extractable lysyl oxidase activity, desmosine content, nor total collagen or elastin were altered from control levels in lungs of weanling Golden Syrian hamsters raised on copper-deficient diets *in utero* and postpartum (Soskel *et al.*, 1984) suggesting that lung tissue in this species is unusually resistant to nutritional copper deficiency. Copper-deficient diets do lower lung elastin content in developing chicks, however, and this effect is somewhat enhanced by zinc-supplementation (LeFevre *et al.*, 1982). The finding of a statistically significant correlation between low levels of copper in drinking water and altered pulmonary function among 297 human subjects (Sparrow *et al.*, 1982) suggests that there may be a human counterpart to these animal models of lung pathology induced by copper insufficiency.

Harris and colleagues have reported a series of studies indicative of a regulatory role for copper in the biosynthesis of lysyl oxidase in addition to its catalytic function as a cofactor for this enzyme (Harris *et al.*, 1982). Thus, the aortic enzyme levels in chicks maintained on a copper-deficient diet decreased to 5% of controls while subsequent administration of $CuSO_4$ (1 mg kg^{-1}) increased aortic enzyme levels 10- to 20-fold within 6 to 20 hours after injection. Since addition of copper to extracts to copper-deficient aortae did not restore activity, it appears that the apoenzyme did not accumulate as a stable product under these conditions. The copper-induced enhancement of activity *in vivo* was largely prevented by prior injection with cycloheximide but not by actinomycin, consistent with a posttranscriptional level of regulation of protein synthesis (Harris, 1976). Similarly, enzyme activity was slowly restored in intact but not in disrupted Cu-deficient aortas in culture medium supplemented with copper salts or a copper–protein fraction isolated from serum (Rayton and Harris, 1979). Restoration of enzyme activity occurred with a 3–5 hr lag time, suggestive of multiple copper transport phenomena coupled with protein biosynthesis. The appearance of a ^{64}Cu-labeled, newly synthesized 60,000-MW protein correlated with induction of the enzyme activity by copper addition. This approximates the expected molecular weight of chick aortic lysyl oxidase previously described by Harris et al. (1974), although more specific evidence that this protein is lysyl oxidase was not available. Thus, these studies reveal that the increase in enzyme activity in copper-deficient chick aorta requires the presence of copper as de novo protein synthesis occurs. These studies have led to the hypothesis that copper may be chelated by one or more specific proteins prior to and/or during its uptake and intracellular transport to the vesicular site of synthesis and activation of lysyl oxidase and that lysyl oxidase synthesis may be induced by such a copper–protein complex (Harris, 1976; Rayton and Harris, 1979; Harris et al., 1980b). It seems that these results do not exclude the alternative possibility that the apoenzyme may be synthesized in the absence of copper but may be more susceptible to proteolytic degradation than the copper-containing holoenzyme. Differentiation between the "induction" or "stabilization" models of copper-dependent increases in enzyme activity should be facilitated by measurement of lysyl oxidase apo- and holoprotein in addition to enzyme activity under these experimental conditions.

While a specific copper-carrying protein has not been directly related to the copper-induced increase in lysyl oxidase activity, Harris and DiSilvestro (1981) have observed a close correlation between levels of aortic lysyl oxidase activity and serum ceruloplasmin, the latter protein known to transport copper between liver and peripheral tissues. Both proteins decreased in concert in copper deficient chicks and both rose in concert upon feeding copper-supplemented diets. The activities of lysyl oxidase and ceruloplasmin each were increased further if copper was given to chicks that had received 17β-estradiol. Ceruloplasmin is thus a potential candidate as a copper-carrying protein involved in lysyl oxidase activation and/or induction. Specific ceruloplasmin receptors have been identified on aortic and cardiac membrane fragments of immature chicks, although these receptors were not correlated with a copper delivery role for ceruloplasmin (Stevens et al., 1984). Further, there may be tissue-specific modes of copper metabolism since isotopically labeled copper was principally bound to a 10,000-MW metal-

lothionein-like protein in liver but to 30,000-MW or greater components in the aorta when administered to copper-deficient chicks. Thus,
these studies point to the existence of multiple, specific, and sequential
events involved in the transport of copper to the site of lysyl oxidase
biosynthesis and/or activation of the nascent apoenzyme to the copper
metalloenzyme. It seems quite possible that defects in connective tissue proteins related to copper metabolism as in Menkes' disease may
find their origins in such pathways.

D. Effects of Ascorbic Acid

Ascorbic acid plays an important role in collagen biosynthesis by its
participation in the enzymatic hydroxylation of certain proline and
lysine residues in collagen precursors (Minor, 1980), although it appears that there are independent modes of regulation of prolyl and
lysyl hydroxylase by ascorbate (Murad *et al.*, 1981). Faris *et al.* (1984)
have implicated an additional role for ascorbate in the regulation of
lysyl oxidase. Thus, both insoluble elastin and lysyl oxidase activity
remained unaltered while collagen accumulation increased considerably when low levels (i.e., 0.5 μg ml^{-1}) of ascorbate were added to ascor-
bate-deprived cultures of rabbit smooth muscle cells. Higher levels of
ascorbate increased collagen content still further but decreased insoluble elastin while lysyl oxidase activity decreased by 25 to 40%. It was
suggested that the apparently coordinated decrease in elastin and enzyme activity may reflect elastin- and collagen-specific enzyme forms.
As noted, however, efforts to demonstrate collagen- and elastin-specific
forms of lysyl oxidase *in vitro* have been unsuccessful, although the
case may differ *in vivo*. Alternatively, the findings of DiSilvestro and
Harris (1981) may impact on the response seen in lysyl oxidase activity
to ascorbate in culture. These investigators observed that intraperitoneal administration of L-ascorbate to copper-deficient chicks 75 min
before or together with administration of CuSO$_4$ lowered the copper-
induced restoration of aortic enzyme activity by 25% while administration of L-ascorbate but not D-isoascorbate 75 min after administration
of copper resulted in a marked stimulation in the copper-induced return of enzyme activity. Thus, ascorbate demonstrates both antago-
nism and stereospecific postabsorption enhancement of the copper-me-
diated effects on enzyme levels. The influence of ascorbate may in part
reflect the ability of this reducing agent to reduce Cu(II) to Cu(I). It
seems possible that the decrease in lysyl oxidase activity in ascorbate-
treated cell cultures seen by Faris *et al.* (1984) might reflect such

chemical effects of ascorbate directly on copper in the growth medium, on copper-transport systems, or on the state of copper at the active site of lysyl oxidase.

E. Lysyl Oxidase during Development and Compensatory Lung Growth

Studies on the quantitative response of lysyl oxidase activity in growth and development appear to be quite limited. Chvapil *et al.* (1974) examined the extractability and activity of lysyl oxidase in granuloma tissue developing within poly(vinylalcohol) sponges subcutaneously implanted in rats. While total enzyme activity decreased with tissue maturation, the proportion of saline-extractable enzyme increased and that of urea-extractable enzyme decreased as the tissue matured.

Parenchymal and pleural urea-extractable enzyme activity of the developing rabbit lung was highest in the first 3 weeks of postnatal life and then decreased by 50% to a level remaining stable for 4 to 10 weeks while airway and aortic enzyme activity remained high during the first 10 weeks and then decreased by 75% (Brody *et al.*, 1979). Shieh and Yasunobu (1976) detected the bulk of lysyl oxidase activity in the parenchyma of bovine lungs with slight activity in the bronchi but no detectable activity in the trachei or pleural tissue. These workers observed that the bovine lung parenchymal enzyme activity continued to increase during the first 2 postnatal years and then remained relatively constant for 6 to 8 years of life. The response of lysyl oxidase activity in development and aging seems both species and organ specific, although it does appear that measurable enzyme activity persists as animals mature. Total insoluble elastin increases markedly in bovine ligament between 150 days of fetal age and birth at 280 days and then remains relatively constant during 10 years of life (Cleary *et al.*, 1967). While total ligament collagen similarly remains relatively constant from birth to adulthood (Cleary *et al.*, 1967), type III collagen increases in bovine ligament during maturation to adulthood (Chambers *et al.*, 1984). In addition to net accumulation of connective tissue proteins during growth, remodeling of at least the collagen component must occur postnatally, further evoking a need for the persistent expression of lysyl oxidase activity during maturation. More definitive studies of this aspect are needed, however, since lysyl oxidase assays in crude extracts of tissue are unavoidably complicated by the potential influence of contaminating saline- or urea-soluble forms of collagen whose concentrations also would be expected to differ with age, since such molecules can interfere with assays against tritiated elastin or collagen substrated *in vitro*.

After pneumonectomy, the remaining lung undergoes rapid compensatory growth, with increases in DNA, connective tissue proteins, and lung size. Lung lysyl oxidase activity of adult Golden Syrian hamsters increased more than twofold within 1 day following pneumonectomy, apparently before the onset of DNA increase (Brody *et al.*, 1979). The lung enzyme in this species also responded to changes in ambient oxygen concentration, with hypoxic conditions (12% oxygen) elevating urea-extractable lung enzyme activity four- to sixfold in pneumonectomized animals and nearly doubling activity in nonpneumonectomized controls. Neither aortic nor tracheal enzyme activity changed under hypoxic conditions while the increase in lung activity appeared to be independent of changes in lung DNA content. Thus, the enzyme in lung appears responsive to organ-specific activation by local or systemic stimuli and in a manner apparently independent of changes in cell number. The specific nature of the chemical stimuli operating in the pneumonectomized or hypoxic animal are not known, nor is it known to what extent increases seen in lysyl oxidase activity reflect activation of enzyme precursors, *de novo* protein synthesis or decreased proteolytic turnover of enzyme protein. Indeed, the latter uncertainty extends to most of the instances cited involving changes in tissue lysyl oxidase activity.

F. Precursors and Secretion of Lysyl Oxidase

Review of the literature before and since the last review of this subject (Siegel, 1979) reveals a general lack of information on the nature of the biosynthetic precursor(s) of lysyl oxidase, possible post-translational modifications, intracellular route of processing, and mechanisms and/or pathways for secretion of the enzyme. The evidence is strong, however, that the enzyme is secreted into the extracellular space, as deduced from studies in cell culture (Layman *et al.*, 1972; Starcher *et al.*, 1977; Royce *et al.*, 1980; Gonnerman *et al.*, 1981). The secretion of enzyme activity generally follows the growth curve of growing cells, increasing with increasing cell number (Layman *et al.*, 1972; Starcher *et al.*, 1977). It is of interest that enzyme secreted into the growth medium from normal and blotchy mouse fibroblasts (Starcher *et al.*, 1977) and from human skin fibroblasts (Layman *et al.*,

1972) becomes maximal as the cells reach confluency while activity then decreases markedly during the next 5 to 7 days in culture. The decrease in soluble enzyme might be accounted for by its increased association with the developing extracellular matrix, and, indeed, approximately 40% of the enzyme in rabbit smooth muscle cell cultures remains in the medium while 60% becomes associated with the matrix in a form requiring 4 M urea for extraction (Gonnerman et al., 1981). In this regard, the extracellular elastic matrix appears to exert feedback control on elastin synthesis by cells in contact with the matrix (Mecham et al., 1984). Thus, the elastic matrix of cells which have differentiated to produce elastin can induce previously undifferentiated cells to express the elastogenic phenotype. Conceivably, such feedback control by the matrix may extend to the biosynthesis and secretion of lysyl oxidase. The results of Gonnerman et al. (1981) suggest that such extracellular signals may influence lysyl oxidase secretion. Thus, replacement of the growth medium of rabbit smooth muscle cell cultures with new aliquots renewed the secretion of enzyme but to a degree which maximally approximated proportionality with the volume of replaced medium, suggesting that the concentration of extracellular enzyme or of another secreted component may control the secretion of lysyl oxidase. A portion of the total enzyme which was secreted into fresh culture medium appeared to represent previously synthesized enzyme present within the cells in a presecretory, "storage" form. Comparison of the molecular properties of this enzyme form with those of the enzyme secreted into the medium has yet to be described although such information should be of particular interest.

Recent studies have identified an unexpectedly large protein of cultured calf aortic smooth muscle cells which is reactive with polyclonal antibody raised against a copurified mixture of the four species of the 32,000-MW bovine aortic enzyme (Bronson et al., 1985). SDS–gel electrophoresis of the immunoprecipitate of newly synthesized proteins released from the cell layer revealed a protein band, the precipitation of which was selectively reduced by the addition of apparently homogeneous 32,000-MW calf aorta lysyl oxidase to the immunoprecipitation mixture. The molecular weight of this band approximated 200,000. Should the enzyme be synthesized as such a large molecular weight precursor, analysis of various possible modes of posttranslational processing to the 32,000-MW product should shed light on what has thus far been the cryptic bases of the unusual solubility properties, ionic variants, and varied molecular weights reported for this enzyme.

VIII. Summary and Prospects

It appears evident that there has been considerable progress made in our understanding of the biological role and properties of lysyl oxidase in recent years. Detailed insights into its participation in crosslinkage biosynthesis in collagen have been provided as have descriptions of its interaction with soluble and insoluble elastin substrates. Progress has been made in methods of purification and assay of the enzyme from various sources, and descriptions of certain key physical and chemical proterties have been provided. Studies with synthetic substrates point toward electrostatic features and vicinal sequence as important components in the enzyme specificity. The activity of the enzyme is clearly deficient in certain genetically related diseases of connective tissue and is often markedly elevated in various fibrotic diseases. β-aminopropionitrile appears to remain as the most promising chemotherapeutic agent for the control of fibrosis by inhibition of lysyl oxidase. Evidence that the enzyme is regulated by hormones, copper availability, and oxygen raises important prospects for research in the control of elastin and collagen biosynthesis at the level of this posttranslational enzymatic step.

Many fundamental aspects of this unusual catalyst remain to be solved, however. Mechanistic possibilities for enzyme function can now be considered although specific testing of such postulates and firm identification of a carbonyl cofactor as well as detailed exploration of the active site remains to be accomplished. The primary and higher levels of structure of isolated forms of lysyl oxidase are similarly unknown as are the structural bases and significance of the enzyme heterogeneity. While some features relating to the control of specificity have been identified, information presently available does not provide a clear answer as to why peptidyllysine oxidase appears to be restricted to elastin and collagen. Conceivably, restriction of the enzyme specificity may reflect compartmentalization and cosecretory relationships between lysyl oxidase and its connective tissue protein substrates yet to be explored. Further, coordinated activation of precursor forms of the enzyme, procollagen, and tropoelastin may also contribute to the specificity of lysine oxidation. Moreover, regulatory subunits may have been separated from the enzyme during its purification which otherwise limit the substrate specificity. Additional areas which remain to be fully explored notably include an understanding of the degree to which protein synthesis, posttranslational modification of enzyme precursors, and proteolytic turnover contribute to the regulation of lysyl oxidase activity *in vivo*. These matters seem of particular importance in view of the many clear examples revealing that lysyl oxidase is highly regulated *in vivo,* responding as it does to various normal physiological and disease-related perturbations. It is expected that the next review of this subject will surely cover progress made on many of these issues and will further report advances in the isolation and sequence analysis of the lysyl oxidase gene.

ACKNOWLEDGMENTS

The author gratefully acknowledges Drs. R. Rucker, E. Harris, K. Kivirikko, F. Ramirez, P. Davison, H. Boedtker, W. Gonnerman, S.-S. Tang, F. Greenaway, and J. Thanassi for providing reports of their work in press and/or for very helpful discussions. The expert assistance of Ms. Susan Calaman in the assemblage of this article is also greatly appreciated. The original research described in this chapter was supported by National Institutes of Health Grants AM 18880, HL 13262, and HL 19717.

REFERENCES

Abraham, P. A., and Carnes, W. H. (1978). *J. Biol. Chem.* **253,** 7993–7995.

Alvarez, O. M., and Gilbreath, R. L. (1982). *J. Trauma* **22,** 20–24.

Andrews, E. J., White, W. J., and Bullock, L. P. (1975). *Am. J. Pathol.* **78,** 199–207.

Arem, A. J., and Misiorowski, R. (1976). *J. Med.* **7,** 239–248.

Arem, A. J., Madden, J. W., Chvapil, M., and Tillema, L. (1975). *Surg. Forum* **26,** 67–69.

Arem, A. J., Misiorowski, R., and Chvapil, M. (1979). *J. Surg. Res.* **27,** 228–232.

Asvadi, S., and Hayes, J. A. (1978). *Am. J. Pathol.* **90,** 89–96.

Baig, K. M., Vlaovic, M., and Anwar, R. A. (1980). *Biochem. J.* **185,** 611–616.

Bailey, A. J., and Fowler, L. J. (1969). *Biochem. Biophys. Res. Commun.* **35,** 672–675.

Bailey, A. J., and Sims, T. J. (1976). *Biochem. J.* **153,** 211–215.

Bailey, A. J., Ranta, M. H., Nicholl, A. C., Partridge, S. M., and Elsden, M. F. (1977). *Biochem. Biophys. Res. Commun.* **78,** 1403–1410.

Bailey, A. J., Sims, T. J., and Light, N. (1984). *Biochem. J.* **218,** 713–723.

Barrow, M. V., Simpson, C. F., and Miller, E. S. (1974). *Q. Rev. Biol.* **49,** 101–128.

Baumgartner, S., Brown, D. J., Salevsky, E., and Leach, R. M. (1978). *J. Nutr.* **108,** 804–811.

Beldekas, J. C., Smith, B., Gerstenfeld, L. C., Sonenshein, G. E., and Franzblau, C. (1981). *Biochemistry* **20,** 2162–2167.

Benson, S. C., and LuValle, P. A. (1981). *Biochem. Biophys. Res. Commun.* **99,** 557–562.

Bhatnager, R. S., Rapaka, S. S. R., Liu, T. Z., and Wolfe, S. M. (1972). *Biochim. Biophys. Acta* **271,** 125–132.

Bing, O. H. L., Fanburg, F. L., Brooks, W. W., and Matsushita, S. (1978). *Circ. Res.* **43,** 632–637.

Bird, T. A., and Levene, C. I. (1982). *Biochem. Biophys. Res. Commun.* **108,** 1172–1180.

Bird, T. A., and Levene, C. I. (1983). *Biochem. J.* **210,** 633–638.

Blum, M., Cunningham, W. C., and Thanassi, J. W. (1976). *Bioorg. Chem.* **5,** 415–424.

Bonewitz, R. F., and Howell, R. R. (1981). *J. Cell. Physiol.* **106,** 339–348.

Bornstein, P., and Traub, W. (1979). *In* "The Proteins" (H. Neurath, ed.), Vol. 4, pp. 411–632. Academic Press, New York.

Bornstein, P., Kang, A. H., and Piez, K. A. (1966). *Proc. Natl. Acad. Sci. U.S.A.* **55,** 417–424.

Boucek, R. J., Gunja-Smith, Z., Noble, N. L., and Simpson, C. F. (1983). *Biochem. Pharmacol.* **32,** 275–280.

Bouissou, H., Julian, M., and Pieraggi, M. T. (1978). *Gerontology* **24,** 250–265.

Brennan, M., and Davison, P. F. (1980). *Biopolymers* **19,** 1861–1873.

Brody, J. S., Kagan, H., and Manalo, A. (1979). *Am. Rev. Respir. Dis.* **120,** 1289–1295.

Bronson, R., Reiss, D., Sonenshein, G., and Kagan, H. (1985). *Fed. Proc.* **44,** 663 (Abstract).

Buckingham, K., Heng-Khoo, C. S., Dubick, M., Lefevre, M., Cross, C., Julian, L., and Rucker, R. (1981). *Proc. Soc. Exp. Biol. Med.* **166,** 310–319.

Buffoni, F. and Raimondi, L. (1981). *Agents Actions* **11,** 38–41.

Buffoni, F., Ignesti, G., and Lodovici, M. (1981). *Ital. J. Biochem.* **30,** 179–189.

Butler, W. T., Miller, E. J., and Finch, J. E., Jr. (1976). *Biochemistry* **15,** 3000–3006.

Byers, P. H., Narayanan, A. S., Bornstein, P., and Hall, J. G. (1976). *Birth Defects* **12,** 293–298.

Byers, P. H., Siegel, R. C., Holbrook, K. A., Narayanan, A. S., Bornstein, P., and Hall, J. G. (1980). *N. Engl. J. Med.* **303,** 61–65.

Cake, M. H., DiSorbo, D. M., and Litwack, G. (1978). *J. Biol. Chem.* **253,** 4886–4890.

Camakaris, J., Mann, J., and Danks, D. M. (1979). *Biochem. J.* **180,** 597–604.

Cannon, D. J., and Davison, P. F. (1978). *Biochem. Biophys. Res. Commun.* **85,** 1373–1378.

Capaldi, M. J., and Chapman, J. A. (1982). *Biopolymers* **21,** 2291–2313.

Carnes, W. H. (1971). *Fed. Proc.* **30,** 995–1000.

Carrington, M. J., Bird, T. A., and Levene, C. I. (1984). *Biochem. J.* **221,** 837–843.

Carter, E. A., McCarron, M. J., Alpert, E., and Isselbacher, K. J. (1982). *Gastroenterology* **82,** 526–534.

Chambers, C. A., Shuttleworth, C. A., Ayad, S., and Grant, M. E. (1984). *Biochem. J.* **220,** 385–394.

Chang, K., Uitto, J., Rowold, E. A., Grant, G. A., Kilo, C., and Williamson, J. R. (1980). *Diabetes* **29,** 778–781.

Chen, T. S. M., and Leevy, C. M. (1975). *J. Lab. Clin. Med.* **85,** 103–112.

Chichester, Co. O., Palmer, K. C., Hayes, J. A., and Kagan, H. M. (1981). *Am. Rev. Respir. Dis.* **124,** 709–713.

Chou, W. S., Savage, J. E., and O'Dell, B. L. (1969). *J. Biol. Chem.* **244,** 5785–5789.

Chou, W. S., Rucker, R. B., Savage, J. E., and O'Dell, B. L. (1970). *Proc. Soc. Exp. Biol. Med.* **134,** 1078–1082.

Chvapil, M. (1975). *Life Sci.* **16,** 1345–1362.

Chvapil, M., and Misiorowski, R. (1980). *Proc. Soc. Exp. Biol. Med.* **164,** 137–141.

Chvapil, M., McCarthy, D. W., Misiorowski, R. L., Madden, J. W., and Peacock, E. E., Jr. (1974). *Proc. Soc. Exp. Biol. Med.* **146,** 688–693.

Chvapil, M., Stith, P. L., Tillema, L. M., Carlson, E. C., Campbell, J. B., and Eskelson, C. D. (1976). *Atherosclerosis* **24,** 393–405.

Chvapil, M., Misiorowski, R., and Eskelson, C. (1981). *J. Surg. Res.* **31,** 151–155.

Clark, J. G., Kostal, K. M., and Marino, B. A. (1982). *J. Biol. Chem.* **257,** 8098–8105.

Cleary, E. G., and Cliff, W. J. (1978). *Exp. Mol. Pathol.* **28,** 227–246.

Cleary, E. G., Sandberg, L. B., and Jackson, D. S. (1967). *J. Cell Biol.* **33,** 469–479.

Cleary, E. G., Fanning, J. C., and Prosser, I. (1981). *Connect. Tissue Res.* **8,** 161–166.

Cohen, I. K., Moncure, C. W., Witorsch, R. J., and Diegelmann, R. F. (1979). *Cancer Res.* **39,** 2923–2927.

Counts, D. F., Evans, J. N., Dipetrillo, T. A., Sterling, K. M., Jr., and Kelley, J. (1981). *J. Pharmacol. Exp. Ther.* **219,** 675–678.

Crabbe, J. C. (1979). *Agents Actions* **9,** 41–42.

Crombie, G., Snider, R., Faris, B., and Franzblau, C. (1981). *Biochim. Biophys. Acta* **640**, 365–367.

Cronlund, A. L. (1983). Ph.D. thesis, Boston University.

Cronlund, A. L., Smith, B. D., and Kagan, H. M. (1985). *Connect. Tissue Res.* **14**, 109–119.

Danks, D. M. (1977). *Inorg. Perspect. Biol. Med.* **1**, 73–100.

Danks, D. M. (1980). *Ciba Found. Symp.* **79**, 209–225.

Danks, P. M. (1983). *In* "The Metabolic Basis of Inherited Disease" (J. B. Stanbury, J. B. Wyngaarden, D. S. Frederickson, J. L. Goldstein, and M. S. Brown, eds.), pp. 1251–1268. McGraw-Hill, New York.

Davis, N. R. (1978). *Biochim. Biophys. Acta* **538**, 258–267.

Deyl, Z., Everitt, A. V., and Rosmus, J. (1967). *Exp. Gerontol.* **7**, 45–51.

Diedrich, D. L., and Schnaitman, C. A. (1978). *Proc. Natl. Acad. Sci. U.S.A.* **75**, 3708–3712.

DiFerrante, N., Leachman, R. D., Angelini, P., Donnelly, P. V., Francis, G., and Almazan, A. (1975a). *Connect. Tissue Res.* **3**, 49–53.

DiFerrante, N., Leachman, R. D., Angelini, P., Donnelly, P. V., Francis, G., Almazan, A., Segni, G., Franzblau, C., and Jordan, R. E. (1975b). *Birth Defects* **11**, 31–37.

DiSilvestro, R. A., and Harris, E. D. (1981). *J. Nutr.* **111**, 1964–1968.

DiSilvestro, R. A., and Harris, E. D. (1983). *Biochem. Pharmacol.* **32**, 343–346.

DiSorbo, D. M., Phelps, D. S., Ohl, V. S., and Litwack, G. (1980). *J. Biol. Chem.* **255**, 3866–3870.

Duine, J. A., and Frank, J. (1981). *Trends Biochem. Sci.* **6**, 278–280.

Dunn, D. M., and Franzblau, C. (1982). *Biochemistry* **21**, 4195–4202.

Erhart, L. A., and Holderbaum, D. (1980). *Atherosclerosis* **37**, 423–432.

Evans, G. W., and Reis, B. L. (1978). *J. Nutr.* **108**, 554–560.

Everitt, A. V., and Delbridge, L. (1972). *Exp. Gerontol.* **7**, 45–51.

Eyre, D. R., and Glunder, M. J. (1973). *Biochem. Biophys. Res. Commun.* **52**, 663–671.

Eyre, D. R., and Oguchi, H. (1980). *Biochem. Biophys. Res. Commun.* **92**, 403–410.

Eyre, D. R., Paz, M. A., and Gallop, P. M. (1984). *Ann. Rev. Biochem.* **53**, 717–748.

Faris, B., Ferrera, R., Toselli, P., Nambu, J., Gonnerman, W. A., and Franzblau, C. (1984). *Biochim. Biophys. Acta* **797**, 71–75.

Feinman, L., Fecher, R., Lue, S. L., and Lieher, C. S. (1979). *Exp. Mol. Pathol.* **30**, 271–278.

Ferrera, R., Faris, B., Mogayzel, P. J., Jr., Gonnerman, W. A., and Franzblau, C. (1982). *Anal. Biochem.* **126**, 312–317.

Fietzek, P. P., and Kuhn, K. (1976). *Int. Rev. Connect. Tissue Res.* **7**, 1–59.

Fietzek, P. P., Breitkreutz, D., and Kuhn, K. (1974). *Biochim. Biophys. Acta* **365**, 305–310.

Fietzek, P. P., Allman, H., Rauterberg, J., and Wachter, E. (1977). *Proc. Natl. Acad. Sci. U.S.A.* **74**, 84–86.

Fisk, D. E., and Kuhn, C. (1976). *Am. Rev. Respir. Dis.* **113**, 787–797.

Fleisher, J. H., Arem, A. J., Chvapil, M., and Peacock, E. E., Jr. (1976). *Proc. Soc. Exp. Med.* **152**, 469–474.

Fleisher, J. H., Misiorowski, R., Owen, J. A., and Chvapil, M. (1981). *Life Sci.* **29**, 2553–2560.

Fleming, W. W., Sullivan, C. E., and Torchia, D. A. (1980). *Biopolymers* **19**, 597–617.

Foster, J. A., Rubin, A. L., Kagan, H. M., and Franzblau, C. (1974). *J. Biol. Chem.* **249**, 6191–6196.

Foster, J. A., Rich, C. B., and Karr, S. R. (1983). *Int. Rev. Connect. Tissue Res.* **10**, 65–96.

Franzblau, C., and Faris, B. (1982). In "Cell Biology of the Extracellular Matrix" (E. D. Hay, ed.), pp. 65–94. Plenum, New York.

Fujii, K., Kajiwara, R., and Kurosu, H. (1979). *FEBS Lett.* **97**, 193–195.

Fujimoto, D., Moriguchi, T., Ishida, T., and Hayashi, H. (1978). *Biochem. Biophys. Res. Commun.* **84**, 52–57.

Fukae, M., and Mechanic, G. L. (1980). *J. Biol. Chem.* **255**, 6511–6518.

Fuller, F., and Boedtker, H. (1981). *Biochemistry* **20**, 996–1006.

Fuller, G. C. (1981). *J. Med. Chem.* **24**, 651–658.

Gallop, P. M., and Paz, M. A. (1975). *Physiol. Rev.* **55**, 418–487.

Geiger, B. J., Steenbock, H., and Parson, H. T. (1933). *J. Nutr.* **6**, 427–442.

Gelman, R. A., Williams, B. R., and Piez, K. A. (1979). *J. Biol. Chem.* **254**, 180–186.

Gibson, M. A., and Cleary, E. G. (1982). *Biochem. Biophys. Res. Commun.* **105**, 1288–1295.

Glanville, R. W., and Fietzek, P. P. (1976). *FEBS Lett.* **71**, 99–102.

Goka, T. J., Stevenson, R. E., Hefferan, P. M., and Howell, R. R. (1976). *Proc. Natl. Acad. Sci. U.S.A.* **73**, 604–606.

Gonnerman, W. A., Toverud, S. U., Ramp, W. K., and Mechanic, G. L. (1976). *Proc. Soc. Exp. Biol. Med.* **151**, 453–456.

Gonnerman, W. A., Ferrara, R., and Franzblau, C. (1981). *Biochemistry* **20**, 3864–3867.

Goodson, W. H., and Hunt, T. K. (1977). *J. Surg. Res.* **22**, 221–227.

Gorski, J., Taft, D. O., Shyamala, G., Smith, D., and Notides, A. (1968). *Recent Prog. Horm. Res.* **24**, 45–80.

Gosline, J. M. (1976). *Int. Rev. Connect. Tissue Res.* **7**, 211–249.

Gotte, L., Giro, M. W., Volpin, D., and Horne, R. W. (1974). *J. Ultrastruct. Res.* **46**, 23–33.

Grant, M. E., Harwood, R., and Williams, I. F. (1976). *J. Physiol.* **257**, 56–57.

Greenaway, F. T., Spacciapoli, P., Young, C. M., and Kagan, H. M. (1984). *Meet. Int. Chem. Congr. Pacific Basin Soc.* (Abstract).

Hamamoto, H., Ueba, Y., Sudo, Y., Sanada, H., Yamamuro, T., and Takeda, T. (1982). *Hand* **14**, 237–247.

Hamilton, G. (1971). *Prog. Bioorgan. Chem.* **1**, 83–157.

Haney, A. F., Peacock, E. E., and Madden, C. W. (1972). *Am. Surg.* **175**, 863–869.

Harris, E. D. (1976). *Proc. Natl. Acad. Sci. U.S.A.* **73**, 371–374.

Harris, E. D., and DiSilvestro, R. A. (1981). *Proc. Soc. Exp. Biol. Med.* **166**, 528–531.

Harris, E. D., and Garcia de Quevedo, M. C. (1978). *Arch. Biochem. Biophys.* **190**, 227–233.

Harris, E. D., Gonnerman, W. A., Savage, J. E., and O'Dell, B. L. (1974). *Biochim. Biophys. Acta* **341**, 332–344.

Harris, E. D., Rayton, J. K., and DeGroot, J. E. (1977). *Adv. Exp. Med. Biol.* **79**, 543–559.

Harris, E. D., Blount, J. E., and Leach, R. M., Jr. (1980a). *Science* **208**, 55–56.

Harris, E. D., Rayton, J. K., Balthrop, J. E., DiSilvestro, R. A., and Garcia de Quevedo, M. (1980b). *Ciba Found. Symp.* **79**, 163–182.

Harris, E. D., DiSilvestro, R. A., and Balthrop, J. E. (1982). In "Inflammatory Diseases and Copper" (J. R. J. Sorenson, ed.), pp. 183–198. Humana Press,

Hayakawa, T., Hino, N., Fuyamada, H., Nagatsu, T., and Aoyama, H. (1976). *Clin. Chim. Acta* **71**, 245–250.

Heathcote, J. G., Bailey, A. J., and Grant, M. E. (1980). *Biochem. J.* **190**, 229–237.

Helseth, D. L., and Veis, A. (1981). *J. Biol. Chem.* **256**, 7118–7128.

Henkel, W., and Glanville, R. W. (1982). *Eur. J. Biochem.* **122**, 205–213.

Higgins, P. J., and Bunn, H. F. (1981). *J. Biol. Chem.* **256**, 5204–5208.

Howarth, D., and Everitt, A. V. (1974). *Gerontologia* **20**, 27–32.
Hunt, D. M. (1974). *Nature* **249**, 852–854.
Hunt, D. M. (1976). *Life Sci.* **19**, 1913–1920.
Iguchi, H., and Sano, S. (1982). *Toxicol. Appl. Pharmacol.* **62**, 126–136.
Iwatsuki, K., Cardinale, G. J., Spector, S., and Udenfriend, S. (1977). *Proc. Natl. Acad. Sci. U.S.A.* **74**, 360–362.
Jackson, S. H. (1973). *Biochim. Biophys. Acta* **45**, 215–217.
Jarvelainen, H., Halme, T., and Ronnemaa, T. (1982). *Acta Med. Scand. Suppl.* **660**, 114–122.
Jordan, R. E., Milbury, P., Sullivan, K. A., Trackman, P. C., and Kagan, H. M. (1977). *Adv. Exp. Med. Biol.* **79**, 531–542.
Kadar, A., Joos, A., and Jellinek, H. (1976). *Arterial Wall* **4**, 165–175.
Kagan, H. M., and Sullivan, K. A. (1982). *In* "Methods in Enzymology" (L. W. Cunningham and D. W. Frederiksen, eds.), Vol. 82, Part A, pp. 637–650. Academic Press, New York.
Kagan, H. M., Crombie, G. D., Jordan, R. E., Lewis, W., and Franzblau, C. (1972). *Biochemistry* **11**, 3412–3418.
Kagan, H. M., Hewitt, N. A., Salcedo, L. L., and Franzblau, C. (1974). *Biochim. Biophys. Acta* **365**, 223–234.
Kagan, H. M., Sullivan, K. A., Olsson, T. A.. 3rd. and Cronlund, A. L. (1979). *Biochem. J.* **177**, 203–214.
Kagan, H. M., Tseng, L., Trackman, P. C., Okamoto, K., Rapaka, R. S., and Urry, D. W. (1980). *J. Biol. Chem.* **255**, 3656–3659.
Kagan, H. M., Raghavan, J., and Hollander, W. (1981a). *Arteriosclerosis* **1**, 287–291.
Kagan, H. M., Tseng, L., and Simpson, D. E. (1981b). *J. Biol. Chem.* **256**, 5417–5421.
Kagan, H. M., Soucy, D. M., Zoski, C. G., Resnick, R. J., and Tang, S. S. (1983a). *Arch. Biochem. Biophys.* **221**, 158–167.
Kagan, H. M., Williams, M. A., Calaman, S. D., and Berkowitz, E. M. (1983b). *Biochem. Biophys. Res. Commun.* **115**, 186–192.
Kagan, H. M., Williams, M. A., Williamson, P. R., and Anderson, J. M. (1984). *J. Biol. Chem.* **259**, 11203–11207.
Kaitila, I. I., Peltonen, L., Kuivaniemi, H., Palotie, A., Elo, J., and Kivirikko, K. I. (1982). *Prog. Clin. Biol. Res.* **104**, 307–315.
Kang, A. H. (1972). *Biochemistry* **11**, 1828–1835.
Kang, A. H., Piez, K. A., and Gross, J. (1969). *Biochemistry* **8**, 3648–3655.
Kao, K. Y. T., Arnett, W. M., and McGavack, T. H. (1969). *Endocrinology* **85**, 1057–1061.
Khalifa, A., and Cohen, M. P. (1975). *Biochim. Biophys. Acta* **386**, 332–339.
Kida, K., and Thurlbeck, W. M. (1980). *Am. Rev. Respir. Dis.* **122**, 467–475.
Kilburn, K. H., and Hess, R. A. (1982). *Teratology* **26**, 1–9.
Kim, C. S., and Hill, C. H. (1966). *Biochem. Biophys. Res. Commun.* **24**, 395–400.
Knapp, T. R., Daniels, R. J., and Kaplan, E. N. (1977). *Am. J. Pathol.* **86**, 47–69.
Kogan, L. L., and Katzen, L. (1983). *Ann. Ophthalmol.* **15**, 842–845.
Kuboki, Y., Takagi, T., Shimokawa, H., Oguchi, H., Sasaki, S., and Mechanic, G. L. (1981). *Connect. Tissue Res.* **9**, 107–114.
Kuhn, C., 3d, and Starcher, B. C. (1980). *Am. Rev. Respir. Dis.* **122**, 453–460.
Kuivaniemi, H., Peltonen, L., Palotie, A., Kaitila, I., and Kivirikko, K. D. (1982). *J. Clin. Invest.* **69**, 730–733.
Kuivaniemi, H., Savolainen, E. R., and Kivirikko, K. I. (1984). *J. Biol. Chem.* **259**, 6996–7003.

Labadie, G. W., Hirschhorn, K., Katz, S., and Beratis, N. G. (1981). *J. Pediatr. Res.* **15,** 257–261.

LaBella, F., and Vivian, S. (1978). *Exp. Gerontol.* **13,** 251–254.

Laurent, P., Janoff, A., and Kagan, H. M. (1983). *Am. Rev. Respir. Dis.* **127,** 189–192.

Layman, D. L., Narayanan, A. S., and Martin, G. R. (1972). *Arch. Biochem. Biophys.* **149,** 97–101.

Leach, R. M., Jr., Rucker, R. B., and Van Dyke, G. P. (1981). *Arch. Biochem. Biophys.* **207,** 353–359.

LeFevre, M., Heng, H., and Rucker, R. B. (1982). *J. Nutr.* **112,** 1344–1352.

Lent, R., and Franzblau, C. (1967). *Biochem. Biophys. Res. Commun.* **26,** 43–50.

LePape, A., Guitton, J. D., and Muh, J. P. (1981). *Biochem. Biophys. Res. Commun.* **100,** 1214–1221.

Lerman, R. H., Apstein, C. S., Kagan, H. M., Osmers, E. L., Chichester, C. O., Vogel, W. M., Connelly, C. M., and Steffee, W. P. (1983). *Circ. Res.* **53,** 378–388.

Levene, C. I. (1961). *J. Exp. Med.* **114,** 295–310.

Levene, C. I., and Gross, J. (1959). *J. Exp. Med.* **110,** 771–790.

Lien, Y. H., Stern, R., Fu, J. C. C., and Siegel, R. C. (1984). *Science* **225,** 1489–1491.

Lobenstein-Verbeek, C. L., Jongejan, J. A., Frank, J., and Duine, J. A. (1984). *FEBS Lett.* **170,** 305–309.

McKusick, V. A. (1982). "Heritable Disorders of Connective Tissue" 4th Ed., pp. 61–223. Mosby, St. Louis.

McPhie, J. L. (1981). *Hepatogastroenterology* **28,** 240–241.

Madia, A. M., Rozovski, S. J., and Kagan, H. M. (1979). *Biochim. Biophys. Acta* **585,** 481–487.

Mann, J. R., Camakaris, J., and Danks, D. M. (1979a). *Biochem. J.* **180,** 613–619.

Mann, J. R., Camakaris, J., Danks, D. M., and Walliczek, E. G. (1979b). *Biochem. J.* **180,** 605–612.

Mann, J. R., Camakaris, J., Francis, M., and Danks, D. M. (1981). *Biochem. J.* **196,** 81–88.

Mecham, R. P., and Foster, J. A. (1979). *Biochim. Biophys. Acta* **577,** 147–158.

Mecham, R. P., Griffin, G. L., Madaras, J. G., and Senior, R. M. (1984). *J. Cell Biol.* **98,** 1813–1816.

Mechanic, G. L. (1977). *Adv. Exp. Med. Biol.* **86B,** 699–708.

Mechanic, G., Gallop, P. M., and Tanzer, M. L. (1971). *Biochem. Biophys. Res. Commun.* **45,** 644–653.

Melet, J., Vianden, G. D., and Bachra, B. N. (1977). *Anal. Biochem.* **77,** 141–146.

Miller, E. J., Martin, G. R., Mecca, C. E., and Piez, K. A. (1965). *J. Biol. Chem.* **240,** 3623–3627.

Miller, E. J., Pinnell, S. R., Martin, G. R., and Schiffman, E. (1967). *Biochem. Biophys. Res. Commun.* **26,** 132–137.

Minor, R. R. (1980). *Am. J. Pathol.* **98,** 226–280.

Mirelman, D., and Siegel, R. C. (1979). *J. Biol. Chem.* **254,** 571–574.

Misiorowski, R. L., and Werner, M. J. (1978). *Biochem. Biophys. Res. Commun.* **85,** 809–814.

Misiorowski, R. L., Ulreich, J. B., and Chvapil, M. (1976). *Anal. Biochem.* **71,** 186–192.

Miyahara, M., Hayashi, K., Berger, J., Tanzawa, K., Njieha, F. K., Trelstad, R. L., and Prockop, D. J. (1984). *J. Biol. Chem.* **259,** 9891–9898.

Moorhead, L. C. (1983). *Am. J. Ophthalmol.* **95,** 97–109.

Mudd, S. H. (1980). *Ciba Found. Symp.* **72,** 239–258.

Muldoon, T. G., and Cidlowski, J. A. (1980). *J. Biol. Chem.* **255,** 3100–3107.

Murad, S., Grove, D., Lundberg, K. A., Reynolds, G., Sivarojah, A., and Pinnell, S. R. (1981). *Biochemistry* **78,** 2879–2882.

Murray, J. C., and Levene, C. I. (1977). *Biochem. J.* **167,** 463–467.

Murray, J. C., Fraser, D. R., and Levene, C. I. (1978). *Exp. Mol. Pathol.* **28,** 301–308.

Myers, B. A., Dubick, M. A., Reynolds, R. D., and Rucker, R. B. (1985). *Biochem. J.* **229,** 153–160.

Nakano, G., Harada, M., and Nagatsu, T. (1974). *Biochim. Biophys. Acta* **341,** 366–377.

Narayanan, A. S., and Page, R. C. (1976). *J. Biol. Chem.* **251,** 1125–1130.

Narayanan, A. S., Siegel, R. C., and Martin, G. R. (1972). *Biochem. Biophys. Res. Commun.* **46,** 745–751.

Narayanan, A. S., Page, R. C., and Martin, G. R. (1974a). *Biochim. Biophys. Acta* **35,** 126–132.

Narayanan, A. S., Siegel, R. C., and Martin, G. R. (1974b). *Arch. Biochem. Biophys.* **162,** 231–237.

Narayanan, A. S., Page, R. C., and Kuzan, F. (1977). *Adv. Exp. Med. Biol.* **79,** 491–508.

Narayanan, A. S., Page, R. C., Kuzan, F., and Copper, C. G. (1978). *Biochem. J.* **173,** 857–862.

Narayanan, A. S., Sandberg, L. B., Jones, K., Coleman, S. S., and Bagley, R. A. (1982). *Exp. Mol. Pathol.* **36,** 107–117.

Newman, R. A., and Cutroneo, K. R. (1978). *Mol. Pharmacol.* **14,** 185–198.

Niewohner, D. E., and Hoidal, J. R. (1982). *Science* **217,** 359–360.

Nimni, M. E. (1968). *J. Biol. Chem.* **243,** 1457–1466.

Numata, Y., Takei, T., and Hayakawa, T. (1981). *Biochem. Pharmacol.* **30,** 3125–3126.

Oda, O., Manabe, T., and Okuyama, T. (1981). *J. Biochem.* **89,** 1317–1323.

O'Dell, B. L., Hardwick, B. C., Reynolds, G., and Savage, J. E. (1961). *Proc. Soc. Exp. Biol. Med.* **108,** 402–405.

O'Dell, B. L., Kilburn, K. H., McKenzie, W. N., and Thurston, R. J. (1978). *Am. J. Pathol* **90,** 413–432.

Ooshima, A., Fuller, G. C., Cardinale, G., Spector, S., and Udenfriend, S. (1974). *Proc. Natl. Acad. Sci. U.S.A.* **71,** 3019–3023.

Opsahl, W., Zeronian, H., Ellison, M., Lewis, D., Rucker, R. B., and Riggins, R. S. (1982). *J. Nutr.* **112,** 708–716.

Opsahl, W., Abbott, U., Kenney, C., and Rucker, R. (1984). *Science* **225,** 440–442.

Osman, M., Cantor, J., Roffman, S., Turino, G. M., and Mandl, I. (1982). *Am. Rev. Respir. Dis.* **125,** 263S (abstract).

Ozasa, H., Tominaga, T., Nishimura, T., and Takeda, T. (1981). *Endocrinology* **109,** 618–621.

Padmanabhan, R. V., Gudapaty, S. R., Liener, I. E., and Hoidal, J. R. (1982). *Environ. Res.* **29,** 90–96.

Page, R. C., and Benditt, E. P. (1966). *Lab. Invest.* **15,** 1643–1651.

Page, R. C., and Benditt, E. P. (1967). *Biochemistry* **6,** 1142–1148.

Partridge, S. M., Elsden, D. F., Thomas, J., Dorfman, A., Telser, A., and Ho, P. (1964). *Biochem. J.* **93,** 30c–33c.

Partridge, S. M., Elsden, D. F., Thomas, J., Dorfman, A., Telser, A., and Ho, P. (1966). *Nature (London)* **209,** 399–400.

Pasquali-Ronchetti, I., Fornieri, C., Castellani, I., Bressan, G. M., and Volpin, D. (1981). *Exp. Mol. Pathol.* **35,** 42–56.

Pasquali-Ronchetti, I., Bressan, G. M., Fornieri, C., Baccarani-Contri, M., Castellani, I., and Volpin, D. (1984). *Exp. Mol. Pathol.* **40,** 235–245.

Paz, M. A., Keith, D. A., and Gallop, P. M. (1982). *Adv. Enzymol.* **82,** 571–587.

Peacock, E. E., Jr., and Madden, J. W. (1969). *Surgery* **66**, 215–223.

Peacock, E. E., Jr., and Madden, J. W. (1978). *Am. J. Surg.* **136**, 600–605.

Peltonen, L., Kuivaniemi, H., Palotie, A., Horn, N., Kaitila, I., and Kivirikko, K. (1983). *Biochemistry* **22**, 6156–6162.

Percarpio, B., and Fischer, J. J. (1976). *Radiology* **121**, 737–740.

Piez, K. A. (1968). *Am. Rev. Biochem.* **37**, 547–570.

Pinnell, S. R., and Martin, G. R. (1968). *Proc. Natl. Acad. Sci. U.S.A.* **61**, 708–718.

Priest, R. E., Moinuddin, J. F., and Priest, J. H. (1973). *Nature* **245**, 264–266.

Prockop, D. J., Kivirikko, K. I., Tuderman, L., and Guzman, N. A. (1979). *N. Engl. J. Med.* **301**, 15–23 and 77–85.

Ranga, V., and Kleinerman, J. (1981). *Am. Rev. Respir. Dis.* **123**, 90–97.

Rankin, L. L., Chvapil, M., Misiorowski, R., Johnson, P., and Weinstein, P. R. (1983). *Exp. Neruol.* **79**, 97–105.

Rauterberg, J., Fietzek, P. P., Rexrodt, F., Becker, U., Stank, M., and Kuhn, K. (1972). *FEBS Lett.* **21**, 75–79.

Rayton, J. K., and Harris, E. D. (1979). *J. Biol. Chem.* **254**, 621–626.

Rigby, B. J., Mitchell, T. W., and Robinson, M. S. (1977). *Biochem. Biophys. Res. Commun.* **79**, 400–405.

Ristelli, J., Kowisto, V. A., Akerblom, H. K., and Kivirikko, K. I. (1976). *Diabetes* **25**, 1066–1070.

Robert, B., Szigeti, M., Derouette, J. C., Robert, L., Bouissou, H., and Fabre, M. T. (1971). *Eur. J. Biochem.* **21**, 507–516.

Robins, S. P. (1983). *Methods Biochem. Anal.* **28**, 329–379.

Robins, S. P., and Bailey, A. J. (1973). *FEBS Lett.* **33**, 167–171.

Robins, S. P., and Bailey, A. J. (1974). *FEBS Lett.* **38**, 334–336.

Rosenberg, L. E., and Scriver, C. R. (1980). *In* "Metabolic Control and Disease" (P. K. Bondy and L. E. Rosenberg, eds.), 8th Ed., pp. 660–667. Saunders, Philadelphia.

Rosenbloom, J., and Cywinski, A. (1976). *FEBS Lett.* **65**, 246–250.

Ross, R., and Bornstein, P. (1969). *J. Cell Biol.* **40**, 366–381.

Ross, R., and Glomset, J. A. (1976). *N. Engl. J. Med.* **295**, 369–377.

Rowe, D. W., McGoodwin, E. B., Martin, G. R., Sussman, M. D., Grahn, D., Faris, B., and Franzblau, C. (1974). *J. Exp. Med.* **139**, 180–192.

Rowe, D. W., McGoodwin, E. B., Martin, G. R., and Grahn, D. (1977). *J. Biol. Chem.* **252**, 939–942.

Royce, P. M., and Danks, D. M. (1982). *IRCS Med. Sci.* **10**, 41.

Royce, P. M., Camakaris, J., and Danks, D. M. (1980). *Biochem. J.* **192**, 579–586.

Royce, P. M., Camakaris, J., Mann, J. R., and Danks, D. M. (1982). *Biochem. J.* **202**, 369–371.

Rucker, R. B., and Dubick, M. A. (1984). *Environ. Health Perspect.* **55**, 179–191.

Rucker, R. B., and Goettlich-Riemann, W. (1972). *Proc. Soc. Exp. Biol. Med.* **139**, 286–289.

Rucker, R. B., and Murray, J. (1978). *Am. J. Clin. Nutr.* **31**, 1221–1236.

Rucker, R. B., and O'Dell, B. L. (1970). *Biochim. Biophys. Acta* **222**, 527–529.

Rucker, R. B., Riggins, R., Laughlin, R., Chan, M. M., and Tom, K. (1975). *J. Nutr.* **105**, 1062–1070.

Rucker, R. B., Roensch, L. F., Savage, J. E., and O'Dell, B. L. (1970). *Biochem. Biophys. Res. Commun.* **40**, 1391–1397.

Sahebjami, H., and Vassallo, C. L. (1979). *Am. Rev. Respir. Dis.* **119**, 443–451.

Salvador, R. A., and Tsai, I. (1973). *Biochem. Pharmacol.* **22**, 37–46.

Sampson, C. E., Chichester, C. O., Hayes, J. A., and Kagan, H. M. (1984). *Am. Rev. Respir. Dis.* **129,** 619–624.

Sanada, H., Shikata, J., Hamamoto, H., Ueba, Y., Yamamuro, T., and Takedo, T. (1978). *Biochim. Biophys. Acta* **541,** 408–413.

Sandberg, L. B., and Wolt, T. B. (1982). *In* "Methods in Enzymology"(L. W. Cunningham and D. W. Frederiksen, eds.), Vol. 82, pp. 657–664. Academic Press, New York.

Sandberg, L. B., Soskel, N. T., and Leslie, J. G. (1981). *N. Engl. J. Med.* **304,** 566–579.

Sandell, L. J., Prentice, H. L., Kravis, D., and Upholt, W. B. (1984). *J. Biol. Chem.* **259,** 7826–7834.

Scheck, M., Siegel, R. C., Parker, J., Chang, Y. H., and Fu, J. C. C. (1979). *J. Anat.* **129,** 645–657.

Schilling, E. D., and Strong, F. M. (1954). *J. Am. Chem. Soc.* **76,** 2848.

Schmidt, C. J., Hamer, D. H., and McBride, J. W. (1984). *Science* **224,** 1104–1106.

Schneir, M., Ramamurthy, N., and Golub, L. (1982). *Diabetes* **31,** 426–431.

Serafini-Fracassini, A., Ventrella, G., Field, M. J., Hinnie, J., Onyezili, N. I., and Griffiths, R. (1981). *Biochemistry* **20,** 5424–5429.

Sheridan, P. J., Kozar, L. G., and Benson, S. C. (1979). *Exp. Mol. Pathol.* **30,** 315–324.

Shieh, J. J., and Yasunobu, K. T. (1976). *Adv. Exp. Med. Biol.* **74,** 447–463.

Shieh, J. J., Tamaye, R., and Yasunobu, K. T. (1975). *Biochim. Biophys. Acta* **377,** 229–238.

Shieh, J. J., Sasaki, T., Minamiura, N., and Yasunobu, K. T. (1977). *Adv. Exp. Med. Biol.* **79,** 509–529.

Shields, G. S., Coulson, W. F., Kimball, D. A., Carnes, W. H., Cartwright, G. E., and Wintrobe, M. M. (1962). *Am. J. Pathol.* **41,** 603–621.

Shoshan, S., and Finkelstein, S. (1976). *Biochim. Biophys. Acta* **439,** 358–362.

Siegel, R. C. (1974). *Proc. Natl. Acad. Sci. U.S.A.* **71,** 4826–4830.

Siegel, R. C. (1976). *J. Biol. Chem.* **251,** 5786–5792.

Siegel, R. C. (1977). *J. Biol. Chem.* **252,** 254–259.

Siegel, R. C. (1979). *Int. Rev. Connect. Tissue Res.* **8,** 73–118.

Siegel, R. C., and Fu, J. C. (1976). *J. Biol. Chem.* **251,** 5779–5785.

Siegel, R. C., and Lian, J. B. (1975). *Biochem. Biophys. Res. Commun.* **67,** 1353–1359.

Siegel, R. C., Page, R. C., and Martin, G. R. (1970a). *Biochim. Biophys. Acta* **222,** 552–555.

Siegel, R. C., Pinnell, S. R., and Martin, G. R. (1970b). *Biochemistry* **9,** 4486–4492.

Siegel, R. C., Fu, J. C., and Chang, Y. (1976). *Adv. Exp. Med. Biol.* **74,** 438–446.

Siegel, R. C., Chen, K. H., Greenspan, J. S., and Aguiar, J. M. (1978). *Proc. Natl. Acad. Sci. U.S.A.* **75,** 2945–2949.

Siegel, R. C., Black, C. M., and Bailey, A. J. (1979). *Biochem. Biophys. Res. Commun.* **88,** 281–287.

Siegel, R. C., Fu, J. C., Uto, N., Horiuchi, K., and Fujimoto, D. (1982). *Biochem. Biophys. Res. Commun.* **108,** 1546–1550.

Silver, F. H. (1981). *J. Biol. Chem.* **256,** 4973–4977.

Silver, F. H., Langley, K. H., and Trelstad, R. L. (1979). *Biopolymers* **18,** 2523–2535.

Smith, D. W., Sandberg, L. B., Leslie, B. H., Wolt, T. B., Milton, S. B., Meyers, B., and Rucker, R. B. (1981). *Biochem. Biophys. Res. Commun.* **103,** 880–885.

Soskel, N. T., Watanabe, S., Hammond, E., Sandberg, L. B., Renzetti, A. D., Jr., and Crapo, J. D. (1982). *Am. Rev. Respir. Dis.* **126,** 316–325.

Soskel, N. T., Watanabe, S., and Sandberg, L. B. (1984). *Chest* **85,** 70S-71S.

Sparrow, D., Silbert, J. E., and Weiss, S. T. (1982). *Am. Rev. Respir. Dis.* **126,** 312–315.

Starcher, B. C. (1969). *Proc. Soc. Exp. Biol. Med.* **132**, 379–382.

Starcher, B. C., and King, G. S. (1980). *Connect. Tissue Res.* **8**, 53–55.

Starcher, B. C., and Mecham, R. P. (1981). *Connect. Tissue Res.* **8**, 255–258.

Starcher, B. C., Madaras, J. A., and Tepper, A. S. (1977). *Biochem. Biophys. Res. Commun.* **78**, 706–712.

Starcher, B., Madaras, J. A., Fisk, D., Perry, E. F., and Hill, C. H. (1978). *J. Nutr.* **108**, 1229–1233.

Stassen, F. L. (1976). *Biochim. Biophys. Acta* **438**, 49–60.

Stevens, M. D., DiSilvestro, R. A., and Harris, E. D. (1984). *Biochemistry* **23**, 261–266.

Sullivan, K. A., and Kagan, H. M. (1982). *J. Biol. Chem.* **257**, 13520–13526.

Sullivan, K., and Kagan, H. (1985). Unpublished results.

Suva, R. H., and Abeles, R. H. (1978). *Biochemistry* **17**, 3538–3545.

Tang, S. S., Trackman, P. C., and Kagan, H. M. (1983). *J. Biol. Chem.* **258**, 4331–4338.

Tang, S. S., Simpson, D. E., and Kagan, H. M. (1984). *J. Biol. Chem.* **259**, 975–979.

Tanzer, M. L. (1965). *Int. Rev. Connect. Tissue Res.* **3**, 91–112.

Tanzer, M. L., and Kefalides, N. A. (1973). *Biochem. Biophys. Res. Commun.* **51**, 775–780.

Thet, L. A., Delaney, M. D., Gregario, C. A., and Massaro, D. (1977). *J. Appl. Physiol.* **43**, 463–467.

Tilson, M. D. (1982). *Arch. Surg.* **117**, 1212–1213.

Tinker, D., and Rucker, R. B. (1985). *Physiol. Rev.* **65**, 605–657.

Trackman, P. C., and Kagan, H. M. (1979). *J. Biol. Chem.* **254**, 7831–7836.

Trackman, P. C., Zoski, C. G., and Kagan, H. M. (1981). *Anal. Biochem.* **113**, 336–342.

Urry, D. W. (1982). *In* "Methods in Enzymology" (L. W. Cunningham and D. W. Frederiksen, eds.), Vol. 82, pp. 673–716. Academic Press, New York.

Urry, D. W., and Long, M. M. (1977). *Adv. Exp. Med. Biol.* **79**, 685–714.

Urry, D. W., Starcher, B., and Partridge, S. M. (1969). *Nature* **222**, 795–796.

Urry, D. W., Sugano, H., Prasad, K., Long, M., and Bhatnager, R. (1979). *Biochem. Biophys. Res. Commun.* **90**, 194–198.

Vannice, J. L., Taylor, J. M., and Rengold, G. M. (1984). *Proc. Natl. Acad. Sci. U.S.A.* **81**, 4241–4245.

Vater, C. A., Harris, E. D., Jr., and Siegel, R. C. (1979). *Biochem. J.* **181**, 639–645.

Viceps-Madore, D., Cidlowski, J. A., Kittler, J. M., and Thanassi, J. W. (1983). *J. Biol. Chem.* **258**, 2689–2696.

Vidal, G. P., Shieh, J. J., and Yasunobu, K. T. (1975). *Biochem. Biophys. Res. Commun.* **64**, 989–995.

Walsh, C. (1979). "Enzymatic Reaction Mechanisms," pp. 451–454. Freeman, San Francisco.

Williamson, P. R., Kittler, J. M., Thanassi, J., and Kagan, H. M. (1986). *Biochem. J.,* in press.

Wimmerova, J., Ledvina, M., Velebny, V., and Hodanova, M. (1980). *Physiologia Bohemoslovaca* **29**, 375–378.

Woessner, J. F., Jr. (1969). *Biochem. J.* **112**, 637–645.

Wolinsky, H. (1972). *Circ. Res.* **30**, 301–309.

Wu, J. J., and Eyre, D. R. (1984a). *Biochemistry* **23**, 1850–1857.

Wu, J. J., and Eyre, D. (1984b). *Biochem. Biophys. Res. Commun.* **123**, 1033–1039.

Wu, V. Y., and Cohen, M. (1982). *Biochem. Biophys. Res. Commun.* **104**, 911–915.

Yamada, H., and Yasunobu, K. T. (1962). *J. Biol. Chem.* **237**, 3077–3082.

Yamada, Y., Kuhn, K., and de Crombrugghe, B. (1983). *Nucleic Acids Res.* **11**, 2733–2744.

Matrix Accumulation and the Development of Form: Proteoglycans and Branching Morphogenesis

Brian S. Spooner

Division of Biology, Kansas State University, Manhattan, Kansas

and

Holly A. Thompson-Pletscher

Department of Chemistry, University of Montana, Missoula, Montana

399

I. INTRODUCTION

The regulation of accumulation of extracellular matrix (ECM) is of fundamental importance to mature tissue and organ function and to understanding an array of connective tissue diseases and organ disorders. In the developing embryo, ECM macromolecules appear to be intimately involved in regulating the morphogenesis of tissues and organs, an activity in addition to simple stromal or supportive matrix functions. Thus, ultimate understanding of morphogenesis will require detailed understanding of the dynamics of ECM regulation in discrete embryonic tissues, including matrix component changes resulting from tissue interactions and molecular interactions between various macromolecules of the ECM.

The large surface area of lungs, mammary and salivary glands, seminal vesicles, kidney collecting tubules, and many other organs is achieved by branching morphogenesis, a process which includes repetitive shape changes in the growing epithelium. Like many other developmental processes, branching morphogenesis requires an interaction between the epithelium and surrounding condensed mesenchyme (reviewed in Grobstein, 1967; Saxen et al., 1976). Early reports that mesenchyme supports epithelial branching even when the tissues are separated by a filter (Grobstein, 1953b; Auerbach, 1960; Golosow and Grobstein, 1962) focused attention on the role of extracellular matrix in branching morphogenesis. There is now ample evidence that matrix components such as proteoglycans, hyaluronic acid, and collagens are involved in this process.

II. BRANCHING MORPHOGENESIS

A. Epithelial–Mesenchymal Interactions

Morphogenesis of most branching epithelia, including lung, pancreas, salivary gland, thymus, prostate gland, and ureteric bud, requires an interaction with mesenchyme (reviewed in Grobstein, 1967; Spooner, 1974; Saxen et al., 1976; Cunha et al., 1981). Such epithelia fail to branch when cultured alone, but resume morphogenetic activity when recombined with mesenchyme. Specificity of the interaction varies greatly between organ systems. Pancreatic epithelium is the least fastidious; mesenchyme from a variety of sources or even an extract of whole chick embryos can support branching activity (Golosow and Grobstein, 1962; Rutter *et al.*, 1964). Although lung and salivary gland epithelia can undergo morphogenesis when recombined with some other mesenchymes (Lawson, 1974, and 1983), branching of these tissues is most active in the presence of homotypic mesenchyme (Spooner and Wessells, 1970a, 1972). The requirement of ureteric bud is quite specific; only metanephric mesenchyme will support morphogenesis (Grobstein, 1955).

More recently, morphogenetic activity of dissociated epithelial cells embedded in three-dimensional collagen matrices has been reported. Primary cultures of normal mammary (Yang *et al.*, 1980) and salivary (Yang *et al.*, 1982) epithelial cells form branched, tubular structures in collagen gels. These observations might suggest that mesenchyme supports branching morphogenesis simply by providing a collagen matrix. However, this is not the case.

Branching morphogenesis is a complex process whereby a small balloon of epithelial cells forms a tissue which has a large surface area but which fits in a compact volume. The characteristic architecture of each organ is established by the pattern of epithelial branching (Fig. 1). Mammalian lung epithelium undergoes a generally bifurcating morphogenesis, with each lobe forming two new lobes. Seminal vesicles form lateral branches off a central elongated tubule. Mature mammary epithelia have clusters of alveoli at the ends of highly branched tubules. Salivary epithelia form similar clusters, but the relatively short tubule system creates a more compact arrangement of alveoli.

The characteristic branching pattern of each organ is specified by the investing mesenchyme. Mammary epithelium acquires a salivary-like architecture when recombined with submandibular gland mesenchyme (Kratochwil, 1969). The branching pattern of mouse lung epithelium is intermediate between mammalian and avian structures when cultured with chick lung mesenchyme (Taderera, 1967) and is salivary-like in the presence of submandibular gland mesenchyme (Lawson, 1983). When salivary epithelium is recombined with lung mesenchyme, it undergoes a transient lung-like lobulation before resuming morphogenesis typical of salivary glands (Lawson, 1974). These examples illustrate the influence of the mesenchyme on the final epithelial architecture. It is clear that mesenchyme must contribute more than a simple enveloping collagen matrix.

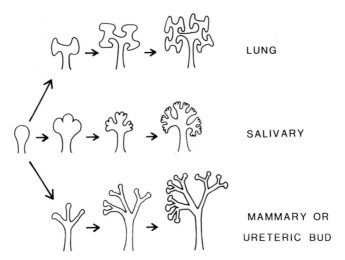

Fig. 1. Schematic illustration of several patterns of epithelial branching morphogenesis. An epithelial bud can undergo dichotomous branching to produce a bronchial "tree," or can balance branch point formation and branch elongation to generate salivary, mammary, and ureteric bud patterns of branching.

Processes which contribute to development of the mature epithelial architecture include (1) growth, (2) epithelial polarization, and (3) cleft formation. It is useful to review what is known about the influence of mesenchyme on each of these processes.

1. Growth

During development, all of the branching epithelia undergo a tremendous increase in size. Both cellular proliferation and active protein synthesis contribute to this growth. The stimulatory effect of mesenchyme on epithelial growth and proliferation has been noted in many systems (Kratochwil, 1969; Ronzio and Rutter, 1973; Masters, 1976; Sakakura *et al.*, 1979). Laswon (1983) reviews the evidence that mesenchyme maintains morphogenetically active regions of epithelium in the cell cycle, while cells in morphogenetically quiescent regions gradually withdraw from mitotic activity.

Although epithelial growth and proliferation are necessary for ongoing branching morphogenesis, these events can be distinguished from lumen and cleft formation. For example, kidney and mammary epithelial cells cultured in a collagen matrix undergo lumen formation even in the presence of inhibitors of DNA, RNA, and protein synthesis (Hall *et al.*, 1982). Similarly, epithelial cleft formation occurs in embryonic salivary glands treated with cycloheximide, even when protein synthesis is inhibited 50% and the lobes are much smaller than those of control rudiments (Spooner *et al.*, 1986). These observations suggest that the control degree of growth is not a necessary prerequisite for either lumen or cleft formation. Conversely, supernumerary buds can be induced on trachea, either by mesenchyme taken from actively branching bronchial buds or by epidermal growth factor embedded in agarose pellets (Wessells, 1970; Goldin and Wessells, 1979; Goldin and Opperman, 1980). In each case, epithelial proliferation is stimulated in the locally treated region of trachea. However, only the bronchial mesenchyme-induced buds form branch points (clefts) and develop further. Thus, for ongoing branching morphogenesis, the stimulation of epithelial growth is a necessary, but not sufficient, process of the tissue interaction.

2. Lumen Formation and Polarization of Epithelial Cells

Epithelia may initially invade the investing mesenchyme as cords of epithelial cells (reviewed in Hogg *et al.*, 1983) or as hollow outpocketings of epithelium. In either case, the tissue rapidly forms a lumen and acquires polarity, with apical cells or ends of cells facing the lumen and basal cells or basal ends of cells forming a basal lamina at the interface with the extracellular matrix. Dissociated epithelial cells from mammary gland, salivary gland, thyroid, or kidney form lumenal structures when cultured in three-dimensional collagen matrices (Yang *et al.*, 1980, 1982; Chambard *et al.*, 1981; Hall *et al.*, 1982). Interactions between the epithelium and collagen substratum promote deposition of basal lamina components (David and Bernfield, 1979, 1981; Ormerod *et al.*, 1983), suggesting that extracellular collagen may trigger the polarization. It is interesting that cells which have been plated on a collagen substratum and allowed to establish polarity undergo reorganization when challenged with collagen overlaid on the "apical" surface of the epithelium; the cells form a lumenal structure with only "basal" surfaces in contact with the collagen (Hall *et al.*, 1982). For lumen formation and polarization of epithelial cells, collagen matrix appears to replace the requirement for mesenchyme.

3. Cleft Formation

Formation of clefts or branch points in the epithelial tubules is necessary to establish the extensive systems of bronchioles in the lung and collecting ducts in the ureteric bud and various glands. Epithelia cultured in the absence of mesenchyme do not form branched structures (Grobstein, 1953a, 1955; Auerbach, 1960; Cunha *et al.*, 1981). Again, recent studies have demonstrated that dissociated epithelial cells or fragments grown in collagen matrices can form systems of branched tubules (Yang *et al.*, 1980, 1982; Bennett *et al.*, 1981; Richards *et al.*, 1982; Foster *et al.*, 1983). None of these developing structures resemble the architecture of the mature epithelium from which the cells were isolated. For example, the structures formed by salivary epithelial cell appear to have undergone far more growth between formation of each new branch point than salivary glands which have developed *in vivo*. The strong similarity between the tubule systems formed *in vitro* by salivary and mammary cells suggest that collagen matrix might induce some type of "archetypal"branching activity in epithelia. Interestingly, the cells which have formed these branched tubules *in vitro* retain the ability to undergo normal morphogenesis. Mammary epithelial cells form glands with normal morphology when removed from the collagen gel, dissociated, and injected back into the mammary fat pads of mice. Similar studies using epithelium from the various embryonic branching organs have not yet been reported. However, it seems clear that the pattern of cleft formation in collagen matrix is atypical and that homotypic mesenchyme provides important morphogenetic cues which are missing in collagen preparations.

Little is known about the signals which terminate arborization of the ductal system and initiate formation of alveoli. One possibility is that the epithelium grows and invades the mesenchyme until it has filled all the available stroma, at which point branching stops. There is some evidence that this occurs in mammary glands (Faulkin and Deome, 1960). Another possibility is that the developing mesenchyme becomes incompetent to stimulate growth or shape changes in the epithelium. There is indirect evidence for this mechanism. When embryonic mammary or salivary gland mesenchyme is transplanted into adult mice, mammary epithelium near the implant begins to proliferate and form branched ducts (Sakakura *et al.*, 1979). Not surprisingly, the branching pattern is dependent on the source of the mesenchyme. The observation that the stimulated epithelium grows into the implanted embryonic mesenchyme but not into the recipient's preexisting stroma suggests that as mesenchyme differentiates, it may lose competence to support epithelial arborization.

In summary, branching morphogenesis requires an interaction between epithelium and investing mesenchyme. At least three processes critical for ongoing morphogenesis can be distinguished. Differences in the relative rates of these processes might be responsible for establishing organs with very different architecture. It will be useful in future studies to delineate the roles of tissue interactions and extracellular matrix components in each of these processes individually.

B. Cell Shape Changes and Epithelial Branch Point Formation

Bending, folding, and formation of branch points (clefts) in epithelia are caused by forces generated within the cells themselves. Mechanical movement of epithelium by the stromal cells has been ruled out by observations that epithelia undergo branching morphogenesis even when separated from mesenchyme by a filter (Grobstein, 1953b, Auerbach, 1960; Golosow and Grobstein, 1962). These morphogenetic movements of the epithelium result from coordinated changes in the shapes of individual cells (Spooner, 1973, 1975). Fig. 2A illustrates schematically how a tissue which consists initially of cuboidal cells can form a lobe by constriction of the apical ends of some of the cells. A cleft forms in the lobe by further coordinated constrictions at apical and basal ends of appropriate groups of cells. The relative rates of mitotic activ-

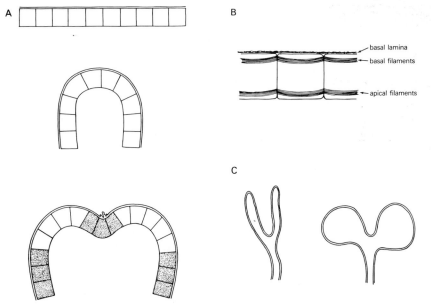

FIG. 2. (A) Changes in cell shape produce morphogenetic movements of an epithelial sheet. Apical constriction of some cells generates a bud, while basal constriction of other cells initiates a cleft or branch point in the bud. (B) Apical and basal arrays of cytoplasmic microfilaments in the epithelial cells are responsible for the changes in individual cell shape. (C) Controlling the areas of proliferation within the epithelium can modulate the structure produced by a single branch point.

ity and changes in cell shape may influence the pattern of branching morphogenesis. More vigorous mitotic activity of the stippled cells would cause elongation of the cleft, resulting in relatively long tubules (Fig. 2C). Conversely, proliferation in the unstippled cells and rapid formation of new clefts would create a more highly branched ductal system.

Cytoplasmic microfilaments provide the motive force for changes in epithelial cell shape. Electron micrographs of embryonic lungs and salivary glands show linear arrays of microfilament bundles at the apical and basal ends of the cells (Bernfield and Wessells, 1970; Spooner and Wessells, 1970b). Microfilament arrays from both tissues stain with heavy meromyosin (Spooner et al., 1973). It has been proposed that the ends of epithelial cells constrict by "purse-string" contractions of the actin-containing filaments (Wessells et al., 1971). Experimental evidence supports this model. In the presence of cytochalasin B, morphogenesis of lungs and salivary glands stops, and all but the oldest (and deepest) clefts are lost (Bernfield and Wessells, 1970; Spooner and Wessells, 1972). The inhibition of branching is correlated with loss of organized apical and basal arrays of microfilaments. Both cleft formation and microfilament organization recover after removal of cytochalasin B, suggesting that the microfilaments are indeed responsible for branching of the epithelium. They appear to be regulated by available calcium, analogous to muscle systems. Papaverine is a smooth muscle relaxant that blocks calcium transport. Embryonic salivary glands cultured in papaverine or in calcium-free medium stop branching and lose existing clefts, although microfilament arrays appear normal ultrastructurally (Ash et al., 1973). Both microfilament structure and function are required for branching morphogenesis.

C. Extracellular Matrix

The interface between epithelium and investing mesenchyme contains abundant extracellular matrix, and so matrix macromolecules are prime candidates for mediators of tissue interactions. Extracellular matrix includes both interstitial matrix and basement membranes. Additionally, a pericellular compartment of extracellular materials has been defined for some systems. It should be emphasized that these compartments are arbitrary designations. In tissues, there is a continuum between intracellular elements, such as cytoskeleton, integral plasma membrane components, pericellular coat, or basement membrane, and the interstitium. Molecules with multiple domains may act as structural or functional bridges between the various compartments.

Extracellular matrix components include collagens, proteoglycans, glycosaminoglycans, and other structural proteins such as laminin and fibronectin. The possible involvement of some of these macromolecules in branching morphogenesis is discussed briefly in this section.

1. COLLAGENS

The field of collagen chemistry has entered a logarithmic phase in the identification of new isotypes. Recent reviews have covered types I through V (Bornstein and Sage, 1980; Linsenmayer, 1981; Miller and Gay, 1982), but as of this writing, at least five new collagens have been described (representative publications: Sage et al., 1980; Schmid and Conrad, 1982; von der Mark et al., 1982; Bentz et al., 1983; Odermatt et al., 1983). Some of these types represent a small percentage of the total collagen produced by the tissue, and the range of cells which synthesize each of the new types has not yet been explored. However, it is useful to take note of some of the collagens which may be involved in developmental events such as branching morphogenesis.

Type I, the most abundant collagen, and type III, originally thought to be a fetal collagen, are interstitial molecules with wide distribution (Bornstein and Sage, 1980; Linsenmayer, 1981). Type IV collagen is almost ubiquitous in basement membranes (Heathcote and Grant, 1981). Types I, III, and IV all appear very early in embryonic development and they have been implicated in morphogenesis and differentiation of many systems (Hay, 1981). Type V collagen is synthesized by many cells, and is interesting because of its unusually close association with the cell surface (discussed in Alitalo et al., 1982). Type VII collagen, isolated from a tissue rich in epithelial basement membrane, forms aggregates in vitro which are intriguingly similar to the anchoring filaments of basement membranes (Bentz et al., 1983). Future studies will undoubtedly uncover important developmental roles for many of these collagen isotypes.

2. COLLAGENS AND BRANCHING MORPHOGENESIS

Mesenchymal tissues associated with branching organs synthesize abundant collagen (Bernfield, 1970). Early attempts to correlate this collagen with branching morphogenesis relied on enzyme degradations: collagenase treatment of embryonic lung, salivary, and ureteric bud epithelium interrupted morphogenesis, caused regression of branch points, and depleted the extraepithelial matrix of fibrous material (Grobstein and Cohen, 1965; Wessells and Cohen, 1968). However, contaminating glycosaminoglycan-degrading activity in the collagenase complicated interpretation of these experiments (Bernfield *et al.*, 1973). More direct evidence for the importance of collagen in branching morphogenesis has been obtained using inhibitors of collagen hydroxylation and secretion. Branching of embryonic salivary and lung rudiments is inhibited by α,α'-dipyridyl and L-azetidine-2-carboxylic acid (Spooner and Faubion, 1980). The inhibition of branching accompanies both a decrease in total collagen synthesis and a substantial depletion of fibrillar collagen in the extracellular matrix. Similarly, administration of the proline analog *cis*-hydroxyproline inhibits ductal and alveolar formation in mammary glands of rats, and the inhibition is correlated with decreased collagen synthesis and diminished type IV collagen in the basement membrane (Wicha *et al.*, 1980).

One possible function for interstitial collagens is that of structural stabilization of morphogenetically quiescent regions of the epithelium, such as ducts and established branch points. The arrangement of collagen fibrils on embryonic lung rudiments provides evidence for this: collagen fibrils are oriented parallel to the long axis of the trachea, but appear more randomly organized at the actively branching bronchial buds (Wessells, 1970). Similarly, collagen is deposited in established clefts of salivary glands (Bernfield *et al.*, 1973), allowing the suggestion that it may stabilize the oldest branch points against loss in the presence of agents which disrupt microfilaments (Spooner and Wessells, 1972). However, depletion of interstitial collagen in the presence of proline analogs does not destabilize established clefts (Spooner and Faubion, 1980).

A second possible function for interstitial collagens is enhancement of deposition of basement membrane components. Culture of mammary epithelial cells on type I collagen increases deposition of heparan sulfate proteoglycan (David and Bernfield, 1981), fibronectin. laminin, and type IV collagen (Ormerod *et al.*, 1983). Culture of cells on an artificial collagen matrix is analogous to the tissue interaction *in vivo*, where interstitial collagen is synthesized by the mesenchyme. Even when tissues are separated by a filter, collagen synthesized by the mesenchyme diffuses across the filter and is deposited at the surface of the epithelium (Kallman and Grobstein, 1965), where it can interact with and stabilize basement membrane components.

Type IV collagen has been implicated in a number of tissue interactions (Ekblom, 1981; Thesleff *et al.*, 1981), including mammary gland development (Wicha *et al.*, 1980). It is likely that basement membrane collagen contributes to stabilization of the basal cell surface. When corneal epithelium is stripped of extracellular matrix, blebs form at the basal cell surfaces, and the underlying cortical mat of microfilaments becomes disorganized. Addition of soluble type IV collagen to the medium results in reorganization of the cortical mat and flattening of the cytoplasmic blebs (Sugrue and Hay, 1981). These observations are particularly interesting because shape changes in branching epithelia appear to be generated by microfilaments.

3. OTHER STRUCTURAL PROTEINS OF THE EXTRACELLULAR MATRIX

More is known about the structure, function, and gene expression of fibronectin than any of the other matrix proteins. Fibronectin is a glycoprotein which is found on cell surfaces, interstitial matrices, and many basement membranes, as well as in blood plasma. The molecule has multiple domains, including binding sites for native and denatured collagens, glycosaminoglycans, proteoglycans, and actin (Hynes and Yamada, 1982), and is an ideal candidate for linking the various extracellular compartments to each other and to intracellular elements. Fibronectin mediates adhesion of cells to types I–V collagen (Kleinman et al., 1981).

Laminin is a large molecular weight glycoprotein found almost ubiquitously in basement membranes (Timpl et al., 1979). Like fibronectin, it has separate binding sites for type IV collagen, proteoglycans, and the cell surface (Kleinman et al., 1984). In vitro, laminin serves as a cell adhesion factor and promotes attachment of epithelial cells to type IV collagen substrate (Kleinman et al., 1981). Other unique matrix components which have been described recently include entactin, connectin, and nidogen. The sulfated glycoprotein entactin is found in many basement membranes (Carlin et al., 1981), including that of mammary gland (Warburton et al., 1984). Entactin is synthesized by both mesenchymal and epithelial cells (Hogan et al., 1982), suggesting that it may be a component of interstitial matrix as well as basement membranes. Nidogen is a glycoprotein which is present in many embryonic and adult basement membranes. It first appears at compaction of the eight cell mammalian embryo, and codistributes with laminin thereafter (Dziadek and Timpl, 1985). Nidogen has several molecular weight forms, and aggregates of the 80,000 form have a characteristic nest-like morphology when examined by electron microscopy (Timpl et al., 1983). The larger molecular weight forms (100,000 and 150,000) complex strongly with laminin (Dziadek and Timpl, 1985). These observations suggest that nidogen may play an important role in the organization of basement membranes. In contrast to the basement membrane glycoproteins, connectin is a cell surface macromolecule. It binds to both laminin and actin (Brown et al., 1983), and may provide a link between cytoskeletal elements and the extracellular matrix.

Fibronectin, laminin, nidogen, and entactin appear very early in embryogenesis (Hynes and Yamada, 1982; Wu *et al.,* 1983; Timpl *et al.,* 1983). The various matrix components have been implicated in epithelial–mesenchymal interactions during development (Brownell *et al.,* 1981; Ekblom, 1981; Thesleff *et al.,* 1981), but it is not yet known how these matrix proteins are involved in epithelial branching morphogenesis. One possibility is that they contribute to stability of the cytoskeleton, thereby permitting appropriate cell shape changes to occur. Like type IV collagen, laminin and fibronectin prevent disorganization of the cortical mat of microfilaments in isolated corneal epithelium (Sugrue and Hay, 1981). The cell surface protein connectin organizes actin filaments into bundles *in vitro* (Brown *et al.,* 1983), and may also do so *in situ.*

III.   Proteoglycans and Hyaluronic Acid

A.   Basic Structure

Glycosaminoglycans (GAGs) are long, unbranched chains of alternating hexosamine and uronic acid (hyaluronic acid, chondroitin sulfates, dermatan sulfate, heparan sulfate, and heparin) or hexosamine and galactose (keratan sulfate) residues. With the possible exception of hyaluronic acid, all of the GAGs are synthesized on a core protein primer. Proteoglycans are a class of macromolecules with remarkably complex and varied structures (reviewed in Hascall, 1981; Hascall and Hascall, 1981). Minimally, they consist of a core protein and at least one covalently bound GAG chain. Proteoglycan complexity is achieved by variations in amino acid sequence and length of the core protein; number, length, and type of GAG chains; and modifications of the GAGs such as epimerization and sulfation. Additionally, many proteoglycans contain asparagine- and serine(threonine)-linked oligosaccharides with structures similar to those of classic glycoproteins (Nilsson *et al.,* 1982; Yanagishita and Hascall, 1983a,b).

Given this potential for structural complexity, it is not surprising that many proteoglycans have multiple functional domains. One example, the predominant cartilage proteoglycan, has at least two functional domains. A globular region of core protein near the amino terminus (Stevens and Hascall, 1986) is responsible for anchoring the proteoglycan monomer to hyaluronic acid, while the chondroitin sulfate chains necessary for maintenance of the mechanical properties of cartilage are bound to an extended region towards the carboxy end of the protein (Hascall and Heinegard, 1974). Similarly, a heparan sulfate proteoglycan synthesized by mammary epithelial cells has both a lipophilic domain, which appears to be anchored in the plasma membrane, and a GAG attachment region (Rapraeger and Bernfield, 1983). The two domains have been reported to bind F-actin and collagen, respectively (Bernfield *et al.*, 1984).

The cartilage chondroitin sulfate proteoglycan and mammary epithelial heparan sulfate proteoglycan illustrate some important points about proteoglycan structure: in addition to providing structural components of tissues, proteoglycans act as organizers of extracellular matrices (reviewed in Muir, 1983) and as intermediaries between cells and the extracellular environment; structural analysis of proteoglycans provides important clues to the functions of these molecules in tissues.

B. Distribution

Proteoglycans have been found in each of the various extracellular compartments, including the cell surface, pericellular matrix, basement membrane, and interstitial matrix. Examples of proteoglycans and GAGs found in each of these compartments are discussed briefly, as an introduction to possible functions of these macromolecules in branching morphogenesis.

1. CELL SURFACE

The ubiquitous distribution of cell surface heparan sulfate proteoglycans originally proposed by Kraemer (1971) has been confirmed in numerous systems, and analogous chondroitin and dermatan sulfate species have been reported more recently (Hedman *et al.*, 1983; Yanagishita and Hascall, 1984a). Some cell surface proteoglycans are anchored in the plasma membrane via hydrophobic regions of the protein core. Studies of liver (Kjellen *et al.*, 1981), mammary gland (Rapraeger and Bernfield, 1983), and ovarian granulosa cells (Yanagishita and Hascall, 1984a,b), summarized briefly here, have revealed similarities between the various integral membrane proteoglycans. During extraction, detergent is necessary to prevent self-association and aggregation of these proteoglycans with other membrane proteins. The detergent-extracted proteoglycans bind to hydrophobic gels and can be inserted into liposomes, whereas release of proteoglycans from cells or liposomes with mild trypsin treatment removes the lipophilic portion of the core and destroys the ability to reintercalate into either lipid vesicles or cell membranes. A second form of proteoglycan, less tightly associated with the cell surface than the membrane-intercalated form, can be released from cells with heparin. Presumably, the heparin-releasable proteoglycans are bound via interactions of the GAG chains with other macromolecules in the membrane. Both the heparin-releasable and membrane-intercalated forms can be removed from the cell surface by mild trypsin treatment.

Ovarian granulosa cells offer an ideal model system for studying cell surface associated proteoglycans. Both a heparan sulfate and a dermatan sulfate species appear on the cell surface as integral membrane components. These molecules become susceptible to release by heparin, probably as a result of a proteolytic clip between extracellular and membrane-intercalated domains of the core, and eventually are released into the medium (Yanagishita and Hascall, 1984a). The medium and cell layer forms of these proteoglycans are identical in terms of GAG and oligosaccharide composition (Yanagishita and Hascall, 1984b). The integral membrane form is an intermediate in the release of newly synthesized proteoglycans from the cells, but not all of the membrane-intercalated form is released. About 70% remains on the cell surface until it is reinternalized and degraded intracellularly. Conversely, not all of the proteoglycans released into the medium are transported via a membrane intercalated intermediate. The granulosa cells also synthesize a distinct, very large dermatan sulfate proteoglycan which does not have a lipophilic form, although it does exist as a cell surface, heparin-releasable intermediate before release into the medium. From observations on this one model system, it is apparent that some proteoglycan species pass through an intermediate, membrane intercalated form before being shed into the extracellular matrix. It is equally apparent that release into the matrix is not obligatory for all integral membrane proteoglycans, and that not all extracellular proteoglycan species pass through a membrane intercalated intermediate.

Another type of cell surface compartment is the "footprint" left behind by fibroblasts cultured on serum-adsorbed plates. These adhesion sites contain cytoskeletal proteins, proteoglycans, hyaluronic acid, and cellular fibronectin (Rollins et al., 1982). Pulse–chase experiments have demonstrated changes in the hyaluronate, chondroitin sulfate, and heparan sulfate proteoglycans during maturation of the adhesion sites (Lark and Culp, 1983, 1984), and these molecules may provide important links between the extracellular matrix and cytoskeletal elements of migrating cells.

2. PERICELLULAR MATRIX

Distinctions between the pericellular matrix and other matrix compartments are somewhat arbitrary. However, the pericellular coat of hyaluronic acid which forms around some cells in culture (Toole, 1981) is clearly a unique compartment of the extracellular matrix. Hyaluronate interacts with a binding protein on the cell surface (Underhill *et al.*, 1983) and builds up a thick coat. In tissues, these pericellular coats might shield individual cells from interactions with other cells or the interstitial matrix, or conversely, they might permit hyaluronate-mediated cell aggregation (Toole, 1981).

Immunolocalization studies suggest that chondrocytes may also have distinct pericellular matrices. Articular cartilage stained with antibodies against the major cartilage proteoglycan shows a generally uniform distribution throughout the interstitial matrix, except for a narrow region of heavily stained matrix around the cells (Poole *et al.*, 1980). These observations suggest the existence of pericellular matrices which are structurally (and perhaps functionally) distinct from either the cell surface or the interstitial matrix.

3. BASEMENT MEMBRANE

Basement membranes are specialized regions of extracellular matrix formed between nonconnective tissues (epithelium, endothelium, muscle, and neuronal cells) and the underlying matrix. They are seen at the light microscopy level by histochemical or immunofluorescent staining. At the electron microscopic level, basement membranes include the lamina densa, a sheet of electron dense material; the lamina lucida interna (or lamina rara externa), a relatively electron lucid zone between the cell membrane and lamina densa; and the lamina lucida externa or reticular lamina (or lamina rara interna), a region of fibrillar material merging with the underlying matrix. There is disagreement in the literature about whether "basal lamina" refers to all three zones or just the lamina densa. The latter convention appears to be useful, since type IV collagen, heparan sulfate proteoglycan, laminin, and fibronectin have been reported to be localized in the lamina densa (Laurie *et al.*, 1982). However, we shall consider the basal lamina as consisting of all three layers, since all have resolvable structure and the lucidae contain anionic sites (see Section VI).

Recognition that proteoglycans are integral components of basement membranes is a surprisingly recent event. Fewer than 10 years ago,

GAGs were dismissed as transient components of embryonic basement membranes or as contaminants of adult basement membrane preparations (Kefalides, 1978). Basement membrane GAGs detected by histochemical and autoradiographic techniques (Trelstad et al., 1974; Bernfield et al., 1973; Hay and Meier, 1974) were thought to be unique to embryonic tissues. However, the demonstration that anionic sites in the kidney glomerular basement membrane contained heparan sulfate (Kanwar and Farquhar, 1979) and the isolation in quantity of a heparan sulfate proteoglycan from a basement membrane-producing tumor (Hassell et al., 1980) fundamentally changed our ideas about these complex structures.

The heparan sulfate proteoglycan first isolated from the Engelbrath-Holm–Swarm (EHS) sarcoma appears to be an almost ubiquitous component of basement membranes. Antibodies which recognize determinants on the protein core of this molecule react with many embryonic and adult basement membranes (Hassell et al., 1980). Although heparan sulfate proteoglycans are more common, chondroitin and dermatan sulfate proteoglycans and hyaluronic acid have been found associated with a variety of embryonic (Bernfield et al., 1973; Trelstad et al., 1974; Cohn et al., 1977; Lau and Ruch, 1983) and adult (Gordon and Bernfield, 1980; Kanwar et al., 1981; Vaccaro and Brody, 1981) basement membranes.

Proteoglycans in the kidney glomerular basement membrane are critical to blood filtration. The highly anionic heparan sulfate chains provide a charge-selective barrier (Kanwar et al., 1980). Similar proteoglycans may function as a permeability barrier in lung alveoli (Vaccaro and Brody, 1981). Specific functions in other systems have not yet been determined, but basement membrane proteoglycans and hyaluronate do appear to be involved in development of many organ systems (Bernfield et al., 1973; Banerjee et al., 1977; Ekblom, 1981; Thesleff et al., 1981; Silberstein and Daniel, 1982a,b).

4. INTERSTITIAL MATRIX

More is known about the interstitial matrix proteoglycans than those of other extracellular compartments. The most complex of these macromolecules is the cartilage-specific proteoglycan, which has both chondroitin sulfate and keratan sulfate GAG chains and asparagine- and serine-linked oligosaccharides (reviewed in Hascall and Hascall, 1981). Dissociative extraction procedures using 4 M guanidine hydrochloride, originally developed for the cartilage system (Sajdera and Hascall, 1969), have proven useful for isolating proteoglycans in intact form from almost any interstitial matrix. Interstitial proteoglycans and hyaluronic acid have been implicated in such diverse developmental events as corneal clearing (Hart, 1976), organization of the cerebral cortex (Nakanishi, 1983), Mullerian duct development and regression (Hayashi et al., 1982), morphogenesis of the metanephric kidney (Belsky and Toole, 1983), and lung alveolar formation (Brody et al., 1982).

C. Synthesis

Proteoglycan biosynthesis is initiated by translation of the core protein in the rough endoplasmic reticulum. It is likely that, analogous to other glycoproteins, the mannose core of asparagine-linked oligosaccharides is added very early, possibly cotranslationally (Hanover et al., 1982). Addition of serine(theronine)-linked GAGs and oligosaccharides occurs relatively late, probably in the Golgi apparatus (Thonar et al., 1983; Fellini et al., 1984). Transport of membrane-intercalated species to the cell surface and secretion of extracellular proteoglycans occur very rapidly after the molecules are completed (Thonar et al., 1983; Yanagishita and Hascall, 1984b).

Synthesis of the O-linked GAGs (chondroitin sulfates, dermatan sulfate, heparin, and heparan sulfates) is initiated by xylosylation of serine residues in the core protein. Sequential actions of xylosyltransferase, galactosyltransferases I and II, and glucuronyltransferase I form the linkage region, shown in Fig. 3. The linkage regions then serve as primers for addition of the alternating hexosamine and uronic acid residues appropriate for each type of GAG. The chains on a single proteoglycan species can be polydisperse with respect to length (Fellini et al., 1981), suggesting that the mechanism for termination of GAG chains is not precise (see discussion in Mitchell and Hardingham, 1982b).

Further steps in the synthesis of proteoglycans include other posttranslational modifications to the core protein, processing of N- and O-linked oligosaccharides, and extensive modification of the GAGs. Both heparan sulfate and heparin undergo stepwise modification which includes removal of the N-acetyl groups from some glucosamine residues, N-sulfation at these positions, subsequent epimerization of nearby glucuronate residues to iduronic acid, stabilization of the iduronate epimer by introduction of O-sulfate groups on C-2, and further O-sulfation at C-6 of the glucosamine residues (Jacobsson and Lindahl, 1980; Riesenfeld et al., 1982; Roden, 1980). Heparin is distinguished from heparan sulfate by its higher charge density, which results from more extensive N- and O-sulfation during biosynthesis (Roden, 1980).

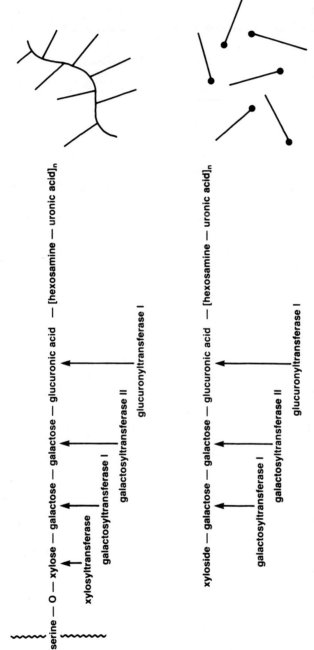

serine — O — xylose — galactose — galactose — glucuronic acid — [hexosamine — uronic acid]$_n$

xylosyltransferase

galactosyltransferase I

galactosyltransferase II

glucuronyltransferase I

xyloside — galactose — galactose — glucuronic acid — [hexosamine — uronic acid]$_n$

galactosyltransferase I

galactosyltransferase II

glucuronyltransferase I

FIG. 3. Scheme illustrating the synthesis of O-linked glycosaminoglycans. Certain serine residues in the core protein are xylosylated, then the linkage region is completed by sequential enzymatic addition of two galactose residues and one glucuronic acid residue. The linkage regions serve as primers for addition of the alternating hexosamine and uronic acid residues appropriate for each type of GAG. Exogenous xylosides compete with xylosylated core protein as substrate for the first galactosyltransferase, leading to the synthesis of xyloside initiated (core protein-free) GAGs.

The chondroitin family of GAGs is generated by modifications to the parent polysaccharide. Chondroitin is O-sulfated primarily at the C-4 or C-6 position of the N-acetylgalactosamine, although hybrid chains containing adjacent 4- and 6-sulfated disaccharides have been isolated (Faltynek and Silbert, 1978). Chondroitin sulfates rich in disulfated disaccharides have also been reported. The most common of these appears to be a disaccharide carrying sulfates on both C-4 and C-6 of the galactosamine (Suzuki et al., 1968; Razin et al., 1982; Seno and Murakami, 1982). Dermatan sulfate, closely related to chondroitin 4-sulfate, is generated by epimerization of glucuronic acid residues to iduronate. Some species of dermatan sulfate also contain disulfated disaccharides (Yanagishita and Hascall, 1983a). Epimerization and sulfation steps during biosynthesis are not independent, but the exact relationship between these events has not yet been determined (Malmstrom, 1984).

There is conflicting evidence as to whether hyaluronic acid synthesis is initiated on a core protein primer. Hyaluronate preparations commonly contain small amounts of protein. Hyaluronate–protein complex isolated from transformed fibroblasts is resistant to disruption by Nonidet P-40 and sodium dodecyl sulfate (Mikuni-Takagaki and Toole, 1981), suggesting that the interaction might be covalent. In cultured chondrocytes, protein is noncovalently bound to newly synthesized hyaluronic acid, but the hydrophobic interaction is strong and requires 4% Zwittergent plus 4 M guanidine hydrochloride for disruption (Mason et al., 1982). It is not clear whether these conflicting observations of hyaluronate–protein complexes are due to very strong, noncovalent interactions which are difficult to disrupt or to differences in the hyaluronate biosynthetic pathways in different cell types. However, it is clear that synthesis of hyaluronic acid is unlike the other GAGs, which are N- or O-glycosidically linked to protein. Alkaline borohydride treatment of hyaluronate does not generate sugar alditols (Varma et al., 1975), ruling out a serine(threonine) linkage. Tunicamycin does not inhibit hyaluronic acid synthesis (Hart and Lennarz, 1978), suggesting that the polysaccharide is not bound via an asparagine linkage. Furthermore, unlike proteoglycans, synthesis of hyaluronic acid is not inhibited by monensin, an ionophore which interferes with Golgi function and secretory pathways (Mitchell and Hardingham, 1982a; Yanagishita and Hascall, 1984b). Thus, in terms of biosynthetic mechanisms, hyaluronate differs significantly from the GAGs which are moieties of proteoglycans.

Modulation of proteoglycan and hyaluronic acid biosynthesis, including both quantitative and qualitative changes, occurs during development and regeneration of tissues (Toole and Gross, 1971; Hart,

1976; Edward *et al.*, 1980; Kapoor and Prehm, 1983; Kolset *et al.*, 1983) and in response to hormonal regulation (Yanagishita *et al.*, 1981; Giraud and Bouchillox, 1983), transformation (Hopwood and Dorfman, 1977) and to the substrate on which cells are grown (Gallagher *et al.*, 1980; Luikart *et al.*, 1983), to mention just a few examples.

Very little is known about the mechanisms which regulate proteoglycan and hyaluronic acid synthesis. Quantitatively, proteoglycan synthesis may be regulated by availability of the core protein. Glycosaminoglycan synthesis is inhibited in the presence of cycloheximide or puromycin. For the xylose-linked GAGs, this inhibition is relieved by providing exogenous initiators of GAG synthesis. Certain derivatives of xylose act as substrates for galactosyltransferase I, bypassing the need for endogenous substrate (xylosylated core protein) and initiating synthesis of free GAG chains (Fig. 3). Xylosides not only relieve the cycloheximide or puromycin inhibition (Robinson and Lindahl, 1981), but in many cell types total GAG synthesis is stimulated above normal levels (Schwartz *et al.*, 1974; Mitchell and Hardingham, 1982b; Thompson and Spooner, 1982), suggesting that initiation by core protein is the limiting step. Consistent with this suggestion is the existence of mutants in chickens and mice which are deficient in the major cartilage specific proteoglycan. Both mutants lack normal core protein, but have the capacity to synthesize large amounts of chondroitin sulfate when provided with xylosides (Stearns and Geotinck, 1979; Kimata *et al.*, 1981; McKeown-Longo and Goetinck, 1982).

D.   *Deposition*

Extracellular matrices, whether pericellular, interstitial, or basal laminar, are supramolecular assemblies of various macromolecules, including proteoglycans, hyaluronic acid, collagens, fibronectin, and other structural proteins. Many of the molecules have multiple domains, with binding sites for self-aggregation and/or interaction with other matrix components. These interacting domains are responsible for the ordered assembly of the various components into functional extracellular matrices. In cartilage, for example, proteoglycans, hyaluronate, and link protein are secreted independently (Bjornsson and Heinegard, 1981; McKeown-Longo *et al.*, 1983). Once outside the cell, they form aggregates which are efficiently trapped by the meshwork of collagen fibrils. Disruption of the structure of any of these components compromises the function of cartilage matrix (Hascall and Hascall, 1981). Clearly, orderly deposition of proteoglycans and hyaluronic acid into matrices is dependent on self-assembly of the various extracellular macromolecules.

IV. PROTEOGLYCANS AND HYALURONATE IN BRANCHING ORGANS

A. Synthesis

During branching morphogenesis, organ rudiments actively synthesize proteoglycans and hyaluronic acid, as demonstrated by histochemical staining, autoradiography, and immunofluorescence. Preliminary characterization of some of these proteoglycans has been reported (Thompson and Spooner, 1983), but the limited amount of material has hampered more detailed structural analysis. Embryonic organs are extremely small and the microdissections required to isolate them are time consuming. However, methodologies appropriate for limited quantities of proteoglycans are currently being developed (for example, Rostand et al., 1982; Yanagishita and Hascall, 1983a,b), and these methodologies will be useful for characterizing the proteoglycans involved in branching morphogenesis.

Synthesis of extracellular matrix components is modulated by interactions between epithelium and the surrounding mesenchyme. Embryonic salivary mesenchyme cultured transfilter from homologous epithelium synthesizes substantially more collagen than mesenchyme cultured alone (Bernfield, 1970). Additionally, tissue interactions can alter the type of collagen synthesized (Ekblom et al., 1981). Because synthesis of extracellular matrix components is modulated both quantitatively and qualitatively, contributions of epithelium and mesenchyme to the pool of proteoglycans and hyaluronate in the matrix are difficult to determine. For example, it is not known whether any macromolecules synthesized by the epithelium are deposited in the matrix around mesenchymal cells. There is some evidence that proteoglycans and hyaluronic acid in the basal lamina are synthesized exclusively by the epithelium. Embryonic salivary epithelium from which the investing mesenchyme and the basal lamina have been removed can deposit a new lamina, even in the absence of mesenchyme. The new structure is indistinguishable from basal lamina synthesized by intact rudiments, on the basis of GAG composition and ultrastructural appearance (Cohn et al., 1977). However, these experiments do not rule out some contribution of basal laminar components from the mesenchyme of intact rudiments, analogous to the mesenchymally derived collagen which is deposited at the epithelial surface (Kallman and Grobstein, 1965).

B. Deposition

Since GAGs are found almost ubiquitously, it is not surprising that various proteoglycan species and hyaluronate are deposited in the extracellular compartments of branching organs, including plasma membrane (Rapraeger and Bernfield, 1983) and mesenchymal interstitial matrix (Cohn et al., 1977). However, GAG is most concentrated at the interface between the epithelium and mesenchyme, a region which includes the basal lamina. The interface regions of developing mammary gland (Silberstein and Daniel, 1982a), seminal vesicle (Cunha and Lung, 1979), salivary gland, lung, and ureteric bud (Bernfield et al., 1973) all stain heavily with Alcian Blue, a cationic dye. Likewise, when embryonic salivary glands have been fixed for electron microscopy in the presence of ruthenium red, light microscopic observation of the intact rudiments show heaviest deposition of the cationic dye at the epithelial–mesenchymal interface (H. A. Thompson, unpublished observations). Newly synthesized GAG labeled with either [^{3}H]glucosamine or [^{35}S]sulfate co-localizes with intense Alcian Blue staining at the basal epithelial surface (Bernfield et al., 1973; Cunha and Lung, 1979; Gordon and Bernfield, 1980; Silberstein and Daniel, 1982a; Spooner et al., 1985).

The basal laminae of branching organ rudiments are rich in GAG. Ultrastructural studies of the basal laminae show beautifully ordered arrays of Ruthenium Red-stained anionic sites (Cohn et al., 1977; Gordon and Bernfield, 1980; Grant et al., 1983). Similar arrays are seen in rudiments stained with polyethyleneimine. The pattern of anionic sites suggests nonrandom insertion of GAG into the basal lamina. Specific interactions between proteoglycans, hyaluronic acid, type IV collagen, laminin, and other macromolecules may be responsible for generating the highly ordered structure of the basal lamina.

Based on removal of Ruthenium Red binding sites with enzymes which degrade GAGs, the anionic sites in basal laminae contain, variously, heparan sulfate, chondroitin sulfates, and hyaluronic acid. Newly synthesized basal laminar GAG from embryonic salivary glands has been isolated and contains approximately half hyaluronate and half chondroitin sulfates (Cohn et al., 1977). At present, there are insufficient data to determine whether differences in reported GAG composition are due to differences between the various organ rudiments, or whether they might also reflect differences in the stages of development at which the basal laminae have been examined.

Integrity of the GAG-rich basal lamina is necessary for maintenance of lobular morphology in embryonic salivary glands. Epithelium freed from the investing mesenchyme and treated briefly with testicular hyaluronidase to remove the basal lamina undergoes dramatic changes. The epithelial cells become more loosely adherent, cytoskeletal elements are disorganized, and microvilli form at the basal cell surfaces (Banerjee et al., 1977), similar to the changes seen in corneal epithelial cells which have been removed from underlying extracellular matrix (Sugrue and Hay, 1981). If denuded salivary epithelium is immediately recombined with mesenchyme, clefts regress and the tissue rounds up. However, if the epithelium is first allowed to regenerate a basal lamina, cellular architecture returns to normal and the lobular morphology is retained after addition of mesenchyme (Banerjee et al., 1977). Thus, intact GAG-rich basal lamina is required for maintenance of the lobular structure of salivary rudiments.

C. Turnover

The basal lamina of branching organ rudiments is a dynamic structure which must accomodate rapid growth and shape changes of the epithelium. Along morphogenetically active regions such as the distal ends of lobes, the basal lamina has numerous interruptions. Cell processes extend across these gaps, providing close contacts between epithelial and mesenchymal cells (Cutler and Chaudhry, 1973; Coughlin, 1975; Bluemink et al., 1976; Grant et al., 1983). The basal lamina is continuous in areas which are stabilized and do not undergo further drastic shape changes. Such relatively stable areas include ducts and interlobular clefts.

Turnover of proteoglycans and hyaluronic acid is critical to the dynamic remodeling of basal lamina during morphogenesis (Bernfield and Banerjee, 1982). At the light microscopic level, GAG accumulation in the basement membrane has been assessed by Alcian Blue staining. Deposition of Alcian Blue along the basement membranes of seminal vesicle, mammary, ureteric bud, lung, and salivary rudiments is not uniform (Bernfield et al., 1973; Cunha and Lung, 1979; Silberstein and Daniel, 1982a). Rather, staining is most intense in morphogenetically quiescent regions. The areas of heaviest GAG accumulation correspond to regions which have intact basal laminar ultrastructure. In contrast, staining of the basement membrane at the distal ends of lobes or end buds is very faint. This paucity of GAG in the basement membrane correlates with the regions of interrupted basal lamina seen ultrastructurally. It is of interest that embryonic seminal vesicles which have been deprived of androgen stimulation show both a uniform GAG accumulation at the basement membrane and inhibition of morphogenesis (Cunha and Lung, 1979). These observations suggest that the pattern of GAG accumulation at the epithelial–mesenchymal interface is important to branching activity of the rudiment.

Newly synthesized GAG in the basement membrane has been localized by labeling rudiments with [³H]glucosamine or [³⁵S]sulfate for several hours. Autoradiograms show more label at the distal ends of lobes than in morphogenetically quiescent regions such as ducts and interlobular clefts (Bernfield et al., 1973; Silberstein and Daniel, 1982a). Thus, deposition of newly synthesized GAG is most active in regions where there is relatively little accumulation of GAG. This apparent discrepancy is due to significant degradation of GAG in these regions. Kinetic studies have demonstrated that, in embryonic salivary glands, GAG is rapidly synthesized and deposited in the basement membrane at the distal ends of lobes, then rapidly degraded (Bernfield and Banerjee, 1982). In contrast, degradation in the interlobular clefts is slow relative to deposition of new material, and basement membrane GAG accumulates in these regions. Coordinate synthesis and degradation of GAG results in dynamic remodeling of the basal lamina.

Both epithelium and mesenchyme contribute to remodeling of the basal lamina. Epithelium produces most or all of the proteoglycan and hyaluronate in the structure (Cohn et al., 1977), but degradation appears to be mediated by the surrounding stroma. This has been tested by incubating living mesenchyme with fixed salivary epithelia which have previously been allowed to generate a basal lamina in the presence of [³H]glucosamine. Mesenchyme releases significant amounts of GAG from the epithelial surface (Smith and Bernfield, 1982), and similar degradative activity in intact rudiments may be responsible for the interrupted basal lamina at the distal ends of lobes. In addition to degrading GAG in active regions, mesenchyme may contribute to stabilization of the basal lamina in morphogenetically quiescent regions. Extracellular matrix in the interlobular clefts and adjacent to ducts, such as primary bronchi, contains abundant fibrillar collagen (Wessells, 1970; Bernfield et al., 1973). In vitro, collagen matrix reduces degradation of the proteoglycans secreted by mammary epithelial cells and promotes deposition of a basal lamina (David and Bernfield, 1981). Similarly, interstitial collagen synthesized by mesenchyme and deposited at the epithelial surface (Kallman and Grobstein, 1965) of morphogenetically quiescent regions may promote accumulation of basal laminar GAG. Thus, remodeling of the basal lamina is likely to include complex interactions between the epithelium and mesenchyme.

A number of observations link proteoglycan and hyaluronic acid in the basal lamina with branching morphogenesis. Integrity of the GAG-rich basal lamina is required for maintenance of lobular structure, presumably a prerequisite for further branching activity. Topographically, rapid turnover of basal laminar GAG is correlated with regions of intense morphogenetic activity. Regional differences in GAG accumulation are absent under conditions which inhibit epithelial branching. One further experiment suggests that the relationship between branching morphogenesis and turnover of proteoglycan and hyaluronate is causal. Silberstein and Daniel (1982b) have implanted pellets of a slow release polymer containing testicular hyaluronidase into the stroma of developing mammary glands. Alcian Blue staining of the epithelial–mesenchymal interface is reduced, and the implants stimulate morphogenesis of nearby epithelial ducts. Taken together, the observations discussed in this section suggest strongly that dynamic remodeling of the basal lamina by the combined activities of the epithelium and surrounding mesenchyme is required for branching morphogenesis.

V. Effects of β-d-Xyloside

A. Branching Morphogenesis

Proteoglycan biosynthesis is disrupted in the presence of certain derivatives of xylose. These β-d-xylosides act as primers, initiating synthesis of xylose-linked GAGs (Fig. 3). In most systems, β-d-xylosides stimulate synthesis of large amounts of free GAG, suggesting that availability of core protein limits GAG production under normal conditions (Okayama et al., 1973; Galligani et al., 1975; Robinson and Lindahl, 1981; Spooner et al., 1983). Because the xylose derivatives compete with endogenous substrate, xylosylated core protein, at the level of the first galactosyltransferase, synthesis of core protein-associated GAG is inhibited at high concentrations of xyloside (Schwartz, 1977; Lohmander et al., 1979; Robinson and Gospodarowicz, 1984). Galactosyltransferase I requires β-d-xylose, and the α-anomers of each xylose derivative provide convenient controls for any nonspecific effects of the aglycone moieties on cell metabolism.

Branching morphogenesis of embryonic mouse salivary glands is inhibited dramatically by chronic exposure to <1 mM of p-nitrophenyl-β-D-xylopyranoside (Thompson and Spooner, 1982), and comparable concentrations of the α-anomer have no effect on morphogenesis. Branching activity can be quantitated by photographing the living rudiments daily, and counting the number of lobes on each submandibular and sublingual gland. Inhibition of morphogenesis is apparent by 24 hr of culture, but becomes more pronounced with longer culture periods (Fig. 4). As shown in Fig. 5, A and B, branching activity is dependent on the concentration of xyloside in the culture medium.

The p-nitrophenyl derivative of β-D-xyloside equilibrates rapidly between extracellular and intracellular compartments (Thompson et al., 1986). If the inhibition of branching is related directly to disruption of GAG synthesis, then morphogenesis should recover following removal of the xyloside. Rudiments cultured for up to 48 hr in 1 mM β-D-xyloside resume branching activity within 24 hr after return to normal medium (Thompson and Spooner, 1982). Thus, the inhibition of branching morphogenesis is dose dependent, specific for the β-anomer, and reversible. These characteristics suggest strongly that the abnormal development of salivary rudiments cultured in the presence of β-D-xyloside is a result of disruption of GAG synthesis.

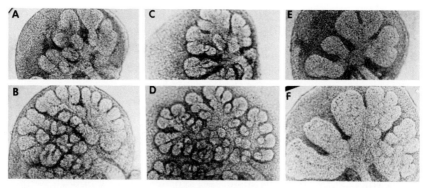

FIG. 4. β-Xylosides inhibit branching morphogenesis of embryonic salivary rudiments. α-Xyloside (1 mM)-treated rudiments (A, B) and untreated rudiments (C, D) undergo extensive branching activity during the 24-hr (A, C) to 48-hr (B, D) culture period. In contrast, treatment with β-xyloside (1.0 mM) dramatically inhibits branching activity from 24 hr (E) to 48 hr (F). Growth and lobule expansion continue, but new branch formation is inhibited (compare F with B and D). A–F, 32×.

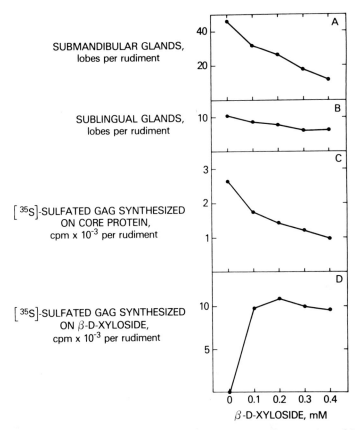

FIG. 5. β-Xyloside dose–response correlations between effects on branching, proteoglycan synthesis, and free glycosaminoglycan synthesis. Increasing β-xyloside concentrations produce increasing inhibition of branching morphogenesis by both submandibular and sublingual salivary rudiments, which correlates with an increasing inhibition of proteoglycan synthesis. Core protein-free GAG synthesis in the presence of β-xyloside does not exhibit a dose–response correlation with the effects on branching. All data at 48 hr of culture.

B.   Proteoglycan and GAG Synthesis

Untreated salivary rudiments synthesize several proteoglycan species (Thompson and Spooner, 1983). Sepharose CL-4B chromatography distinguishes three size classes of GAG-bearing molecules (Fig. 6, solid circles). Peak I contains chondroitin or dermatan sulfate proteoglycan. This material is excluded on CL-4B and may be either a very large extracellular species or a membrane-intercalated species which forms large aggregates in the absence of detergents. Examples of such

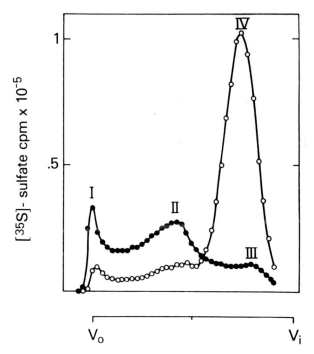

FIG. 6. Sulfated glycosaminoglycan size classes synthesized by 48-hr salivary rudiments, as resolved by Sepharose CL-4B chromatography. Control rudiments (solid circles) synthesize two proteoglycan size classes (peaks I and II) and a small (peak III) amount of apparently core protein-free GAG. β-Xyloside (0.5 mM)-treated rudiments (open circles) synthesize reduced amounts of the two proteoglycan size classes and a large amount of xyloside-initiated (core protein-free) GAG (peak IV). See text.

dermatan sulfate proteoglycans have been well characterized in other systems (Yanagishita and Hascall, 1983a, 1984a). Peak II contains both heparan sulfate and chondroitin or dermatan sulfate proteoglycans. Peak III appears to be a species with a single GAG chain (Thompson and Spooner, 1983) and probably represents an intermediate of intracellular degradation (Yanagishita and Hascall, 1984a,b).

In the presence of 0.5 mM β-D-xyloside, total proteoglycan synthesis is inhibited by about 50%, although the proteoglycan species appear to be qualitatively similar to those isolated from control cultures (Thompson and Spooner, 1983). Xyloside also initiates synthesis of large amounts of free GAG (Fig. 6, peak IV), predominantly chondroitin or dermatan sulfate. As a result, the total accumulation of newly synthesized GAG in treated cultures is severalfold higher than in controls.

To determine whether the inhibition of branching morphogenesis is related to the inhibition of proteoglycan synthesis or to the presence of abnormally high levels of free GAG, rudiments were cultured in the presence of various concentrations of the xylose derivative. Even at the lowest dose, 0.1 mM, synthesis of xyloside-initiated GAG is already maximally stimulated (Fig. 5D). It is likely that this lack of dose–response of xyloside-initiated GAG synthesis in the range of 0.1–0.4 mM reflects some rate-limiting step in the GAG synthesizing system. Further, it suggests that the dose-responsive inhibition of branching activity (Fig. 5A and B) does not result from the presence of large amounts of xyloside-initiated GAG in the cultures. Rather, the effect on morphogenesis is directly correlated with a dose-dependent inhibition of core protein-initiated GAG synthesis (Fig. 5C). Thus, synthesis of proteoglycan is required for normal branching morphogenesis.

C. Proteoglycan Deposition

Metabolic labeling of submandibular salivary rudiments with [^{3}H]glucosamine, followed by fixation, sectioning, and processing for light microscopic autoradiography, demonstrates deposition of labeled material at the basal epithelial surface that is sensitive to GAG degradative enzymes (Bernfield and Banerjee, 1972, 1982). The deposition of this newly synthesized GAG can be accomplished by the epithelium alone (Banerjee *et al.*, 1977), and analysis of the radiolabeled material demonstrates that it is about 50% hyaluronic acid and 50% sulfated GAG, i.e., proteoglycan (Cohn *et al.*, 1977). Furthermore, the bulk of the deposited proteoglycan contains chondroitin/dermatan sulfate GAG chains and only small amounts of heparan sulfate-like material (Cohn *et al.*, 1977).

When 48-hr cultures are pulse-labeled for 2 hr with [^{35}S]sulfate (thus excluding visualization of newly synthesized hyaluronate) prior to processing for autoradiography, a similar deposition of radioactivity is observed (Spooner *et al.*, 1985). The basal epithelial surface at the epithelial–mesenchymal interface is intensely labeled. The bulk of the radioactivity is sensitive to testicular hyaluronidase and chondroitin ABC lyase, confirming the conclusion of Cohn *et al.* (1977) that the GAG composition of the newly synthesized and deposited proteoglycan is principally chondroitin/dermatan sulfate. Autoradiographic analysis of rudiments incubated in the continuous presence of 0.5 mM β-xyloside, but otherwise identically cultured and [^{35}S]sulfate labeled, demonstrates a dramatic decrease in radioactivity localized to the basal epithelial surface (Spooner *et al.*, 1985). Figure 7 illustrates the decreased radioactivity deposited at the epithelial–mesenchymal tis-

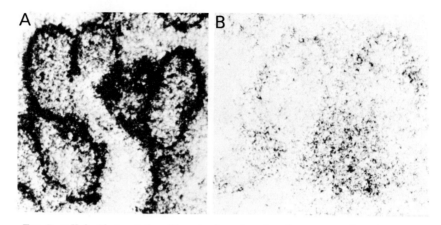

FIG. 7. β-Xyloside-treated rudiments deposit reduced amounts of sulfated glyco-saminoglycan at the basal epithelial surface. Control (A) and 0.5 mM β-xyloside-treated rudiments (B) were cultured for 48 hr, pulse-labeled with [³⁵S]sulfate for 2 hr, fixed, embedded, sectioned, and processed for light microscopic autoradiography. The reduced deposition is of sulfated GAG since the deposited radioactivity of both control and treated rudiments is sensitive to GAG degradative enzymes. See text. 200 ×.

sue interface, compared to control deposition. Although the amount of radioactivity is sharply reduced, the majority of it, as in controls, is sensitive to GAG degradative enzymes. The large amounts of ³⁵S-labeled GAG, initiated on xyloside rather than on xylosylated core protein, are found in the medium of these β-xyloside-treated rudiments and do not tissue localize. These data demonstrate that inhibition of proteoglycan biosynthesis, in the presence of β-xyloside, results in a sharp reduction of proteoglycan deposition at the basal epithelial surface, at the level of the basal lamina, and correlates with inhibition of branching morphogenesis.

D. Proteoglycan Turnover

The [³H]glucosamine-labeled material that is deposited at the epithelial–mesenchymal tissue interface of pulse-labeled salivary rudiments is differentially lost during subsequent incubation in nonradioactive medium (Bernfield and Banerjee, 1982). The pattern is that radioactivity is most rapidly lost from the tips of lobes and more slowly disappears from the clefts between lobes. This turnover results from mesenchyme-induced degradation (Smith and Bernfield, 1982), preferentially at lobule tips. The correlation is that turnover of basal epithelial surface-associated, i.e., basal laminar, GAG is most rapid at sites where the next clefts or branch points will form. Lobule growth and expansion appear to be integral components of this process, since inhibition of cell proliferation with inhibitors of DNA synthesis results in inhibition of lobule expansion and cessation of branching, which correlates with a marked decrease in the rate of labeled GAG loss (Bernfield and Banerjee, 1982).

A similar turnover pattern is observed when 48-hr cultures of salivary rudiments are pulse-labeled with [^{35}S]sulfate and then chased in nonradioactive medium (Spooner *et al.*, 1985). Label loss occurs over an 8-hr chase period, initially from the tips of lobes and more slowly from clefts between lobes. Since the bulk of the deposited ^{35}S radioactivity is sensitive to testicular hyaluronidase and chondroitin ABC lyase, the turnover observed by autoradiography of these pulse–chased rudiments is of chondroitin/dermatan sulfate proteoglycan. A similar proteoglycan turnover pattern is observed when the 48-hr culture period, 2-hr labeling period, and the chase periods are conducted in the continuous presence of 0.5 mM β-xyloside. Although less [^{35}S]sulfate-labeled material is initially deposited at the epithelial–mesenchymal interface, its pattern and rate of loss is equivalent to controls, with rapid preferential disappearance from the tips of lobes and slower incomplete loss from clefts between lobes over an 8-hr chase period. If lobule expansion is a key event in proteoglycan turnover, this result is not surprising, since lobule expansion continues in the presence of β-xylosides. Although lobule expansion and differential proteoglycan turnover may be necessary for branching morphogenesis, they are clearly insufficient, since both occur in β-xyloside-treated rudiments, but branching morphogenesis is still inhibited. Thus, β-xylosides inhibit proteoglycan synthesis, resulting in decreased proteoglycan deposition (without apparent effects on subsequent turnover patterns) at the level of the basal lamina, which correlates with a dramatic inhibition of branching morphogenesis. The data suggest that the basal lamina, which is still structurally intact (Thompson and Spooner, 1983), is quantitatively deficient in proteoglycan, a condition incompatible with epithelial branching morphogenesis.

VI.   BASAL LAMINA IN BRANCHING MORPHOGENESIS

A.   *Effects of Removal and Resynthesis*

Removal of the mesenchyme from submandibular rudiments can be accomplished by treatment with collagenase preparations that are free of protease and GAGase activities combined with mechanical separation, resulting in isolated epithelia that are still covered by a morphologically intact and GAG-rich basal lamina (Bernfield *et al.*, 1972). The basal lamina can be subsequently removed by treatment with testicular hyaluronidase. Mesenchyme-free epithelia, with or without a basal lamina, will not undergo morphogenesis without recombination with mesenchyme. While recombination of epithelia possessing a basal lamina with mesenchyme results in cultures that maintain epithelial shape and continue morphogenesis, recombination and culture using basal lamina denuded epithelia gives dramatically different results (Bernfield *et al.*, 1972). The epithelium loses its branched morphology, assuming a ball-like shape, and fails to continue morphogenesis. After about 24 hr, branching morphogenesis resumes in these recombinants, coincident with the reappearance of GAG-rich material at the basal epithelial surface.

These important experiments demonstrated a basal lamina requirement for epithelial stability and continuing morphogenesis. These same investigators also demonstrated that the denuded epithelium alone would resynthesize a basal lamina during a 2-hr period *in vitro*, and that recombination of such epithelia, possessing regenerated basal laminae, with submandibular mesenchyme, resulted in retention of epithelial morphology and uninterrupted morphogenesis (Banerjee *et al.*, 1977). The failure of basal lamina-free epithelia to resynthesize a lamina, retain shape, and continue morphogenesis when immediately recombined with mesenchyme appears to result from mesenchyme-mediated degradative activities. If a basal lamina is already present, dynamic remodeling occurs by a balance between epithelial synthesis and deposition of basal lamina components and mesenchyme-dependent regionally specific degradation of basal lamina components (Bernfield and Banerjee, 1982; Smith and Bernfield, 1982). If a basal lamina is not already present, mesenchyme retards basal lamina reappearance, presumably by virtue of degradative activities in excess of the epithelial synthesis and deposition activities.

Thus, the submandibular basal lamina is principally a product of the epithelium, is subject to dynamic remodeling by the mesenchyme, and is necessary for morphogenesis.

B. Presence when Branching is Inhibited

Branching morphogenesis does not take place in the absence of a basal lamina. However, basal lamina presence is insufficient to assure branching activities, a fact that emphasizes the multiplicity of balanced requirements involved in regulation of branching morphogenesis. It is worth noting a number of experimental situations where submandibular epithelial branching is inhibited, even though a basal lamina is present, to illustrate the complexity of the process. Culture of intact rudiments, containing both epithelium and mesenchyme, in the presence of cytochalasin B inhibits branching morphogenesis. Such treatment disrupts the arrays of cytoplasmic microfilaments present in the epithelial cells (Spooner and Wessells, 1970, 1972), which are composed of actin (Spooner et al., 1973, 1978) and are responsible for the epithelial cell shape changes that generate clefts or branch points in the epithelium (Spooner and Wessells, 1972; Spooner, 1974, 1975). In such inhibited rudiments, transmission electron microscopy reveals a normal appearing epithelial–mesenchymal tissue interface, containing both interstitial collagen and a morphologically intact basal lamina (Spooner and Wessells, 1970, 1972; Spooner, 1973). Similarly, branching is inhibited by culture of rudiments in either papaverine or calcium-free medium (Ash et al., 1973; Spooner, 1973), conditions that implicate extracellular calcium in branching activity, possibly by regulation of microfilament contractility. Electron microscopic observations again demonstrate a normal appearing basal lamina (Ash et al., 1973), though branching is stopped. Perturbation of collagen and proteoglycan synthesis also inhibits branching morphogenesis. In the presence of proline analogs, collagen synthesis and secretion are inhibited, leading to depletion of interstitial collagen from the extracellular matrix and inhibition of submandibular epithelial branching. Nevertheless, a morphologically intact basal lamina is still observed by transmission electron microscopy (Spooner and Faubion, 1980). Furthermore, when proteoglycan synthesis is inhibited with β-xylosides (Thompson and Spooner, 1983), leading to reduced proteoglycan deposition at the basal epithelial surface (Spooner et al., 1985) and inhibition of branching morphogenesis (Thompson and Spooner, 1982, 1983), a normal appearing basal lamina is still observed by transmission electron microscopy (Thompson and Spooner, 1983). Finally, when the isolated salivary epithelium is recombined in culture with salivary mesenchyme on one side and bronchial mesenchyme on the other, the epithelium branches only where it is adjacent to, and interacting with, salivary mesenchyme (Spooner and Wessells, 1972). Nevertheless, electron microscopy demonstrates that the epithelial cells have normal arrays of cytoplasmic microfilaments and that a normal appearing epithelial–mesenchymal interface is established between the submandibular epithelium and the bronchial mesenchyme, with interstial collagen and an intact basal lamina covering the epithelium (Spooner and Wessells, 1972; Spooner, 1974), though the epithelium fails to branch.

Thus, although the basal lamina is required, its mere morphological presence is insufficient. In addition, it seems clear that microfilaments must be present and functionally regulated in the epithelial cells, that interstial collagen must be present, that proteoglycan must be deposited in the basal lamina, and that the lamina, at least with respect to its GAG components, must be dynamically remodeled, presumably under the influence of the appropriate homologous mesenchyme. Perturbation of any one of these components or events appears to interfere with branching morphogenesis, demonstrating an essential interrelationship between them all.

C. Anionic Sites in the Presence of β-Xyloside

A most intriguing feature of proteoglycans is their highly anionic character, a property due to the high net negative charge of their component GAG chains. This anionic condition is a function both of sulfate groups and of free carboxy groups of uronic acid residues. The use of cationic probes such as Ruthenium Red in electron microscopic analyses demonstrates arrays of anionic sites in the basal lamina of numerous organ systems, including the embryonic submandibular rudiment (Cohn et al., 1977) and the embryonic lung (Grant et al., 1983). Although proteoglycans are clearly components of anionic sites, other macromolecules are also potentially involved. The nonprotein-linked GAG hyaluronic acid, although not sulfated, is highly anionic due to free carboxy groups of uronic acid residues and will bind cationic probes. Sulfated glycoproteins are also anionic molecules. There is evidence for the presence of sulfated glycoproteins such as entactin in basal laminae (Warburton et al., 1984), and data supporting hyaluronate presence in the basal lamina also exist (Cohn et al., 1977).

Electron microscopic demonstration of anionic sites in the basal lamina of the embryonic salivary rudiment, using Ruthenium Red and polyethyleneimine as cationic probes reveals an ordered array of sites. A double row of anionic sites is present (Fig. 8), with one row of particles present in the lamina lucida interna, between the lamina densa and the epithelial plasma membrane, and the other row of particles associated with the outer surface of the lamina densa, predominantly located in the lamina lucida externa. Pretreatment with testicular hyaluronidase or chondroitin ABC lyase eliminates the anionic sites, suggesting that they are a function of chondroitin/dermatan sulfate proteoglycan and/or hyaluronic acid. Ruthenium Red and polyethele-

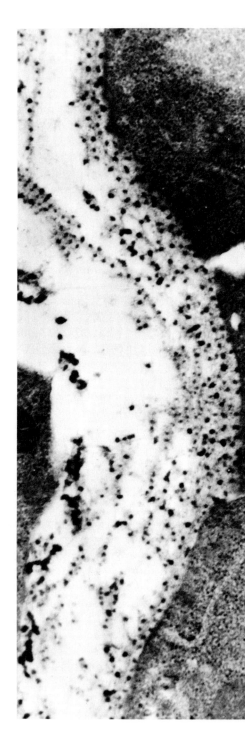

FIG. 8. Anionic sites in the basal lamina of the embryonic submandibular rudiment. Rudiments were cultured for 48 hr, then treated with the cationic probe polyethyleneimine (PEI) and processed for transmission electron microscopy. PEI-binding sites are resolved as electron-dense particles, present in the basal lamina and the extended matrix and associated with interstitial collagen. Basal lamina anionic sites appear as a double row of particles, with the lamina densa between the two rows of particles. 34,500×.

neimine also resolve anionic sites in 0.5 mM β-xyloside-treated rudiments. Again, a double row of particles is observed, sensitive to GAG degradative enzymes, with no immediately evident differences from control observations. Careful analysis of the micrographs suggests a 15–25% decrease in anionic sites in the presence of β-xyloside, as determined by center particle spacing average increases.

The small difference in anionic sites appears to be inconsistent with the 50% inhibition of proteoglycan synthesis, resolved biochemically, and dramatic reduction of proteoglycan deposition, resolved by autoradiography, in the presence of β-xylosides, if the anionic sites are, in fact, exclusively proteoglycan in nature. On the other hand, if half the anionic sites were proteoglycan and half were hyaluronic acid, a 50% decrease in proteoglycan synthesis and deposition would only result in a maximum 25% overall reduction in the total number of anionic sites, consistent with the decrease that we observe. Although direct evidence that hyaluronic acid accounts for some 50% of the basal lamina anionic sites does not exist, it is interesting that the GAG composition of the newly synthesized basal lamina of the submandibular epithelium is 50% hyaluronic acid and 50% sulfated GAG (i.e., proteoglycan).

Thus, β-xyloside inhibition of proteoglycan synthesis and deposition results in a small (~20%) decrease in basal lamine anionic sites, a condition that correlates with inhibition of branching morphogenesis.

D. Consideration of Structural and Functional Basal Lamina Criteria

The importance of the basal lamina in epithelial morphogenesis is established, but recognition of a defective basal lamina presents a problem. On the one hand, such recognition is possible if the defect results in a structural alteration. By conventional transmission electron microscopy, abnormal gaps in, or even absence of, a basal lamina would be detected. Similarly, absence of normally occurring gaps (Grant et al., 1984), abnormal thickening, or spacing from the epithelial plasma membrane could be recognized. Using cationic probes, major increases or decreases in anionic sites could also be determined at the electron microscopic level. Recognition of a functionally inadequate basal lamina, however, might not be detected at the ultrastructural level, since the absence of a functionally crucial molecule or class of molecules would not necessarily alter the transmission electron microscopic image of the basal lamina. Basal laminae generally appear to be composed of basement membrane collagen, laminin, and proteoglycan, and possibly hyaluronate, fibronectin, and other glycoproteins. It is not clear that the absence of any one component would after the conventional electron microscopic image of the lamina, although lamina function could be dramatically changed. β-Xyloside inhibition of proteoglycan deposition, for example, does not alter the conventional electron microscopic image of the basal lamina, and anionic site distribution changes are not even readily apparent. Similarly, changes in basement membrane collagen or proteoglycan types, for example, would not necessarily alter the electron microscopically resolved structure of the basal lamina, although function might be dramatically changed. Such changes have been observed by immunofluorescence in several systems during normal development (Ekblom, 1981; Bernfield et al., 1984).

Thus, a functionally deficient basal lamina might not be recognizable as defective by current structural criteria. Immunoelectron microscopy, using antibodies against specific basal lamina components, may ultimately provide a better assessment of abnormally constructed or component-deficient basal laminae, but, at present, that technology does not possess sufficient resolving power.

VII. POSSIBLE FUNCTIONS OF PROTEOGLYCANS IN BRANCHING MORPHOGENESIS

Although proteoglycans appear to be necessary for branching morphogenesis, their precise functions are not understood. Possibilities include both stimulatory and inhibitory effects on the synthesis of other extracellular matrix components by the epithelium and/or the mesenchyme, mitogenic activities (perhaps in conjunction with other matrix molecules), particularly on the epithelium, physical interactions with other matrix components (both in the basal lamina and in the interstitial matrix), and cation binding activities, due to their anionic character. Physical coupling between the extracellular matrix and intracellular structures is also an intriguing possibility, in light of the demonstration that an apparently integral membrane heparan sulfate proteoglycan has an interstitial collagen binding domain on the GAG chain-containing end of the molecule, which would extend from the cell surface into the matrix, and an actin filament binding domain on the end of the molecule which would be expected to face to cytoplasm.

Ultimate understanding of the role of proteoglycans in branching morphogenesis will be best achieved through a comprehensive understanding of the multiple requirements for this process. Since a number of the requirements are known for branching morphogenesis of the embryonic submandibular epithelium, it is useful to enumerate them, and then to consider a comprehensive model that would include all the known requirements. There are eight such requirements that should be listed and commented on.

1. *Epithelial–mesenchymal tissue interactions.* The epithelium alone will not branch (Grobstein, 1953). Furthermore, interaction with nonsalivary mesenchyme results in failure to branch (Spooner and Wessells, 1972) or in retarded and transiently altered branching (Lawson, 1974, 1983).

2. *Interstitial collagen.* Experimental inhibition of collagen synthesis and secretion, leading to elimination of interstitial collagen from the extracellular matrix, inhibits branching morphogenesis (Spooner and Faubion, 1980). Whether basement membrane collagen is also required is not known for the submandibular system, since the basal lamina is still intact in these experiments and specific collagen types have not been analyzed. Basement membrane collagen does appear to be required in the analogous mammary gland system (Wicha *et al.,* 1980).

3. *Basal lamina.* Removal of the GAG-rich basal lamina causes loss of epithelial shape and branching activity (Bernfield *et al.,* 1972), while resynthesis of the GAG-rich basal lamina by the epithelium results in retention of epithelial shape and continuation of branching activity (Banerjee *et al.,* 1977).

4. *Proteoglycan synthesis and deposition.* Inhibition of proteoglycan synthesis (Thompson and Spooner, 1983) and deposition (Spooner *et al.,* 1985) in the basal lamina results in the reversible inhibition of branching morphogenesis. Decreased numbers of basal lamina anionic sites are observed under these conditions.

5. *Proteoglycan and GAG turnover.* Basal epithelial surface-associated (basal laminar) GAG turns over rapidly at lobule tips (Bernfield and Banerjee, 1982) due to mesenchyme-mediated degradation (Smith and Bernfield, 1982), coincident with regions where epithelial clefts will form. When the rate of GAG turnover is decreased by inhibition of lobule expansion, branching is stopped (Bernfield and Banerjee, 1982). Equivalent turnover is observed when only sulfated GAG, i.e., proteoglycan, is monitored. Whether turnover of other basal lamina components occurs or is required is not yet known.

6. *Mitosis and lobule expansion.* Inhibition of epithelial mitosis with inhibitors of DNA synthesis inhibits expansion of epithelial lobules and stops branching activity (Bernfield and Banerjee, 1982). This correlates with a reduced rate of GAG degradation. The lobule expan-

sion–GAG turnover requirement is distinguishable from the proteoglycan synthesis and deposition requirement, since when the latter events are inhibited lobule expansion and proteoglycan turnover continue, even though branching activity ceases (Spooner et al., 1985).

7. *Intracellular epithelial microfilaments.* Disruption of the arrays of cytoplasmic microfilaments in the epithelial cells reversibly blocks branching morphogenesis (Spooner and Wessells, 1970, 1972). These actin filament arrays (Spooner et al., 1973, 1978) are required for the epithelial cell shape changes that generate clefts or branch points in the epithelium (Spooner and Wessells, 1972; Spooner, 1973, 1974, 1975, 1978).

8. *Extracellular calcium ions.* Branching morphogenesis is reversibly blocked by culturing rudiments in the absence of exogenous calcium ions or in the presence of papaverine, a smooth muscle relaxant thought to act by interfering with extracellular calcium influx (Ash et al., 1973; Spooner, 1973). Although direct demonstration of an extracellular calcium requirement is lacking, these experiments are consistent with that possibility.

Consideration of all these requirements allows proposition of an integrated model that could explain regulation of branching activity. The principal events leading to generation of a cleft or branch point in the epithelium are schematically illustrated in Fig. 9. Since branching morphogenesis is a repetitive process, epithelial–mesenchymal instructions are continuous as the sequence of events is repeated. One contribution of the mesenchyme is interstitial collagen (Bernfield, 1970), which polymerizes in the epithelial–mesenchymal tissue interface, near the epithelial surface (Kallman and Grobstein, 1975). The epithelium produces the basal lamina, including its proteoglycan component. One function of the *interstitial collagen* may be to promote deposition of basal lamina components (David and Bernfield, 1979, 1981). Of particular interest is that proteoglycan secreted by epithelial cells is found in the culture medium rather than being cell-layer (basal lamina?) localized, in the absence of an interstitial collagen substratum. A possible collagen function in stabilization of deep epithelial clefts has also been proposed (Bernfield and Wessells, 1970) but appears not to be absolutely necessary (Spooner and Faubion, 1980). The *basal lamina* itself is, however, necessary for retention of epithelial shape (Bernfield et al., 1972; Banerjee 1977). *Proteoglycan* synthesis and deposition in the basal lamina is required (Thompson and Spooner, 1983; Spooner et al., 1985) and results in an anionic site-rich basal lamina. In this model, it is the cation-binding ability of the basal

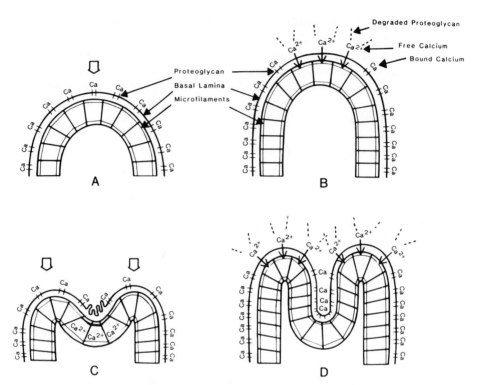

FIG. 9. Model for proteoglycan involvement in the regulation of epithelial branching morphogenesis. (A) Basal lamina proteoglycan (‖) binds calcium (Ca). Arrow indicates future cleft site. (B) Cell division causes lobule expansion, which activates mesenchymal degradation of proteoglycan (⁝) at lobule tip. This results in locally free calcium ions (Ca²⁺), which enter the local (i.e., lobular tip) epithelial cells. (C) Elevated free Ca²⁺ in the epithelial cells activates microfilament contraction that narrows the basal ends of those cells and generates a cleft. The overlying basal lamina is thrown into folds. Arrows indicate where the next clefts will form. (D) The sequence is repeated. Lobular cell division, lobule expansion, mesenchymal degradation of proteoglycan, and production of free Ca²⁺ at lobule tips which enters the epithelial cells. Microfilaments can now generate two new clefts. The original cleft has deepened and proteoglycan has been redeposited in the basal lamina.

lamina proteoglycan (and possibly hyaluronate), organized as symetrically distributed anionic sites, that is crucial to branching activity. The proposal is that *extracellular calcium* ions are localized near the basal epithelial surface by binding to basal lamina proteoglycan. The scheme does not require proteoglycan distribution differences, so that calcium localization can be equivalent over the entire basal epithelial surface. *Cell division* in the epithelium, which is more rapid in lobules than at the base of clefts (Bernfield *et al.*, 1972), results in *lobule expansion* and, incidentally, in the deepening of clefts on either side of lobules (Spooner and Wessells, 1972). As lobule tips expand distally, they stimulate GAG degradative activity by the local mesenchyme. The mesenchyme-mediated *degradation of basal lamina proteoglycan* at the tips of lobules causes a sharp local decrease in calcium binding capacity and, therefore, a local increase in free calcium ions at the tips of lobules. Free calcium influx into the epithelial cells activates acto-myosin *microfilament contraction* at the basal ends of those cells, changing cell shape and generating a cleft.

The crucial function of basal lamina proteoglycan deposition and turnover, in this model, is regulation of intracellular microfilament contractility via control of calcium ion availability. Whether calcium entry into the epithelial cells would require a membrane depolariza-tion event is not known, but, if necessary, could result from mesenchy-mal perturbation of the basal epithelial surface. Whether this model is correct or not remains to be determined. However, for the present, it does accommodate the existing data and provides a possible explana-tion of various experiments demonstrating inhibition of branching morphogenesis. Thus, when lobule expansion is inhibited, decreasing GAG and proteoglycan turnover rates at lobule tips, the prediction is that insufficient calcium is released to enter the epithelium and acti-vate the contractile apparatus. On the other hand, when insufficient proteoglycan deposition in the basal lamina is caused by β-xyloside inhibition of proteoglycan synthesis, the calcium-binding capacity of the lamina is reduced. Although lobule expansion and proteoglycan turnover continue, the prediction is that the reduced amount of bound calcium that becomes free to enter the epithelial cells is inadequate to activate microfilament contraction. Interestingly, this effect would ap-pear to require only a 20% decrease in basal lamina anionic sites. The interstitial collagen requirement might operate at the same level. That is, when interstitial collagen is reduced, insufficient proteoglycan might be deposited in the basal lamina, an effect functionally equiva-lent to β-xyloside treatment. It would be of interest to examine anionic site distribution under reduced interstitial collagen conditions to test this possibility.

In summation, branching morphogenesis of embryonic epithelia is a complex process involving epithelial–mesenchymal tissue interac-tions, extracellular matrix macromolecules, and intracellular struc-tures controlling cell shape. Proteoglycans appear to be essential mole-cules in this morphogenetic activity, whose crucial function is intimately interrelated with the other essential components of this process.

ACKNOWLEDGMENTS

We thank Mark Sullins and Ken Bassett for assistance in preparation of figures, and Dr. Marie Dziadek for sharing data on nidogen prior to publication. H.A.T. expresses appreciation to Dr. Vincent Hascall, in whose laboratory she was a postdoctoral fellow during the period when much of the writing of this manuscript was accomplished. This research was supported by NIH Postdoctoral Fellowship F32HL06696 (H.A.T.) and NIH Grant HL25910 (B.S.S.).

REFERENCES

Alitalo, K., Myllylä, R., Sage, H., Pritzl, P., Vaheri, A., and Bornstein, P. (1982). *J. Biol. Chem.* **257**, 9016–9024.
Ash, H. F., Spooner, B. S., and Wessells, N. K. (1973). *Dev. Biol.* **33**, 463–469.
Auerbach, R. (1960). *Dev. Biol.* **2**, 271–284.
Banerjee, S. D., Cohn, R. H., and Bernfield, M. R. (1977). *J. Cell Biol.* **73**, 445–463.
Belsky, E., and Toole, B. P. (1983). *Cell Differ.* **12**, 61–66.
Bennett, D. C., Armstrong, B. L., and Okada, S. M. (1981). *Dev. Biol.* **87**, 193–199.
Bentz, H., Morris, N. P., Murray, L. W., Sakai, L. Y., Hollister, D. W., and Burgeson, R. E. (1983). *Proc. Natl. Acad. Sci. U.S.A.* **80**, 3168–3172.
Bernfield, M. R. (1970). *Dev. Biol.* **22**, 213–231.
Bernfield, M. R., and Banerjee, S. D. (1982). *Dev. Biol.* **90**, 291–305.
Bernfield, M. R., and Wessells, N. K. (1970). *Dev. Biol. (Suppl.)* **4**, 195–249.
Bernfield, M. R., Banerjee, S. D., and Cohn, R. (1972). *J. Cell Biol.* **52**, 674–689.
Bernfield, M. R., Cohn, R. H., and Banerjee, S. D. (1973). *Am. Zool.* **13**, 1067–1083.
Bernfield, M. R., Banerjee, S. D., Koda, J. E., and Rapraeger, A. C. (1984). *In* "The Role of Extracellular Matrix in Development" (R. L. Trelstad, ed.), 545–572. Liss, New York.
Björnsson, S., and Heinegard, D. (1981). *Biochem. J.* **199**, 17–29.
Bluemink, J. G., Van Maurik, P., and Lawson, K. A. (1976). *J. Ultrastruct. Res.* **55**, 257–270.
Bornstein, P., and Sage, H. (1980). *Annu. Rev. Biochem.* **49**, 957–1003.
Brody, J. S., Vaccaro, C. A., Gill, P. J., and Silbert, J. E. (1982). *J. Cell Biol.* **95**, 394–402.
Brown, S. S., Malinoff, H. L., and Wicha, M. S. (1983). *Proc. Natl. Acad. Sci. U.S.A.* **80**, 5927–5930.
Brownell, A. G., Bessem, C. C., and Slavkin, H. C. (1981). *Proc. Natl. Acad. Sci. U.S.A.* **78**, 3711–3715.
Carlin, B., Jaffe, R., Bender, B., and Chung, A. E. (1981). *J. Biol. Chem.* **256**, 5209–5214.
Chambard, M., Gabrion, J., and Mauchamp, J. (1981). *J. Cell Biol.* **91**, 157–166.
Cohn, R. H., Banerjee, S. D., and Bernfield, M. R. (1977). *J. Cell Biol.* **73**, 464–478.
Coughlin, M. D. (1975). *Dev. Biol.* **43**, 123–139.
Cunha, G. R., and Lung, B. (1979). *In Vitro* **15**, 50–71.
Cunha, G. R., Shannon, J. M., Neubauer, B. L., Sawyer, L. M., Fujii, H., Taguchi, O., and Chung, L. W. K. (1981). *Hum. Genet.* **58**, 68–77.
Cutler, L. S., and Chaudhry, A. P. (1973). *Dev. Biol.* **33**, 229–240.
David, G., and Bernfield, M. R. (1979). *Proc. Natl. Acad. Sci. U.S.A.* **76**, 786–790.
David, G., and Bernfield, M. (1981). *J. Cell Biol.* **91**, 281–286.
Dziadek, M., and Timpl, R. (1985). *Dev. Biol.* **111**, 372–382.
Edward, M., Long, W. F., Watson, H. H. K., and Williamson, F. B. (1980). *Biochem. J.* **188**, 769–773.
Ekblom, P. (1981). *J. Cell Biol.* **91**, 1–10

Ekblom, P., Lehtonen, E., Saxén, L., and Timpl, R. (1981). *J. Cell Biol.* **89**, 276–283.

Faltynek, C. R., and Silbert, J. E. (1978). *J. Biol. Chem.* **253**, 7646–7649.

Faulkin, L. J., and Deome, K. B. (1960). *J. Natl. Cancer Inst.* **24**, 953–963.

Fellini, S. A., Kimura, H. J., and Hascall, V. C. (1981). *J. Biol. Chem.* **256**, 7883–7889.

Fellini, S. A., Hascall, V. C., and Kimura, J. H. (1984). *J. Biol. Chem.* **259**, 4643–4641.

Foster, C. S., Smith, C. A., Dinsdale, E. A., Monaghan, P., and Neville, A. M. (1983). *Dev. Biol.* **96**, 197–216.

Gallagher, J. T., Gasiunas, N., and Schor, S. L. (1980). *Biochem. J.* **190**, 243–254.

Galligani, L., Hopwood, J., Schwartz, N. B., and Dorfman, A. (1975). *J. Biol. Chem.* **250**, 5400–5406.

Giraud, A., and Bouchilloux, S. (1983). *Biochem. Biophys. Res. Commun.* **111**, 353–359.

Goldin, G. V., and Opperman, L. A. (1980). *J. Embryol. Exp. Morphol.* **60**, 235–243.

Goldin, G. V., and Wessells, N. K. (1979). *J. Exp. Zool.* **208**, 337–346.

Golosow, N., and Grobstein, C. (1962). *Dev. Biol.* **4**, 242–255.

Gordon, J. R., and Bernfield, M. R. (1980). *Dev. Biol.* **74**, 118–135.

Grant, M. M., Cutts, N. R., and Brody, J. S. (1983). *Dev. Biol.* **97**, 173–183.

Grant, M. M., Cutts, N. R., and Brody, J. S. (1984). *Dev. Biol.* **104**, 469–476.

Grobstein, C. (1953a). *J. Exp. Zool.* **124**, 383–404.

Grobstein, C. (1953b). *Nature* **172**, 869–871.

Grobstein, C. (1955). *J. Exp. Zool.* **130**, 319–339.

Grobstein, C. (1967). *Natl. Cancer Inst. Monogr.* **26**, 279–299.

Grobstein, C., and Cohen, J. (1965). *Science* **150**, 626–628.

Hall, H. G., Farson, D. A., and Bissell, M. J. (1982). *Proc. Natl. Acad. Sci. U.S.A.* **79**, 4672–4676.

Hanover, J. A., Elting, J., Mintz, G. R., and Lennarz, W. J. (1982). *J. Biol. Chem.* **257**, 10172–10177.

Hart, G. W. (1976). *J. Biol. Chem.* **251**, 6513–6521.

Hart, G. W., and Lennarz, W. J. (1978). *J. Biol. Chem.* **253**, 5795–5801.

Hascall, V. C. (1981). *In* "Biology of Carbohydrates" (V. Ginsburg and P. Robbins, eds.), pp. 1–49. Wiley, New York.

Hascall, V. C., and Hascall, G. K. (1981). *In* "Cell Biology of Extracellular Matrix" (E. D. Hay, ed.), 39–63. Plenum, New York.

Hascall, V. C., and Heinegard, D. (1974). *J. Biol. Chem.* **249**, 4232–4241.

Hassell, J. R., Gehron-Robey, P., Barrach, H.-J., Wilczek, J., Rennard, S. I., and Martin, G. R. (1980). *Proc. Natl. Acad. Sci. U.S.A.* **77**, 4494–4498.

Hay, E. D. (1981). *In* "Cell Biology of Extracellular Matrix" (E. D. Hay, ed.), pp. 379–409. Plenum, New York.

Hay, E. D., and Meier, S. (1974). *J. Cell Biol.* **62**, 889–898.

Hayashi, A., Donahoe, P. K., Budzik, G. P., and Trelstad, R. L. (1982). *Dev. Biol.* **92**, 16–26.

Heathcote, J. G., and Grant, M. E. (1981). *Int. Rev. Connect. Tissue Res.* **9**, 191–264.

Hedman, K., Christner, J., Julkunen, I., and Vaheri, A. (1983). *J. Cell Biol.* **97**, 1288–1293.

Hogan, B. L. M., Taylor, A., Kurkinen, M., and Couchman, J. R. (1982). *J. Cell Biol.* **95**, 197–204.

Hogg, N. A. S., Harrison, C. J., and Ticle, C. (1983). *J. Embryol. Exp. Morphol.* **73**, 39–57.

Hopwood, J. J., and Dorfman, A. (1977). *J. Biol. Chem.* **252**, 4777–4785.

Hynes, R. O., and Yamada, K. M. (1982). *J. Cell Biol.* **95**, 369–377.

Jacobsson, I., and Lindahl, U. (1980). *J. Biol. Chem.* **255**, 5094–5100.

Kallman, F., and Grobstein, C. (1965). *Dev. Biol.* **11**, 169–183.

Kanwar, Y. S., and Farquhar, M. G. (1979). *Proc. Natl. Acad. Sci. U.S.A.* **76**, 1303–1307.

Kanwar, Y. S., Linker, A., and Farquhar, M. G. (1980). *J. Cell Biol.* **86,** 688–693.

Kapoor, R., and Prehm, P. (1983). *Eur. J. Biochem.* **137,** 589–595.

Kefalides, N. A. (1978). *In* "Biology and Chemistry of Basement Membranes" (N. A. Kefalides, ed.), pp. 215–228. Academic Press, New York.

Kimata, K., Barrach, H.-J., Brown, K. S., and Pennypacker, J. P. (1981). *J. Biol. Chem.* **256,** 6961–6968.

Kjellen, L., Pettersson, I., and Höök, M. (1981). *Proc. Natl. Acad. Sci. U.S.A.* **78,** 5371–5375.

Kleinman, H. K., Klebe, R. J., and Martin, G. R. (1981). *J. Cell Biol.* **88,** 473–485.

Kleinman, H. K., McGarvey, M. L., Hassell, J. R., Martin, G. R., Baron-van Evercooren, A., and Dubois-Dalcq, M. (1984). *In* "The Role of Extracellular Matrix in Development" (R. L. Trelstad, ed.), pp. 123–143. Alan R. Liss, Inc., New York.

Kolset, S. O., Kjellén, L., Seljelid, R., and Lindahl, U. (1983). *Biochem. J.* **210,** 661–667.

Kraemer, P. M. (1971). *Biochemistry* **10,** 1437–1455.

Kratochwil, K. (1969). *Dev. Biol.* **20,** 46–71.

Lark, M. W., and Culp, L. A. (1983). *Biochemistry* **22,** 2289–2296.

Lark, M. W., and Culp, L. A. (1984). *J. Biol. Chem.* **259,** 212–217.

Lau, E. C., and Ruch, J. V. (1983). *Differentiation,* **23,** 234–242.

Laurie, G. W., Leblond, C. P., and Martin, G. R. (1982). *J. Cell Biol.* **95,** 340–344.

Lawson, K. A. (1974). *J. Embryol. Exp. Morphol.* **32,** 469–493.

Lawson, K. A. (1983). *J. Embryol. Exp. Morphol.* **74,** 183–206.

Linsenmayer, T. F. (1981). *In* "Cell Biology of Extracellular Matrix" (E. D. Hay, ed.), pp. 1–37. Plenum, New York.

Lohmander, L. S., Hascall, V. C., and Caplan, A. I. (1979). *J. Biol. Chem.* **254,** 10551–10561.

Luikart, S. D., Maniglia, C. A., and Sartorelli, A. C. (1983). *Proc. Natl. Acad. Sci. U.S.A.* **80,** 3738–3742.

McKeown-Longo, P. J., and Goetinck, P. F. (1982). *Biochem. J.* **201,** 387–394.

McKeown-Longo, P. J., Velleman, S. G., and Goetinck, P. F. (1983). *J. Biol. Chem.* **258,** 10779–10785.

Malmström, A. (1984). *J. Biol. Chem.* **259,** 161–165.

Mason, R. M., d'Arville, C., Kimura, J. H., and Hascall, V. C. (1982a). *Biochem. J.* **207,** 445–457.

Mason, R. M., Kimura, J. H., and Hascall, V. C. (1982b). *J. Biol. Chem.* **257,** 2236–2245.

Masters, J. R. W. (1976). *Dev. Biol.* **51,** 98–108.

Mikuni-Takagaki, Y., and Toole, B. P. (1981). *J. Biol. Chem.* **256,** 8463–8469.

Miller, E. J., and Gay, S. (1982). *In* "Methods in Enzymology" (L. W. Cunningham and D. W. Frederiksen, eds.), Vol. 82, pp. 3–32. Academic Press, New York.

Mitchell, D., and Hardingham, T. (1982a). *Biochem. J.* **202,** 249–254.

Mitchell, D., and Hardingham, T. (1982b). *Biochem. J.* **202,** 387–395.

Muir, H. (1983). *Biochem. Soc. Trans.* **11,** 613–622.

Nakanishi, S. (1983). *Dev. Biol.* **95,** 305–316.

Nilsson, B., De Luca, S., Lohmander, S., and Hascall, V. C. (1982). *J. Biol. Chem.* **257,** 10920–10927.

Odermatt, E., Risteli, J., Van Delden, V., and Timpl, R. (1983). *Biochem. J.* **211,** 295–302.

Okayama, M., Kimata, K., and Suzuki, S. (1973). *J. Biochem.* **74,** 1069–1073.

Ormerod, E. J., Warburton, M. J., Hughes, C., and Rudland, P. S. (1983). *Dev. Biol.* **96,** 269–275.

Poole, R., Pidoux, I., Reiner, A., Tang, L.-H., Choi, H., and Rosenberg, L. (1980). *J. Histochem. Cytochem.* **28,** 621–635.

Rapraeger, A. C., and Bernfield, M. (1983). *J. Biol. Chem.* **258**, 3632–3636.

Razin, E., Stevens, R. L., Akiyama, F., Schmid, K., and Austen, K. F. (1982). *J. Biol. Chem.* **257**, 7229–7236.

Richards, J., Guzman, R., Konrad, M., Yang, J., and Nandi, S. (1982). *Exp. Cell. Res.* **141**, 433–443.

Riesenfeld, J., Höök, M., and Lindahl, U. (1982). *J. Biol. Chem.* **257**, 421–425.

Robinson, H. C., and Lindahl, U. (1981). *Biochem. J.* **194**, 575–586.

Robinson, J., and Gospodarowicz, D. (1984). *J. Biol. Chem.* **259**, 3818–3824.

Rodén, L. (1980). *In* "The Biochemistry of Glycoproteins and Proteoglycans" (W. J. Lennarz, ed.), pp. 267–371. Plenum, New York.

Rollins, B. J., Cathcart, M. K., and Culp, L. A. (1982). *In* "The Glycoconjugates" (M. I. Horowitz, ed.), Vol. III, pp. 289–329. Academic Press, New York.

Ronzio, R. A., and Rutter, W. J. (1973). *Dev. Biol.* **30**, 307–320.

Rostand, K. S., Baker, J. R., Caterson, B., and Christner, J. E. (1982). *J. Biol. Chem.* **257**, 703–707.

Rutter, W. J., Wessells, N. K., and Grobstein, C. (1964). *Natl. Cancer Inst. Monogr.* **13**, 51–65.

Sage, H., Pritzl, P., and Bornstein, P. (1980). *Biochemistry* **19**, 5747–5755.

Sajdera, S. W., and Hascall, V. C. (1969). *J. Biol. Chem.* **244**, 77–87.

Sakakura, T., Sakagami, Y., and Nishizuka, Y. (1979). *Dev. Biol.* **72**, 201–210.

Saxén, L., Karkinen-Jääskeläinen, M., Lehtonen, E., Nordling, S., and Wartiovaara, J. (1976). *In* "The Cell Surface in Animal Embryogenesis and Development" (G. Poste and G. L. Nicolson, ed.), pp. 331–407. North-Holland Publ., New York.

Schmid, T. M., and Conrad, H. E. (1982). *J. Biol. Chem.* **257**, 12444–12450.

Schwartz, N. B. (1977). *J. Biol. Chem.* **252**, 6316–6321.

Schwartz, N. B., Galligani, L., Ho, P.-L., and Dorfman, A. (1974). *Proc. Natl. Acad. Sci. U.S.A.* **71**, 4047–4051.

Seno, N., and Murakami, K. (1982). *Carbohydrate Res.* **103**, 190–194.

Silberstein, G. B., and Daniel, C. W. (1982a). *Dev. Biol.* **90**, 215–222.

Silberstein, G. B., and Daniel, C. W. (1982b). *Dev. Biol.* **93**, 272–278.

Smith, R. L., and Bernfield, M. (1982). *Dev. Biol.* **94**, 378–390.

Spooncer, E., Gallagher, J. T., Krizsa, and Dexter, T. M. (1983). *J. Cell Biol.* **96**, 510–514.

Spooner, B. S. (1973). *Am. Zool.* **13**, 1007–1022.

Spooner, B. S. (1974). *In* "Concepts of Development" (J. Lash and J. R. Whittaker, eds.), pp. 213–240. Sinauer, Stamford, Conn.

Spooner, B. S. (1975). *Bioscience,* **25**, 440–451.

Spooner, B. S., and Faubion, J. M. (1980). *Dev. Biol.* **77**, 84–102.

Spooner, B. S., and Wessells, N. K. (1970a). *J. Exp. Zool.* **175**, 445–454.

Spooner, B. S., and Wessells, N. K. (1970b). *Proc. Natl. Acad. Sci. U.S.A.* **66**, 360–364.

Spooner, B. S., and Wessells, N. K. (1972). *Dev. Biol.* **27**, 38–54.

Spooner, B. S., Ash, J. F., Wrenn, J. T., Frater, R. B., and Wessells, N. K. (1973). *Tissue Cell,* **5**, 37–46.

Spooner, B. S., Ash, J. F., and Wessells, N. K. (1978). *Exp. Cell Res.* **114**, 381–387.

Spooner, B. S., Bassett, K., and Stokes, B. (1985a). *Dev. Biol.* **109**, 177–183.

Spooner, B. S., Thompson, H. A., Stokes, B., and Bassett, K. (1986). *In* "Cell Surface in Development and Cancer" (M. Steinberg, ed.). Plenum, New York (in press).

Stearns, K., and Goetinck, P. F. (1979). *J. Cell. Physiol.* **100**, 330–38.

Stevens, J., and Hascall, V. C. (1986). In preparation.

Sugrue, S. P., and Hay, E. D. (1981). *J. Cell Biol.* **91**, 45–54.

Suzuki, S., Saito, H., Yamagata, T., Anno, K., Seno, N., Kawai, Y., and Furuhashi, T. (1968). *J. Biol. Chem.* **243**, 1543–1550.

Taderera, J. V. (1967). *Dev. Biol.* **16,** 489–512.

Thesleff, I., Barrach, H.-J., Foidart, J. M., Vaheri, A., Pratt, R. M., and Martin, G. R. (1981). *Dev. Biol.* **81,** 182–192.

Thompson, H. A., and Spooner, B. S. (1982). *Dev. Biol.* **89,** 417–424.

Thompson, H. A., and Spooner, B. S. (1983). *J. Cell Biol.* **96,** 1443–1450.

Thompson, H. A., Yanagishita, M., and Hascall, V. C. (1986). In preparation.

Thonar, E. J.-M. A., Lohmander, L. S., Kimura, J. H., Fellini, S. A., Yanagishita, M., Hascall, V. C., and Rodbard, D. (1983). *J. Biol. Chem.* **258,** 11564–11570.

Timpl, R., Rohde, H., Gehron Robey, P., Rennard, S. I., Foidart, J.-M., and Martin, G. R. (1979). *J. Biol. Chem.* **254,** 9933–9937.

Timpl, R., Dziadek, M., Fujiwara, S., Nowack, H., and Wick, G. (1983). *Eur. J. Biochem.* **137,** 445–465.

Toole, B. P. (1981). *In* "Cell Biology of Extracellular Matrix" (E. D. Hay, ed.), pp. 259–294. Plenum, New York.

Toole, B. P., and Gross, J. (1971). *Dev. Biol.* **25,** 57–77.

Trelstad, R. L., Hayashi, K., and Toole, B. P. (1974). *J. Cell Biol.* **62,** 815–830.

Underhill, C. B., Chi-Rosso, G., and Toole, B. P. (1983). *J. Biol. Chem.* **258,** 8086–8091.

Vaccaro, C. A., and Brody, J. S. (1981). *J. Cell Biol.* **91,** 427–437.

Varma, R., Varma, R. S., Allen, W. S., and Wardi, A. H. (1975). *Biochim. Biophys. Acta* **399,** 139–144.

Von der Mark, K., van Menxel, M., and Wiedemann, H. (1982). *Eur. J. Biochem.* **124,** 57–62.

Warburton, M. J., Monaghan, P., Ferns, S. A., Rudland, P. S., Perusinghe, N., and Chung, A. E. (1984). *Exp. Cell Res.* **152,** 240–254.

Wessells, N. K. (1970). *J. Exp. Zool.* **175,** 455–466.

Wessells, N. K., and Cohen, J. H. (1968). *Dev. Biol.* **18,** 294–309.

Wessells, N. K., Spooner, B. S., Ash, J. F., Bradley, M. O., Ludueñna, M. A., Taylor, E. L., Wrenn, J. T., and Yamada, K. M. (1971). *Science* **171,** 135–143.

Wicha, M. S., Liotta, L. A., Vonderhaar, B. K., and Kidwell, W. R. (1980). *Dev. Biol.* **80,** 253–266.

Wu, T.-C., Wan, Y.-J., Chung, A. E., and Damjanov, I. (1983). *Dev. Biol.* **100,** 496–505.

Yanagishita, M., and Hascall, V. C. (1983a). *J. Biol. Chem.* **258,** 12847–12856.

Yanagishita, M., and Hascall, V. C. (1983b). *J. Biol. Chem.* **258,** 12857–12864.

Yanagishita, M., and Hascall, V. C. (1984a). *J. Biol. Chem.* **259,** 10260–10269.

Yanagishita, M., and Hascall, V. C. (1984b). *J. Biol. Chem.* **259,** 10270–10283.

Yanagishita, M., and Hascall, V. C. (1981). *Endocrinology,* **109,** 1641–1649.

Yang, J., Richards, J., Guzman, R., Imagawa, W., and Nandi, S. (1980). *Proc. Natl. Acad. Sci. U.S.A.* **77,** 2088–2092.

Yang, J., Larson, L., and Nandi, S. (1982). *Exp. Cell Res.* **137,** 481–485.

Index

A

Adult respiratory distress syndrome
neutrophil elastase and, 299–300
α_1-proteinase inhibitor and, 300
African lungfish pancreatic elastase, 225, 232, 276
Aging, elastin accumulation, 206–207
4-Aminophenyl mercuric acetate (APMA)
collagenase–inhibitor complex
dissociation, 58, 73
procollagenase conformation, 59–60
Aminopropeptides
amino acid sequence, 105
cleavage from procollagen, 105–106
distribution in body fluids and tissues, 106
in fibrotic diseases, 114 (table)
collagen synthesis and, 113–115
in pN-collagens, 103–104
preparation from calf skin, 107
from procollagen type I and III, inhibition of
collagen mRNA translation in cell-free system, 111–113
collagen synthesis in skin fibroblasts, 110–111
retaining by collagen
in dermatosparaxis, animal, 108
in Ehlers–Danlos syndrome type VII, human, 108
stability *in vivo,* 106
structure in collagen types, 103–105
β-Aminopropionitrile (BAPN)
lathyrism induction, 322, 338, 352
lysyl oxidase inhibition, 322, 331, 339–340
in fibrosis, 377–378
mechanism of, 352–354
treatment of
hypertension, rat, 373
pulmonary fibrosis, hamster, 375

Androgen
collagen metabolism regulation in
aortic wall, 153–154
male accessory sex organs, 154
Aneurysm, aortic, in mottled mouse, 369–369
β_1-Anticollagenase, serum, 75–76
Antiinflammatory drugs
human leukocyte elastase inhibition, 259–260
α_1-Antitrypsin, *see* α_1-Proteinase inhibitor
Aorta
collagen metabolism
estrogen and, 380
glucocorticoids and, 142
elastin abundance, warm-blooded vertebrates, 181
copper deficiency and, 198–199
developmental regulation, 198–199
elastin synthesis, regulation by glucocorticoids
in chicken embryonic culture, 156–157
in hypertensive rat, 157
sex hormones, rat, 159–160
hypertension and, 160
Aortic smooth muscle cells
collagen metabolism, estrogen and, 155
glucocorticoid effects on
collagen and noncollagen protein synthesis, 149
proliferation, 149
APMA, *see* 4-Aminophenyl mercuric acetate
Arachidonic acid
collagenase production in macrophages and, 88
prostaglandin E_2 production in macrophages and, 88
Ascorbic acid
elastin synthesis *in vitro* and, 204

445

R